Practical Fracture Treatment

Commissioning Editor: Mike Parkinson
Project Development Manager: Fiona Conn
Project Manager: Frances Affleck
Designer: Erik Bigland

Practical Fracture Treatment

Ronald McRae FRCS (Eng) FRCS (Glas) AIMBI
Max Esser FRCS Ed FRCS Ed (Orth) FRACS (Orth)

Original drawings by Ronald McRae

FOURTH EDITION

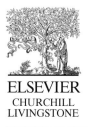

ELSEVIER
CHURCHILL
LIVINGSTONE

EDINBURGH LONDON NEW YORK OXFORD PHILADELPHIA ST LOUIS SYDNEY TORONTO 2002

CHURCHILL LIVINGSTONE
An imprint of Elsevier Limited

First edition 1981
Second edition 1989
Third edition 1994
Fourth edition 2002

ISBN 0 443 07038 5
   Reprinted 2003 (twice), 2004 (twice), 2005, 2006 (twice)
International Student Edition ISBN 0 443 07037 7
   Reprinted 2003 (twice), 2004 (twice), 2005

British Library Cataloguing in Publication Data
A catalogue record for this book is available from the British
Library

Library of Congress Cataloguing in Publication Data
A catalogue record for this book is available from the Library
of Congress

Note
Medical knowledge is constantly changing. As new
information becomes available, changes in treatment,
procedures, equipment and the use of drugs become
necessary. The authors and the publishers have taken care to
ensure that the information given in this text is accurate and
up to date. However, readers are strongly advised to confirm
that the information, especially with regard to drug usage,
complies with the latest legislation and standards of practice.
                                          The Publisher

 your source for books,
journals and multimedia
in the health sciences
www.elsevierhealth.com

Working together to grow
libraries in developing countries
www.elsevier.com | www.bookaid.org | www.sabre.org
ELSEVIER   BOOK AID International   Sabre Foundation

Printed in China
N/07/06

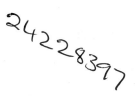
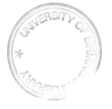

The
publisher's
policy is to use
**paper manufactured
from sustainable forests**

CONTENTS

PREFACE AND ACKNOWLEDGEMENTS TO THE FOURTH EDITION

In this edition changes have been made in most sections to reflect the continued expansion of the use of internal fixation methods in the treatment of many fractures. At the same time, and where appropriate, the details of conservative treatment have been retained.

I have taken the opportunity that a new edition has afforded of re-working all of the drawings in the previous edition, and adding a number of new ones. These I have digitised, tidied up where necessary, and used a variety of grey fills to improve their clarity.

The features in a number of the radiographs in the previous edition were in places not as clear as might be desired. This has been addressed in a number of ways. A new paper has been chosen to improve the quality of reproduction and minimise 'see through' from the other side. In many cases I have digitised the original slides and used a number of computer enhancement techniques to improve the images. In places I have added arrows to draw attention to areas where the pathology may not be obvious on first inspection.

In the third edition Max Esser made a number of invaluable suggestions which I included in that work. (Max is presently Consultant Orthopaedic Surgeon at the Alfred and Cabrini Hospitals in Melbourne, and has an academic appointment at the Monash University Department of Surgery.) He brought to the book his knowledge of attitudes to current fracture treatment in the United Kingdom, the United States and Australia.

In this edition he has been much more extensively involved, contributing information from his own experience and sourcing relevant recent publications, details of materials, radiographs and scans. (He acknowledges the additional help he has had from his colleagues in the appended list.) I have incorporated this new material through the many alterations I have made to the original text.

I trust that the reader finds these many changes to be of value.

RM, Gourock 2001

Acknowledgements

I wish to acknowledge the help I have had from my colleagues at the Alfred Hospital: in particular Mr Greg Hoy and Mr Owen Williamson of the Orthopaedic Service; Mr Ross Snow, Urologist; Dr Peter Blombery, Vascular Physician; Dr Will MacLaurin, Radiologist and Medical Administration. I would like to record the help I also have had from Dr Terence Lim, Rehabilitationist, and Mr Gary Nattrass, Orthopaedic Surgeon at the Royal Children's Hospital in Melbourne.

I am grateful for the excellent technical help I have had from the Department of Audio-visual Services, Alfred Hospital, particularly from Gavin Hawkins and Caroline Hedt. I would like to thank Kaye Lionello, my secretary who has been a constant source of help and efficiency.

ME, Melbourne 2001

PREFACE TO THE FIRST EDITION

This book has been written primarily for the medical student, and the introductory section assumes little prior knowledge of the subject. The second part, which deals with particular fractures, is set in places at a more advanced level; it is hoped that the book will thereby continue to prove of value to the student when he moves to his first casualty or registrar post.

In planning this volume, I have paid particular attention to two points. Firstly, the details of each fracture and a good deal of the introductory section have been arranged in a linear sequence. The material has been divided into small packets of text and illustration in order to facilitate comprehension and learning. These packets have been set out in a logical sequence which in most cases is based on the relative importance of the initial decisions which must be made in a case, and the order in which treatment procedures should be carried out. This format is in a few places restrictive, with an imbalance in the amount of information carried by either text or illustration. This must be accepted because of spatial and subject limitations. Generally, however, text and illustration will be found to complement one another. The text, although of necessity brief, is concise and, it is hoped, to the point.

Secondly, fracture treatment has been given in an uncommon amount of practical detail. As there is such a variety of accepted treatments for even the simplest of fractures, this has the danger of attracting the criticism of being controversial and didactic. This is far from my intention, and I have tried to avoid this in several ways. Firstly, as minor fractures and most children's fractures (together forming the bulk of all fractures) are most frequently treated conservatively, the conservative approach I have employed for these injuries should on the whole receive general approval. Secondly, in the more controversial long bone fractures in adults, and in fractures involving joints, I have on the whole pursued a middle course between the extremes of conservative and surgical management. The methods I have singled out for description are those which I consider safest and most reliable in the hands of the comparatively inexperienced. Where alternative methods appear to me to be equally valid I have generally included these. To conceal my own whims I have not always placed these in the order of personal preference. In consequence, I hope that any offence given by the methods described will be restricted to the most extreme quarters.

R.M.

HOW TO USE THIS BOOK

The basic principles of fractures and their treatment are dealt with in the first part of this book. The AO Classification of fractures (pp. 21–23), Trauma scoring (pp. 42–45) and the Mangled Extremity Severity Score (pp. 51–52) may be noted but do not require detailed study by the undergraduate.

The second part of the book is arranged on a regional basis and may be used as a guide for the handling of specific fractures. Detailed study is not required by the undergraduate, but a superficial reading should consolidate knowledge of the basic principles, and indicate how they are applied in practice.

The following conventions are used in the illustrations and text:

1. Where two sides are shown for comparison, the patient's *right* side is the one affected.
2. As a general rule, when a procedure is being illustrated, the patient is shown for clarification in a lighter tone of grey than the surgeon and his assistants.
3. Where several conditions are described, and only one illustrated, the first mentioned is the one shown, unless followed by the abbreviation 'Illus.'.
4. Most cross references within a chapter are made by quoting the relevant frame number. Elsewhere, page numbers are given.

Abbreviations

A = anterior
Illus. = illustrated
L = lateral or left
M = medial
N = normal
P = posterior
R = right

SECTION

A
GENERAL PRINCIPLES

CHAPTER

1

Pathology and healing of fractures

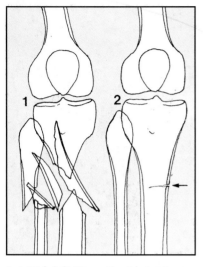

1. Initial definitions: Fracture: A fracture is present when there is loss of continuity in the substance of a bone. The term covers all bony disruptions, ranging from the situation when (1) a bone is broken into many fragments (multifragmentary or comminuted fracture) to (2) hairline and even microscopic fractures. To the layman the word 'fracture' implies a more severe injury than a simple break in the bone, but in the strict medical sense there is no difference between these terms.

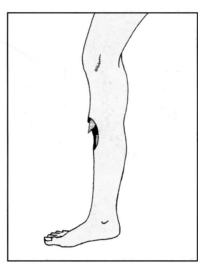

2. Open fracture: All fractures are either *closed* or *open*. In an open fracture there is a wound in continuity with the fracture, and the potential exists for organisms to enter the fracture site from outside. All open fractures therefore carry the risk of becoming infected. In addition, blood loss from external haemorrhage may be significant. (Note: the term 'compound' is still frequently used to describe a fracture which is open; the term 'simple', to describe a closed fracture, may lead to confusion, and is now largely abandoned.)

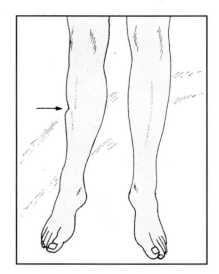

3. Closed fracture: In a closed fracture the skin is either intact, or if there are any wounds these are superficial or unrelated to the fracture. So long as the skin is intact, there is no risk of infection from outside (blood-borne infection of closed fractures being extremely rare). Any haemorrhage is internal.

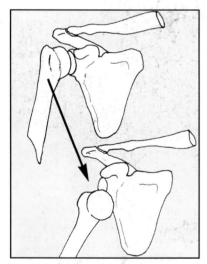

4. Dislocation: In a dislocation there is complete loss of congruity between the articulating surfaces of a joint. The bones taking part in the articulation are displaced relative to one another. For example, in a dislocated shoulder the head of the humerus loses all contact with the glenoid; in the common anterior dislocation, the head of the humerus is displaced anteriorly.

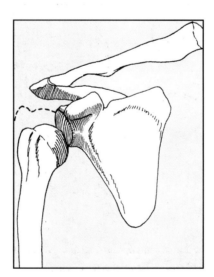

5. Subluxation: In a subluxation, the articulating surfaces of a joint are no longer congruous, but loss of contact is incomplete. The term is often used to describe the early stages in a condition which may proceed to complete dislocation (e.g. in a joint infection or in rheumatoid arthritis).

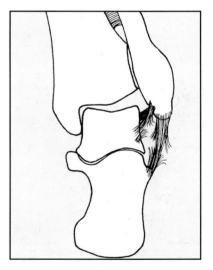

6. Sprain: A sprain is an incomplete tear of a ligament or complex of ligaments responsible for the stability of a joint, e.g. a sprain of the ankle is a partial tear of the external ligament and is not associated with instability (as distinct from a complete tear). The term sprain is also applied to incomplete tears of muscles and tendons.

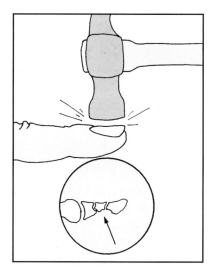

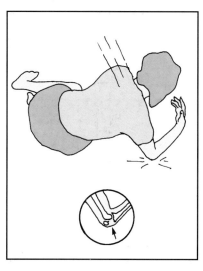

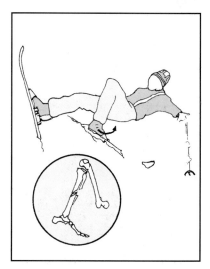

7. Causes of fracture: Direct violence (a): Fractures are caused by the application of stresses which exceed the limits of strength of a bone. Violence is the commonest cause. In the case of *direct* violence, a bone may be fractured by being struck by a moving or falling object, e.g. a fracture of the terminal phalanx of a finger by a hammer blow.

8. Direct violence (b): A bone may also be fractured if *it* forcibly strikes a resistant object. For example, a fall on the point of the elbow may fracture the olecranon.

9. Indirect violence: Very frequently, fractures result from *indirect* violence. A twisting or bending stress is applied to a bone, and this results in its fracture at some distance from the application of the causal force. For example, a rotational stress applied to the foot may cause a spiral fracture of the tibia. Indirect violence is also the commonest cause of dislocation.

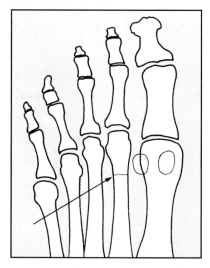

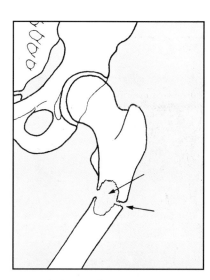

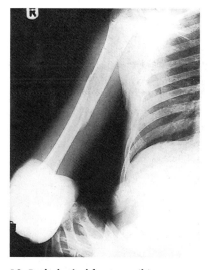

10. Fatigue fractures: Stresses, repeated with excessive frequency to a bone, may result in fracture. This mechanism is often compared with fatigue in metals which break after repeated bending beyond their elastic limit. The commonest of these fractures involves the second metatarsal – the 'march fracture' (so-called because of its frequency in army recruits).

11. Pathological fractures (a): A pathological fracture is one which occurs in an abnormal or diseased bone. If the osseous abnormality reduces the strength of the bone then the force required to produce fracture is reduced, and may even become trivial. For example, a secondary tumour deposit may lead to a pathological fracture of the subtrochanteric region of the femur – a common site.

12. Pathological fractures (b): Pathological fractures may also occur at the site of simple tumour, e.g. a fracture of the humerus in a child with a simple bone cyst. *The commonest causes of pathological fracture are osteoporosis and osteomalacia.*

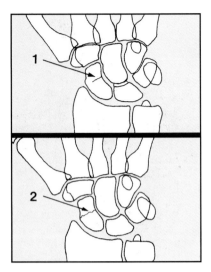

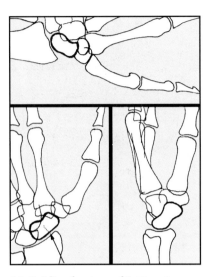

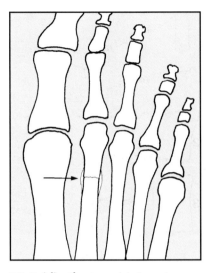

13. Fracture patterns and their significance: Hairline fractures (a): Hairline fractures result from minimal trauma, i.e. trauma which is just great enough to produce a fracture but not severe enough to produce any significant displacement of the fragments. Such fractures may be (1) incomplete or (2) complete.

14. Hairline fractures (b): These fractures may be difficult to detect on the radiographs, and where there are reasonable clinical grounds for suspecting a fracture, the rules are quite clear: 1. Additional oblique radiographic projections of the area may be helpful; 2. Do not accept poor quality films; 3. Films repeated after 7–10 days may show the fracture quite clearly (due to decalcification at the fracture site).

15. Hairline fractures (c): *Stress fractures* are generally hairline in pattern and are often not diagnosed with certainty until there is a wisp of subperiosteal callus formation, or increased density at the fracture site some 3–6 weeks after the onset of symptoms. Hairline fractures generally heal rapidly, requiring only symptomatic treatment, **but** the scaphoid and femoral neck are notable exceptions.

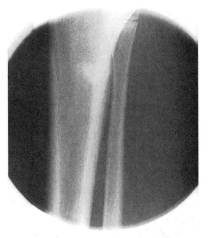

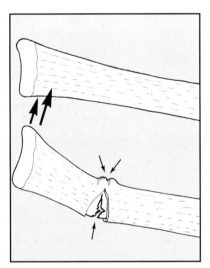

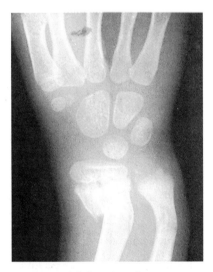

16. Hairline fractures (d): Radiograph of upper tibia of an athletic adolescent with a 7 week history of persistent leg pain. Previous radiographs were reported as normal. Note the coned view to obtain optimal detail and the incomplete hairline fracture revealed by bone sclerosis and subperiosteal callus. A crepe bandage support only was prescribed, and the symptoms settled in a further 6 weeks.

17. Greenstick fractures (a): Greenstick fractures occur in children, but not all children's fractures are of this type. The less brittle bone of the child tends to buckle on the side opposite the causal force. Tearing of the periosteum and of the surrounding soft tissues is often minimal.

18. Greenstick fractures (b): This radiograph illustrates a more severe greenstick fracture of the distal radius and ulna. Note that although there is about 45° of angulation at the fracture site, there is no loss of bony contact in either fracture. The clinical deformity is clearly suggested by the soft tissue shadow.

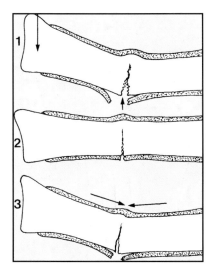

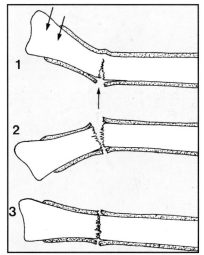

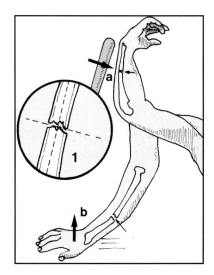

19. Greenstick fractures (c): Reduction of a greenstick fracture is facilitated by the absence of displacement and by the intact tissues on the concavity of the fracture. Angulation may be corrected by supporting the fracture and applying pressure over the distal fragment (1 & 2). The elastic spring of the periosteum may however lead to recurrence of angulation (3). Particular attention must therefore be taken over plaster fixation and aftercare.

20. Greenstick fractures (d): In the forearm in particular, where angulation inevitably leads to restriction of pronation and supination, some surgeons deliberately overcorrect the initial deformity (1). This tears the periosteum on the other side of the fracture (2). This reduces the risks of secondary angulation (3). Healing in all greenstick fractures is rapid.

21. Simple transverse fractures (a): Transverse fractures run either at right angles to the long axis of a bone (1), or with an obliquity of less than 30°. They may be caused by *direct* violence, when the bone fractures immediately beneath the causal force (e.g. the ulna fracturing when warding off a blow (a)). They may also result from *indirect* violence, when the bone is subjected to bending stresses by remotely applied force (e.g. a fracture of the forearm bones resulting from a fall on the outstretched hand (b)).

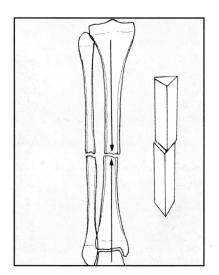

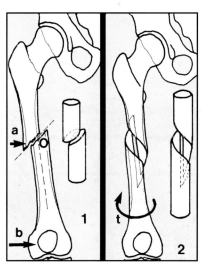

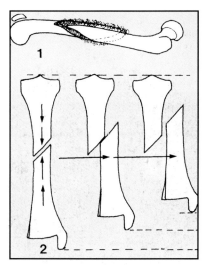

22. Simple transverse fractures (b): The inherent stability of this type of fracture (illustrated by the model on the right) reduces the risks of shortening and displacement. In the tibia, as a result, weight bearing may be permitted at a comparatively early stage. On the other hand, the area of bony contact is small, requiring very strong union before any external support can be discarded. (NB: The term 'simple' used to describe this and the following fractures means that the fracture runs circumferentially round the bone with the formation of only two main fragments.)

23. Simple oblique fractures (a): In an oblique fracture (1) the fracture runs at an oblique angle of 30° or more (O). Such fractures may be caused by (a) direct or (b) indirect violence. In *simple spiral* fractures (2) the line of the fracture curves round the bone in a spiral. Simple spiral fractures result from indirect violence, applied to the bone by twisting (torsional) forces (t).

24. Simple oblique and spiral fractures (b): In spiral fractures, union can be rapid (1) as there is often a large area of bone in contact. In both oblique and spiral fractures, unopposed muscle contraction or premature weight bearing readily lead to shortening, displacement and sometimes loss of bony contact (2). (Note: In the AO classification of fractures (see later) simple spiral, oblique and transverse fractures are classified as Type A fractures.)

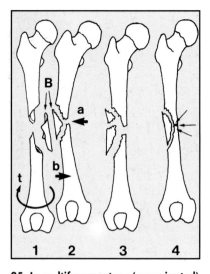

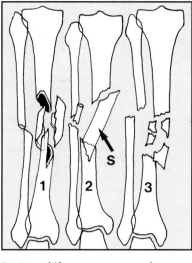

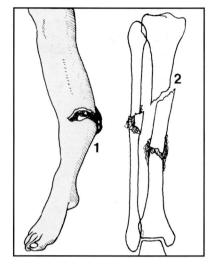

25. In multifragmentary (comminuted) fractures there are more than two fragments. The *spiral wedge* fracture (1) is produced by torsional forces (t), and the *bending wedge* fracture (2) by direct (a) or indirect (b) violence. The fragment (B) is often called a butterfly fragment (because of its shape). With greater violence, a *fragmented (comminuted) wedge* fracture (3) results. (All these fractures are in Type B in the AO classification (see later) and their characteristic is that after reduction there is still bony contact between the main fragments (4)).

26. In multifragmentary complex fractures (a further division of comminuted fractures) there is no contact between the main fragments after reduction. In *complex spiral* fractures (1) there are two or more spiral elements; in *complex segmental* fractures (sometimes called *double fractures*) (2) there is at least one quite separate complete bone fragment (S). In *complex irregular* fractures (3) the bone lying between the main elements is split into many irregular fragments. (All these fractures are classified as Type C in the AO classification.)

27. Multifragmentary fractures are generally the result of greater violence than is the case with most simple fractures, and consequently there is an increased risk of damage to neighbouring muscle, blood vessels and skin (1). The fractures tend to be unstable, and delayed union and joint stiffness are common. Segmental fractures are often difficult to reduce by closed methods, and direct exposure may threaten the precarious blood supply to the central segment. Non-union at one level is not uncommon in these fractures (2).

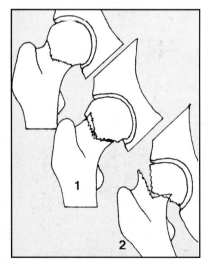

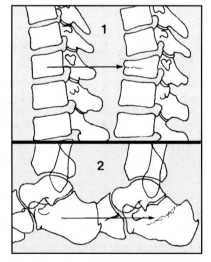

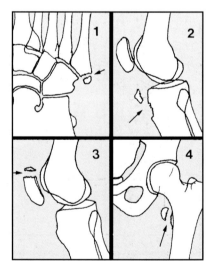

28. Impacted fractures: A fracture is impacted when one fragment is driven into the other (1). Cancellous bone is usually involved and union is often rapid. The *stability* of these fractures varies and is more implied than real. Displacement will occur if the fracture is subjected to deforming forces, e.g. without fixation, impacted femoral neck fractures frequently come adrift (2).

29. Compression (or crush) fractures: Crush fractures occur in cancellous bone which is compressed beyond the limits of tolerance. Common sites are (1) the vertebral bodies (as a result of flexion injuries) and (2) the heels (following falls from a height). If the deformity is accepted, union is invariably rapid. In the spine, if correction is attempted, recurrence is almost inevitable.

30. Avulsion fractures (a): An avulsion fracture may be produced by a sudden muscle contraction, the muscle pulling off the portion of bone to which it is attached. Common examples include:
(1) Base of fifth metatarsal (peroneus brevis).
(2) Tibial tuberosity (quadriceps).
(3) Upper pole of patella (quadriceps).
(4) Lesser trochanter (iliopsoas).
(These are all AO Type A fractures.)

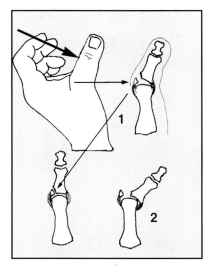

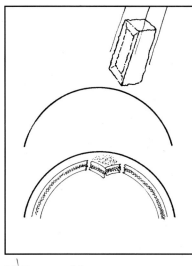

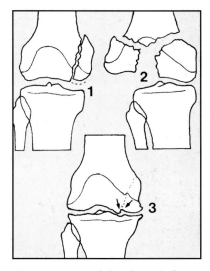

31. Avulsion fractures (b): Avulsion fractures may also result from traction on a ligamentous or capsular attachment: these are often witness of *momentary dislocation*, e.g. (1) an abduction force may avulse the ulnar collateral ligament attachment, with spontaneous reduction. *Late subluxation* (2) is common with this ('gamekeeper's thumb') and other injuries and is especially serious in the case of the spine.

32. Depressed fracture: Depressed fractures occur when a sharply localised blow depresses a segment of cortical bone below the level of the surrounding bone. Although common in skull fractures, this pattern is only rarely found in the limbs, where the tibia in the upper third is probably most frequently affected. Healing is rapid; complications are dependent on the site.

33. Fractures involving the articular surfaces of a joint: In *partial articular* fractures (1) part of the joint surface is involved, but the remainder is intact and solidly connected to the rest of the bone (AO Type B fracture). In *complete articular* fractures (2) the articular surface is completely disrupted and separated from the shaft (AO Type C fracture). When a fracture involves the articular surfaces, any persisting irregularity may cause secondary osteoarthritis (3). Stiffness is a common complication; this may be minimised by early mobilisation.

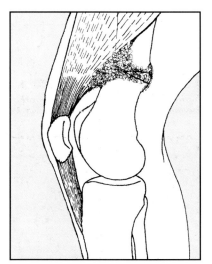

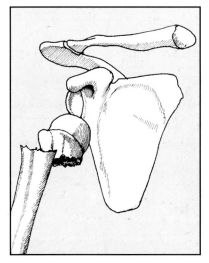

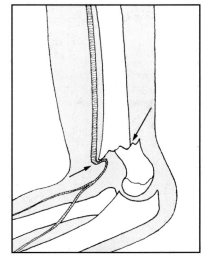

34. Fracture close to a joint: When a fracture lies close to a joint, stiffness may also be a problem due to tethering of neighbouring muscles and tendons by spread of callus from the healing fracture, e.g. in fractures of the femur close to the knee, the quadriceps may become bound down by the callus, resulting in difficulty with knee flexion.

35. Fracture–dislocation: A fracture–dislocation is present when a joint has dislocated and there is in addition a fracture of one of the bony components of the joint. Illustrated is a fracture–dislocation of the shoulder, where there is an anterior dislocation with a fracture of the neck of the humerus. Injuries of this kind may be difficult to reduce and may be unstable. Stiffness and avascular necrosis are two common complications.

36. Complicated fractures: A fracture is described as *complicated* if there is accompanying damage to major neighbouring structures. The diagram is of a complicated supracondylar fracture of the humerus. (Such an injury might also be described as a supracondylar fracture complicated by damage to the brachial artery.)

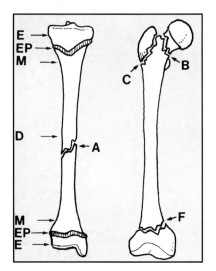

37. Describing the level of a fracture
(a): The *anatomical divisions* of a long bone include the epiphysis (E), epiphyseal plate (EP), and diaphysis or shaft (D). Between the latter two is the metaphysis (M). A fracture may be described as lying within these divisions, or involving a distinct anatomical part, e.g. A = fracture of the tibial diaphysis; B = fracture of the femoral neck; C = fracture of the greater trochanter; F = supracondylar fracture of the femur.

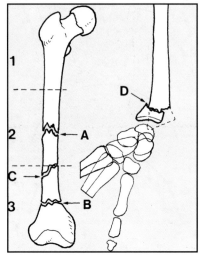

38. Describing the level of a fracture
(b): For descriptive purposes a bone may be divided arbitrarily into thirds. In this way, A = fracture of the mid third of the femur; B = fracture of the femur in the distal third; C = fracture of the femur at the junction of the middle and distal thirds. The level of a fracture in some cases may be made quite clear by an eponym, e.g. a Colles fracture (D) involves the radius, and occurs within an inch (2.5 cm) of the wrist.

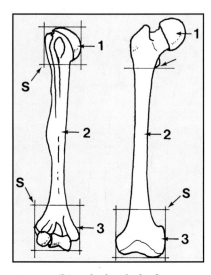

39. Describing the level of a fracture
(c): In AO terminology, long bones are divided into three unequal segments: a *proximal* segment (1), a central *diaphyseal* segment (2), and a *distal* segment (3). The boundaries between these segments are obtained by erecting squares (S) which accommodate the widest part of the bone ends. In the special case of the femur the diaphysis is described as commencing at the distal border of the lesser trochanter.

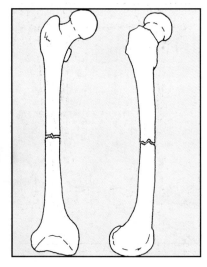

40. Describing the deformity: If there is no deformity, i.e. if the violence which has produced the fracture has been insufficient to cause any movement of the bone ends relative to one another, then the fracture is said to be in anatomical position. Similarly, if a perfect position has been achieved after manipulation of a fracture, it may be described as being in anatomical position.

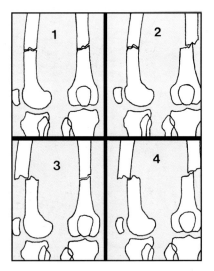

41. Displacement (a): Displacement (or translation) is present if the bone ends have shifted relative to one another. The direction of displacement is described in terms of movement of the distal fragment. For example, in these fractures of the femoral shaft at the junction of the middle and distal thirds, there is (1) no displacement, (2) lateral displacement, (3) posterior displacement, (4) both lateral and posterior displacement.

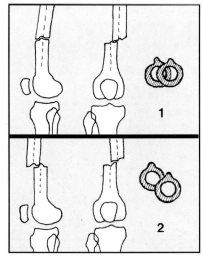

42. Displacement (b): Apart from the direction of displacement, the degree must be considered. A rough estimate is usually made of the percentage of the fracture surfaces in contact, e.g. (1) 50% bony apposition, (2) 25% bony apposition. Good bony apposition encourages stability and union.

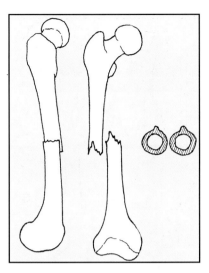

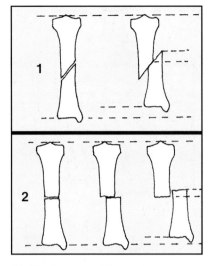

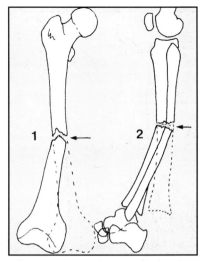

43. Displacement (c): Where none of the fracture surfaces is in contact, the fracture is described as having 'no bony apposition' or being 'completely off-ended'. Off-ended fractures are: 1. Potentially unstable; 2. Liable to progressive shortening; 3. Liable to delay or difficulty in union; 4. Often hard to reduce, sometimes due to trapping of soft tissue between the bone ends.

44. Displacement (d): (1) Displacement of a spiral or oblique fracture will result in shortening. Displacement of transverse fractures (2) will result in shortening only after loss of bony contact. The amount of shortening may be assessed from the radiographs (if an allowance is made for magnification). Speaking generally, displacement, whilst undesirable, is of much less significance than angulation.

45. Angulation (a): The accepted method of describing angulation is in terms of the position of the *point* of the angle, e.g. (1) fracture of the femur with medial angulation, (2) fracture of the tibia and fibula with posterior angulation (both are midshaft fractures). This method can on occasion give rise to confusion, especially as deformity is described in terms of the distal fragment.

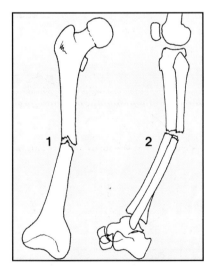

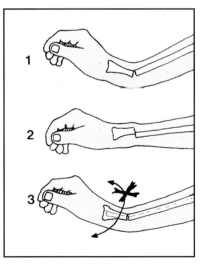

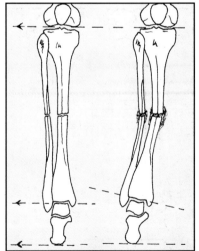

46. Angulation (b): Equally acceptable, and perhaps less liable to error, would be to describe these fractures in the following way: (1) a fracture of the middle third of the femur with the distal fragment tilted laterally, (2) a fracture of the tibia and fibula in the middle thirds, with the distal fragment tilted anteriorly.

47. Angulation (c): Significant angulation must always be corrected for several reasons. Deformity of the limb will be conspicuous (1) and regarded (often correctly) by the patient as a sign of poor treatment. Deformity from displacement (2) is seldom very obvious. In the upper limb, function may be seriously impaired, especially in forearm fractures where pronation/supination may be badly affected (3).

48. Angulation (d): In the lower limb, alteration of the plane of movements of the hip, knee or ankle may lead to abnormal joint stresses, leading to the rapid onset of secondary osteoarthritis.

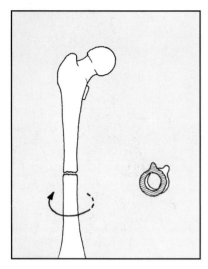

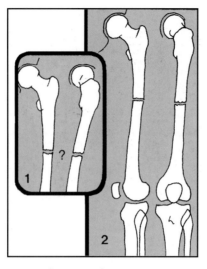

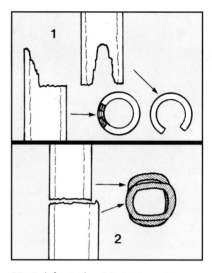

49. Axial rotation (a): A third type of deformity may be present; this is when one fragment rotates on its long axis, with or without accompanying displacement or angulation. This type of deformity may be overlooked unless precautions are taken and the possibility of its occurrence kept in mind.

50. Axial rotation (b): Radiographs which fail to show both ends of the bone frequently prevent any pronouncement on the presence of axial rotation (1). When both ends of the fractured bone are fully visualised on one film rotation may be obvious (2). The moral is that in any fracture both the joint above and the one below should be included in the examination.

51. Axial rotation (c): Axial rotation may also be detected in the radiographs by noting (1) the position of interlocking fragments (displaced fracture with 90° axial rotation illustrated). If a bone is not perfectly circular in cross-section at the fracture site, differences in the relative diameters of the fragments may be suggestive of axial rotation (2). Axial rotation is of particular importance in forearm fractures.

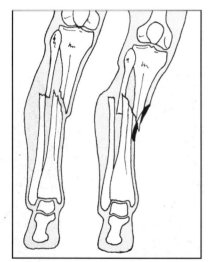

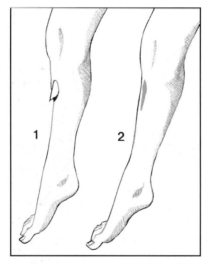

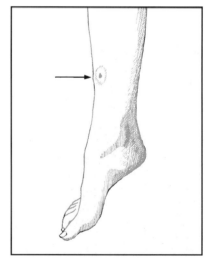

52. Open fractures: *Open* (compound) fractures are of two types: those which are open from *within out*, and others which are open from *without in*. In fractures which are open from *within out*, the skin is broached by the sharp edge of one of the bone ends. This may occur at the time of the initial injury, or later from unguarded handling of a closed fracture.

53. Fractures open from within out: (1) The case may be first seen with bone obviously still penetrating the skin which may be tightly stretched round it. (2) More commonly, the fracture, having once broken the skin, promptly spontaneously reduces, so that what is seen is a wound at the level of the fracture.

54. Technically open fracture: Occasionally the skin damage is minimal, with a small area of early bruising, in the centre of which is a tiny tell-tale bead of blood issuing from a puncture wound; this bead of blood reappears as soon as it is swabbed. The risks of infection are much less in open from *within out* fractures than in those from *without in*. This is especially so in the technically open fracture just described.

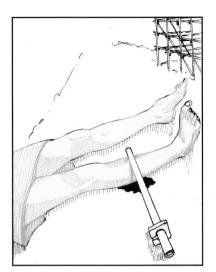

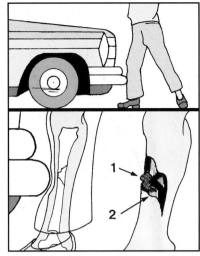

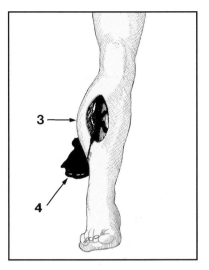

55. Fractures open from without in (a): This type of injury is caused by direct violence; the causal force breaks the skin and fractures the underlying bone. Causes include injuries from falling objects (e.g. in the construction industry, mining, rock falls in mountaineering, etc.) and motor vehicle impacts.

56. Open from without in (b): The risks of infection are greater in this type of open fracture as: (1) dirt and fragments of clothing, etc. may be driven into the wound, (2) the skin is often badly damaged; skin may even be lost. In either case, wound healing may be in jeopardy. Difficulty in closure must be anticipated.

57. Open from without in (c): Here the skin and soft tissue damage may be more extensive (3) leading to oedema, compartment syndromes, problems with wound cover, and greater haemorrhage (4) and shock. The associated fractures are more frequently comminuted, leading to difficulty in reduction and fixation. There may be vascular and/or neurological complications. *The initial assessment of any open fracture must consider neurovascular and significant muscle and tendon damage as well as the fracture itself.*

SELF-TEST (answers on page 24)

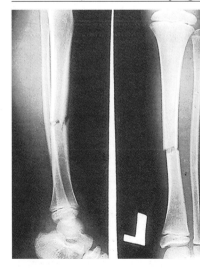

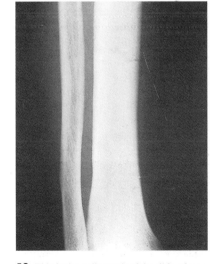

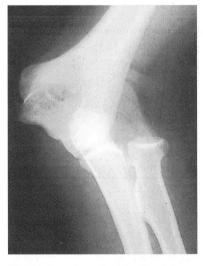

58. Describe the level and pattern of this child's fracture.

59. This is the radiograph of the tibia of a young man who was kicked whilst playing rugby. What is the pattern of fracture? What observations would you make regarding the detection of such a fracture?

60. This is a radiograph of the elbow of an adult injured in a fall. There is obvious clinical deformity. What is the injury?

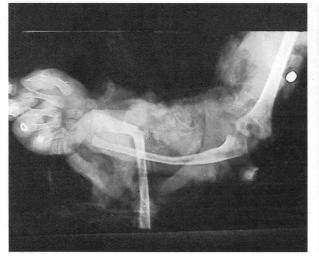

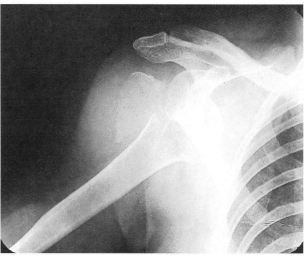

61. This is a radiograph of the arm of a child severely crushed in a run-over road traffic accident. Describe the injury.

62. What is the pattern of this injury?

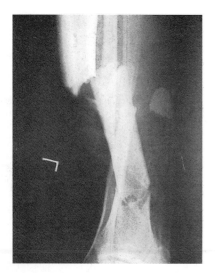

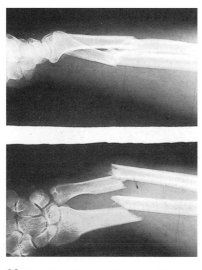

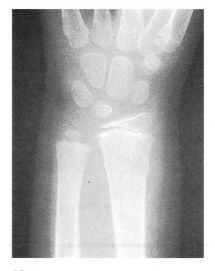

63. Describe this fracture. What problems might you anticipate with it?

64. Describe the level and any angulation or displacement that you see in this fracture.

65. Can you detect any abnormality in this AP radiograph of the wrist and forearm of a child?

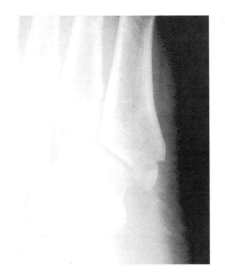

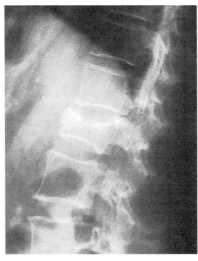

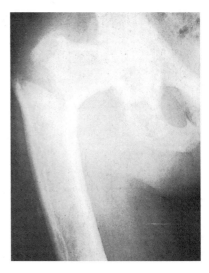

66. This is the radiograph of a patient who complained of pain in the side of the foot following a sudden inversion injury. Where is the fracture, and what is the pattern of injury?

67. The history in this case is of pain in the back following a fall. What is the pattern of fracture?

68. This radiograph is of the hip of an elderly lady who complained of pain after a fall. What deformity is present? Have you any observations to make regarding any factors contributing to the fracture?

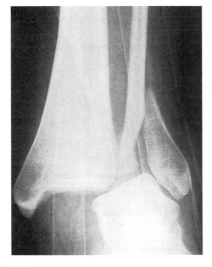

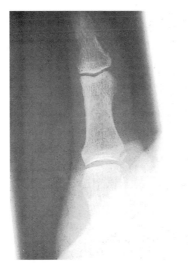

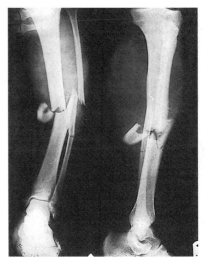

69. What is this pattern of fracture? What is the importance of accurate reduction in this case?

70. What pattern of injury is illustrated in this thumb radiograph? What is its significance?

71. This injury was sustained in a road traffic accident. Describe the pattern of injury and the deformity.

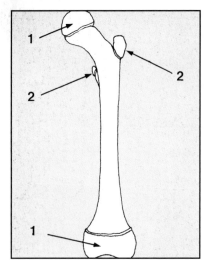
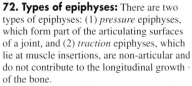

72. Types of epiphyses: There are two types of epiphyses: (1) *pressure* epiphyses, which form part of the articulating surfaces of a joint, and (2) *traction* epiphyses, which lie at muscle insertions, are non-articular and do not contribute to the longitudinal growth of the bone.

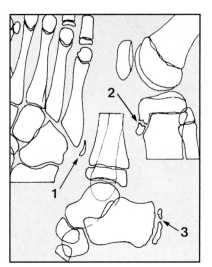

73. Traction epiphyses cntd: Injuries to the traction epiphyses are nearly always avulsion injuries. The sites commonly affected include (1) the base of the fifth metatarsal, (2) the tibial tuberosity, (3) the calcaneal epiphysis. Traction injuries are probably the basic cause of Osgood Schlatter's and Sever's disease (2 & 3). Other sites include the lesser trochanter, ischium and the anterior iliac spines.

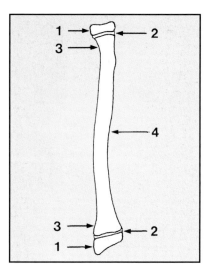

74. Pressure epiphyses (a): Pressure epiphyses are situated at the ends of the long bones and take part in the articulations. The corresponding epiphyseal plates are responsible for longitudinal growth of the bone (circumferential growth is controlled by the periosteum). *Note:* (1) epiphysis, (2) epiphyseal plate, (3) metaphysis, (4) diaphysis.

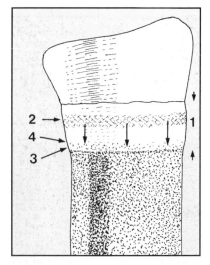

75. Pressure epiphyses (b): Within the epiphyseal plate (1) is a layer of active cartilage cells (2). The newly formed cells undergo hypertrophy. Calcification and transformation to bone occur near the metaphysis (3). When there is an epiphyseal separation, it occurs at the weakest point, the layer of cell hypertrophy (4). The active region (2) remains with the epiphysis.

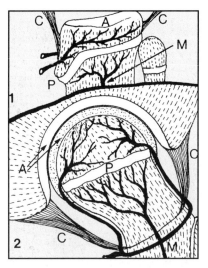

76. Pressure epiphyses (c): The metaphyseal side of the plate is nourished by vessels from the shaft (M). In the tibia (1) the epiphysis is supplied by extra-articular vessels. Vessels to the femoral head (2) lie close to the joint space and epiphyseal plate (P). There is a variable (up to 25%) contribution from the ligamentum teres. Epiphyseal displacements may lead to avascular necrosis or growth arrest. The head of radius is similarly at risk. C = capsule, A = articular cartilage.

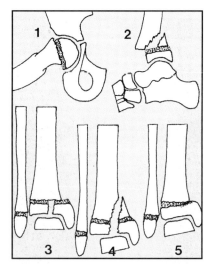

77. Epiphyseal plate injuries
(Salter–Harris classification):
Type 1: The whole epiphysis is separated from the shaft.
Type 2: The epiphysis is displaced, carrying with it a small, triangular metaphyseal fragment (the commonest injury).
Type 3: Separation of part of the epiphysis.
Type 4: Separation of part of the epiphysis, with a metaphyseal fragment.
Type 5: Crushing of part or all of the epiphysis.

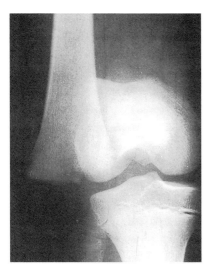

78. Type 1 injuries (a): The epiphysis is separated from the shaft without any accompanying fracture. This may follow trauma in childhood (illustrated is a traumatic displacement of the distal femoral epiphysis) or result from a birth injury. It may occur secondary to a joint infection, rickets or scurvy. Reduction by manipulation is usually easy in traumatic lesions, and the prognosis is good unless the epiphysis lies wholly within the joint.

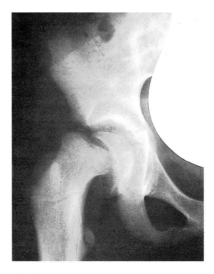

79. Type 1 injuries (b): An endocrine disturbance is thought to be an important factor in the common forms of slipped upper femoral epiphysis. Avascular necrosis is not uncommon, especially if forcible reduction is attempted after a delay in diagnosis. Growth arrest is seldom a problem (as it occurs in adolescence towards the end of growth, and as most femoral growth is at the distal end).

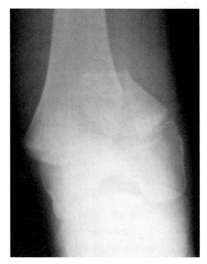

80. Type 2 injuries: The epiphysis displaces, carrying with it a small triangular fragment of the metaphysis (illustrated here in the distal femur). It is caused by trauma and is the commonest of epiphyseal injuries. Its highest incidence is in early adolescence. Growth disturbance is relatively uncommon. Reduction must be early – it becomes difficult after 48 hours by closed methods.

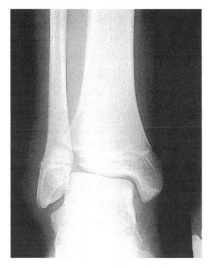

81. Type 3 injuries: Part of the epiphysis is separated. Accurate reduction is necessary in this type of injury to restore the smoothness and regularity of the articular surface. The prognosis is generally good unless the severity of the initial displacement has disrupted the blood supply to the fragment. The lower and upper tibial epiphyses are most commonly affected (note separated portion of tibial epiphysis behind lateral malleolus).

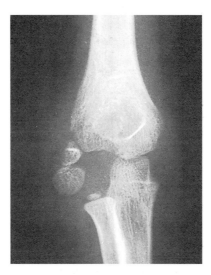

82. Type 4 injuries: Separation of part of the epiphysis with a metaphyseal fragment. The lateral condyle of the humerus is most commonly affected and must be accurately reduced – open reduction is usually necessary. Failure of reduction leads to bone formation in the gap and marked disturbance of growth.

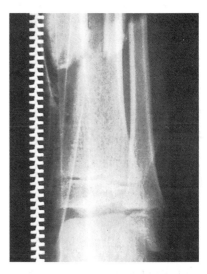

83. Type 5 injuries: Crushing or other damage to the epiphyseal plate. This radiograph of a child who was dragged along the road by a car shows the medial malleolus, part of the epiphyseal plate and the adjacent tibia have been removed by abrasion (the tibia is also fractured). The epiphyseal plate may also be crushed in severe abduction and adduction injuries of the ankle.

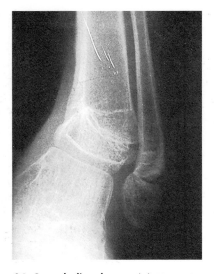

84. Growth disturbances (a): If growth is arrested over part of the epiphyseal plate only, there will be progressive angulatory deformity affecting the axis of movement of the related joint. There will be a little overall shortening. This radiograph shows the tilting of the plane of the ankle joint which occurred in the last case, with deformity of the foot and ankle. In the elbow, injuries of this type may lead to cubitus varus or valgus.

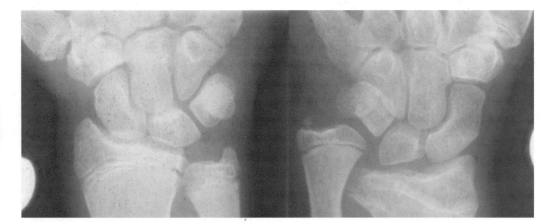

85. Growth disturbances (b): If the whole epiphyseal plate is affected, growth will be arrested, leading to greater shortening of the bone. The final result will depend on the age at which epiphyseal arrest occurred, and the epiphysis involved; obviously the younger the child, the greater is the growth loss. Arrest of one epiphysis in paired bones will lead to joint deformity. In the case illustrated, the radial epiphysis on the right has suffered complete growth arrest following a displaced lower radial epiphysis. The ulna has continued to grow at its usual rate; its distal end appears prominent on the dorsum of the wrist, and there is obvious deformity and impairment of function in the wrist. The normal left side is shown for comparison.

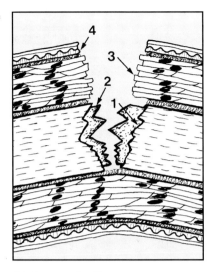

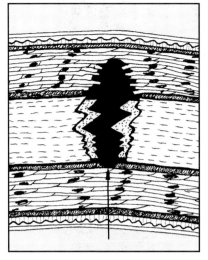

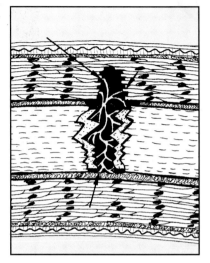

86. Fracture healing: As a result of the injury, (1) the periosteum may be completely or partly torn, (2) there is disruption of the Haversian systems with death of adjacent bone cells, (3) there may be tearing of muscle, especially on the convex side of the fracture, and damage to neighbouring nerves and blood vessels, and (4) the skin may be broached in compound injuries, with risk of ingress of bacteria.

87. Fracture haematoma (a): Bleeding occurs from the bone ends, marrow vessels and damaged soft tissues, with the formation of a fracture haematoma which clots. (A closed fracture is illustrated.)

88. Fracture haematoma (b): The fracture haematoma is rapidly vascularised by the ingrowth of blood vessels from the surrounding tissues, and for some weeks there is rapid cellular activity. Fibrovascular tissue replaces the clot, collagen fibres are laid down and mineral salts are deposited.

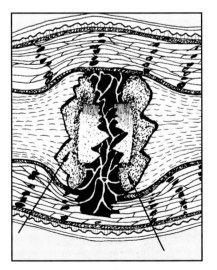

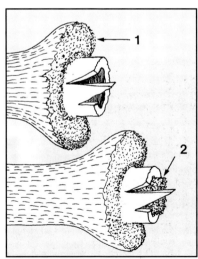

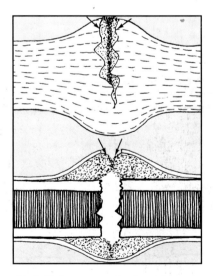

89. Subperiosteal bone: New woven bone is formed beneath the periosteum at the ends of the bone. The cells responsible are derived from the periosteum, which becomes stretched over these collars of new bone. If the blood supply is poor, or if it is disturbed by excessive mobility at the fracture site, cartilage may be formed instead and remain until a better blood

90. Primary callus response: This remains active for *a few weeks* only (1). There is a much less vigorous formation of callus from the medullary cavity (2). Nevertheless, the capacity of the medulla to form new bone remains indefinitely throughout the healing of the fracture.

91. Bridging external callus (a): If the periosteum is incompletely torn, and there is no significant loss of bony apposition, the primary callus response may result in establishing external continuity of the fracture ('bridging external callus'). Cells lying in the outer layer of the periosteum itself proliferate to reconstitute the periosteum.

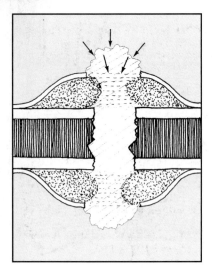

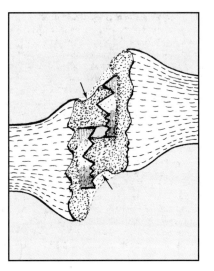

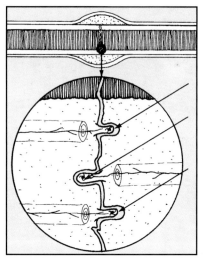

92. Bridging external callus (b): If the gap is more substantial, fibrous tissue formed from the organisation of the fracture haematoma will lie between the advancing collars of subperiosteal new bone. This fibrous tissue may be stimulated to form bone ('tissue induction'), again resulting in bridging callus. The mechanism may be due to a change of electrical potential at the fracture site or to a (hypothetical) wound hormone.

93. Bridging external callus (c): If the bone ends are offset, the primary callus from the subperiosteal region may unite with medullary callus. The net result of the three mechanisms just described is that the fracture becomes rigid, function in the limb returns and the situation is rendered favourable for endosteal bone formation and remodelling.

94. Endosteal new bone formation (a): If there is no gap between the bone ends, osteoclasts can tunnel across the fracture line in advance of ingrowing blood vessels and osteoblasts, which form new Haversian systems. Dead bone is revascularised and may provide an invaluable scaffolding and local mineral source. This process cannot occur if the fracture is mobile.

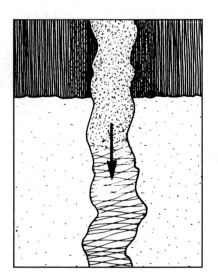

95. Endosteal new bone formation (b): The formation of new cortical bone, with re-establishment of continuity between the Haversian systems on either side, cannot occur if fibrous tissue remains occupying the space between the bone ends. If this is present, it must be removed and replaced with woven bone. This is generally achieved by ingrowth of medullary callus which remains active through the healing phase.

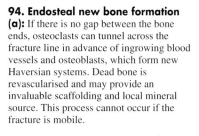

96. Endosteal new bone formation (c): Where the bone ends are supported by rigid internal fixation, there is no functional requirement for external bridging callus: as a result external bridging callus may not be seen, or be minimal. Healing of the fracture occurs slowly through the formation of new cortical bone between the bone ends. It is therefore essential that internal fixation devices are retained until this process is complete.

Remodelling: After clinical union, new Haversian systems are laid down along the lines of stress. In areas free from stress, bone is removed by osteoclasts. Eventually little trace of external bridging callus will remain. The power to remodel bone in this way is great in children, but not so marked in the adult. In a child, most or all traces of fracture displacement (including even off-ending) will disappear. There is also some power to correct angulation, although this becomes progressively less as the child approaches adolescence. Any axial rotation, however, is likely to remain. In the adult, there is virtually no correction of axial rotation or angulation. It is, therefore, important that axial rotation deformity is always corrected, and that angulation, particularly in adults, should not be accepted.

Bone morphogenic proteins (BMP): These make up a family of proteins which have osteogenic facility. At least 14 (BMP 2–15) have been identified; they have been purified, cloned and sequenced into human recombinant forms. They function by inducing mesenchymal cells to transform – first into cartilage and then into bone cells. They may produce and mineralise osteoid, influence angiogenesis, and play a part in bone remodelling. They may also have a role to play in articular cartilage repair.

BMP are being evaluated for effectiveness and safety in the treatment of non-unions, bone segmental defects and avascular necrosis, especially of the femoral head.

97. The classification of fractures

There is no fracture of any bone which has escaped an attempt at classification. Sometimes this has been done on the basis of region and pattern, sometimes through a concept of the stresses to which the bone has been subjected, and usually with an eye on some understanding of the severity of the injury and its prognosis. Unfortunately not everyone has the same ideas regarding the relative importance of the various factors concerned, and as time progresses and knowledge expands the number of classifications that exist has been continuing to grow.

The result is that in nearly every area there is a wealth of classifications, usually with grades, degrees or numbers attached to the originator's name. This bewilders the newcomer, and causes much confusion in those who are attempting to assess the results of various treatments, as the injuries classified by one author may not be easily compared with those described by another. There is, too, the problem of how to ascribe certain fractures which have been inconsiderate enough to adopt a pattern that does not quite fit within the classification.

No surgeon is able to master the wealth of classifications outside his own specialist area, and for purposes of communication, as far as single injuries are concerned, a fracture is described mainly by its site and pattern, along the lines already detailed. In such circumstances classifications are only mentioned if they have become familiar through long usage, and in some cases classifications of this type may be archaic.

After many years' work the AO Group have evolved a classification which aims to encompass all fractures, actual or theoretical, and is of particular value for research purposes.

THE AO CLASSIFICATION OF FRACTURES OF LONG BONES

The following points should be noted:

1. This is *not* a classification of injuries: it is a classification of fractures.
2. It does not include dislocations, unless they have an associated fracture.
3. It does not differentiate between undisplaced and displaced fractures of the shafts of the long bones (but it does so in the case of certain fractures of the bone ends).
4. It does not give any indication of the relative frequency of particular fractures.
5. The sorting of fractures (beyond the area of the bone involved) depends on the AO Group's assessment of the severity of the fracture; this they define as 'the morphological complexity, the difficulty in treatment, and the prognosis'. In areas this may reflect a preference for the use of internal fixation rather than conservative methods of treatment.
6. The classification results in an alpha-numeric code which is suitable for computer sorting, and which allows for research purposes (e.g. in assessing the results of any treatment, wherever carried out) the comparison of like with like.
7. Because of the format, it is not descriptive in a verbal sense, and is not suitable for conveying information about the nature of an individual fracture (e.g. over the telephone).

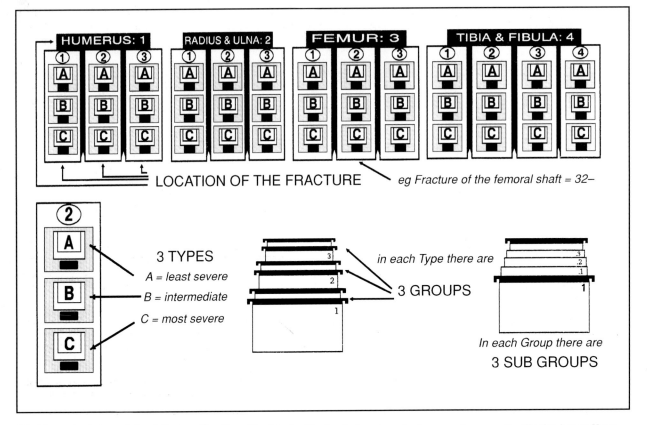

eg Fracture of the femoral shaft = 32–

3 TYPES

A = least severe

B = intermediate

C = most severe

in each Type there are

3 GROUPS

In each Group there are

3 SUB GROUPS

98. The principles of the AO classification: The AO classification for long bone fractures may be grasped by likening it to an X-ray storage system, with numbered blocks of filing cabinets: one block for each bone. Within each block, each filing cabinet (which is also numbered) represents a particular area of each bone: cabinet number 1 stores fractures of the proximal segment, number 2 the diaphysis or shaft, and number 3 the distal segment. In the case of the tibia, there is a fourth cabinet to deal with fractures of the malleoli. (The junction between the segments is determined in the way described on p. 10, Frame 39.)

When a fracture bridges the junction between two segments, the segment under which it is classified is determined by the site of the mid-point of the line of the fracture. In practice, therefore, a two digit code determines the **location** of a fracture: e.g. under 22– would be stored all fractures of the shafts of the radius, or the ulna, or of both these bones.

In *each cabinet* all the radiographs for a single location of fracture are divided into fracture **Types** (represented by the three drawers); the least severe go in drawer A (Type A fractures), those of intermediate severity in B (Type B), and the most severe in C (Type C). Some of the criteria used to differentiate between the three types of fracture have already been indicated (Frames 25, 26, 33), but see Footnote.

Any type of fracture can be put in one of three **groups** (represented by folders, and numbered 1–3). The methods of selection are again described later. Within each **group** fractures may be further sorted into **subgroups** (represented by partitions). Each of these subgroups has a numerical representation (.1, .2, .3). (If an even more detailed classification is needed, fractures within each **subgroup** can have added **qualifications**. These can be described by a single number (or two numbers separated by a comma) added in parentheses after the main coding. The first digit in the range 1–6 is used to amplify the description of a fracture's location and its extent, while the second is purely descriptive. The number 7 is reserved to describe partial amputations, 8 for total amputation, and 9 for loss of bone stock.)

As an example of the AO classification, a simple oblique fracture of the proximal part of the femoral shaft distal to the trochanters would be coded 32–A2.1, as follows:

3 = the *bone*: the femur } the **location**
2 = the *segment*: the diaphysis } of the fracture
– = separator between **location** and **type**
A = the **type**: A is the least severe type of fracture, with two bone fragments only
2 = the **group**: group 2 includes all oblique fractures
.1 = **subgroup**: subgroup 1 includes fractures in the proximal part of the diaphysis where the medullary cavity is wider than in the more central part of the bone.

Footnote: the criteria employed in sorting fractures into their appropriate types, groups and subgroups are given in a little more detail in the section on Regional Injuries.

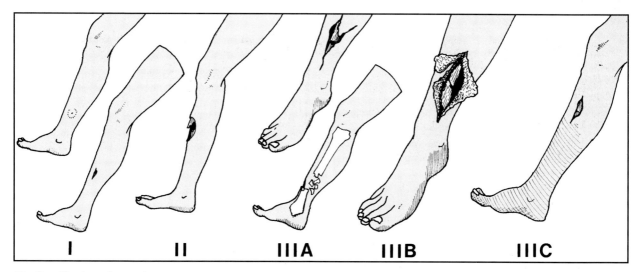

| I | II | IIIA | IIIB | IIIC |

99. Classification of open fractures (a):

The classification of Gustilo et al is well established and in common use. It is a practical classification which relates well to the common patterns of injury and their prognosis. Three types are described, with the third being subdivided to allow a more precise grading:

Type I: An open fracture with a wound which is (a) less than 1 cm and (b) clean.

Type II: An open fracture with a wound which is (a) more than 1 cm long and (b) not associated with extensive soft tissue damage, avulsions, or flaps.

Type IIIA: An open fracture where there is adequate soft tissue coverage of bone in spite of (a) extensive soft tissue lacerations or flaps or (b) high energy trauma irrespective of the size of the wound.

Type IIIB: An open fracture with extensive soft tissue loss, periosteal stripping and exposure of bone. Massive contamination is usual.

Type IIIC: An open fracture associated with an arterial injury which requires repair.

100. Classification of open fractures (b):

The AO Group use separate classifications for closed and open skin injuries and for injuries to muscle; they employ a separate fourth classification for nerve and vascular injuries. The classification is more complex and is given here for completeness:

Skin lesions in closed fractures (Integuments, Closed):

IC1 = Skin undamaged
IC2 = Contusion of skin
IC3 = Local degloving
IC4 = Extensive (but closed) degloving
IC5 = Skin necrosis resulting from contusion

Skin lesions in open fractures (Integuments, Open):

IO1 = Skin broken from *within out*
IO2 = Skin broken from *without in*, with contused edges but less than 5 cm in length

IO3 = In excess of 5 cm of skin broken, with devitalised edges and local degloving
IO4 = Full thickness contusion, abrasion, skin loss
IO5 = Extensive degloving

Muscle and tendon injuries in fractures:

MT1 = No muscle injury
MT2 = Local muscle injury, one muscle group only
MT3 = Extensive muscle injury with involvement of more than one group
MT4 = Avulsion or loss of entire muscle groups, tendon lacerations
MT5 = Compartment syndrome; Crush syndrome

Neurovascular injuries in fractures:

NV1 = No neurovascular injury
NV2 = Isolated nerve injury

NV3 = Isolated vascular injury
NV4 = Combined neural and vascular injury
NV5 = Subtotal or total amputation

Note that for data storage purposes the above AO soft tissue classifications are appended to their alpha-numeric fracture classification, e.g. a segmental fracture of the tibia in which there was a small skin wound, no obvious muscle damage, but an associated drop foot would be classified 42–C2/IO2–MT1–NV2: this is *not* a classification for committing to memory!

Note the very approximate correlations between the Gustilo and AO classifications:

Gustilo Type I equivalent to IO1
Gustilo Type II equivalent to IO2
Gustilo Type IIIA equivalent to IO3
Gustilo Type IIIB equivalent to IO4
Gustilo Type IIIC equivalent to IO3–5 + NV2

ANSWERS TO SELF-TEST

58. Transverse fracture of the tibia in the middle third. Simple transverse fracture of the tibia in the middle third (or simple transverse fracture of the tibial diaphysis). There is no significant displacement or angulation, and the fibula is intact. The fracture is of adult pattern and is not a greenstick fracture.

59. Hairline fracture of the tibial diaphysis (or of the tibia in the lower mid third). Coned-down views are often helpful; if the initial radiographs appear normal, they should be repeated after an interval if there is continued suspicion that a fracture is present. CAT scans of the suspect area are also often useful.

60. Dislocation of the elbow. The radius and ulna are displaced laterally in relation to the humerus (and also posteriorly, although this is not shown on the single radiograph).

61. This injury cannot be anything but *open* as the right-angled angulation of the greenstick fracture of the radius (at the junction of its middle and lower thirds) indicates. The mottling of the soft tissue shadows due to air is confirmatory. In addition, there is a greenstick fracture of the ulna in its middle third (note the posterior angulation) and dislocation of the elbow (the ulna appears lateral and the humerus AP). Both fractures are of the diaphysis.

62. Fracture–dislocation of the shoulder. The head of the humerus is not congruous with the glenoid. Lateral to it is a large fragment of bone, the avulsed greater tuberosity of the humerus.

63. Segmental (double) fracture of the tibia (complex segmental fracture). The proximal fracture is virtually transverse and in the middle third. The distal fracture is also transverse and situated in the distal third. The fibula is fractured, and the tibia displaced medially. Bony apposition has probably been lost in the proximal fracture. Problems with reduction, fixation and non-union at one level are to be anticipated.

64. Fracture of the radius and ulna in the distal third. In the lateral projection, there is some slight anterior (volar) angulation (posterior (or dorsal) tilting) of the ulna. In the AP view, there is lateral (or radial) displacement of the distal fragments which are virtually off-ended. There is some medial (ulnar) angulation (or the distal fragments are tilted laterally). The radial fracture is oblique with a slight spiral element. The ulnar fracture is transverse.

65. There is a greenstick fracture of the radius. Note the ridging of the radius both medially and laterally just proximal to the epiphysis.

66. Fracture of the base of the fifth metatarsal. This is an avulsion fracture, produced by the peroneus brevis which is inserted into the fifth metatarsal base.

67. The radiograph shows deformity of the body of the first lumbar vertebra which has been reduced in height anteriorly. This is an anterior compression or crush fracture.

68. There is a simple oblique fracture of the proximal femur, running between the lesser and greater trochanters, with a coxa vara deformity (the distal femur is tilted medially). The hip is arthritic and the disturbance in bone texture in the pelvis and femur is typical of Paget's disease (i.e. this is a pathological fracture).

69. There is a simple oblique fracture of the fibula, which is displaced laterally, accompanied by the talus. The distal end of the fibula is tilted laterally (medial angulation). Unless accurately reduced, this fracture involving a joint is liable to lead to secondary osteoarthritis.

70. The small fragment of bone detached from the base of the proximal phalanx has been avulsed by the ulnar collateral ligament of the MP joint. It indicates that the thumb has been dislocated, and that there is potential instability at this level.

71. There is a fragmented wedge fracture of the tibial diaphysis. There are four fragments, and the main butterfly fragment of a bending wedge fracture remains in contact and alignment with the main distal fragment. There is a segmental (double) fracture of the fibula. Both fractures are in the middle third. Soft tissue shadows indicate, as might be anticipated, that this is an open fracture. There is lateral angulation (i.e. the distal fragment is tilted medially). During the taking of the AP and lateral radiographs there has been some alteration of position of the fracture: note that in the lateral projection there is considerable *axial rotation* (the foot is lateral, but the upper tibia is almost in the AP plane). Axial rotation is not a feature of the AP projection.

CHAPTER

2

The diagnosis of fractures and principles of treatment

HOW TO DIAGNOSE A FRACTURE

1. HISTORY

In taking the history of a patient who may have a fracture, the following points may prove to be helpful, especially when there has been a traumatic incident.

1. What activity was being pursued at the time of the incident (e.g. taking part in a sport, driving a car, working at a height, etc.)?
2. What was the nature of the incident (e.g. a kick, a fall, a twisting injury, etc.)?
3. What was the magnitude of the applied forces? For example, if a patient was injured in a fall, it is helpful to know how far they fell, if the fall was broken, the nature of the surface on which they landed, and how they landed. Trivial violence may lead one to suspect a pathological fracture; severe violence makes the exclusion of multiple injuries particularly important.
4. What was the point of impact and the direction of the applied forces? In reducing a fracture, one of the principal methods employed is to reduplicate the causal forces in a reverse direction. If a fracture occurs close to the point of impact, additional remotely situated fractures must be excluded.
5. Is there any significance to be attached to the incident itself? For example, if there was a fall, was it precipitated by some underlying medical condition, such as a hypotensive attack, which requires separate investigation?
6. Where is the site of any pain, and what is its severity?
7. Is there loss of functional activity? For example, walking is seldom possible after any fracture of the femur or tibia; inability to weight bear after an accident is of great significance.
8. What is the patient's age? Note that while a young person may sustain bruising or a sprain following moderate trauma, an incident of comparative magnitude in an older patient may result in a fracture.

Diagnosis In some cases the diagnosis of fracture is unmistakable, e.g. when there is gross deformity of the central portion of a long bone or when the fracture is visible, as in certain compound injuries. *In the majority of other cases, a fracture is suspected from the history and clinical examination, and confirmed by radiography of the region.*

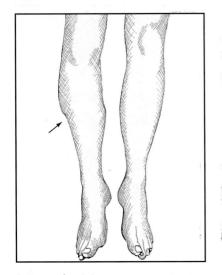

2. Inspection (a): Begin by inspecting the limb most carefully, comparing one side with the other. Look for any *asymmetry of contour*, suggesting an underlying fracture which has displaced or angled.

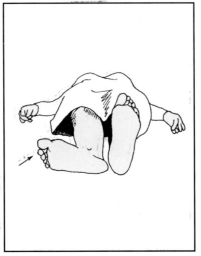

3. Inspection (b): Look for any persisting *asymmetry of posture* of the limb, e.g. persisting external rotation of the leg is a common feature in disimpacted fractures of the femoral neck.

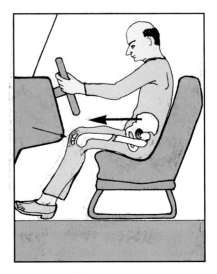

4. Inspection (c): Look for local bruising of the skin suggesting a *point of impact* which may direct your attention locally or to a more distant level. For example, bruising over the knee from dashboard impact should direct your attention to the underlying patella, and also to the femoral shaft and hip.

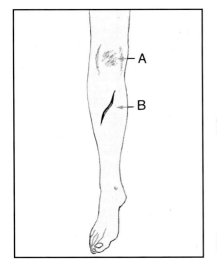

5. Inspection (d): Look for other tell-tale skin damage. For example (A) grazing, with or without ingraining of dirt in the wound, or friction burns, suggests an impact followed by rubbing of the skin against a resistant surface. (B) Lacerations suggest impact against a hard edge, tearing by a bone end, or splitting by compression against a hard surface.

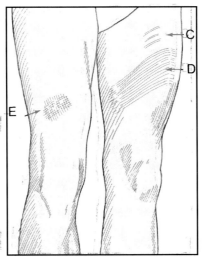

6. Inspection (e): Note the presence of: (C) skin stretch marks, (D) band patterning of the skin, suggestive of both stretching and compression of the skin in a run-over injury, (E) pattern bruising, caused by severe compression which leads the skin to be imprinted with the weave marks of overlying clothing. Any of these abnormalities should lead you to suspect the integrity of the underlying bone.

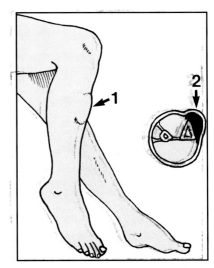

7. Inspection (f): If the patient is seen shortly after the incident, note any localised swelling of the limb (1). Later, swelling tends to become more diffuse. Note the presence of any haematoma (2). A fracture may strip the skin from its local attachments (degloving injury); the skin comes to float on an underlying collection of blood which is continuous with the fracture haematoma.

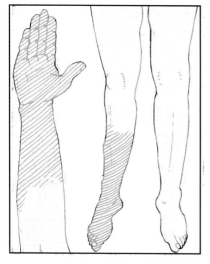

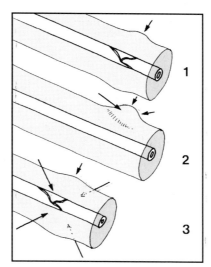

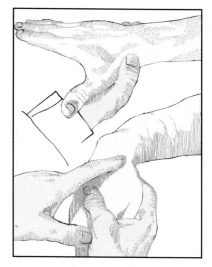

8. Inspection (g): Note the colour of the injured limb, and compare it with the other. Slight cyanosis is suggestive of poor peripheral circulation; more marked cyanosis suggests venous obstruction; and whiteness may indicate disturbance of the arterial supply. Feel the limb and note the temperature at different levels, again comparing the sides. Check the pulses and the rapidity of pinking-up after tissue compression.

9. Tenderness (a): Look for tenderness over the bone suspected of being fractured. Tenderness is invariably elicited over a fracture (1), but tenderness will also be found over any traumatised area, even though there is no underlying fracture (2). The important distinguishing feature is that in the case of a fracture tenderness will be elicited when the bone is palpated on *any* aspect (3).

10. Tenderness (b): In eliciting tenderness, once a tender area has been located the part should be palpated at the same level from another direction. For example, in many sprained wrists tenderness will be elicited in the anatomical snuff-box – but not over the dorsal and palmar aspects of the scaphoid, which are tender if a fracture is present.

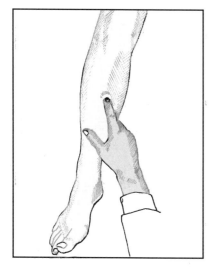

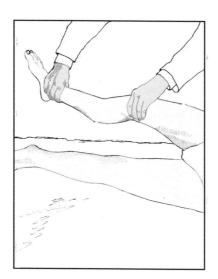

11. Palpation: The sharp edge of a fracture may be palpable. Note also the presence of localised oedema. This is a particularly useful sign over hairline and stress fractures. The development of oedema may however take some hours to reach detectable proportions.

12. Other signs: If the fracture is mobile, moving the part may produce angulation or crepitus from the bone ends rubbing together. In addition, the patient will experience severe pain from such movement. These signs may be inadvertently observed during routine examination of the patient, but should not be sought unless the patient is unconscious and the diagnosis is in doubt.

13. Radiographic examination: In every case of suspected fracture, radiographic examination of the area is mandatory. Radiographs of the part will generally give a clear indication of the presence of a fracture and provide a sound basis for planning treatment. In the case where there is some clinical doubt, radiographs will reassure patient and surgeon and avert any later medicolegal criticism.

Radiographers in the United Kingdom receive thorough training in the techniques for the satisfactory visualisation of any suspect area, but it is essential that they in turn are given clear guidance as to the area under suspicion. The request form must be quite specific, otherwise mistakes may occur. At its simplest, the request must state both the *area to be visualised* and the *bone suspected of being fractured*. It is desirable to include the joints above and below the fracture. It need hardly be stressed that a thorough clinical examination should precede the completion of the radiographic request if repetition and the taking of unnecessary films are to be avoided.

The following table lists some of the commonest errors made in the filling in of request forms.

Area suspected of fracture	Typical request	Error	Correct request
Scaphoid	'X-ray wrist, ? fracture'	Fractures of the scaphoid are difficult to visualise: a minimum of 3 specialised views is required. A fracture may not show on the standard wrist projections	'X-ray scaphoid, ? fracture'
Calcaneus	'X-ray ankle, ? fracture' 'X-ray foot, ? fracture'	A tangential projection, with or without an additional oblique (along with the usual lateral), is necessary for satisfactory visualisation of the calcaneus. These views are not taken routinely when an X-ray examination of the foot or ankle is called for	'X-ray calcaneus, ? fracture'
Neck of femur	'X-ray femur, ? fracture'	Poor centring of the radiographs may render the fracture invisible	'X-ray hip, ? fracture neck of femur' or 'X-ray to exclude fracture of femoral neck'
Tibial table or tibial spines	'X-ray tibia, ? fracture'	Poor centring may render the fracture invisible, or the area may not be included on the film	'X-ray upper third tibia to exclude fracture of tibial table'

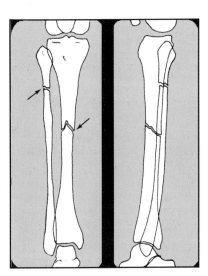

14. The standard projections: These are an *anteroposterior (AP)* and *lateral*. Ideally the beam should be centred over the area of suspected fracture, with visualisation of the proximal *and* distal joints. This is especially important in the paired long bones where, e.g., a fracture of the tibia at one level may be accompanied by a fibular fracture at another.

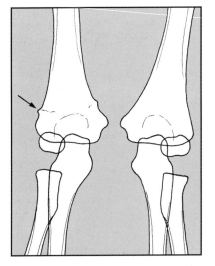

15. Comparison films: Where there is some difficulty in interpreting the radiographs (e.g. in the elbow region in children, where the epiphyseal structures are continually changing, or where there is some unexplained shadow or a congenital abnormality) films of the other side should be taken for direct comparison.

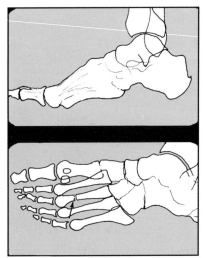

16. Oblique projections: In the case of the hand and foot, an oblique projection may be helpful when the lateral gives rise to confusion due to the superimposition of many structures. Such oblique projections may have to be specifically requested when they are not part of an X-ray department's routine.

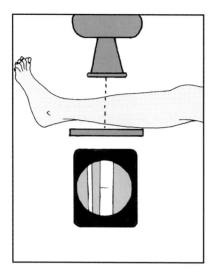

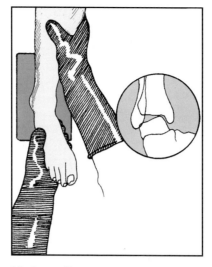

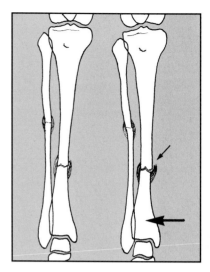

17. Localised views: Where there is marked local tenderness but routine films are normal, coned-down localised views may give sufficient gain in detail to reveal a hairline fracture. If such films are also negative, the radiographs should be repeated after an interval of 10–14 days if the symptoms are persisting (see also Hairline Fractures p. 6).

18. Stress films (a): Stress films can be of value in certain situations, e.g. when a complete tear of a major ligament is suspected. Where the lateral ligament of the ankle is thought to be torn, for example, radiographs of the joint taken with the foot in forced inversion may demonstrate instability of the talus in the ankle mortice. (Local or general anaesthesia may be required in fresh injuries.)

19. Stress films (b): Stress films may also be used where there is some doubt as to stability of a uniting fracture. They may also be employed where the possibility of refracture arises.

CAT (CT) scans   These can show tissue slices in any plane, but characteristically in median sagittal, parasagittal, coronal and, most importantly, transverse planes. The last projection cannot be readily obtained with plain X-rays, and can often provide useful additional information which is not otherwise available. In addition, in the CAT scan there is a greater range of grey-scale separation, allowing a greater differentiation of tissue types. It is of particular value in:

1. Vertebral fractures, to show the relationship between bony fragments and the spinal canal.
2. Acetabular floor fractures, to clarify the degree of disturbance of the articular surface.
3. Pelvic fractures, to show the number of elements involved and their relationship. In some cases it may be possible to display and rotate informative 3D reconstructions.
4. Calcaneal and other fractures involving joints, to visualise the position of the elements and the degree of joint disturbance.

AP and lateral tomography   In this X-ray technique the tube and film are rotated (or slid) in opposite directions during the exposure. Their position relative to one another and the part being examined determines the tissue slice being clearly visualised. The results are inferior to those obtained by CAT scanning, but may be helpful if the latter is not available.

Technetium bone scans   Technetium tagged methylene diphosphate (^{99}Tc^{m}-methylene diphosphate (MDP)) can be used 48 hours after an injury to demonstrate bone activity at a fracture site, and confirm the presence of a fracture when other methods of detection have failed.

MRI scans   These avoid any exposure to X-radiation and produce image cuts as in CAT scans with a greater ability to distinguish between different soft tissues. In the trauma field they are of particular value in assessing neurological structures within the skull and spinal canal, and meniscal and ligamentous structures about the knee and shoulder.

Ultrasound   Ultrasound imaging is of great sensitivity and of value in assessing the abdominal cavity and soft tissues such as the shoulder cuff, the patellar ligament and the calcaneal tendon.

DIAGNOSTIC PITFALLS

A number of fractures are missed with great regularity – sometimes with serious consequences. You should always be on the look-out for the following:

1. An elderly patient who is unable to weight bear after a fall must be examined most carefully. The commonest cause by far is a fracture of the femoral neck, and this must be eliminated in every case. If the femoral neck is intact, look for a fracture of the *pubic rami*. Note that, on the rare occasion, a patient with an impacted fracture of the femoral neck may be able to weight bear, albeit with pain.

2. If a car occupant suffers a fracture of the patella or femur from a dashboard impact, always eliminate the presence of a silent dislocation of the hip.

3. If a patient fractures the calcaneus in a fall, examine the other side most carefully. Bilateral fractures are extremely common, and the less painful side may be missed.

4. If a patient complains of a 'sprained ankle' always examine the foot as well as the ankle. Fractures of the base of the fifth metatarsal frequently result from inversion injuries, and are often overlooked. The mistake of not performing a good clinical examination in these circumstances is compounded by requesting radiographs of the ankle (which do not show the fifth metatarsal bone).

5. In the unconscious patient, injuries of the cervical spine are frequently overlooked. It pays to have routine screening films of the neck, chest and pelvis in the unconscious patient.

6. Impacted fractures of the neck of the humerus are often missed, especially when one view only is taken. Conversely, in children, the epiphyseal line is often wrongly mistaken for fracture.

7. Posterior dislocation of the shoulder may not be diagnosed when it should be at the initial attendance. This is because the humeral head comes to lie directly behind the glenoid, and is not detected if only a single AP projection is taken. If there is a strong suspicion of injury, and especially if there is deformity of the shoulder, a second projection is *essential* if no abnormality is noted on the AP film. (Two views should be taken routinely in all injuries, but in many departments the shoulder, for no good reason, is excluded from this rule.)

8. Apparently isolated fractures of either the radius or ulna should be diagnosed with caution. The Monteggia and Galeazzi fracture–dislocations are still frequently missed. In the same way, it is unwise to diagnose an isolated fracture of the tibia until the whole of the fibula has been visualised; fracture of the tibia close to the ankle is, for example, often accompanied by fracture of the fibular neck.

9. At the wrist, greenstick fractures of the radius in children are often overlooked due to lack of care in studying the radiographs.

10. In adults, fractures of the radial styloid or Bennett's fracture may be missed or treated as suspected fractures of the scaphoid. Complete tears of ulnar collateral ligament of the MP joint of the thumb are frequently overlooked, sometimes with severe resultant functional disability.

THE TREATMENT OF FRACTURES

PRIMARY AIMS

The primary aims of fracture treatment are:
1. The attainment of sound bony union without deformity.
2. The restoration of function, so that the patient is able to resume their former occupation and pursue any athletic or social activity they wish.

To this might be added 'as quickly as possible' and 'without risk of any complications, whether early or late'. These aims cannot always be achieved, and in some situations are mutually exclusive. For example, internal fixation of some fractures may give rapid restoration of function, but at the expense of occasional infection. The great variations that exist in fracture treatment are largely due to differences in interpretation of these factors and their relevance in the case under consideration; they are in constant flux, with on the one hand the development of more sophisticated methods of fracture fixation and new antibiotics, and on the other the emergence of antibiotic resistant organisms.

STAGES OF TREATMENT

A number of systems have been devised to divide the time elapsing from the occurrence of a fracture into stages, within each of which it is the aim to complete a recognised phase of treatment. This is of especial importance in the management of multiple injuries. In one such scheme three stages are recognised: these follow vital resuscitation.

Primary This lasts for 72 hours. During this period the fracture and any accompanying injuries should be investigated to a conclusion and treated accordingly. Within this time scale it is usually possible to carry out definitive fracture treatment (e.g. open reduction and internal fixation), discarding any initial splintage.

Secondary This covers the period 3–8 days post-injury. If the patient's condition during the primary phase is too poor to allow time-consuming procedures (such as the internal fixation of both forearm bones or complex joint reconstructions), then these should performed during this period. At this time secondary wound closures, soft tissue reconstructions, and the reduction and fixation of facial fractures should be carried out.

Tertiary After 8 days, assuming that the patient's general condition is stable, additional procedures may be required. These include bone grafting of massive defects, secondary closure of amputations, soft tissue reconstructions, and any procedures postponed from the secondary period.

RESUSCITATION

If a limb fracture is a patient's sole injury, resuscitation is less frequently required, so that it is often possible to proceed with treatment without undue delay (although unfitness for anaesthesia may sometimes upset this ideal). If, however, a fracture is complicated by damage to other structures, or involvement of other systems, then treatment of the fracture usually takes second place. Immediate action must be taken to correct any life-endangering situation which may be present or anticipated.

Advanced trauma life support (ATLS) It is recognised that a well organised trauma team can give the best treatment to a severely injured patient. The core trauma team will normally consist of ten staff: a team leader, an anaesthetist and his assistant, a general surgeon, an orthopaedic surgeon, an emergency department physician, two nurses, a radiographer, and a note-taker (scribe). Each member has his own specific areas of responsibility. The team leader should not normally touch the patient, but orchestrate the team. Additional staff will include porters, blood bank staff including a haematologist, and a biochemist. A neurosurgeon, thoracic surgeon, plastic surgeon, and radiologist should also be available at short notice.

To maintain such a team with its equipment makes heavy demands, and is only possible in a few hospitals which have the necessary work load and resources. In most situations, especially away from large centres, smaller teams are involved and assessment and management follow a more linear approach (as adopted below).

INITIAL MANAGEMENT

Some general principles in the initial management of cases of multiple injuries are well established, and may be summarised with the mnemonic **ABCDE(F)**.

A = Airway

1. Any blood, mucus or vomit must be removed from the upper respiratory passages by suction or swabbing. Dentures should be looked for and extracted. In the more minor situations, respiratory obstruction may be avoided by support of the jaw, a simple airway, and turning the patient on their side.
2. An endotracheal tube may have to be passed:
   (a) in the unconscious patient with an absent gag reflex
   (b) where inhalation of mucus or vomit has already taken place (or is suspected), for clearing of the respiratory passages under vision
   (c) where there is bleeding from the upper airway
   (d) for the more effective management of cases where there is respiratory difficulty or evidence of hypoxia, e.g. in cases of flail chest. Where there is need for intubation in a patient with a suspected cervical spine injury, the procedure should be carried out with great care, avoiding excessive cervical spine extension; naso-tracheal intubation should be used. Confirm placement by auscultation (and/or by a radiograph).

B = Breathing

1. Ventilate with 100% oxygen. Check the breath sounds. After intubation assess the arterial blood gas levels so that if these remain impaired the appropriate steps may be taken (e.g. reviewing the diagnosis and noting the situations described below).
2. An open chest wound must be immediately covered to reduce the risks of tension pneumothorax. A vaseline gauze dressing, covered with a swab, and firmly secured to the skin with broad adhesive tape is usually quite adequate in the emergency situation.
3. If there is evidence of a tension pneumothorax (hyper-resonance and decreased breath sounds on the affected side, or tracheal shift to the other), or of pneumothorax or haemothorax, the appropriate chest cavities should be drained by intercostal catheters connected to water seal drains. A routine radiograph of the chest will usually confirm the diagnosis, but if this remains in doubt, the chest should be tapped in the fifth interspace in the mid-axillary line.
4. If there is evidence of paradoxical respiration due to flail rib segments, blood gas levels should be estimated. Normal values are given below:

pO$_2$	75–100 mmHg
pCO$_2$	35–45 mmHg
pH	7.38–7.44
Oxygen content	15%–23%
Oxygen saturation	95%–100%
Bicarbonate	22–25 millequivalent/L

Slight impairment of respiratory function may be managed by giving oxygen by inhalation and analgesics with caution. When the blood gas levels are seriously disturbed, and especially in the presence of a concurrent head injury, some form of assisted respiration is usually the best method of management.

C = Circulation

1. Any severe external haemorrhage must be brought under rapid control. This can almost always be achieved with local padding or packing along with firm bandaging. The use of a tourniquet is best avoided except in the rarest of circumstances; then one should be used only in circumstances where its retention for excessive periods cannot occur. A tourniquet must be properly applied: too little pressure will increase the blood loss by preventing venous return, and too great a pressure will endanger underlying nerves. A pneumatic tourniquet should always be applied in preference to any other type.
2. Remove blood for grouping and cross-matching, and the establishment of baseline parameters including haemoglobin and haematocrit.

3. Set up two large bore (14–16 gauge) intravenous lines, performing if necessary a rapid cut-down and insertion of a large bore intravenous cannula under vision.

4. Make an assessment of the circulatory state. Initially, the blood pressure and pulse are the most useful familiar guides to the state of the circulation, but note that tachycardia and a low blood pressure may sometimes be absent in those suffering from hypovolaemic shock, requiring the exercise of clinical judgement. The *need* for replacement depends on an assessment of loss and the circulatory state. The *amount and type* of replacement is dependent on the nature and extent of the loss. The *rate* of infusion is largely determined by the response to replacement.

Classification of haemorrhage A 70 kg male has a circulatory volume of 5 L of blood (equivalent to 25 units of packed red blood cells).

Class I: loss of up to 15% of blood volume (equivalent to 4 units of packed red cells) normally does not cause a change in blood pressure or pulse.

Class II: loss of 15–30% of blood volume (equivalent to 4–8 units of packed red cells) normally leads to tachycardia, but no significant disturbance of the blood pressure.

Class III: loss of 30–40% of blood volume (about 2 L in a 70 kg man) results in tachycardia and lowering of the blood pressure.

Class IV: loss of more than 40% of blood volume leads generally to severe tachycardia and lowering of the blood pressure.

Estimating blood loss The following gives a crude guidance in anticipating potential blood loss:

- Closed fracture of the femoral shaft: 1 L
- Open book fractures of the pelvis: 2–3 L (potentially much greater where there is a sacroiliac disruption).
- Intra-abdominal haemorrhage: 2–3 L
- Haemothorax: 1–2 L
- Closed head injury: blood loss is insubstantial and hypotension does not occur unless the patient is close to death

5. If there is blood loss accompanied by tachycardia or hypotension rapidly run in crystalloids such as normal saline or Ringer-lactate. (In children, give 20 mL/kg body weight initially, and up to 60 mL/kg.) Use of warmed solutions has been shown to reduce mortality and help preserve the haemostatic mechanisms, and should be routine. **If the response is inadequate after 2 L, other measures will be required.** These include the administration of packed red blood cells or whole blood, and possibly surgery (see later.) Temporary splintage of limb fractures will reduce local haemorrhage whether the fracture is open or closed.

(Note that crystalloids are poorly retained in the intravascular space. Some prefer the use of plasma or synthetic colloids which do not suffer from this disadvantage, but others claim that these have no advantage in the trauma setting. Fresh frozen plasma does have the advantage of covering any tendency to hypofibrinogenanaemia and factor V and factor VII deficiencies, but takes 20–30 minutes to thaw. Two units of fresh frozen plasma should be given where bleeding is continuing and there are coagulation factor deficiencies present.)

D = Drugs, allergies, disabilities   Carry out a rapid screening of the patient, and note any information (e.g. on warning cards, bracelets or lockets, or from relatives) of any relevant problem.

E = Eating and exposure   Obtain, if possible, information on the patient's intake of fluids and solids in case general anaesthesia is required. Where applicable, remove clothing to allow inspection of the entire patient to avoid overlooking any additional injuries.

F = Foley catheter   In cases of multiple injury, and where no urinary tract damage is suspected, insert a catheter to allow monitoring of urinary output (and hence the adequacy of the blood pressure in maintaining renal function).

FURTHER ASSESSMENT

Screening films   At an early stage in the assessment of a patient with multiple injuries, screening films of the cervical spine, chest and pelvis should be obtained. Where there is the possibility of an abdominal injury with intra-abdominal haemorrhage an ultrasound examination should be carried out. If the circumstances dictate and allow, the opportunity may be taken at this stage to arrange an X-ray examination of any limb injury, or any injury to the skull or facial bones.

Fluid replacement   If the patient fails to be stabilised by the administration of crystalloids, then blood will be required. Normally, blood will also be required if the haemoglobin falls below 9 g/dL. Note the following points:

1. If the patient is exsanguinated, and will die unless blood is administered immediately, give two units of Group O Rhesus negative blood pending supply of cross-matched blood. The latter should ideally should become available not more than 20 minutes after the patient's blood sample is submitted to the blood bank.
2. Thereafter, or if the situation is less acute, administer cross-matched packed red cells. If bleeding continues, then whole blood becomes more appropriate.

The volume of the replacement required can vary enormously, and therefore must be judged by the response: see the following flow chart (Fig. 2.1) for a summary of replacement management.

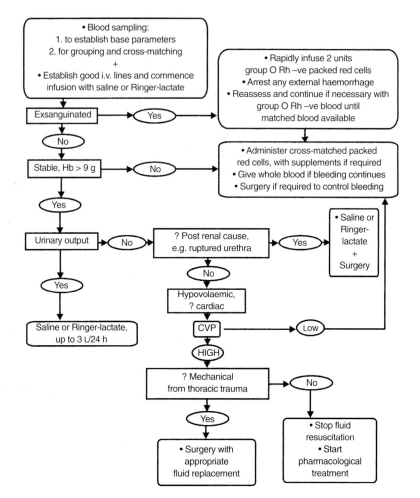

Fig 2.1: Flow chart summarising fluid replacement management.

Assessing the response to replacement There is varying opinion on the best methods of assessing the stability of the circulation and the success of resuscitation. In all, the degree and maintenance of a positive response to treatment is more important than the reading of isolated values. Many methods are advocated including the following:

1. **Pulse and blood pressure**. In spite of some unreliability, these remain the most valuable guides. The initial aim should be to restore the pulse rate to less than 140, and to obtain a blood pressure in excess of 90 mm systolic and rising.

2. **Urinary output.** Aim at 0.5 mL/kg body weight per hour in an adult (ie. 6 mL every 10 minutes in a 70 kg man) and 1.0 mL/kg body weight in a child (i.e. twice the rate per kg).

3. **Central venous pressure (CVP)**. This allows the monitoring of atrial filling pressures. (Normal value = less than 10 mmHg.)

4. **Haemoglobin.** If the Hb level reaches 10 g/dL and remains there, further blood is not usually required. (Below 9 g/dL, blood will usually be required, and virtually invariably below 7 g/dL. When the Hb lies between 7–10 g/dL, and there is doubt, the P_vO_2 and ER (see below) may be helpful in defining transfusion requirements). In the absence of continuing bleeding, one unit of packed red blood cells would be expected to raise the Hb level by 1g/dL.

Less common investigations include

5. **Pulmonary Artery Pressure (PAP):** A pulmonary artery catheter allows the measurement of pulmonary artery pressure and has been particularly advocated in the elderly patient. (Normal values: systolic = 15–28 mmHg; diastolic = 5–16 mmHg.)
6. **Pulmonary Capillary Wedge Pressure (PCWP):** (Normal value, mean = 6–12 mmHg.)
7. **Cardiac output:** (Normal value = 4–7 L/min.)
8. **Cardiac index (CI):** This represents the circulating blood volume per minute. (Normal value = 2.8–4.2 L/min.)
9. **Systemic vascular resistance (SVR):** (Normal value = 11–18 mmHg.)
10. **Arterial-alveolar oxygen difference (AaDO$_2$):** (Normal = 10 mmHg.)
11. **Peripheral/body core temperature difference:** This gives a useful assessment of prolonged shock.
12. **Mixed venous partial pressure of oxygen (P_vO_2):** This is a guide to the tissue oxygen supply and is normally 6 kPa, 45 mmHg. If the patient's condition is stable no treatment is indicated until a critical level of 3 kPa, 23 mmHg is reached.
13. **Extraction ratio (ER):** This is the ratio of oxygen consumption to oxygen delivery, and normally is around 25%. It equals:

$$\frac{C_aO_2 - C_vO_2}{C_aO_2}$$

where C_aO_2 = arterial oxygen; C_vO_2 = venous oxygen.

COMPLICATIONS OF TRANSFUSION

1. Hypocalcaemia. Transfused blood contains citrate which binds the patient's ionised calcium. Usually this is not a problem as the healthy liver can metabolise (to bicarbonate) the citrate in one unit of blood in 5 minutes. Where transfusion rates are rapid, however, excessive calcium binding may itself lead to hypotension, and also to tetany. To avoid citrate toxicity it has been common practice to give 1g of calcium chloride (or 4 g calcium gluconate) for every 4 units of blood administered. It is recommended, as better practice, to avoid the administration of calcium unless there are clinical or biochemical indications (e.g. by the assessment of the ionised calcium levels).

2. Hyperkalaemia. This is not usually a problem unless very large amounts of blood are transfused. It is more usual to find hypokalaemia as the metabolic activity of the red cells begins and the tissues begin to take up potassium. Attempts at correction are only indicated if the serum electrolytes or the ECG are disturbed.

3. Acid/base disturbances. After large transfusions any residual disturbance is dependent on the quality of tissue perfusion, the rate of administration, and the effectiveness of citrate metabolism in the liver. The need for correction is determined by regular serum sampling.

4. Defects of clotting. It has been suggested that 8 units of platelet concentrate and 2 units of fresh frozen plasma should be transfused routinely with every 12 units of packed red blood cells (1 unit (50 mL) of platelet concentrate should raise the platelet count by 10 000). Nevertheless, during the administration of large replacements it is preferable that there should be regular monitoring of the platelet count, prothrombin time, partial prothromboplastin time and fibrinogen levels, and appropriate replacements given only where clearly indicated. (Fresh frozen plasma should be given if the prothrombin or partial prothromboplastin exceed 1.5 times the control levels. Cryoprecipitate (1.0–1.5 units) is given for fibrinogen levels less than 0.8 g/L.)

5. Transmission of disease. The risks of HIV and hepatitis B transmission are small (said to be in the order of 1 in 200 000 in the US), but are higher in the case of Hepatitis C (c. 1 in 5000). Septic reactions are rare, but commoner with platelet concentrates which are stored at room temperature.

6. Reactions. Acute haemolytic reactions from mismatched blood require immediate cessation of blood administration and a full investigation, which should include a haematocrit to check for the presence of haemolysis, culture of the patient's and donor's blood to exclude bacterial contamination, repeat cross-matching, a full blood count and examination of red cell morphology, and a Coombs' test. The donor blood should be returned to the blood bank and advice sought from the haematologist regarding any further investigation thought desirable. All aspects should be rigorously documented. The urinary output must be carefully monitored while an attempt is made to obtain a brisk diuresis. Severe reactions can occur from 30 mL of mismatched blood, are life threatening, and may require dialysis. Non-haemolytic reactions, often with severe associated urticaria, usually occur after administration of larger quantities of whole blood or packed cells, and may often be controlled with intravenous benadryl. Washed red cells may be given if further transfusion is required.

PERSISTING CIRCULATORY IMPAIRMENT

Where rapid, appropriate transfusion fails to control the situation, the commonest cause is continued bleeding. In most cases the site is obvious.

1. External haemorrhage accompanying limb injuries should be readily controlled if this has not already been done.

2. Continuing blood loss from intrathoracic injuries should be obvious. Assuming that a haemothorax has been diagnosed and treated by the insertion of a chest drain, the quantity and rate of loss may be evaluated by monitoring the volumes in the collection bottle(s). This may be used to assess the need for exploration to control persisting haemorrhage.

3. Massive bleeding from within the abdominal cavity usually requires immediate laparotomy, but it is essential to be sure that the bleeding is not from the pelvis. (An unstable fracture of the pelvis and a negative abdominal ultrasound would be a contraindication for laparotomy.)

The commonest causes of intra-abdominal haemorrhage are tearing of the liver, spleen or mesentery, and all are potentially amenable to surgery.

4. Haemorrhage accompanying fractures of the pelvis. This is most common in unstable fractures involving the sacroiliac joints; the bleeding may be from the pelvic plexus of veins or from damage to the iliac arteries. In the first instance, especially if there is little sacroiliac disruption, an external pelvic fixator should be employed, and replacement efforts renewed. If the sacroiliac joint is disrupted and the situation fails to resolve, a (posterior) C-clamp should be applied. If circulatory instability persists, then exploration may be needed as a last resort. Diffuse bleeding from the pelvic venous plexus is generally best controlled by packing. On rare occasions selective embolisation or ligature of the iliac arteries may be necessary.

5. Haemorrhage from the urinary tract is seldom very severe, but nevertheless may be a problem. It should be suspected if there is a haematuria or some other indication (such as the presence of a fracture of the pelvis of appropriate pattern). The diagnosis may be clarified by an intravenous pyelogram, a cystogram, or a urethrogram.

SECONDARY SURVEY TO ESTABLISH PRIORITIES OF TREATMENT

The presence of other matters of importance may well have been noted in the initial survey, but their management may have to be deferred until resuscitation is under way. Note the following:

Head injury

1. Where there is a head injury the following procedures should be followed:

(a) The unconscious patient should be intubated to minimise the risks of cerebral hypoxia.

(b) A complete neurological examination must be carried out and the results charted, using a suitable set of protocols (such as the Glasgow Coma Scale, see p. 40); the examination should be repeated at regular intervals. Of particular significance is (i) a history of a post-traumatic lucid interval; (ii) a history of progressive deterioration in the level of consciousness; (iii) focal neurological signs; (iv) a rising blood pressure and falling pulse rate.

(c) Where there is evidence of increased intracranial pressure further investigation with a CAT scan should be carried out. If an extradural haematoma is discovered its immediate evacuation should be undertaken. If a subdural haematoma is found this also should be promptly removed. If there is evidence of diffuse cerebral oedema, surgery is contraindicated, and an infusion of a hyperosmolar solution of mannitol may be commenced.

Where appropriate, monitoring of the intracranial pressure may be carried out using a catheter inserted into the lateral ventricle.

As far as the treatment of fractures accompanying a head injury is concerned, the following points should be noted.

- Where the head injury requires urgent investigative procedures or operative intervention (e.g. an extradural haemorrhage with deterioration in the level of consciousness) this will take priority over the local treatment of most fractures.
- A combined procedure may often be planned with advantage but certainly in all cases some estimate should be made as to when definitive treatment of the fracture is likely to be possible.
- Depending on that interval there is the choice of a variety of initial procedures which may include the application of sterile dressings or light packing of open wounds, supporting an injured limb with sandbags or an

---

Glasgow Coma Scale

A patient is defined as being comatose if they do not open their eyes, if they do not obey commands, and if they do not utter recognisable words. The severity of the coma may be assessed by assigning a value to the eye, motor and verbal responses, and summing these. By repeating the examinations at regular intervals progress may be monitored, and any deterioration (suggesting intracranial complications) recognised at an early stage.

Variable	Score
Eye-opening (E)	
Spontaneous	4
To speech	3
To pain	2
Nil	1
Best motor response (M)	
Obeys	6
Localises	5
Withdraws	4
Abnormal flexion	3
Extensor response	2
Nil	1
Verbal response (V)	
Oriented	5
Confused conversation	4
Inappropriate words	3
Incomprehensible sounds	2
Nil	1

The coma score = E+M+V, with a value of 3 being the worst possible response and 15 the best. A value of less than 7 indicates severe coma, 8–12 moderate and 13–14 mild. Severe injuries are infrequent, and most patients who develop haematomas requiring surgery are classified as moderate or minor on admission.

---

inflatable splint in such a position that the distal circulation is maintained, or the use of light temporary plaster splintage.

2. Where there is a head injury in which the immediate prognosis is hopeless any temporary splintage of the fracture should be retained but no fresh treatment planned.

3. Where no active neurosurgical treatment is contemplated and the prognosis regarded as very poor but not absolutely hopeless, it is usually possible to devise some simple measures to give reasonable support to the

injured part but at the same time permitting more definitive treatment in the near future should unexpected improvement occur.

Cardiac tamponade: intrathoracic rupture of the aorta

Prompt drainage of an intrapericardial haematoma may be a life-saving measure and aortic rupture may not be immediately fatal. Widening and squaring-off of the mediastinal shadow on the chest radiograph and cardiac distress should alert suspicion of these injuries. Further investigation may be required by echocardiography, angiography or CAT scan. Thoracotomy may be required (with by-pass facilities in the case of intrathoracic rupture of the aorta). Thoracotomy may also be indicated where there is a tracheal, bronchial or oesophageal injury, or a penetrating injury to the mediastinum.

Visceral complications

Most require exploration and surgical correction. Injury to the liver, spleen and kidneys may give rise to severe intra-abdominal haemorrhage. Haemorrhage may also follow mesenteric tears and ruptures of the stomach and intestine with which the problems of perforation are also associated. Intra-abdominal haemorrhage is best diagnosed by ultrasound. Perforation may be suspected in the absence of bowel sounds and where there is loss of liver dullness. Plain lateral recumbent abdominal radiographs may be of some help, but peritoneal lavage is often invaluable: the presence of bile or digestive contents may be diagnostic. CAT scans are sometimes helpful, especially in diagnosing injuries to the pancreas. Rupture of the diaphragm is often missed in cases of blunt abdominal trauma. Its presence may be concealed if there is an accompanying chest injury. Diagnosis may require chest films taken while a contrast medium is administered by nasogastric tube. In the case of the urinary tract examination of the urine for blood; an intravenous pyelogram and cystogram, and in certain pelvic fractures a urethrogram may also be employed (see Complications of Pelvic Fractures).

Eye and faciomaxillary injuries

Perforating injuries of the eye and major facial injuries require immediate surgery at the beginning of the primary period. Minor facial soft tissue injuries and fractures may be delayed till later during the primary period. Unstable facial fractures are generally stabilised during the primary period, with major reconstructive procedures being delayed until facial swelling has subsided.

Spinal fractures

Where there is an unstable fracture with no neurological involvement, or incomplete neurological involvement, stabilisation of the fracture is essential during the primary period to prevent deterioration. Where there is evidence of progressive neurological involvement (e.g. from compression of the cord by bone or disc fragments), surgery is also indicated in the primary phase. (See under Spine, p. 241).

Vascular injuries In the presence of continuing blood loss or ischaemia, further investigation may be required prior to exploration if the nature and extent of any injury is not apparent. (See p. 98.)

EVALUATION OF PATIENTS WITH MULTIPLE INJURIES
Trauma scoring; hospital trauma index; injury severity
score Several systems have been developed in an attempt to assess the severity of injuries. These may be used as an alert for the need for prompt and expert treatment; they may give an indication of the prognosis; and over a period they may be used statistically to evaluate the performance of a team, unit or hospital, or to draw attention to some injury pattern where treatment efforts might be profitably concentrated.

The two main systems in use are the Abbreviated Injury Scale (AIS), and the Hospital Trauma Index (HTI). Both classifications are largely comparable, and for normal working purposes grade injuries into five degrees of severity:

0 = None
1 = Minor
2 = Moderate
3 = Major, but not life-threatening
4 = Severe, life-threatening, but survival probable
5 = Critical, survival uncertain

Where the injury is *isolated* (i.e. the case is not one of multiple injuries), there is no problem and the grade into which the injury falls is used as required. Where there are *multiple injuries* the addition of the values obtained from the AIS or HTI tables does not give an accurate indication of severity, being overly pessimistic regarding outcome. It has been found, however, that if the grade figures are manipulated, a figure is reached which can be used with some measure of accuracy as a prognostic indicator in cases of multiple injury.

In practice, the patient's three worst injuries are assessed and the relevant grade numbers are each squared before being added together. If several injuries lie within the same area, only the worst is selected. The break point for the resultant sum is in the area of 50. The following points may be noted:

- Score < 10: death rare in any patient under the age of 50
- Score 10–20: mortality 4–30%, depending on age
- Score > 50: only rare survival, and only in exceptional circumstances and with prompt treatment by specialised staff. In this group nearly all the deaths occur within the first week, and half within the first hour.

In all groups the mortality rate rises with age; for example when the score lies between 10–19, the mortality rate in the 70+ age group is more than 8 times the rate for those under 50 years. The effects of age are somewhat paradoxically most noticeable when the injury severity scores are comparatively low.

- Score 10–15: the response to treatment of cases within this band does most to throw light on the evaluation of the standard of medical care offered by any team or department. Cases within this group are sufficiently ill to be adversely affected by poor care, but they are not so ill that no matter how expert the treatment they cannot survive.

Summary of hospital trauma index Six areas must be considered when using this method of assessment: Respiratory, Cardiovascular, Nervous system, Abdominal, Extremities, Skin and Subcutaneous. A seventh area of Complications can be included for assessments which are made at a late stage.

Respiratory

1	(minor)	Chest discomfort – minimal findings
2	(moderate)	Simple rib or sternal fracture, chest wall contusion with pleuritic pain
3	(major)	Multiple rib or first rib fracture, haemothorax, pneumothorax
4	(severe)	Open chest wound, flail chest, tension pneumothorax with normal BP, simple laceration of diaphragm
5	(critical)	Acute cyanotic respiratory failure, aspiration, tension pneumothorax with lowered BP, complicated laceration of diaphragm

Cardiovascular

1	(minor)	Less than 500 mL blood loss (less than 10% blood volume) with no change in perfusion
2	(moderate)	Blood loss of 500–1000 mL (10–20% blood volume), decreased skin perfusion but normal urinary output, myocardial contusion with normal BP
3	(major)	Blood loss of 1000–1500 mL (20–30% blood volume), decreased skin perfusion, slight decrease in urinary output, tamponade, BP 80 mmHg
4	(severe)	Blood loss of 1500–2000 mL (30–40% blood volume), decreased skin perfusion, urinary output less than 10 mL per hour, tamponade, conscious, BP less than 80 mmHg
5	(critical)	Blood loss in excess of 2000 mL (40–50% blood volume), restless, coma, cardiac contusion or arrhythmia, BP unrecordable. (Note that previously described classification of haemorrhage into 4 grades has been slightly altered for this 5 point scoring system.)

Nervous system

1	(minor)	Head injury with or without scalp laceration, but no loss of consciousness or skull fracture
2	(moderate)	Head injury with unconsciousness of under 15 minutes, skull fracture, cervical pain with minimal findings, one facial fracture

3	(major)	Head injury with coma of more than 15 minutes, depressed skull fracture, cervical spine fracture or dislocation with positive neurological findings, multiple facial fractures
4	(severe)	Head injury with coma in excess of 1 hour or with positive neurological findings, cervical spine fracture or dislocation with paraplegia
5	(critical)	Head injury with coma and no response to stimuli up to 24 hours, cervical spine fracture or dislocation with quadriplegia

Abdominal

1	(minor)	Mild abdominal wall, flank or back pain with tenderness but no peritoneal signs
2	(moderate)	Acute flank, back or abdominal discomfort and tenderness, fracture of a 7th to 12th rib
3	(major) kidney,	Isolated injury to liver (minor), small bowel, spleen,
		body of pancreas, mesentery, ureter, urethra, fractures of ribs 7–12
4	(severe)	Two major injuries: rupture of the liver, bladder, head of pancreas, duodenum, colon, or mesentery
5	(critical)	Two severe injuries: crushing of liver, major vascular – including thoracic or abdominal aorta, vena cava, iliacs, hepatic veins

Extremities

1	(minor)	Minor sprain or fracture not involving a long bone
2	(moderate)	Closed fracture of humerus, clavicle, radius, ulna, tibia, fibula, involvement of a single nerve
3	(major)	Multiple moderate fractures, open moderate, closed femur, stable pelvis, major dislocation, major nerve injury
4	(severe)	Two major long bone fractures, open fracture of femur, crushing or amputation of limb, unstable pelvic fracture
5	(critical)	Two severe or multiple major fractures

Skin and subcutaneous

1	(minor)	Less than 5% burns, abrasions, contusions, lacerations
2	(moderate)	Burns of 5–15%, extensive contusions, avulsions 8–15 cm, lacerations totalling 30 cm in length
3	(major)	Burns of 15–30%, avulsions of 30 cm
4	(severe)	Burns of 30–45%, avulsion of leg or arm
5	(critical)	Burn of 45–60%

Complications

1	(minor)	Minor wound infection, atelectasis, cystitis, superficial thrombophlebitis, temperature of >38.5°C
2	(moderate)	Major wound infection, atelectasis, pyelonephritis, septic or deep thrombophlebitis, temperature of >38.5°C
3	(major)	Intraperitoneal abscess, pneumonia, anuria or oliguria with raised serum urea, jaundice, less than 6 units of

Case example

A man aged 30 years has been admitted after being injured in a gas explosion. He was rendered unconscious for about half an hour, but skull films show no fracture and there is no sign of any intracranial damage. He has 35% superficial burns of the face, chest and abdomen. Radiographs of the chest have confirmed multiple rib fractures with a one-sided pneumothorax, but there is no immediate respiratory difficulty. He has also sustained a closed fracture of the left tibia.

Injury Severity Score

Nervous system: 3	square = 9
Skin: 4	square = 16
Respiratory: 3	square = 9
Extremities: 2	square = 4

Only the three most severe injuries are summed, so that the Injury Severity Score would be 34. Age in this case is not a further disadvantage, but nevertheless he will require prompt, expert treatment; with this his chances of survival are good. In treating him, priority would be given to the management of his chest injury (e.g. by confirming the presence of a good airway, administering oxygen, inserting a chest drain, and estimating the blood gases) and by prevention or treatment of oligaemic shock (e.g. by removal of blood for grouping, cross-matching, assessment of haemoglobin and haematocrit; and by the establishment of a good intravenous line, with monitoring of a pulse, blood pressure, and urinary output (after insertion of a catheter)).

The tibial fracture should be splinted at an early stage to help relieve pain and reduce local haemorrhage. The progress of the head and chest injuries must be closely monitored and the fluid replacement programme will require careful supervision. The large area that has been burned will in itself demand heavy and appropriate fluid replacement.

Once the emergency procedures have been instituted and the immediate situation brought under control, thought can be given to how to deal with the burns and the limb injury; this will be dictated by the exact nature of both these injuries.

		gastrointestinal (GI) haemorrhage, respiratory distress syndrome for less than 1 day
4	(severe)	Septicaemia, empyema, peritonitis, pulmonary embolism with normal BP, renal failure with dialysis of less than 1 week, more than 6 units of GI haemorrhage, less than 3 days of respiratory distress syndrome
5	(critical)	Septicaemia with fall in BP, pulmonary embolism with fall in BP, renal failure for 7–40 days, GI haemorrhage of more than 12 units, respiratory arrest, more than 3 days of respiratory distress syndrome on ventilator

TREATMENT OF THE FRACTURE

The initial stages are clear:

1. Undue movement at the fracture site should be prevented by the use of temporary splintage until radiographic and any other examination is complete. This will reduce pain and haemorrhage and minimise the chances of a closed fracture becoming open. In the case of the lower limb, support with pillows and sandbags may be adequate. In both the upper and the lower limbs inflatable splints are invaluable.

2. If the deformity is so great that the fracture or dislocation is seriously endangering the viability of the overlying skin, it is usually advisable to do something to correct this; in many cases gentle repositioning of the distal part of the limb is sufficient; the use of Entonox may be required.

3. If the fracture is an open one, a bacteriological swab should be taken and the wound covered with sterile dressings. Firm bandaging may be required if brisk bleeding is continuing. If a polaroid photograph is taken of the wound prior to covering it, this will eliminate the need for the removal of dressings for repeated inspection by other members of staff. Antibiotic therapy should be commenced immediately; the choice of therapy is dependent on the current status of bacterial flora in wound infections occurring in the particular local situation.

4. The fracture should be fully assessed by clinical and radiological examination: the site, pattern, displacement and angulation should be noted. Involvement of the skin, and damage to related structures such as important nerves or blood vessels should be assessed.

With this information the following key decisions must be made:

- Does the fracture require reduction?
- If reduction is required, how is it planned to carry this out?
- What support is required till union occurs?
- If the fracture is open, how will this influence treatment?
- Does the patient require admission to hospital, and what rehabilitation will be required?
- If reduction is required, Apley's summary of 'reduce, maintain, rehabilitate' is apposite.

Some observations about these decisions will be made in sequence.

Does the fracture require reduction?   It is obvious that an undisplaced fracture does not require reduction, but unfortunately one still sees fractures in anatomical position subjected to manipulation, although only rarely are they displaced as a result of this.

If a fracture is only slightly displaced, reduction may nevertheless be highly desirable, as for example in fractures involving the ankle joint, where even slight persisting deformity may lead to the development of osteoarthritis. In other situations, some displacement may often be accepted, depending on:

1. the site involved,
2. where good remodelling may be anticipated (especially in children)
3. if the patient is very old, when the risks of anaesthesia, etc. may be considered to outweigh a problematical improvement.

If the fracture is appreciably angled or rotated, reduction is generally essential for cosmetic and functional reasons (but see under appropriate fractures).

If the fracture requires reduction, how is it planned to carry this out?

1. The commonest method is by the application of traction, followed by manipulation of the fracture, under general anaesthesia. General anaesthesia has most to offer in terms of muscle relaxation, duration and overall versatility, but for minor procedures regional anaesthesia and intravenous diazepam are popular and useful measures, with the advantage that waiting time may be reduced.

2. Continuous traction is used to achieve a reduction in fractures of the femur and fracture dislocations of the cervical spine. It is used less commonly for a number of other fractures.

3. Open reduction of the fracture is carried out:

(i) as an obvious part of the treatment of an open fracture, i.e. debridement of the wound exposes the fracture which may be reduced under vision

(ii) where conservative methods have failed to give a satisfactory reduction

(iii) where it is considered that the best method of supporting the fracture involves internal fixation, and exposure of the fracture is a necessary part of that procedure.

What support is required until union of the fracture occurs?

Non-rigid methods of support   Arm slings, bandages and adhesive strapping may be used, and serve some of the following purposes.

1. Firm support, e.g. in the form of crepe bandaging or circular woven bandaging, may help to limit swelling and oedema, and restrict the spread of haematoma.

2. Slings are often employed for elevation purposes, especially to limit gravitational swelling of the hand and fingers in upper limb injuries.

3. Pain may be relieved by the restriction of movement.

4. By restriction of limb movement, forces acting on the bone ends may be reduced to a level at which relative movement is unlikely, or insufficient to interfere with healing. This applies particularly to impacted fractures.

Continuous traction   Traction may be maintained for several weeks, while holding a fracture in reduction. Fractures of the femoral shaft are frequently treated by this method. Traction may be effected through the skin (skin traction) by, for example, adhesive strapping, or through bone (skeletal traction) by, e.g., a Steinman pin.

Plaster fixation   Plaster of Paris, generally in the form of plaster-impregnated bandages, is the commonest method of supporting a fracture. The plaster is carefully moulded to fit the contours of the limb, and the quick-setting properties of the plaster allow the limb to be held without undue strain in the correct position until setting has occurred. For a plaster to achieve its purpose, care must be taken over its application and subsequent supervision. A disadvantage of plaster splints is that they soften if they are allowed to become wet. There are a number of plaster substitutes now available to overcome this problem, but none as yet combine the unique properties of plaster with moderate cost.

Internal fixation   Internal fixation is indicated:

1. Where a fracture cannot be reduced by closed methods (e.g. a fracture of the tibia with soft tissue between the bone ends, or many fractures of the forearm bones).

2. Where a reduction can be achieved but it cannot be satisfactorily held by closed methods (e.g. fractures of the femoral neck, certain fractures of the tibial and humeral shaft).

3. Where a higher quality of reduction and fixation is required than can be obtained by closed methods (e.g. some fractures involving articular surfaces).

4. In the case of multiple injuries involving the lower extremities, where the risks of acute respiratory distress syndrome (ARDS), fat embolism and other serious post-injury complications are considerably reduced by early operative stabilisation of lower extremity (especially femoral) fractures. (Respiratory function is improved when the patient can sit up, reducing abdominal pressure on the diaphragm with its risks of atelectasis; and less analgesia is required for fracture pain, with less respiratory depression resulting.)

The present tendency in dealing with patients with multiple injuries is to stabilise (with internal or external fixation) all major lower limb fractures as soon as the patient's general condition will allow, and preferably as part of the initial treatment on the day the injuries are sustained.

In addition, there is a controversial area where the risks of internal fixation in a particular set of circumstances are outweighed, in the experience and opinion of the surgeon in charge, by the advantages. Some of the factors involved may include:

1. The possibility of achieving and maintaining a high quality reduction.

2. Earlier mobilisation of joints, with less risk of permanent stiffness, disuse osteoporosis, etc.

3. Earlier discharge from hospital, and earlier return to full function (including work, athletic activities, etc.).

Some of the disadvantages of internal fixation are:

1. The possibility of introducing infection. The consequences may be serious (e.g. chronic bone infection with non-union, which may sometimes necessitate amputation).

2. Internal fixation techniques require a degree of mechanical aptitude and experience on the part of the surgeon if the occasional serious failure is to be avoided.

3. To cover a wide range of fracture situations, a fairly formidable number of instruments and fixation devices will be required.

4. As on the whole the time under anaesthesia is much longer than when conservative measures are employed, the patient's general condition and health is of greater concern: the services of an expert anaesthetist are more frequently required.

The methods of achieving internal fixation include the use of a wide range of devices (screws, nails, plates, etc.).

External skeletal fixation With this method, the bone fragments are held in alignment with pins inserted percutaneously. Two common methods of placing the pins are used; in one, each pin is passed through the skin and a bone fragment, and exits through the skin on the other side. More commonly, a cantilever system is used, with rigid pins which are screwed into a bone fragment and protrude from one side of the limb only. One to six pins are fixed in each bone fragment. The fracture is reduced with the pins in situ (at open operation, or by using an image intensifier). The pins are then held in proper relation to one another by a rigid external support. The ends of the pins are normally connected together with clamps; in emergency situations plaster bandages may be used for this purpose.

Such systems are of particular value in the management of open fractures where the state of the skin and other factors may make the use of internal fixation devices undesirable. Cantilever (one-sided) systems give the best access for the dressing of open wounds.

In the Ilizarov method of external fixation, control of the major fragments of the shaft of a bone is obtained by fine wires passed through skin and bone, and held under tension on metal toroidal frames encircling the limb. Two or more frames are used for each major fragment, and these are held in alignment by threaded spacers.

Hybrid systems (such as the Sheffield system) are of particular value in treating fractures of the ends of long bones involving the related joints. Wires under tension are held in an Ilizarov type frame which is linked to pins inserted in the shaft.

The use of external fixators is sometimes followed, even in the case of closed fractures, by pin track infections. The quality of the fixation is also dependent on the pins remaining tight in the bone, and there is some risk of non-union.

Cast bracing Cast bracing techniques are sometimes employed some weeks after the initial conservative management of a fracture. The method is used particularly in the treatment of fractures of the femur and tibia. In the case of fractures of the femur, one method employs two supports – one for the thigh and one for the leg below the knee – linked together by hinges at the side of the knee. Sufficient fixation may be achieved thereby to allow early ambulation.

Plastic splints A number of off-the-shelf plastic splints are available for the immediate or delayed support of certain fractures (e.g. of the humeral shaft), and have hygienic advantages. Some incorporate hinges.

If the fracture is open, how will this influence treatment?
The following points will require separate consideration:

1. As debridement of the wound will almost certainly be needed, general anaesthesia and theatre facilities are essential. Pulsatile lavage may be used to reduce the amount of bacterial contamination, bearing in mind the adage 'the solution to pollution is dilution'.

2. In every case, potential difficulty in skin closure and cover of the fracture must be anticipated, and at least one possible line of treatment worked out prior to the patient being taken to theatre.

3. If the wound is badly soiled, and the skin damage substantial, the use of large implants is discouraged. The wider stripping of the tissues required for the insertion of some internal fixation devices may disseminate any infecting organisms and cause further (albeit local) tissue damage. The presence of inert material in the tissues may act as a nidus for infection, so that it is difficult for any local infection to be overcome. The bulk of an internal fixation device may make wound closure more difficult, and subsequent swelling is more likely to lead to sloughing of devitalised skin over any prosthesis. If intramedullary nailing is to be employed, reaming of the medullary canal should be avoided.

If wound contamination is judged to be slight, and if good cover of the fracture can be obtained, internal fixation of the fracture is often carried out where it is felt to contribute to the chances of union and a successful outcome. Where there is much tissue damage, and the risks of infection are high, the use of an external fixator should be considered.

4. Open fractures are usually associated with greater damage to surrounding soft tissues than closed fractures. Postoperative swelling is invariable, is often severe, and may lead to circulatory impairment in the limb. Special precautions must be taken over the type of splintage used, and the limb must be elevated. Admission for observation of the patient and of the limb circulation is almost invariably required.

In some cases there is serious elevation of pressure within the closed fascial compartments of the limb giving rise to one or several recognised compartment syndromes: these may be suspected on clinical grounds, and be confirmed by manometry. (In performing this an electronic transducer-tipped catheter gives the most accurate results.) In those situations where the clinical findings are difficult to assess (e.g. in the unconscious patient or in the presence of multiple injuries), and where particular compartments are at risk, continuous prophylactic monitoring may have to be considered. In weighing up the findings, the diastolic blood pressure should be taken into account. A *differential pressure* (diastolic blood pressure minus the intracompartmental pressure) of 30 mmHg or less is regarded as an indication for surgical decompression (by fasciotomy). (See also p. 99.)

5. As a rule, open fractures are associated with greater violence, more initial deformity and more direct soft tissue damage. Neurological and vascular damage is more common, and should be looked for; if found, then the appropriate additional treatment will be required.

6. The majority of open fractures have microbial contamination which may be of both gram negative and gram positive organisms. The risk of the development of infection is closely related to the degree of soft tissue injury. There are special risks from organisms acquired from farmyards, fresh water contamination, and hospital environments (e.g. *Clostridium perfringens*, *Pseudomonas aeruginosa*, penicillin-resistant staphylococci). It is considered that the duration of antibiotic courses should be short to reduce the risks of the emergence of resistant strains. Swabs should be taken from wounds on admission.

Gustilo et al recommend the following:

- **Type I fractures:** a single dose of 2.0 g of cephalosporin on admission followed by 1.0 g every 6–8 h for 48–72 h
- **Type II or Type III injuries:** gram negative and gram positive prophylaxis is necessary, as well as cephalosporin in the previously recommended dosage. The patient should be given aminoglycosides (tobramycin), 1.5 mg per kg body weight on admission, and 3.0–5.0 mg per kg body weight daily thereafter in divided doses. This must be adjusted if there is renal insufficiency. If there is risk of clostridial infection, 10 million units of penicillin should also be given. If any secondary procedure (e.g. internal fixation, delayed wound closure) is being performed, the antibiotic courses should be repeated.

Attention should also be paid to tetanus prophylaxis.

If wound contamination is judged to be slight, antibiotics may or may not be given, depending to some extent on the assessment of the particular circumstances of the case and of unit policy. (See Chapter 4 for details of local treatment.)

7. In the most severe open injuries, where there is perhaps much comminution of bone, extensive crushing of muscle, gross wound contamination and neurological damage, primary amputation may have to be considered. The decision to amputate is not an easy one to make, especially in a climate where success in the re-attachment of severed limbs is not unusual. Nevertheless, it must be borne in mind that even with the most sophisticated techniques, requiring perhaps many operations spread over months or years, there may be ultimate failure; when amputation is then carried out, and an artificial limb fitted, the rapidity of rehabilitation may tempt the previously demoralised patient to wish that the decision to amputate had been made at the beginning.

Mangled Extremity Severity Score Such an irrevocable line of treatment as amputation should not of course be suggested to a patient without the backing of a second, independent, senior opinion. In coming to a decision it may be helpful to consider the **Mangled Extremity Severity Score**

MESS factors

1. Skeletal/soft tissue injury
- Low energy injury (stab wound, closed fracture, low velocity gunshot wound)   1
- Medium energy injury (open fracture, multiple fractures, dislocation)   2
- High energy injury (shotgun wound, high velocity gunshot wound, crush injury)   3
- Very high energy injury (as above, but with gross contamination, soft tissue avulsion)   4

2. Limb ischaemia
- Pulse reduced or absent, normal perfusion:
  - less than 6 hours   1
  - more than 6 hours   2
- Pulseless, paraesthesiae, reduced capillary refill:
  - less than 6 hours   2
  - more than 6 hours   4
- Cool, paralysed, insensate limb:
  - less than 6 hours   3
  - more than 6 hours   6

3. Shock
- BP more than 90 mm   0
- Transient hypotension   1
- Persistent hypotension   2

4. Age
- <30 years   0
- 30–50 years   1
- >50 years   2

Case examples

1. A man aged 25 years involved in a road traffic accident 3 h previously is found to have an open fracture of the tibia, with reduced tissue perfusion and absent distal pulses; he is normotensive. The Mangled Extremity Severity Score would be 4 (age score = 0, open tibial fracture = 2, circulatory impairment = 2, shock = 0), so that other things being equal, primary amputation would not be considered, but an aggressive attempt to save the limb should be made (e.g. by fixation of the fracture and arterial reconstruction).

2. A man of 60 is brought in with a gunshot fracture of the femur sustained 8 h previously. The limb is cold and paralysed, and the sensation absent. There is transient hypotension. The Mangled Extremity Severity Score would be 12 (age = 2, gunshot wound = 3, ischaemia = 6, shock = 1) and primary amputation would be advised.

(Johansen et al). This scheme has been devised to give a quantitative assessment of the severity of injury to a limb, and to offer a guide in making the difficult decision as to whether it is worth striving to save a limb or to minimise losses and advise a primary amputation.

In applying the scheme, four factors are considered and the scores for each are added together to obtain a total. A score of 7 or more is considered a highly reliable guide to the need for amputation. (In a large series no false positives were found, i.e. in no case where the score was 7 or more was there ultimate survival of the limb.) On the other hand, as might be expected, a score of less than 7 does not necessarily guarantee that amputation may not eventually be required. The scoring emphasises the great importance of the early restoration of good tissue perfusion. The four factors and their scoring are as follows.

Does the patient require admission to hospital? In most cases the decision is an easy one, being related to the seriousness of the injury, the nature of the treatment and the need for continuous observation. The main criteria for admission very frequently overlap, and include the following:

1. **Admission dictated by treatment**. Admission may be dictated by problems associated with anaesthesia – undue delay before anaesthesia, a prolonged anaesthetic, or where the anaesthetic is administered very late at night and recovery would be occurring at an inconvenient time in the early morning. Admission will also obviously be required if the patient is being treated by continuous traction, partly because of the continuous use of special equipment, and partly because of the expert supervision required. Most commonly, admission will be required when as a result of his injury the patient must be confined to bed.

2. **Admission for observation.** Where there is appreciable risk of complications developing, admission may be required for continuous observation. This is obvious in the case of associated head injury, abdominal injury, or in the case of general multiple trauma. Of particular relevance is admission for observation of the circulation in an injured limb. The majority of tibial fractures in adults, and ideally all supracondylar fractures in children, should be admitted for elevation of the limb and observation of the

circulation. After open injuries (with the possible exceptions of fingers and toes) admission is advisable so that any developing infection can be detected and dealt with as early as possible.

3. **Admission for general nursing care.** Many fracture cases may or may not require special treatment, but are nevertheless completely dependent on good nursing care. This applies particularly to fractures of the pelvis and spine where the patient is confined to bed. It also applies to other less obvious situations, such as the patient with fractures of both arms, who may be rendered virtually helpless with two comparatively minor injuries.

4. **Admission for mobilisation.** Admission may be required for a period until the patient adapts to the limitations of the fracture and its splintage, e.g., until a patient becomes sufficiently adept in the use of crutches that they can manage in their own home.

5. **Admission for social reasons.** Many elderly and infirm people, living alone or with equally affected relatives, may just be able to cope with life prior to injury. Even a minor fracture may render them unable to return to their normal environment. Admission is a necessity if no other help is available, and of course treatment is aimed at getting them fit to return home. Opportunity may be taken of their admission to investigate and treat any concurrent physical problem. If recovery is poor, assistance from hospital and domiciliary occupational therapists, social workers or geriatricians may be required.

6. **Admission in the case of suspected child abuse.** Where there is the possibility of non-accidental physical injury ('battered baby' syndrome), a child returned to the home environment may be put at risk of further injury which might be life-threatening, and admission is mandatory under such circumstances.

SUSPECTED CHILD ABUSE

The possibility of child abuse should always be kept in mind, especially in dealing with injuries sustained by children under the age of 3 years (80% of cases lie within this age group). The other factors which might alert you include the following:

1. The presence of a fracture with no history of injury, or a vague history which is not in keeping with the nature or the extent of the injury.
2. The presence of multiple fractures or other injuries, especially when these are at different stages of healing, indicating that they have occurred as the result of separate incidents.
3. The presence of multiple soft tissue injuries, including swellings, bruises, burns, welts, lacerations and scars. There may be hand infections secondary to local burns; again, the appearance of these having occurred with a time interval between them is of importance.
4. If there is a head injury, radiographs of the skull may show evidence of fracture or widening of sutures, possibly from raised intracranial pressure secondary to cerebral oedema or subdural haematoma (which is found in about 25% of child abuse victims).
5. Evidence of failure to thrive, growth retardation, fever, anaemia or seizures. The commonest fractures that are found, in order of frequency, are of the ribs, humerus, femur, tibia and skull, and in the average case 3–4 fractures are present. In the case of the long bones, the shafts are now recognised as being most commonly involved: in the older lesions there may be gross deformity and exuberant callus (due to lack of fixation). The

presence of multiple lesions in varying states of healing is pathognomonic.

In the metaphyseal region, the fractures may be impacted with copious new bone formation, there may be buckling of the bone without much in the way of new bone formation, or there may be irregular deformity with new bone appearing in layers as a result of repeated trauma. In some cases there is periosteal avulsion with marked local tenderness; this may not be detected on the initial films, but may show up if the radiographs are repeated after 10 days (with the formation of subperiosteal new bone). Injuries to the epiphyses and the growth plates are very uncommon in cases of child abuse (whereas this pattern of injury is seen frequently in other forms of trauma).

Apart from admission and the carrying out of treatment appropriate to the fractures or other injuries, further investigations should usually include the following:

1. Review of the records of previous admissions.
2. Observations of the child's weight and height.
3. Obtaining an X-ray skeletal survey, including the skull.
4. Obtaining clinical photographs.
5. Most importantly, informing the Social Services so that the child's home background can be looked into, and the appropriate action taken to safeguard the child should the diagnosis of child abuse seem likely.

CHAPTER

3

Closed reduction and casting techniques in fracture management

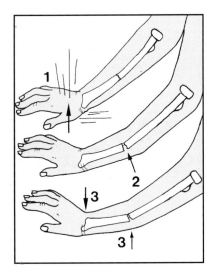

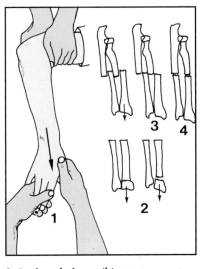

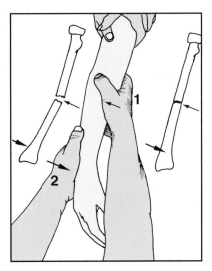

1. Closed reduction of fractures: Basic techniques (a): The direction and magnitude of the causal force (1) and the deformity (2) are related, and may be worked out from the history, the appearance of the limb and the radiographs. Any force required to correct the displacement of a fracture is applied in the opposite direction (3).

2. Basic techniques (b): The first step in most closed reductions is to apply traction – generally in the line of the limb (1). Traction will lead to the disimpaction of most fractures (2) and this may occur almost immediately in the relaxed patient under general anaesthesia. Traction will also lead to reduction of shortening (3), and in most cases to reduction of the deformity (4).

3. Basic techniques (c): Any residual angulation following the application of traction may be corrected by using the heel of the hand under the fracture (1) and applying pressure distally with the other (2).

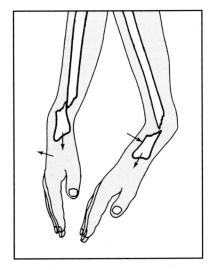

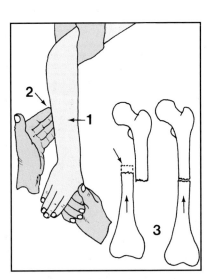

4. Basic techniques (d): In some fractures there may be difficulty in reduction due to prominent bony spikes or soft tissue interposition. Reduction may sometimes be achieved by initially increasing the angulation prior to manipulation. This method of unlocking the fragments must be pursued with care to avoid damage to surrounding vessels and nerves.

5. Basic techniques (e): The effectiveness of reduction may be assessed by noting the appearance of the limb (1), by palpation, especially in long bone fractures (2), by absence of telescoping (i.e. axial compression along the line of the limb does not lead to further shortening) (3), and by check radiographs.

6. Basic techniques (f): After reduction of the fracture it must be prevented from redisplacing until it has united. The methods include the following:
- Plaster fixation (see p. 57).
- Skin and skeletal traction (see p. 309).
- Thomas splint (see p. 310).
- Cast bracing (see pp. 314, 350).
- External fixation (see p. 78).

For common methods of internal fixation see Chapter 4.

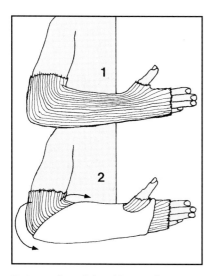

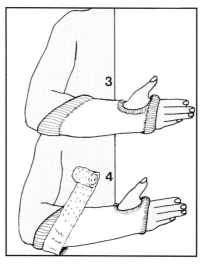

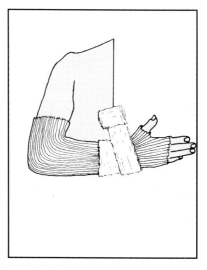

7. Protection of the skin: Stockinet: A layer of stockinet is usually applied next to the skin (1). This has several functions: it helps prevent the limb hairs becoming caught in the plaster; it facilitates the conduction of perspiration from the limb; it removes any roughness caused by the ends of the plaster; and it may aid in the subsequent removal of the plaster. After the plaster has been applied, the stockinet is turned back (2).

8. Stockinet cntd: After the stockinet has been reflected, excess is removed, leaving 3–4 cm only at each end (3). The loose edge of stockinet is then secured with a turn or two of a plaster bandage (if a complete plaster is being applied) or with the encircling gauze bandage in the case of a slab.

9. Wool roll: A layer of wool should be used to protect bony prominences (e.g. the distal ulna). In complete plasters, where swelling is anticipated, several layers of wool may be applied over the length of the limb; the initial layer of stockinet may be omitted. A layer of wool may also be substituted for stockinget under a slab, and indeed many like to use a layer of wool under any type of cast. Wool roll is also advisable where an electric saw is used for plaster removal.

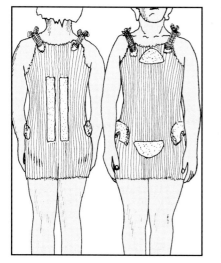

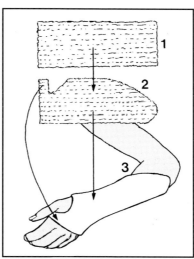

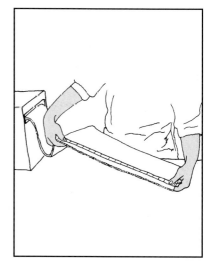

10. Felt: Where friction is likely to occur over bony prominences, protection may be given with felt strips or felt cut-outs, fashioned to isolate the area to be relieved (e.g. the vertebral and iliac spines, the pubis and manubrium in plaster jackets). Adhesive felt should not be applied directly to the skin if skin eruptions are to be avoided.

11. Plaster slabs (a): These consist of several layers of plaster bandage and may be used for the treatment of minor injuries or where potentially serious swelling may be anticipated in a fracture. In their application, slabs are cut to length (1), and trimmed as required (2) to fit the limb before being applied (3). Slabs may also be used as foundations or reinforcements of complete plasters.

12. Plaster slabs (b): If a slab dispenser is available, measure the length of slab required and cut to length. A single slab of six layers of bandage will usually suffice for a child. In a large adult, two slab thicknesses may be necessary. In a small adult, one slab thickness may be adequate with local reinforcement.

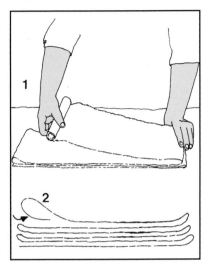

13. Plaster slabs (c): Alternatively, manufacture a slab by repeated folding of a plaster bandage, using say 8–10 thicknesses in an adult and six in a child as described (1). Turn in the end of the bandage (2) so that when the slab is dipped the upper layer does not fall out of alignment.

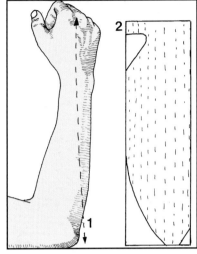

14. Plaster slabs (d): Ideally, the slab should be trimmed with plaster scissors so that it will fit the limb without being folded over. For example, a slab for an undisplaced greenstick fracture of the distal radius should stretch from the metacarpal heads to the olecranon. It may be measured (1) and trimmed as shown, with a tongue (2) to lie between the thumb and index.

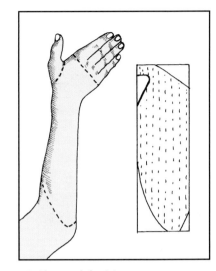

15. Plaster slabs (e): In a Colles fracture, where the hand should be placed in a position of ulnar deviation, the slab should be trimmed to accommodate this position, a stage that is often omitted in error. The preceding two plaster slabs are examples of dorsal slabs.

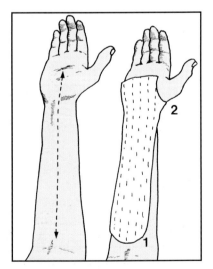

16. Plaster slabs (f): An anterior slab may be used as a foundation for a scaphoid plaster, or to treat an injury in which the wrist is held in dorsiflexion (measuring from a point just distal to the elbow crease, with the elbow at 90°, to the proximal skin crease in the palm). The proximal end is rounded (1) while the distal lateral corner is trimmed for the thenar mass (2).

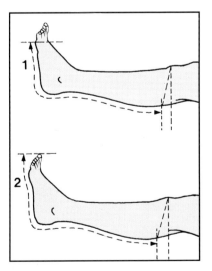

17. Plaster slabs (g): For the ankle (1) a plain untrimmed slab may be used, measuring from the metatarsal heads to the upper calf, 3–4 cm distal to a point behind the tibial tubercle. For the foot (2) where the toes require support, choose the tips of the toes as the distal point.

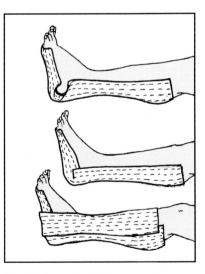

18. Plaster slabs (h): Owing to the abrupt change in direction of the slab at the ankle, the slab requires cutting on both sides so that it may be smoothed down with local overlapping. A back slab may be further strengthened by a long U-slab with its limbs lying medially and laterally.

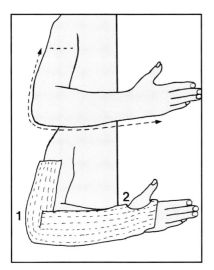

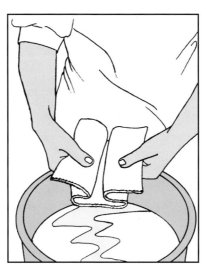

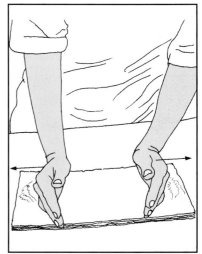

19. Plaster slabs (i): The same technique of side cutting is required for long arm plaster slabs (1). These are measured as indicated from the upper arm to the metacarpal heads, with a cut-out at the thumb as in a Colles plaster slab (2).

20. Plaster slabs (j): Wetting the slab: hold it carefully at both ends, immerse completely in tepid water, lift out and momentarily bunch up at an angle to expel excess water. Plaster-setting time is decreased by both hot and soft water.

21. Plaster slabs (k): Now consolidate the layers of the slab. If a plaster table is available, quickly place the slab on the surface and, with one movement with the heels of the hands, press the layers firmly together. (Retained air reduces the ultimate strength of the plaster and leads to cracking or separation of the layers).

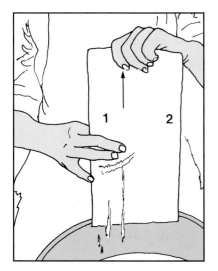

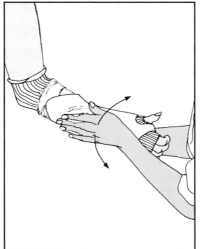

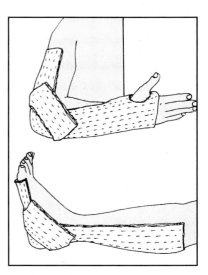

22. Plaster slabs (l): Alternatively, consolidate the layers by holding the plaster at one end and pulling between two adducted fingers (1). Repeat the procedure from the other edge (2).

23. Plaster slabs (m): Carefully position the slab on the limb and smooth out with the hands so that the slab fits closely to the contours of the limb without rucking or the formation of sore-making ridges on its inferior surface.

24. Plaster slabs (n): At this stage any weak spots should be reinforced. Where there is a right-angled bend in a plaster – for example at the elbow or the ankle – two small slabs made from 10 cm (4″) plaster bandages may be used as triangular reinforcements at either site. A similar small slab may be used to reinforce the back of the wrist.

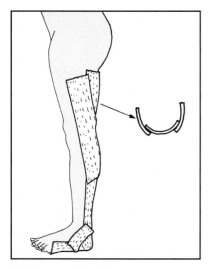

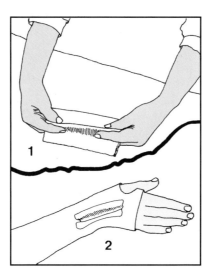

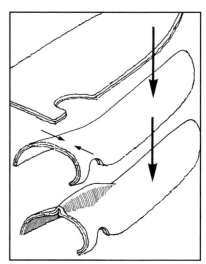

25. Plaster slabs (o): In the case of a long leg plaster slab, additional strengthening at the thigh and knee is always necessary, and this may be achieved by the use of two additional 15 cm (6″) slabs.

26. Plaster slabs (p): Where even greater strength is required, the plaster may be girdered. For example, for the wrist, make a small slab of six thicknesses of 10 cm (4″) bandage and pinch up in the centre (1). Dip the reinforcement, apply, and smooth down to form a T-girder over the dorsum (2).

27. Plaster slabs (q): Girdering may also be achieved without a separate onlay. The basic plaster slab is pinched up locally after being applied to the limb. Care must be taken to avoid undue ridging of the interior surface.

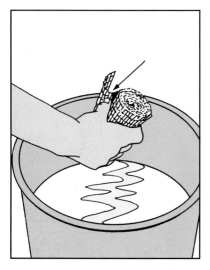

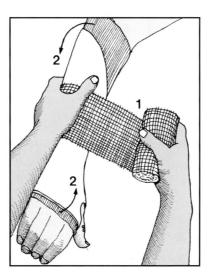

28. Bandaging (a): Bandages used to secure plaster slabs should be of open weave (cotton or muslin) and be thoroughly wetted. This is to avoid tightening from shrinkage after coming in contact with the slab. Secure the end of the bandage between the thumb and fingers, and squeeze several times under water.

29. Bandaging (b): Apply to the limb firmly, but without too much pressure (1). Do not use reverse turns, which tend to produce local constrictions. The ends of the underlying stockinet may be turned back and secured with the last few turns of the bandage (2). On completion, secure the bandage with a small piece of wetted plaster bandage.

30. Complete POP technique: The skin should be protected as previously described using, where applicable, stockinet, wool roll and felt. The following sizes of plaster bandage are recommended for normal application:

Upper arm and forearm	15 cm (6″)
Wrist	10 cm (4″)
Thumb and fingers	7.5 cm (3″)
Trunk and hip	20 cm (8″)
Thigh and leg	20 cm (8″)
Ankle and foot	15 cm (6″)

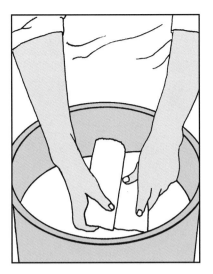

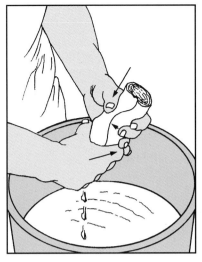

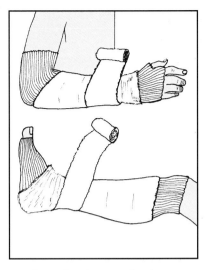

31. Plaster bandage wetting (a):
Plaster bandages should be dipped in tepid water. Secure the end of the bandage with one hand to prevent the end becoming lost in the mass of wet bandage. Hold the bandage lightly with the other without compression. Immerse at an angle of 45°, and keep under water until bubbles stop rising.

32. Plaster bandage wetting (b):
Remove excess water by gently compressing in an axial direction and twisting slightly. Alternatively, pull the bandage through the encircled thumb and index while lightly gripping the bandage.

33. Plaster bandage application (a):
Most moulding of the plaster will be required at the wrist in upper limb plasters, and at the ankle in lower limb plasters. It is often useful to apply the more proximal parts first, so that moulding can be more profitably carried out against a set or nearly set cuff of plaster on the forearm or calf (i.e. start a forearm plaster at the elbow, and a below-knee plaster at the tibial tubercle).

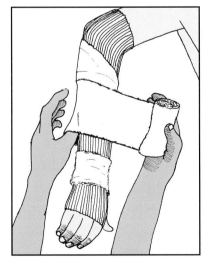

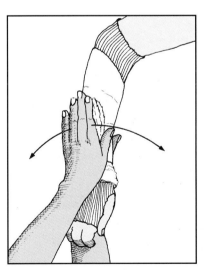

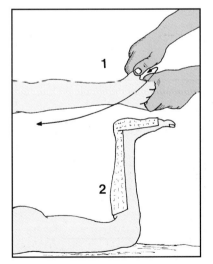

34. Plaster bandage application (b):
Roll each bandage without stretching if there is no wool beneath; if there is a layer of wool, and no swelling is anticipated, a little even pressure may be applied to compress the wool to half thickness. Plain tucks may be used distally to ensure a smooth fit, but figure-of-eight or reverse turns should not be used if local constriction is to be avoided.

35. Plaster bandage application (c):
After the application of each bandage smooth the layers down to exclude any trapped air and consolidate the plaster. A second and, if necessary, third bandage may be applied to complete the proximal portion. Each bandage should extend 2–3 cm distal to the previous, and be well smoothed down. The distal part may then be completed, and the hand or foot portion moulded before setting is complete.

36. Plaster bandage application (d):
Where possible, the assistant should hold the limb in such a way that the surgeon has a clear run while applying the plaster (1). Where support must be given to a part included in the plaster, the flats of the hands should be used, and the hands eased proximally and distally to avoid local indentation. Where slabs are used, try to let gravity assist rather than hinder (2).

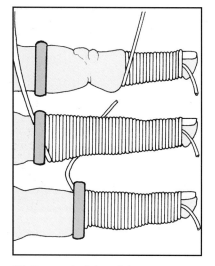

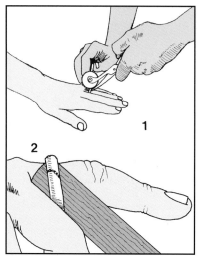

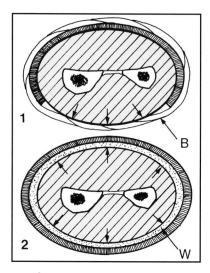

37. Removal of rings (a): Wherever possible rings should be removed in case finger swelling leads to distal gangrene. A tight ring can generally be coaxed from a finger if it is well coated with olive oil or a similar lubricant. If this fails, the finger may sometimes be sufficiently compressed by binding it with, for example, macramé twine to allow removal as shown.

38. Removal of rings (b): Otherwise a ring may be cut with a ring cutter (1) or a saw cut may be made with a fine tooth hacksaw on to a spatula (2) to spring the ring. Ring removal is nevertheless sometimes obsessively pursued. If significant swelling is unlikely, the ring loose below the knuckle, the patient intelligent and the potential danger is indicated, it may be retained with acceptable safety.

39. Plaster precautions (a): After an acute injury, if much swelling is anticipated (1) use a plaster slab in preference to a complete plaster. The retaining bandages have more 'give' than plaster, and are more readily cut in an emergency. (2) If a slab does not give sufficient support, then allow for swelling with a generous layer of wool beneath the plaster. (W = wool; B = bandage.)

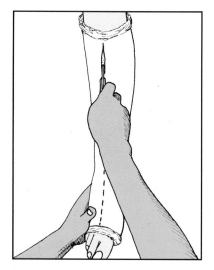

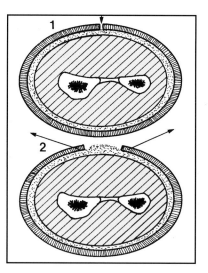

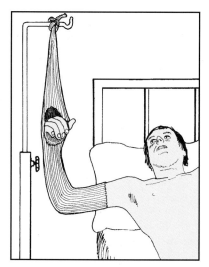

40. Plaster precautions (b): Consider splitting any complete plaster. This should be done *routinely* after any operative procedure when swelling may be considerable (from tourniquet release, postoperative oedema, etc.). Use a sharp knife and cut down through the plaster to the underlying wool (the wool protects the skin). This should be done immediately after application of the plaster before it has had time to dry out.

41. Plaster precautions (c): Be sure the plaster has been *completely* divided down to the wool along its whole length (1). (Any remaining strands will act dangerously as constricting bands.) You should be able to see the wool quite clearly. The plaster edges should spring apart by 5–10 mm or they may be eased apart by the handle of the knife, thereby dynamically relieving any underlying pressure (2).

42. Elevation (a): Wherever possible, the injured limb should be elevated. In the case of the hand and forearm in a patient who has been admitted, the limb may be secured in stockinet (or in a roller towel using safety pins) attached to a drip stand at the side of the bed. Elevation should be maintained at least until swelling is beginning to resolve.

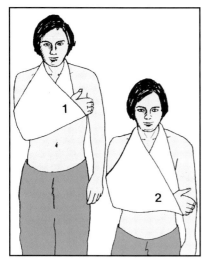

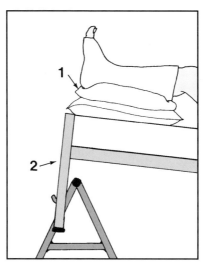

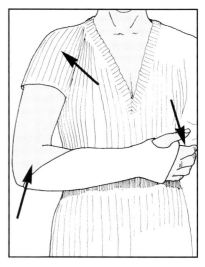

43. Elevation (b): In the case of the ambulant patient a sling may be used, provided the arm is kept high enough (1). If the sling is too slack the arm will hang down, encouraging oedema (2).

44. Elevation (c): In the case of the lower limb, the leg may be elevated on pillows (1). The end of the bed may be raised on an A-frame or on chairs (2). The ambulant patient should be advised to keep the foot as high as possible on a couch or chair whenever they are at rest.

45. Exercise: Those parts free of plaster should be exercised as frequently as possible, e.g. the fingers in a Colles fracture (and later the elbow and shoulder). The patient should be shown how they should curl the fingers into full flexion and then fully extend them. They should be given clear instructions as to how frequently to perform these exercises (e.g. for 5 minutes every waking hour).

Instructions for Patients in Plaster of Paris Splints

A. (1) If fingers or toes become swollen blue, painful or stiff, raise limb.

(2) If no improvement in half an hour call in Doctor or return to hospital immediately.

B. (1) Exercise all joints not included in plaster—especially fingers and toes

(2) If you have been fitted with a walking plaster walk in it.

(3) If plaster becomes loose or cracked—report to hospital as soon as possible.

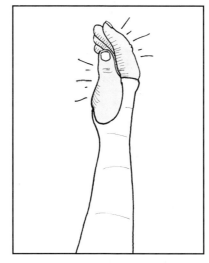

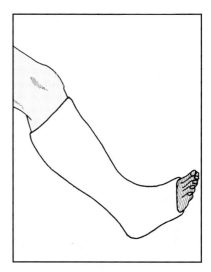

46. The patient who is being allowed home must be given clear warnings to return should the circulation appear in any way to be impaired. Inform the patient or, where appropriate, a relative who will be looking after the patient. It is also useful to reinforce this by pasting an instruction label (such as the one illustrated) directly to the plaster.

47. Aftercare of patients in plaster (a): *Is there swelling?* Swelling of the fingers or toes is common in patients being treated in plaster, but the patient must be examined carefully for other signs which might suggest that circulatory impairment is the cause, rather than the local response to trauma. If there is no evidence of circulatory impairment, the limb should be elevated and movements encouraged.

48. Aftercare (b): *Is there discoloration of the toes or fingers?* Compare one side with the other; bluish discoloration, especially in conjunction with oedematous swelling distally, suggests that swelling of the limb within the plaster has reached such a level as to impair the venous return, and appropriate action must be taken.

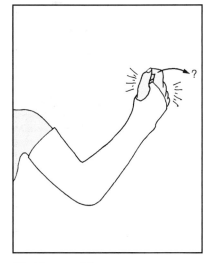

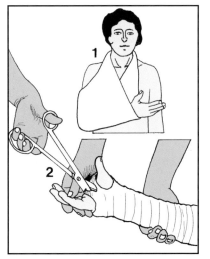

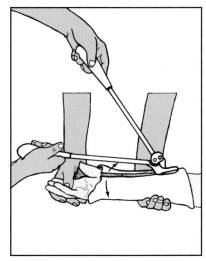

49. Aftercare (c): *Is there any evidence of arterial obstruction?* Note the five Ps: intense **pain, paralysis** of finger or toe flexors, **paraesthesiae** in fingers or toes, **pallor** of the skin with disturbed capillary return, and 'perishing cold' feel of the fingers and toes. Arterial obstruction requires *immediate*, positive action. (Clinical findings of a similar nature, along with pain on passive movements of the fingers or toes, is found in the compartment syndromes: see p. 99.)

50. Treatment of suspected circulatory impairment (a): Elevate the limb (1). In the case of a plaster slab, cut through the encircling bandages and underlying wool (2) until the *skin is fully exposed*, and ease back the edges of the plaster shell until it is apparent that it is not constricting the limb in any way.

51. Treatment (b): Where the plaster is a complete one, split the plaster throughout its entire length. *Ease* back the edges of the cast to free the limb on each side of the midline. *Divide* all the overlying wool and stockinet and turn it back till skin is exposed. The same applies to any dressing swabs hardened with blood clot.

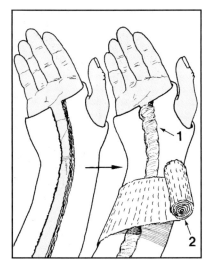

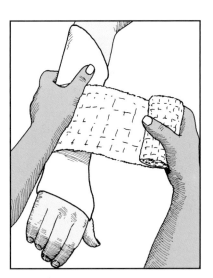

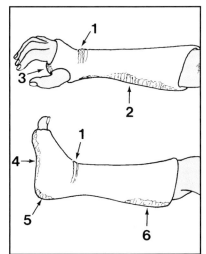

52. Treatment (c): If the circulation has been restored, gently pack wool between the cut edges of the plaster (1) and firmly apply an encircling crepe bandage (2). If this is not done, there is risk of extensive skin ('plaster') blistering locally. If the circulation is not restored, reappraise the position of the fracture and suspect major vessel involvement. *On no account adopt an expectant and procrastinating policy.*

53. Aftercare (d): *Can the plaster be completed?* If the plaster consists of a back-slab or shell, completion depends on your assessment of the present swelling, and your prediction of any further swelling. Most plasters may be completed after 48 hours; but if swelling is very marked completion should be delayed for a further 2 days, or until it is showing signs of subsiding.

54. Aftercare (e): *Is the plaster intact?* Look for evidence of cracking, especially in the region of the joints (1). In arm plasters, look for anterior softening (2) and softening in the palm (3). In the leg, look for softening of the sole piece (4), the heel (5) and calf (6). Any weak areas should be reinforced by the application of more plaster locally.

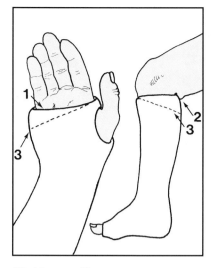

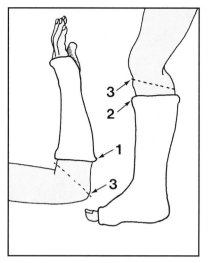

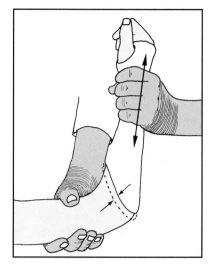

55. Aftercare (f): *Is the plaster causing restriction of movement?* Look especially for encroachment of the palm piece on the ulnar side of the hand, restricting MP joint flexion (1). In forearm plasters, look also for restriction of elbow movements. In below-knee plasters, note if the plaster is digging in when the knee is flexed (2). Trim the plaster as appropriate (3).

56. Aftercare (g): *Is the plaster too short?* Note especially the Colles-type plaster with inadequate grip of the forearm (1); note the below-knee plaster which does not reach the tibial tuberosity (2) and which, apart from affording unsatisfactory support of an ankle fracture, will inevitably cause friction against the shin. Extend the defective plasters where appropriate (3).

57. Aftercare (h): *Has the plaster become too loose?* A plaster may become loose as a result of the subsidence of limb swelling and from muscle wasting. If a plaster is slack, then the support afforded to the underlying fracture may become inadequate. Assess looseness by attempting to move the plaster proximally and distally, while noting its excursion in each direction.

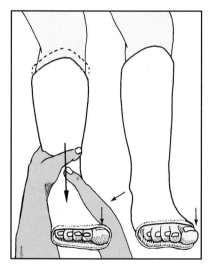

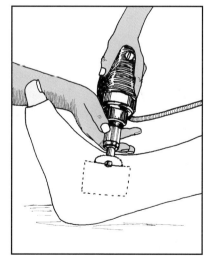

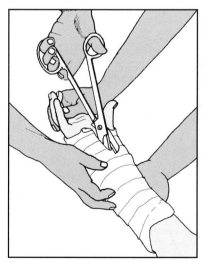

58. Aftercare (i): *Has the plaster become too loose? cntd* In the leg, grasp the plaster and pull it distally; note how far the toes disappear into the plaster. If a plaster is loose, it should be changed unless (i) union is nearing completion and risks of slipping are minimal or (ii) a good position is held and the risks of slipping while the plaster is being changed are thought to be greater than the risks of slipping in a loose plaster.

59. Aftercare (j): *Is the patient complaining of localised pain?* Localised pain, especially over a bony prominence, may indicate inadequate local padding, local pressure and pressure sore formation. In a child it may sometimes suggest a foreign body pushed in under the plaster. In all cases, the affected area should be inspected by cutting a window in the plaster and replacing it after examination.

60. How to remove a plaster – plaster slabs: Plaster shells or slabs are easily removed by cutting the encircling open weave bandages which hold them in position. Care must be taken to avoid nicking the skin, and Bohler scissors are helpful in this respect.

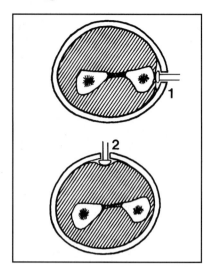

**61. Removing complete plasters –
Using shears (a):** The heel of the shears
must lie between the plaster and the limb.
Subcutaneous bony prominences such as the
shaft of the ulna (1) should be avoided to
lessen the risks of skin damage and pain.
Instead, the route of the shears should be
planned to lie over compressible soft tissue
masses (2).

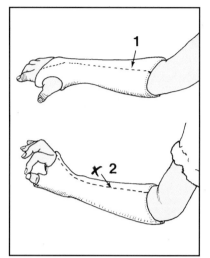

62. Using shears (b): If possible, avoid
cutting over a concavity. If the wrist is in
moderate palmar flexion, as in a Colles
plaster, the plaster should be removed by a
dorsal cut (1). In a scaphoid plaster, the
dorsal route should be avoided (2) and the
plaster removed anteriorly.

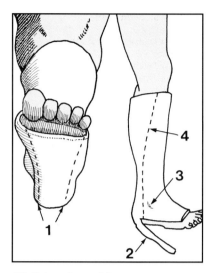

63. Using shears (c): Where there is the
right-angled bend of the ankle to negotiate, it
is often helpful to make two vertical cuts
down through the sole piece (1) and turn it
down (2). This then gives access for the
shears to make a vertical cut behind the
lateral malleolus (3) and then skirt forwards
over the peronei (4). The remaining plaster
may then be sprung open.

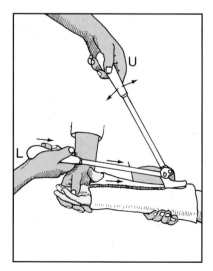

64. Using shears (d): Keep the lower
handle (L) parallel to the plaster, or even a
little depressed. Lift up the upper handle
(U); push the shears forward with the lower
handle so that the plaster fills the throat of
the shears. Maintaining a slight pushing
force – all the cutting action may be
performed with the upper handle, moving it
up and down like a beer pump.

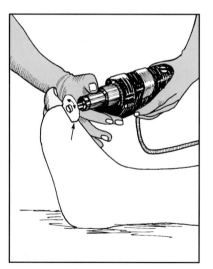

65. Using a plaster saw (a): Plaster
saws may be used for removing or cutting
windows in plasters, but they should be used
with caution and treated with respect. Do not
use a plaster saw unless there is a layer of
wool between the plaster and the skin. Do
not use it over bony prominences and do not
use if the blade is bent, broken or blunt.
Note: the blade does not rotate but oscillates.

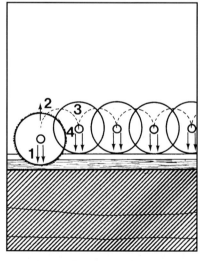

66. Using a plaster saw (b): Electric
saws are noisy, and the apprehensive patient
should be reassured. Cut down through the
plaster at one level (1); the note will change
as soon as it is through. Remove the saw (2)
and shift it laterally about 2.5 cm (3), and
repeat (4). *Do not* slide the saw laterally in
shallow cuts; the cutting movement should
be up and down.

67. Polymer resin casts: Most use bandages of cotton (e.g. Bayer's Baycast®), fibreglass (Smith & Nephew's Dynacast XR®) or polypropylene (3M's Primacast®), impregnated with a resin which hardens on contact with water. Advantages include: 1. Strength combined with lightness. 2. Rapid setting (5–10 min) and curing, reaching maximum strength in 30 min (cf. plasters whose slow 'drying out' period of about 48 hours may lead, if unprotected, to cracking). 3. Water resistance combined with porosity (although wetting of the inner layers should still be avoided). 4. Radiolucence.

Disadvantages include: 1. High item cost – but their durability reduces demands on staff and transport. 2. They generally mould less well than plaster, and are more unyielding.

After acute injuries, where further swelling is likely, plaster is generally the more suitable casting material: it can be carefully moulded to the part giving particularly good support, and where necessary it can be applied in the form of a slab. When swelling subsides, and the stability of the fracture is not in doubt, a resin cast may be substituted. Where little swelling is anticipated in a stable fresh fracture, a resin cast may be used from the outset. Where a cast is likely to be abused (e.g. in wet weather where an extroverted teenager requires support for an ankle injury) there is much to be said for using a resin cast, and of course it is possible to reinforce an ordinary plaster cast with an outer resin bandage.

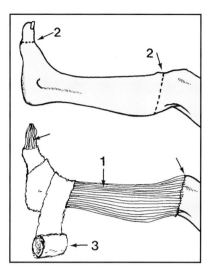

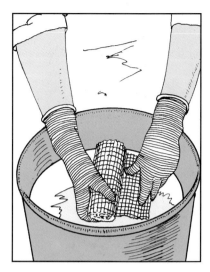

68. Application (a): Apply conforming stockinet (1) to the limb: ensure that it extends 3–5 cm (1–2″) beyond the proposed limits of the cast itself (2). Next, apply a layer of padding (3), paying particular care to protect the bony prominences. Where it is necessary to resist exposure to water or to moisture, a synthetic water-resistant orthopaedic padding may be used (e.g. Smith & Nephew's Soffban®).

69. Application (b): Open each bandage pack only as required to avoid premature curing. Wear gloves to prevent the resin adhering to your skin or causing sensitisation. Immerse the bandage in warm water for 2–5 seconds, squeezing it two to four times to accelerate setting. Fewer bandages will be required than with plaster, e.g. a below-knee cast in an adult may be applied with two 7.5 cm (3″) and one to two 10 cm (4″) bandages. Use the smaller sizes for the areas requiring a high degree of conformity (e.g. the ankle).

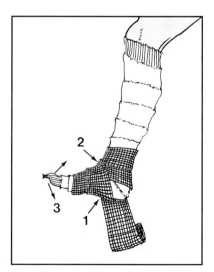

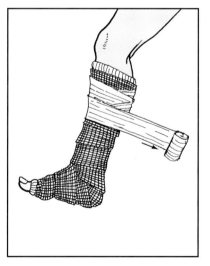

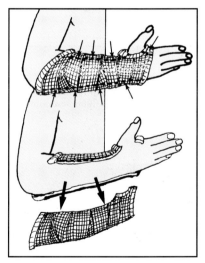

70. Application (c): Ensure the limb is correctly positioned, and apply each turn so that it overlaps the one beneath by half a width (1). It is permissible to use a figure-of-eight (2) round the ankle, elbow and knee to assist the bandage to lie neatly in conformity with the contours of the limb beneath. Turn back the stockinet (3) before applying the top layers of the bandage, and make quite certain that there will be no sharp or hard cast edges which can cause ulceration of the skin.

71. Application (d): In some cases close moulding of the cast may be encouraged by the temporary application of a firm external bandage. For this a thick cotton or crepe bandage may be used. This is first wetted, and then wrapped tightly round the limb. This will also be found helpful in retaining the last turn or two of the resin bandages, which often have a disturbing tendency to peel away before they set. Remove the wet overbandage once the cast has set.

72. Removal of resin casts: Because of their inherent springiness, resin casts cannot be cracked open after they have been cut down one side, as can plasters. In most cases it is necessary to bivalve by cutting down both sides. In the case of leg casts, it is best to turn down the sole piece first. Either shears or an oscillating saw may be used; in the latter case, a dust extractor should be employed to avoid the inhalation of resin dust. Resin casts are less likely to break after windowing than plasters.

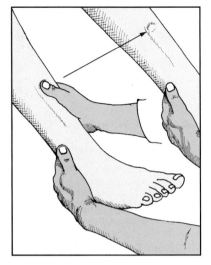

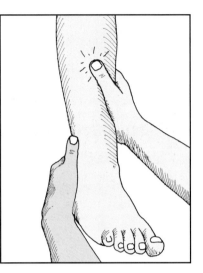

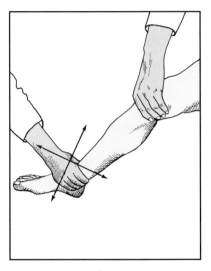

73. Assessment of union (a): Union in a fracture cannot be expected until a certain amount of time has elapsed, and it is pointless to start looking too soon. (See individual fractures for guidelines.) When it is reasonable to assess union, the limb should be examined out of plaster. Persistent oedema at the fracture site suggests union is incomplete.

74. Assessment of union (b): Examine the limb carefully for tenderness. Persistent tenderness localised to the fracture site is again suggestive of incomplete union.

75. Assessment of union (c): Persistent mobility at the fracture site is certain evidence of incomplete union. Support the limb close to the fracture with one hand, and with the other attempt to move the distal part in both the anterior and lateral planes. In a uniting fracture this is not a painful procedure.

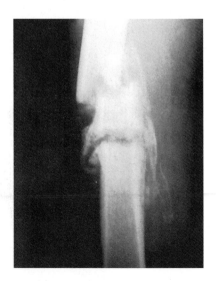

76. Assessment of union (d): Although clinical assessment is often adequate in many fractures of cancellous bone, it is advisable, in the case of the shafts of the femur, tibia, humerus, radius and ulna, to have up-to-date radiographs of the region. The illustration is of a double fracture of the femur at 14 weeks. In the proximal fracture, the fracture line is blurred and there is external bridging callus of good quality; union here is fairly far advanced. In the distal fracture, the fracture line is still clearly visible, and bridging callus is patchy. Union is incomplete, and certainly not sufficient to allow unprotected weight bearing.

In assessing radiographs for union, be suspicious of unevenly distributed bridging callus, of a persistent gap, and of sclerosis or broadening of the bone ends. Note that where a particularly rigid system of internal fixation has been employed, bridging callus may be minimal or absent, and endosteal callus may be very slow to appear.

If in doubt regarding the adequacy of union, continue with fixation and re-examine in 4 weeks.

Note that in all cases you must assess whether the forces the limb is exposed to will result in displacement or angulation of the fracture, or cause such mobility that union will be prevented. You must therefore balance the following equation:

External forces < (degree of union + support supplied by any internal fixation device and/or external splintage).

CHAPTER

4

Open fractures: internal fixation

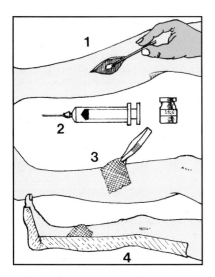

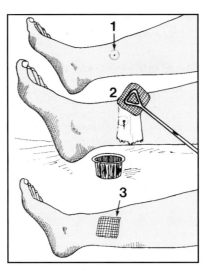

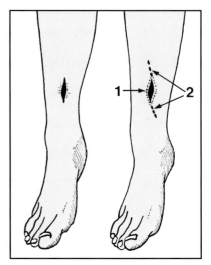

1. Open fractures – immediate care:
When the case first presents, ensure that the following procedures are carried out in every case: (1) Take a bacteriology swab from the wound. (2) Commence a short course of appropriate antibiotics (see p. 50). (3) Cover the wound with care, using sterile dressings (to reduce the risks of secondary (hospital) infection). (4) Apply temporary splintage (e.g. a plaster back shell or, if appropriate, an inflatable splint).

2. Type I, technically open fractures:
(1) The risks of infection are slight and are unlikely to be lessened by wide exposure (although this is advocated by some). The wound should be thoroughly cleaned (2) and a sterile dressing applied locally (3). Thereafter the method of supporting the fracture must be decided (see p. 79 and also Regional Injuries). If a plaster cast is being applied there *must* be allowance for swelling, e.g. by using a backshell or by splitting a cast applied over copious wool.

3. Type I, open from within out: The wound is small with clean or minimally bruised, viable edges (1). The skin edges may be minimally excised, and the wound extended (2) to allow a thorough inspection of the soft tissues and bone ends. It is unlikely that much will be required in the form of excision of contaminated or avascular tissue to achieve a thorough debridement. *Advantage may be taken of the exposure to allow an accurate open reduction of the fracture.*

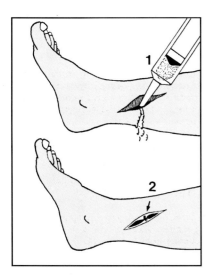

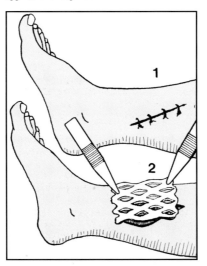

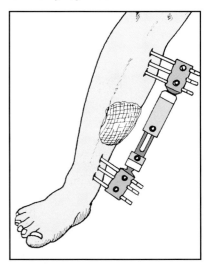

4. Type I cntd: Carry out a thorough (preferably pulsatile) wound lavage. Up to 10 L of normal saline may be used (followed, by some, with 2 L of bacitracin-polymyxin solution) (1). Primary closure of the skin is not advisable, but it may be helpful to use subcutaneous anchoring sutures (2) to prevent undue retraction and aid secondary suture. Apply a dressing which ensures the tissues remain moist (e.g. saline-soaked swabs over vaseline gauze). Attention must then be paid to fixation of the fracture.

5. Type I cntd: Inspect the wound after 48 hours; if necessary, perform any secondary debridement. If the wound remains clean, the aim should be to carry out a (delayed primary) wound closure under repeat antibiotic cover at 5 days (1). If the wound cannot be closed without tension, any remaining defect should be covered with a split-skin meshed graft (2) (which allows the escape of exudate). If the wound is dirty, then it should be treated by radical excision of all necrotic and infected tissue every 2–3 days until clean and ready to be grafted.

6. Type II open fractures: These should be managed along similar lines. In **Type III** injuries perform a rigorous lavage and debridement (with, if needed, wound enlargement): all foreign material must be removed along with any completely devitalised tissue (including small bone fragments). The wound should be left open but dressed so as to prevent drying out. To facilitate wound management (conducted as in Frame 5) an external fixator or locked intramedullary nail may be the best way to hold the fracture.

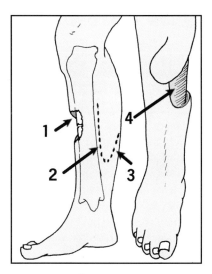

7. Type III cntd: If bone is exposed, the aim should be to get it covered within five days, to reduce the risks of secondary infection. Split skin grafts will only survive if applied to a vascular bed, therefore they cannot be used over open joints, bone devoid of periosteum, and tendons without paratenon. Thought must be given to future access (e.g. for bone grafting should union fail). In these circumstances other methods of cover must be employed. These should only be undertaken by a surgeon experienced in plastic surgical techniques, and *consultation*

with a plastic surgeon prior to the initial procedure, with later transfer to a plastic surgical unit, is highly desirable.

The local fasciocutaneous flap: This is the commonest and most useful technique. These flaps include skin and fascia, but not muscle. (Skin flaps in the lower limb which do not include the fascial layer have a poor record of success.) Distally based flaps are sometimes used to cover defects in the distal third of the leg. Careful planning of the flap is required. In the example (left) of the defect (1) to be covered, the anterior limb (2) of the flap to be raised is placed 1–2 cm posterior to the posteromedial border of the tibia. The posterior limb (3) may cross the midline. After the flap has been raised and swung (4), the resulting defect is covered with split skin grafts.

8. Type III cntd: Other plastic surgical techniques include the following:

Muscle flaps: These are generally reliable, but may result in functional loss.
(a) The gastrocnemius myocutaneous flap: this provides particularly good cover round the knee and in the proximal third of the tibia. Either the medial or lateral head may be used. (The muscle belly is isolated from soleus, its attachment to the Achilles tendon divided, and it is freed from its other head before the flap is swung.)
(b) The soleal myocutaneous flap: this may be used for cover in the middle third of the tibia.

(The muscle is detached 1 cm distal to its musculotendinous junction, transposed, and anchored distally.) Added length may be obtained by making several transverse incisions in its sheath. At a suitable time, its outer surface may be covered with split skin grafts.

Free microvascular flaps: The commonest and most useful sources are from the latissimus dorsi or rectus abdominis. The techniques are highly specialised, and careful planning must extend to dealing with the secondary defect. Failure is generally due to vascular problems or infection at the recipient site.

Where **bone grafting** is required this should be carried out as soon as it is safe to do so. In the case of *Type I and Type II open fractures,* this can be considered 2–3 weeks after wound healing. In the case of *Type III open fractures,* grafting should be delayed for 6 weeks after healing has been obtained. Where there is extensive bone loss, future reconstruction may be possible using an Ilizarov bone transport technique.

Type IIIc open fractures have the highest failure and amputation rate, due to vascular difficulties or infection. In handling these cases the fracture must be soundly fixed and any arterial repair (e.g. by an interpositional graft) achieved within 4–6 hours; the vascular problem should be dealt with by an experienced vascular surgeon, and not delegated. Prophylactic fasciotomies should be carried out.

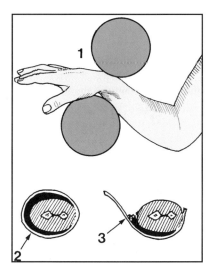

9. Degloving injuries (a): In a degloving injury, an extensive area of skin is torn from its underlying attachments and thereby deprived of its blood supply. In the hand or arm it is commonly caused by the limb being crushed between rollers (1); in the leg it may result from the shearing effect of a vehicle wheel passing over the limb in a run-over accident.

10. Degloving injuries (b): The skin may remain unbroken (2 in Frame 9), in which case the limb feels like a fluid-containing bag, owing to the presence of an extensive haematoma between the skin and fascia. If the skin is torn (3 in Frame 9), the effect is the creation of a large flap of full-thickness skin. In either case, massive sloughing is likely unless the injury is properly managed. A number of plastic surgical procedures are available:

1. If the skin is in good condition it may be de fatted and re applied immediately as a full thickness graft (although failure is not uncommon).

2. If the skin is damaged, split skin grafts may be taken from it (prior to its excision); these may be used immediately if the site is suitable, or stored for a secondary procedure.

3. The flap may be marked for later orientation and excised. After refrigeration storage in a sterile container (storage temperature is important), it is replaced after 1–2 weeks as a single sheet graft, after the deeper layers have been removed using special equipment.

In any open injury it is vital to keep in mind the risks of serious, life-threatening infections, particularly tetanus and gas gangrene, and the appropriate protective measures must be taken.

11. PRINCIPLES OF INTERNAL FIXATION AND COMMON FIXATION METHODS

When it is intended to implant materials for the treatment of fractures, the following criteria must be satisfied:

1. **Freedom from tissue reaction:** It is self-evident that if foreign material is being implanted in the tissues it should be biologically inert, and not give rise to toxic reactions, local inflammatory changes, fibrosis, foreign body giant cell reactions, etc., which in turn are likely to produce local pain, swelling and impairment of function. There is evidence of an extremely low but apparently clear incidence of local, and possibly distal, metal-induced neoplasia. In consequence, in the younger patient (under age 40), internal fixation devices are removed routinely once they have served their purpose.

2. **Freedom from corrosion:** Implanted materials should not corrode. Where stainless steel is used it should be of an accepted grade and free from impurities; steps should be taken to avoid the initiation of corrosion problems by fretting occurring at the point of contact between the separate components of an implant. It is essential to avoid electrolytic degradation, and in practice this means that if more than one implant is used at the same side (e.g. a plate and screws), identical materials are employed.

3. **Freedom from mechanical failure:** Implants must satisfy the purposes for which they are intended. To withstand the forces to which they will be subjected demands a satisfactory compromise between the materials used and the design of the implant. In the treatment of fractures, implants generally must have great mechanical strength in association with small physical bulk; consequently most are made of metal. Of the suitable metals, the most frequently employed are:

- Certain stainless steels
- Alloys of chromium, cobalt and molybdenum (e.g. Vitallium®, Vinertia®)
- Titanium.

The chrome–cobalt alloys are biologically very inert, but are difficult to machine so that most implants, including screws, are microcast using the lost wax technique; this adds to their cost. The stainless steels are less inert, but are easier to machine and are cheaper. In the case of titanium, the favourable combination of high strength, light weight, high fatigue strength, low modulus of elasticity and relative inertness, allows the fabrication of thinner plates and stronger intramedullary nails. It also produces fewer artefacts in CAT and MRI scans, allowing for example, earlier and better detection of avascular necrosis in femoral neck fractures.

In certain situations other materials are sometimes used, e.g. in fractures of the femur in the region of the stems of hip replacements it is possible to employ nylon plates held in position with nylon cerclage straps. At the ankle, biodegradable plastic dowels may be used to treat certain malleolar fractures, and have the advantage that their slow absorption obviates any need for their later removal. Sensitivity to these implants (in the form of a low grade inflammatory response) is, however, a not uncommon occurrence. Where it is desirable to have a certain amount of flexibility in a plate to encourage the formation of some external bridging callus, carbon fibre plates are sometimes used.

FIXATION DEVICES AND SYSTEMS

Fractures vary enormously in pattern; bones vary in their size, texture and strength. To cope with even the most common situations and be a match for every subtle variation of circumstance requires an impressive range of devices and instruments for their insertion. The design of fixation devices has in the past been somewhat haphazard, and aimed at the treatment either of one fracture or the solution of a single fixation problem. There have been attempts to produce integrated systems of fracture fixation: sets of devices which can contend with any fracture situation. The most outstanding system, now firmly established, is that developed by the Association for the Study of Internal Fixation (ASIF or AO (Arbeitsgemeinschaft für Osteosynthesefragen). This group of general and orthopaedic surgeons was founded in 1956 by Maurice E. Müller to research certain concepts propounded by Robert Danis). As a result of their work, apart from the development of a series of screws, plates and other devices, and the corresponding instrumentation, the Association is responsible for some change in emphasis in the philosophy of fracture treatment. They feel that the common aim – a return to full function in the shortest time – can often best be achieved by the use of internal fixation devices, of such strength and design that external splintage can frequently be discarded, permitting immediate joint freedom, early weight bearing, short-term hospitalisation, and early return to work and other activities. These ideals are often achieved, but it must be stressed that optimum results cannot be obtained without the necessary technical knowledge of the system and a degree of mechanical aptitude, both of which can be acquired by appropriate training and experience.

With any form of internal fixation great importance must always be placed on recognising which cases are best treated in this way. It is equally important to recognise which cases are not suited to treatment by internal fixation, and those which may be dealt with either surgically or conservatively. It is in the last group that there is often some difficulty, and it is important to remember the hazards of infection; even though it may be uncommon, it must always be a feared complication which, on occasion, can turn a comparatively minor fracture into a disaster. In certain situations the risks of infection may be reduced and fracture fixation achieved by using minimally invasive techniques (such as closed intramedullary nailing). Disturbance of the fracture haematoma is best avoided if at all possible as this may delay or prevent union; the risks may be reduced by the use of Wave or Less Invasive Plate Systems (see p. 76).

As in many branches of surgery, the core problem is in deciding how many excellent results are required to balance the occasional serious failure, and the compromise to be made between the particulars of a case and the outlook and judgement of the surgeon.

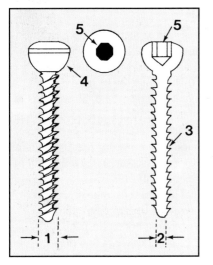

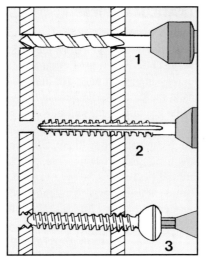

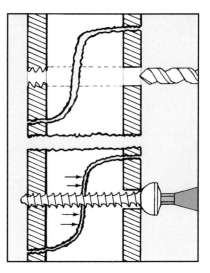

12. Principles of internal fixation and common devices: Cortical bone screws (a): The AO cortical bone screw enjoys widespread use and is probably the commonest of all internal fixation devices. The standard screw has an outside diameter of 4.5 mm (1) and a core diameter of 3.0 mm (2). The thread form is a modified buttress (3), of 1.75 mm pitch (*c.* 15 TPI). The large head has a hemispherical undersurface (4) and contains a hexagon socket (5) which is used for its insertion.

13. Cortical bone screws (b): To insert an AO screw, the bone is drilled with a 3.2 mm drill (1), preferably using a guide to maintain its perpendicularity. The hole is then tapped (2) and sized, so that the correct length of screw (from a wide range) can be chosen. This is then inserted using a hex screwdriver (3). In certain circumstances it is necessary to use smaller screws (e.g. in dealing with phalangeal fractures) and screws of 3.5, 2.7, 2.0 and 1.5 mm are available in the AO range.

14. Cortical bone screws (c): When two bone fragments are being approximated with a screw, it is usually desirable to do so in such a manner that the adjacent surfaces are compressed one against the other – this improves the quality of the fixation, reduces the risks of non-union, and may be essential if the fracture will otherwise be unsupported (e.g. if a cast is not being applied). To do this, a clearance (or gliding) hole is drilled in the nearest fragment; tightening the screw draws the two fragments together: the so-called lag screw principle.

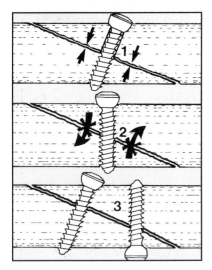

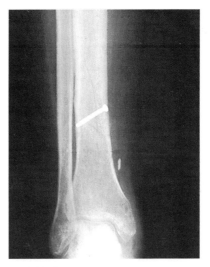

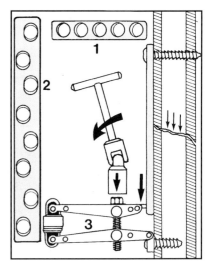

15. Cortical bone screws (d): *Placing the screws.* Two mutually exclusive screw positionings may be used. To obtain the most effective compression, and to avoid side thrusts which might displace the alignment of bone fragments, screws should be inserted at right angles to the plane of the fracture (1). To offer the maximum resistance to torsional forces, screws should be inserted at right angles to the cortex (2). In practice, a combination of these two placements may be employed with effect (3).

16. Cortical bone screws (e): In long bones, one or more screws may be used to hold a fracture in perfect alignment (Illus.). Such an arrangement can seldom suffice without additional support: this may be in the form of plaster cast, but commonly a plate is used to neutralise any torsional or bending stresses that the fracture might be subjected to (neutralising plate). Note that if the stresses are great (e.g. unsupported weight bearing), some of the load *must* be carried by the bone, otherwise eventual fatigue fracture of the plate is likely.

17. Common devices: Plates (a): There are many different types of plate. Some are quite lightweight and occupy little space (1), being used only to hold major bone fragments in alignment, while others are heavy (2) and sufficiently rigid to allow all external splintage to be discarded. For these to be successful and to encourage endosteal callus formation, the bone surfaces should be brought together under a degree of compression. One way of doing this is to use a tensioning device (3) before inserting the screws on the second side of the fracture.

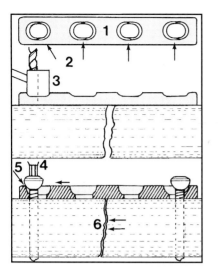

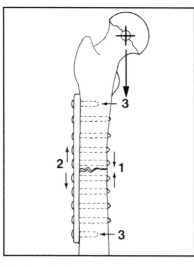

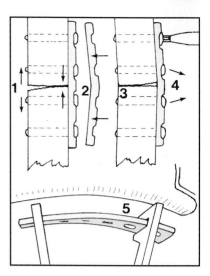

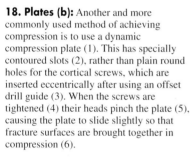

18. Plates (b): Another and more commonly used method of achieving compression is to use a dynamic compression plate (1). This has specially contoured slots (2), rather than plain round holes for the cortical screws, which are inserted eccentrically after using an offset drill guide (3). When the screws are tightened (4) their heads pinch the plate (5), causing the plate to slide slightly so that fracture surfaces are brought together in compression (6).

19. Plates (c): Plates should be placed so that compression loads are taken by bone (1), and tension effects are neutralised by the plate (2). In practice this means that plates should be applied to the convex surface (e.g. the lateral side of the femur). However, in the tibia, plates are often fixed to the anteromedial surface. In the case of the femur, tibia and humerus ideally 8 cortices should be engaged in each major fragment (6 in the forearm). End screws engaging a single cortex (3) may be used to relieve stress.

20. Plates (d): When a flat plate is applied to a bone using any system to obtain compression, this tends to occur in an uneven manner; the far side may open up as compression occurs on the nearside (1). To avoid this, it is common practice to pre-bend the plate at the level of the fracture (2). Then the far side compresses first (3), before the rest of the fracture line becomes involved, with the plate tending to straighten out (4). Note too that with the use of appropriate clamps plates may be individually bent to fit snugly against the contours of a bone (5).

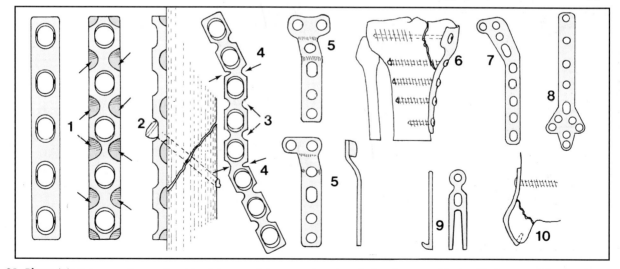

21. Plates (e): Plates come in a great variety of shapes and sizes; some have been designed to cope with a specific fracture, while others have been developed to overcome certain inherent problems associated with the use of plates of a standard pattern.

- The *low-contact dynamic compression plate (LC-DCP)* is relieved on its undersurface (1) so that the bone with which it is in direct contact is reduced in area: this minimises the amount of periosteum and bone which may be deprived of its blood supply by pressure from the plate. The screw slots are shaped in such a manner that interfragmentary bone compression screws (e.g. lag screws) may be inserted at angles up to 40° (2).
- *Reconstruction plates* have V-cuts (3) between the screw holes which allow the plates to be bent in zig-zag fashion (4) (as well as in other planes) so that they can be used in special situations (e.g. in certain pelvic fractures).
- *T- and L-buttress plates* (5) are of particular value in dealing with fractures of the proximal tibia (6).
- *Lateral tibial head (hockey stick)* plates (7) are also used in the proximal tibial area.
- *Cloverleaf* (8) plates are used mainly for the distal tibia.
- *Hook plates* (e.g. Zuelzer (9), AO) may be used when one fragment is not particularly suited to receiving a screw (e.g. fractures of the medial malleolus (10) or certain spinal fractures).
- *Carbon fibre plates* (which can only be contoured at the time of manufacture) are slightly flexible and allow the formation of bridging callus.

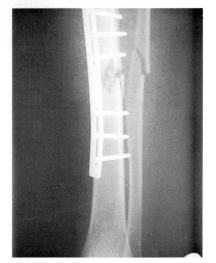

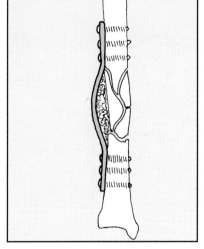

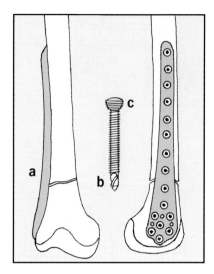

22. Plates (f): The *Eggar plate*, now only occasionally used, is a lightweight plate which is readily contoured to fit the bone to which it is being applied. Additional support (e.g. with an external plaster cast) is generally required. The plate is fixed to the bone with self-tapping screws which are not fully tightened. This permits slight axial movement, so that as bone absorption at the fracture site occurs the bone ends are not kept apart and union is thereby encouraged.

23. Plates (g): The *wave plate* has a substantial concavity in its middle third. This allows the easier ingrowth of blood vessels into any cancellous bone onlay grafts which may be placed between the plate and the bone surface. The wave plate also spreads stress concentrations over a wider area, thereby reducing the risks of fatigue fracture. In certain situations it may also act as a tension band.

24. Plates (h): *Liss* (less invasive stabilisation system) *plates* are made of titanium, and are of particular value in osteoporotic bone and for periprosthetic fractures. In the distal femur a precontoured range ensures a good fit (a). The plate is introduced through a small distal incision, and secured with screws whose tips (b) are self-drilling. Their caps (c) screw into the holes in the plate which are threaded to take them. Proximal screws are inserted through small incisions using a jig.

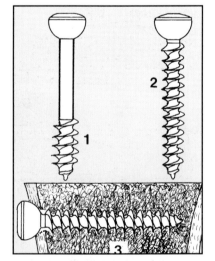

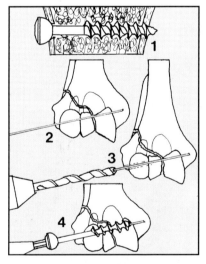

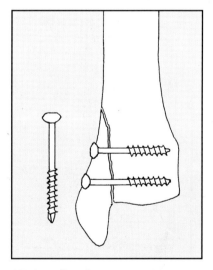

25. Cancellous bone screws (a): Screws designed for insertion in cancellous bone have a coarse pitch and a narrow thread angle, a combination which at its extremes produces auger forms. AO cancellous bone screws (with diameters of 6.5 or 4.0 mm) may be *partially threaded* (for use as lag screws) (1), or *fully threaded* (2) (when used to fix plates in the metaphyseal regions of long bones). The near cortex only is usually tapped, the screw cutting its own path in the cancellous bone (3).

26. Cancellous bone screws (b): In the metaphyseal regions cancellous screws get the best grip if they engage the thin bone of the opposite cortex (which may have to be tapped) (1). If a reduction has been held with a Kirschner wire (2), *cannulated* 3.5 and 6.5 mm screws may be used when premature removal of the wire might threaten the reduction. The near cortex is drilled with a cannulated drill (3) and the screw inserted (4) over the wire which is then removed.

27. Cancellous bone screws (c): Partially threaded *malleolar screws* have been designed to secure small malleolar bone fragments by getting a purchase on the firm cancellous bone of the distal tibial metaphysis. They have an outside diameter of 4.5 mm and have fluted self-tapping tips. Because of this they are generally inserted without preliminary tapping.

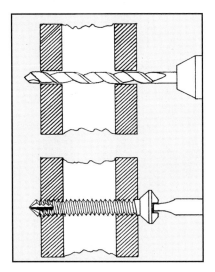

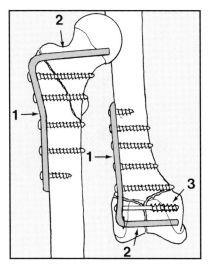

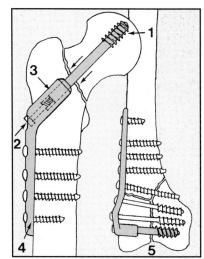

28. Self-tapping screws: Where the bone cortex is very thin, self-tapping screws get a better grip than tapped screws. (Note also that prior to the development of the AO range of bone screws, self-tapping screws were in universal use for all forms of internal fixation; their main disadvantage was that they could be difficult to insert in dense cortical bone.) With the Sherman screw (9/64″, 3.6 mm OD) a pilot hole marginally larger than the core diameter (in practice 7/64″, 2.8 mm) is drilled before insertion of the screw.

29. Blade plates: These are most commonly used at either end of the femur when there is insufficient bone on the epiphyseal side of a fracture to allow an ordinary plate to be used. Blade plates come in a variety of angles and forms: the plate portion (1) is screwed to the shaft of the bone after the blade or spline (2) has been inserted into the bone. Cancellous bone screws (3) may be used for interfragmentary compression.

30. Dynamic hip screw/dynamic condylar screw: This device uses a large diameter cancellous bone screw (1) which can be drawn (with a small screw (2)) into the sleeve (3) of a plate which is screwed to the shaft of the femur (4). In the femoral neck the soft bone of the head is gripped and the fracture can be compressed; at the distal end of the femur (5) it is of particular value in treating T- or Y-fractures, allowing the articular fragments to be drawn together (a blade plate in such circumstances is harder to insert and less effective).

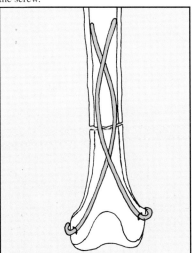

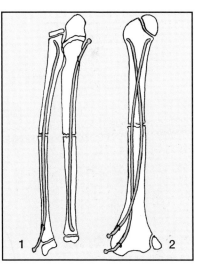

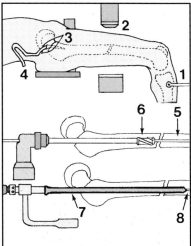

31. Intramedullary nails (a): These are used to treat diaphyseal fractures, and take a number of forms. *Rush pins* are of solid stainless steel, come in a range of lengths and diameters, and have hooked ends to prevent their migration into the bone cavity. They may be used singly and straight as supplied (e.g. in the ulna), but in the femur (Illus.), tibia and humerus they may be *bent* to obtain a measure of 3-point fixation, and *paired*, to provide better support and some control of rotation.

32. Intramedullary nails (b): *Nancy nails* are sometimes used in treating long bone fractures in children. They are made of titanium, are flexible, and of small diameter. Singly, they may be used in the radius and ulna (1), but in the humerus (2), tibia and femur they are employed in pairs. The nails are bent so that they provide dynamic 3-point fixation. Their sharp ends penetrate the cancellous bone of the metaphysis, thereby providing rotational and axial stability.

33. Intramedullary nails (c): *Tubular, solid* or *clover leaf* pattern nails are often used to treat shaft fractures of the tibia, femur and humerus in adults. In many cases the operation can be performed without exposing the fracture. Reduction is obtained, sometimes with skeletal traction (1) under intensifier control (2). Through a proximal incision (3) the medullary canal is located (4). A rod (5) is passed across the fracture, followed by a reamer (6) to allow the later passage of a close-fitting nail (7) over a guide rod (8).

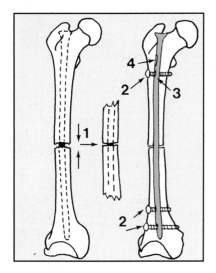

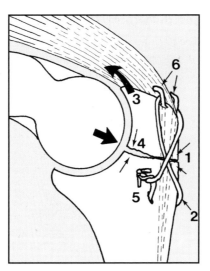

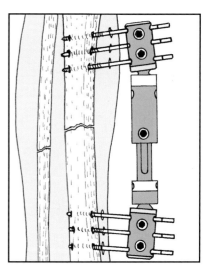

34. Intramedullary nails (d):
Interlocking of the fragments, a well-reamed canal and a close-fitting nail may suffice to resist torsional forces which might jeopardise the fixation. Bone absorption at the fracture site is usually taken up by telescoping (1). If torsional control is poor, an interlocking nail may be used; this employs transversely running locking bolts (2) which pass through holes (3) or slots (4) in the nail. Where reaming is undesirable (e.g. in certain open fractures) solid intramedullary nails (e.g. of titanium) may be used.

35. Tension band wiring: This is used most frequently in olecranon and patellar fractures. The surfaces away from the articular side of the fracture (1) are drawn together and pre-loaded with a high tensile wire (2), while muscle pull (3) acting against the fulcrum of the coronoid (or femoral condyle) brings the rest together (4). The wire is twisted to tighten it (5), and Kirschner wires (6) may be used if required to preserve longitudinal alignment.

36. External fixators (a): There are many types to deal with a wide range of bone sizes. *The pins* (2 or preferably 3 in each main fragment) must be rigid (e.g.flat-threaded Schanz pins) and are inserted through 'safe' areas to avoid damage to underlying nerves or blood vessels. Single-side (unilateral or cantilever) systems give the best access for dressing open wounds, with bilateral systems now being reserved mainly for arthrodeses. Meticulous care must be taken to avoid pin-track infections.

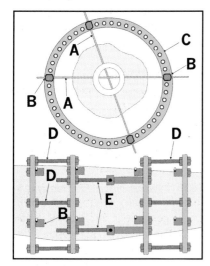

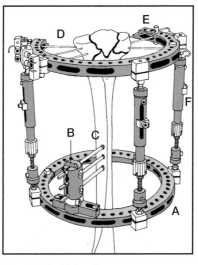

37. (b) Ilizarov fixation: Fine (1.5 or 1.8 mm diameter) Kirschner wires (A) are passed percutaneously through carefully selected sites. Two or more are used at each level. They are generally tensioned and held with wire fixation bolts (B) to a ring (C) which encircles the limb. (The ring may be hinged or have a removable segment to ease application.) Two or more rings are applied to each main bone fragment. They are connected together using threaded rods (D) or adjustors (E).

38. (c) Hybrid fixation: This technique is particularly helpful in dealing with metaphyseal fracture. In the Orthofix*™ hybrid system (shown here being used to hold a tibial metaphyseal fracture) a lower or distal ring (A) is secured by means of a Sheffield clamp (B) and three Schanz pins (C) inserted into the tibial diaphysis. The metaphyseal fragments are held with tensioned wires (D), clamped to a second ring (E) which is connected to the other with three reduction units (F).

39. **INTERNAL FIXATION IN OPEN FRACTURES**

The use of internal fixation devices in open fractures is a controversial subject, but cases which pose real difficulty for the uncommitted are in practice rather uncommon. The following points should be noted:

1. In children, internal fixation seldom needs to be considered; in most fractures, if angulation and axial rotation are controlled, the remarkable powers of remodelling can usually be relied upon, and an anatomical reduction is only occasionally required. It is useful to remember, as in the adult, that if the wound is more than technical, advantage should be taken of it to reduce the fracture under vision; a stable reduction is often attainable.

2. In the adult, where a fracture is undisplaced, conservative methods of treatment can generally be followed without difficulty; once skin healing has occurred, any secondary procedure can be carried out with comparative security.

3. Where a fracture is unstable, and is open from *within out* with minimal tissue contamination (Type I open fractures), internal fixation may be carried out in reasonable safety once the wound has been adequately dealt with.

    In the case of the tibia, intramedullary nailing with reaming may be undertaken without especial risk of infection in Type II open fractures. In Type III open fractures, the use of intramedullary nails is said to carry no greater risks than other methods of treatment, although many would advocate the use of a solid intramedullary nail without reaming, or seek an alternative method of holding the fracture (such as with an external fixator).

    In the case of the femur, intramedullary nailing with reaming may be attempted in both Type I and II fractures; but this procedure carries a very high risk of serious infection in Type III injuries, and therefore is contraindicated.

4. Where there has been extensive skin and soft tissue damage or loss, and the wound has been badly contaminated, as a general rule internal fixation should be avoided; the fracture should be supported by a plaster cast or preferably by an external fixator. In the case of the femur, skeletal traction in a Thomas splint may be used. Note that if an external fixator has been applied, and there is no sign of pin-track infection, it may be possible to convert this (if considered to be to the patient's advantage) to intramedullary nail fixation within the first week without there being a greatly enhanced risk of infection. If there *has* been a pin-track infection, reamed secondary intramedullary nailing is generally contraindicated, the risks of infection being unacceptably high. However, in a few cases, if the pins are removed, pin site debridements carried out, antibiotics administered, and full skin healing obtained and held for some weeks, intramedullary nailing may be reconsidered. Generally speaking, however, when an external fixator is employed, it should be retained until the fracture is united or until a supporting plaster cast can be substituted; alternatively, conversion to Ilizarov fixation may be a possibility, the fine wires being relatively well tolerated.

Difficulty tends to occur in the handling of the unstable fracture where skin cover is perhaps poor and/or the risks of infection are appreciable but not certain. *Against* the use of internal fixation in these circumstances is:

1. The risk of wider dissemination of infection into uncontaminated tissue by the greater exposure required for the insertion of some internal fixation devices.
2. The greater risks of wound breakdown.
3. The greater difficulty in obtaining healing if infection becomes established, because of the presence of the fixation device acting as a foreign body.

In favour of internal fixation are the following:

1. The chance of obtaining a good reduction.
2. The possibility of holding that reduction for as long as required.
3. The better prospects of securing bone union and soft tissue healing.

It is also important to note that in the case of *multiple injuries* the prognosis is best when the circumstances allow early rigid fixation of all lower limb long bone fractures. (This is mainly due to the avoidance of respiratory complications by early mobilisation.) The eventual decision rests on the particular circumstances of the case, and the surgeon's individual assessment of the factors discussed.

40. GUNSHOT WOUNDS

The pattern of injury and the treatment required is dependent on the type of missile; the general principle is that of delayed suture and early split skin grafting.

Low velocity gunshot wounds (for example, handgun wounds)

The principles of treatment of uncomplicated wounds are:

1. The margins of the entry and exit wounds should be excised.
2. The track should be thoroughly irrigated with saline or hydrogen peroxide.
3. A saline-soaked gauze swab should, if possible, be passed through and through, and then removed.
4. The track should be lightly packed open with vaseline gauze.
5. The wound should then be covered with saline soaked dressings, dry gauze and wool, secured with crepe bandages.
6. The wound should then be inspected at about 5 days and, if clean, sutured.

If there is a bullet in the tissues, the need for its removal should be carefully balanced against the risks of exploration. It should be noted that if a bullet remains in a joint, the toxicity of its metallic elements will have a disastrous effect on the articular cartilage. It is strongly advised that the affected joint should be thoroughly irrigated and every attempt made to remove the foreign body.

Plastic bullets These tend to produce localised blunt injuries, and seldom cause fractures; if by any chance there is an accompanying fracture, this can usually be dealt with by normal closed methods of treatment.

High velocity gunshot wounds These are characterised by small entry and large exit wounds. Shock waves may cause extensive tissue destruction and even fracture at a distance from the direct track of the missile. A temporary wave of negative pressure within the wound may suck in clothing and other debris. If bone is struck, a multifragmentary fracture results.

These injuries must be treated with great respect along the lines of other Type IIIB open fractures. A full exploration with removal of all devitalised tissues is essential, and primary closure is contraindicated. In many cases prophylactic compartmental fasciotomies are advisable. The fracture is often best fixed with an external fixator applied in such a way as to give good access to the wound. (If it is likely that a myocutaneous or other flap will be required, the pins must be positioned so that this is possible, and a preliminary consultation with a plastic surgeon is often helpful.)

Explosions The severity of the injuries is inversely proportional to the distance between the victim and the source; the initial shock wave is followed by a short-lived fireball, but the accompanying blast wave causes most of the damage. Death or traumatic amputation may result; there may also be accompanying respiratory and auditory damage, and falling masonry or flying debris may cause crush or other injuries. The variety of tissue damage knows no limits, and the treatment is dependent on the exact nature of the injuries sustained.

Where there are multiple casualties, Major Incident or Disaster Routines are generally followed where the most important principles include the establishment of good communications so that the size of the emergency and the call-out can be determined, and in the hospital, differentiating between minor cases (which do not require immediate treatment), severely injured cases (where resources should be concentrated), and the dead and dying: this initial triage would normally be carried out by the most experienced surgeon present. In the Belfast explosion experience (unlike certain other disaster situations) site medical teams have been thought to hinder rather than help the smooth running of the Police, Fire and Ambulance services.

Resuscitative procedures, as always, precede formal investigation of injuries and arrangements for definitive treatment.

CHAPTER

5

Factors affecting healing; complications; pathological fractures

FACTORS AFFECTING THE RATE OF HEALING OF A FRACTURE

1. TYPE OF BONE

Cancellous bone (spongy bone) Healing in cancellous bone is generally well advanced 6 weeks from the time of the injury, and protection of the fracture can almost invariably be abandoned by that time. This applies to fractures of bones which are composed principally of cancellous tissue, and also to fractures involving the cancellous bone to be found at the ends of long bones. This rule is illustrated in the following examples:

1. Weight bearing after a fracture of the calcaneus may be permitted after about 6 weeks.
2. A patient with a traumatic wedge fracture of a vertebral body may commence full mobilisation after 6 weeks.
3. Plaster fixation may be discarded after 5–6 weeks following a Colles fracture.
4. Weight may be allowed through the leg 6 weeks after a fracture of the tibial table.
5. Bed rest for 6 weeks is usually advised for any fracture of the pelvis involving those parts through which weight transmission is mediated.

Cortical bone (compact bone) Endosteal callus may take many months to become reasonably well established, and many uncomplicated long bone fractures may take 9–18 weeks to unite. In some cases, however, abundant external bridging callus may allow an earlier return of function. For example:

1. The average time to union of a fracture of the tibial shaft treated conservatively is 16 weeks
2. Fractures of the humeral shaft can often be left unsupported after 10 weeks.
3. On the other hand, fractures of the metatarsals, metacarpals and phalanges, where external bridging callus is usually substantial, are usually quite firm in 4–5 weeks.

2. PATIENT AGE

In children, union of fractures is rapid. The speed of union decreases as age increases until skeletal maturity is reached. There is then not a great deal of difference in the rate between young adults and the elderly. For example, in a child, union may be expected in a fractured femur a little after the number of weeks equivalent to its numerical age have passed, i.e. a fractured femur in a child of 3 years is usually united after 4 weeks; a fractured femur in a child of 8 years is usually sound after 9 weeks. In contrast, a fracture of the femoral shaft in an adult may take 3–6 months to unite.

Apart from great rapidity of union it should be noted that children have remarkable powers of remodelling fractures. These powers are excellent as far as displacement is concerned, and are often good for slight to moderate angulation. Remodelling is poor in the case of axial rotation in both adults and children. The power to remodel decreases rapidly once adolescence is reached and epiphyseal fusion is imminent.

3. MOBILITY AT FRACTURE SITE

Excessive mobility persisting at the fracture site (due, for example, to poor fixation) may interfere with vascularisation of the fracture haematoma; it may lead to disruption of early bridging callus and may prevent endosteal new bone growth. One of the main aims of all forms of internal and external splintage is to reduce mobility at the fracture site, and hence encourage union. If splintage is inadequate, union may be delayed or prevented.

4. SEPARATION OF BONE ENDS

Union will be delayed or prevented if the bone ends are separated, for this interferes with the normal mechanisms of healing. (The converse is also true, namely that compression of the fracture facilitates union.) Separation may occur under several circumstances:

1. **Soft tissue interposition.** For example, in fractures of the femoral shaft, one of the bone ends may become isolated from the other by herniating through some of the surrounding muscle mass, thereby delaying or preventing union. Fractures of the medial malleolus may fail to unite due to infolding of a layer of periosteum between the fragments.
2. **Excessive traction.** Excessive traction employed in the maintenance of a reduction may lead to separation of the bone ends and non-union. This may occur, for example, in femoral shaft fractures, particularly those treated by skeletal traction.
3. **Following internal fixation.** In some situations where internal fixation is used to hold a fracture, resorption of bone may occur at the fracture site; the fixation device may continue to hold the bone fragments in such a way that they are prevented from coming together, and mechanical failure may ensue. A bulky internal fixation device may in itself interfere with the local blood supply and the fracture haematoma. Where possible, steps should be taken to avoid this (e.g. by employing a wave plate or a LISS plate).

5. INFECTION

Infection in the region of a fracture may delay or prevent union. This is especially the case if, in addition, movement is allowed to occur at the fracture. Infection of the fracture site is extremely rare in conservatively treated closed fractures; infection, if it occurs, follows either an open injury or one treated by internal fixation. Where infection becomes well established in the presence of an internal fixation device, it is often difficult to achieve healing without removal of the device, which acts as a foreign body and a nidus for persisting infection. This is especially the case if there is breakdown of the overlying skin and the establishment of a sinus. Not infrequently the situation arises where cast fixation alone is unable to provide the degree of fixation necessary for union if the device is removed, and where infection is likely to remain if it is not. In such circumstances it is usually wiser to retain the fixation device until union is reasonably well advanced, or to consider using an external fixator. In some cases, where sound healing can be obtained and maintained after removal of an internal fixation device, it may be possible to repeat the internal fixation in the sterile environment that has been obtained.

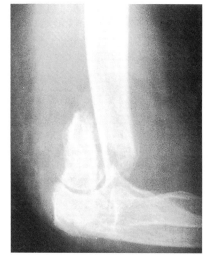

1. Supracondylar fracture of humerus with soft tissue between bone ends.

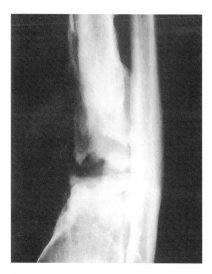

2. Chronic bone infection and failure of union of tibia following plating (plate removed).

6. DISTURBANCE OF BLOOD SUPPLY

It is obvious that for the normal multiplication of bone cells and their precursors an adequate blood supply is required. Where the blood supply to an area is reduced, or where there is interference with the blood supply to both major fragments – e.g. in radionecrosis of bone – healing may be interfered with. On the other hand, reduction of the blood supply to one fragment, especially if cancellous bone is involved, may not interfere with union; indeed, in some situations it may apparently stimulate it. The most striking examples of this are fractures of the femoral neck and scaphoid, where the phenomenon of avascular necrosis is most frequently discovered in soundly united fractures. Interference with the blood supply to one fragment at the time of injury leads to immediate bone death; this is frequently followed by sound union of the fracture. Collapse of necrotic bone beyond the level of union is observed at a later date.

Again, a bulky internal fixation device may in itself interfere with the local blood supply and the fracture haematoma, delaying union. Where possible this should be avoided by choosing the most appropriate device.

7. PROPERTIES OF THE BONE INVOLVED

Fracture healing is also affected by a number of imperfectly understood factors which lead to variations in the speed of union. The clavicle is a spectacular example; non-union is extremely rare, the time to clinical union is unexcelled by any other part of the skeleton, yet movement at the fracture site cannot be controlled with any efficiency. Union of the tibia is often slow to a degree that is difficult to explain even when the influence of its nutrient artery and fracture mobility are taken into account.

8. OTHER FACTORS

- **Effects of smoking.** Smoking has a deleterious effect on fracture union, often being a significant factor in the rate and quality of union.
- **Joint involvement.** When a fracture involves a joint, union is occasionally delayed. This may be due to dilution of the fracture haematoma by synovial fluid.
- **Bone pathology.** Many of the commonest causes of pathological fracture do not seem to delay union in a material way. (Union may progress quite normally in, for example, osteoporosis, osteomalacia, Paget's disease and most simple bone tumours.) Some primary and secondary malignant bone tumours may delay or prevent union (see pp. 105–108).

COMPLICATIONS OF FRACTURES

Complications which may occur in a patient who has suffered a fracture or dislocation may be grouped in the following way:

1. GENERAL COMPLICATIONS OF ANY TISSUE DAMAGE

These include:
1. Internal and external haemorrhage, oligaemic shock, etc.
2. Infection (in open or compound injuries)
3. Electrolyte shifts, protein breakdown and other metabolic responses of trauma.

2. **COMPLICATIONS OF PROLONGED RECUMBENCY**

These include:
1. Hypostatic pneumonia.
2. Pressure sores.
3. Deep venous thrombosis and pulmonary embolism.
4. Muscle wasting and stiffening of joints, making subsequent mobilisation more difficult and prolonged.
5. Skeletal decalcification and the formation of urinary tract calculi.
6. Urinary tract infections.
7. Neurological complications such as: (i) Common peroneal nerve palsy. This sometimes results from a less than ideal posture of the leg when external rotation leads to pressure in the region of the fibular neck, or it sometimes occurs from pressure against a splint. (ii) Ulnar neuropathy, from the patient repeatedly trying to change position using downwards pressure of the elbows against the bed when use of a so-called monkey pole would avoid this.
8. Cardiovascular complications, such as cardiac failure due to weakening of the cardiac muscle and poor venous return.
9. Psychiatric complications such as depression.

Avoiding these complications, as well as the costs of protracted in-patient treatment, are the main reasons for the continuing trend towards the operative management of many fractures. In the case of multiple injuries, internal fixation is of considerable help to the nursing staff in their care of the patient.

3. **COMPLICATIONS OF ANAESTHESIA AND SURGERY**

These include:
1. Atelectasis and pneumonia.
2. Blood loss leading to anaemia or shock with their secondary effects.
3. Wound infection, mechanical failure of internal fixation devices, etc.

4. **COMPLICATIONS PECULIAR TO FRACTURES**

These include:
1. Disorders involving the rate and quality of union.
2. Joint stiffness.
3. Sudeck's atrophy.
4. Avascular necrosis.
5. Myositis ossificans.
6. Infections.
7. Neurological, vascular and visceral complications.
8. Implant complications.

The last group will be considered in more detail.

Slow union   In slow union, the fracture takes longer than usual to unite, but passes through the stages of healing without any departure from normal, clinically or radiologically.

Delayed union   In delayed union, union fails to occur within the expected time. As distinct from slow union, radiographs of the part may show abnormal bone changes. Typically there is absorption of bone at the level of the fracture, with the production of a gap between the bone ends.

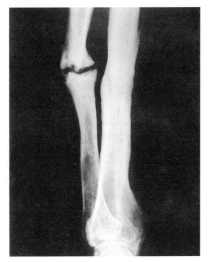

3. Hypertrophic non-union of the ulna.

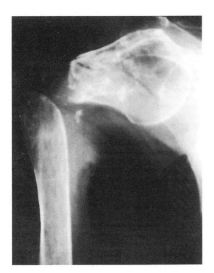

4. Atrophic non-union of the humerus.

External bridging callus may be restricted to a localised area and be of poor quality. There is, however, no sclerosis of the bone ends.

Non-union In non-union, the fracture has failed to unite, and there are radiological changes which indicate that this situation will be permanent, i.e. the fracture will never unite, unless there is some fundamental alteration in the line of treatment. Two types of non-union are recognised:

1. In **hypertrophic non-union** the bone ends appear sclerotic, and are flared out so that the diameter of the bone fragments at the level of the fracture is increased ('elephant's foot' appearance). The fracture line is clearly visible, the gap being filled with cartilage and fibrous tissue cells. The increase in bone density is somewhat misleading, and conceals the fact that the blood supply is good.
2. In **atrophic non-union** there is no evidence of cellular activity at the level of the fracture. The bone ends are narrow, rounded and osteoporotic; they are frequently avascular.

Treatment

Slow union Assuming that the fracture is adequately supported, patience should ultimately be rewarded with sound bony union.

Delayed union The difficult problem in this field is to differentiate between delayed union which is going to proceed with proper encouragement to union, and delayed union which is going to go on to non-union. The only sure arbiter is time, but the disadvantage of delay is that it tends to encourage irreversible stiffness in those joints which are immobilised with the fracture (besides frequently creating problems from prolonged hospitalisation and absence from work).

If union has not occurred within the time normally required (or certainly if the fracture is ununited by 4 months) or if gross mobility is still present at 2 months there should be a careful appraisal of the radiographs and the methods of fixation. As the commonest cause of delayed union is inadequate fixation, particular attention should be paid to this aspect of the case. If the radiographs show the changes of slow or delayed union, but none of the changes of non-union, and the fracture is well supported, immobilisation should be continued and the situation re-assessed, with further radiographs, in 4–6 weeks. Improvement in the radiological appearance will then be an encouraging sign, suggesting that persistence in the established line of treatment will lead to union. If there is no change, or if there is deterioration, this is an indication for more active treatment (e.g. rigid internal fixation).

Hypertrophic non-union If the fracture can be fixed with absolute rigidity by mechanical means (which substitute for the primary bridging callus which is wanting) the cartilaginous and fibrous tissue between the bone ends will mineralise and be converted to bone (by induction). In the femur, this may be accomplished by careful reaming of the medullary canal and the introduction of a stout, large-diameter intramedullary nail. The bone ends are not disturbed. In the tibia and the other long bones, good fixation may usually be obtained by compression plating or intramedullary nailing. If the fibula has united or is otherwise acting as a tether, preventing the tibial fracture surfaces from coming in contact, it may as an initial measure have to be divided.

There is some evidence that the process of induction which results in the conversion of the tissue at the fracture into bone may also be stimulated by the creation of small electric currents in the gap between the bone ends. This may be achieved by embedding percutaneous electrodes in the fracture gap, or by placing field coils round the limb. Treatment by this method is lengthy (extending over several months) but can often be administered on an out-patient basis and is particularly indicated where it is desirable to avoid surgery (e.g. in the presence of continued infection).

Ultrasound has also been claimed to accelerate union, as has the use of bone morphogenic protein.

Atrophic non-union Treatment for atrophic non-union is less easy or reliable, and involves four important aspects:
1. The fracture must be held rigidly: this usually implies internal fixation (e.g. the use of a large-diameter intramedullary nail or a rigid compression plate).
2. Fibrous tissue should be removed from between the bone ends which should be 'freshened' by a limited local trimming with an osteotome.
3. The bone ends should be decorticated from the level of the fracture back to healthy bone; fine interrupted cuts are made in the outer surface of the bone cortex until it has a feathered or shingled appearance.
4. The area round the fracture is packed circumferentially with cancellous bone grafts.

Malunion In theory, the term malunion could be applied to any fracture which has united in less than anatomical position. In practice, it is used in the following circumstances:
1. Where a fracture has united in a position of persistent angulation or rotation which is of a degree that gives the limb a displeasing appearance or affects its function. For example, malunion in a Colles fracture may lead to undue prominence of the distal ulna. The cosmetic effect may cause the patient some distress, although functionally the result may be good. Again, persistent angulation in a fracture of the femur may not be particularly conspicuous, but will lead to impairment of function in the limb as a result of shortening and the effects of abnormal stresses on the knee and hip (leading ultimately, perhaps, to secondary osteoarthritis in these joints). This effect is most marked when the angulation deformity is situated close to a joint.
2. Where a fracture has united with a little persistent deformity in a situation where even the slightest displacement or angulation is a potential source of trouble. This applies particularly to fractures involving joints. For example, slight persistent deformity in a fracture of the ankle may predispose to early secondary osteoarthritis.

Treatment In treating fractures, one of the main objectives is adequate reduction and avoidance of malunion. Regrettably, malunion is sometimes a sign of poor management. Fracture return clinics must be undertaken with the greatest care so that if any loss of position occurs this is detected and assessed as to whether it has reached an unacceptable level. If found at a very early stage, simple re-manipulation and the application of a close fitting cast may correct the problem, leading to a better result (and even avoiding litigation). This approach is often useful in a slipped Colles fracture. Similarly, rotational deformity in a long bone fracture treated by intramedullary nailing may be corrected with cross screws; a Smith's fracture may be treated by an anterior plate; and a conservatively treated ankle fracture which has moved may be reduced and treated by internal fixation. At a later stage, but before union has become complete, angulation

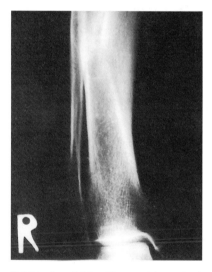

5. Malunion of tibia with potential stressing of ankle joint.

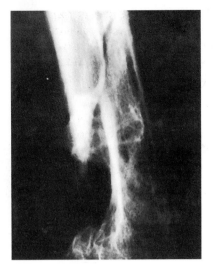

6. Malunion of femur leading to shortening.

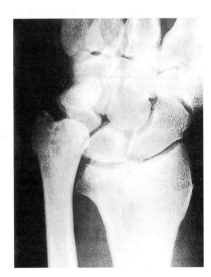

7. Traumatic epiphyseal arrest of radius leading to shortening.

may sometimes be corrected by wedging of a plaster (see p. 349) or forcible manipulation under anaesthesia, i.e. manipulation which refractures the limb through the early callus. If union is already complete, an osteotomy may be considered if the deformity is particularly severe.

Shortening This is generally a sequel of malunion. It occurs in transverse fractures which are off-ended (i.e. where there is complete lateral displacement or translation with loss of bony contact at the fracture site), and often in spiral or oblique fractures which are displaced. It also results from marked angulation of a fracture.

In children, bone growth is always accelerated in the injured limb, presumably as a result of the epiphyses being stimulated by the increased blood supply. Any discrepancy in limb length is usually quickly made up. For example, a fracture of the femoral shaft in a child may heal with the fragments overlapping and with perhaps 3–4 cm of shortening. After a year, the leg lengths may be equal – or the injured leg may even be a little longer than the other.

In adults, shortening in the lower limb is seen most frequently after fractures of the tibial shaft. It is also seen after fractures of the shaft of the femur, and of the femoral neck where there is persistent coxa vara. Shortening of 1.5 cm is easily tolerated, being compensated for by tilting of the pelvis. Shortening in excess of this should be dealt with by alteration of the footwear: for example, 3.5 cm of shortening may be corrected by a 2 cm raise to the affected heel, most or all of which can usually be given by a cork lift within the shoe. Where shortening is due to severe persistent angulation of a fracture, a corrective osteotomy may be indicated not only to correct the shortening but also to reduce abnormal stresses on the related joints.

In the upper limb, shortening seldom causes any problem other than to the patient's tailor. (Note, however, that shortening of either the radius or the ulna, while leading to little overall shortening, may cause severe disability at the wrist or elbow.)

Traumatic epiphyseal arrest The epiphyseal plate may be damaged as a result of trauma. If the whole width of the plate is affected, then growth may be arrested at that level, leading to progressive shortening of the limb. The final discrepancy in limb lengths is dependent on the epiphysis affected and the child's age at the time of injury; obviously the younger the child, the greater are the potential growth and potential shortening.

More commonly, the epiphyseal plate is incompletely affected so that growth continues more or less normally at one side while at the other it may be severely retarded or arrested. This irregularity of growth leads to some shortening of the limb and to distortion of the associated joint which can only be partly corrected by remodelling. In practice there may be progressive tilting of the axis of movement of the joint. For example, a supracondylar fracture may be followed by a cubitus varus deformity as a result of a degree of malunion. This deformity may become more severe as (uneven) growth continues. Traumatic epiphyseal arrest also occurs after open (compound) injuries, where the delicate epiphyseal plate is damaged, especially by friction. This is seen in road traffic accidents when a child is dragged along by a vehicle, sustaining skin loss and progressive abrasion of the deeper tissues by friction against the road surface.

In all cases of suspected epiphyseal damage a careful follow-up is necessary. The child should be seen every 6–12 months, and any residual deformity carefully assessed by clinical and radiological measurement. In the upper limb, if the deformity is progressive it may produce an unsightly appearance and may be responsible for delayed neurological involvement. In the lower limb, abnormal stresses may be produced in the weight bearing joints, ultimately giving rise to pain, stiffness, instability and often a rapidly progressive secondary osteoarthritis.

Treatment It is sometimes possible to treat this problem with an epiphyseolysis. In this procedure the abnormal block of bone bridging the epiphyseal plate is excised, and the defect plugged with fat or bone wax to prevent recurrence. In late cases, a corrective osteotomy may be indicated.

Joint stiffness This is a common complication. It must be borne in mind at every stage of fracture treatment in order that its effects may be minimised. Stiffness may result from a combination of factors which include pathology:
1. Within the joint
2. Close to the joint
3. Remote from the joint.

Intra-articular causes of stiffness

1. Intra-articular adhesions: fibrous adhesions may form within a joint as a result of: (i) Organisation of a haemarthrosis or fracture haematoma produced, for example, when a fracture runs into a joint. (ii) Damage to the articulating (cartilaginous) surfaces with subsequent organisation within the joint. (iii) Prolonged immobilisation leading to degenerative changes in articular cartilage.
2. Mechanical restrictions: (i) The fracture may disrupt the joint to such an extent that there is mechanical restriction of movement, e.g. bony fragments may block part of the range of movements in a joint. (ii) Movements may be restricted by the formation of loose bodies, and in their turn loose bodies may abrade the articular surfaces leading rapidly to osteoarthritis.
3. Osteoarthritis (osteoarthrosis): joint movements may be restricted as a result of (secondary) osteoarthritis. This may be caused by: (i) irregularity of the joint surfaces (caused, for example, by displacement of a fracture which runs into a joint; it may also follow damage to subchondral bone, which may not show on routine radiographs but be detectable by MRI scans). (ii) Avascular necrosis (produced as result of damage to the blood supply of an intra-articular fragment of bone). (iii) Malunion of a fracture (leading to abnormal stresses on the joint from persistent angulation).

Peri-articular causes of stiffness

1. Joint capsules and musculotendinous cuffs may become functionally impaired, leading to joint stiffness. There are many causes which include: (i) Fibrosis resulting from direct injury, passive stretching or disuse. (ii) Oedema, often encouraged by dependency, disuse, or Sudeck's atrophy (post-traumatic osteodystrophy, see later).
2. Persistent displacement of a fracture lying close to a joint may lead to a mechanical block to movement.
3. Persistent angulation of a fracture lying close to a joint may lead to loss of part of a range of movements (sometimes with a corresponding gain elsewhere). For example, persisting anterior angulation in a Colles fracture will result in loss of some palmar flexion. There is sometimes a corresponding gain in dorsiflexion.

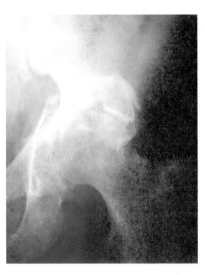

8. Malunion of acetabular fracture causing joint stiffness and secondary osteoarthritis.

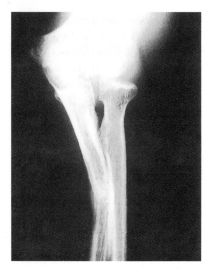

9. Malunion of fracture–dislocation of elbow (Monteggia) leading to loss of pronation and supination.

4. In a fracture lying close to a joint, movement may be restricted by adhesions forming between the fracture and overlying muscle or tendon. This leads to tethering of these structures with inevitable restriction of movements. As a general rule, the closer a fracture is to a joint, the greater the danger of movements being restricted in this way. Restriction of movements by tendon tethering is a particular problem in phalangeal fractures.

5. Myositis ossificans, if present, will act as a mechanical block to movement.

Stiffness from causes remote from a joint

1. Stiffness may result from tethering or entrapment of muscle by adhesions forming between a fracture and overlying muscle. This is commonly seen in fractures of the femoral shaft where the quadriceps muscle may become tethered to the bone, and may sometimes be aggravated by surgery, where exposure of the fracture requires further muscle division. This effect may be minimised by early mobilisation.

2. Muscle ischaemia, followed by replacement fibrosis and contractures, may occur when there is a vascular injury accompanying the fracture. Deformity of the distal parts is common, and there may be restriction of passive as well as active movements (e.g. Volkmann's ischaemic contracture of the forearm or calf leading to restriction of movements in the hand and foot respectively).

Avoidance of stiffness Some of the basic principles in the avoidance of joint stiffness are as follows:

1. Accurate reduction of the fracture wherever possible.
2. Splintage of the minimal number of joints compatible with security.
3. Splintage of the fracture for the shortest time compatible with the relief of pain and fracture healing.
4. Urgent mobilisation of all unsplinted joints in the limb, e.g. a patient with a Colles fracture should practise finger, elbow and shoulder movements from the day of injury.
5. Elevation of the injured part during the initial stages to decrease joint oedema.
6. Where applicable, supporting the joints in such a position that restoration of movement on discarding splintage will be encouraged.
7. Where a fracture involves articular surfaces, early movement becomes particularly important if an adequate range is to be regained.
8. Where stiffness is present or anticipated, physiotherapy, and where appropriate, occupational therapy should be started as early as possible.
9. Anticipate complications and avoid procrastination, especially with regard to non-union.
10. When internal fixation is being contemplated, there is some merit in selecting techniques and devices which will support the fracture to such an extent that the limb may be exercised without external support while avoiding movement at the fracture site, with the enhanced risk of non-union. This particularly valid in fractures lying close to, or involving, a joint (e.g. supracondylar fractures of the humerus and the distal femur in adults). Physiotherapy and early movements of related joints are essential in the management of fractures treated by internal fixation, and measures may have to be taken to reduce the limiting effects of wound pain in the early days following surgery.

Complex regional pain syndrome There are a number of imperfectly understood overlapping conditions where there is post-traumatic pain associated with disturbances to the local sympathetic nerve supply. The pain component is often severe, and appears disproportionate to the injury. The terminology for this group of conditions is confusing, and in an attempt to simplify this, the term 'complex regional pain syndrome' has been suggested. This syndrome is subdivided into two groups.

In the smaller **Group II** are those cases where there has been an injury to a major peripheral nerve (e.g. to the sciatic nerve following a gunshot wound or amputation). They are characterised by severe unremitting pain (often described as burning in character), increased skin temperature and sweating in the territory of the nerve, and vascular effects with alterations in skin colour (usually to blue or dusky red). Pain may follow light touch (such as by the contact of bed clothes) and is often out of proportion to the stimulus. Later on, trophic changes may occur, with the skin often becoming smooth and shiny; the nails may be fast-growing and brittle and hair growth in the limb stimulated. Those conditions described as major and minor causalgia fall within this group.

The larger **Group I** of complex regional pain syndrome includes a number of closely related conditions with largely synonymous titles (Sudeck's atrophy, reflex sympathetic dystrophy, pseudodystrophy, post-traumatic osteodystrophy, reflex algodystrophy). In these conditions there is sensitisation of pain pathways and of the sympathetic nervous system, but these features do not follow the course of a peripheral nerve; the clinical findings are in general similar to those described above in Group II.

This complication is seen most frequently after Colles fractures of the wrist. It may present shortly after the initial manipulation, and an associated compressive neuropathy (e.g. the median nerve in the carpal tunnel) may potentiate it. In most cases however it is not recognised until removal of the plaster at the end of the normal 4–6 week period of immobilisation. There is swelling of the hand and fingers, and the skin is warm, pink and glazed in appearance. There is striking restriction of movements in the fingers, and diffuse tenderness over the wrist and carpus. This tenderness may at first suggest that the fracture is ununited, but check radiographs will show that this is not the case. Typically the radiographs demonstrate union of the fracture, with diffuse, osteoporotic mottling of the carpus. Although seen most frequently after Colles fractures, it may follow a scaphoid fracture or indeed any injury about the wrist whether accompanied by a fracture or not. The condition is also seen in the lower limb, the foot being similarly affected after, for example, an ankle fracture or even a sprain. About the knee, the effects can be particularly severe.

The causal mechanisms of the condition, where there is an unusual sympathetic response to trauma, are uncertain. It may follow the use of splintage which is too tight or too slack; it may occur in association with prolonged elevation of pressure within the muscle compartments of a limb; it may appear when the affected part has had a prolonged period of dependence. It is usually self-limiting, with the abnormalities of circulation and decalcification resolving slowly over a period of 4–12 months. Nevertheless, restriction of movements may be permanent; to minimise this, intensive physiotherapy is usually prescribed and continued to resolution. In the more severe cases additional treatment may be advised.

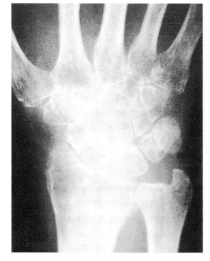

10. Sudeck's atrophy: note the patchy decalcification.

Diagnosis The diagnosis is not often in doubt, but a number of tests are considered to be of value for confirmation, especially if aggressive forms of treatment are being contemplated. These include:

1. 3-phase radionuclide scintigraphy (which may show asymmetrical blood flow and increased periarticular uptake; this seems to be of greatest value in the early stages of the disease).
2. Thermography.
3. The measurement of vasomotor and sudomotor responses.
4. The measurement of skin potentials and resistance.
5. Synovial biopsy (which may show non-specific subsynovial fibrosis with synovial proliferation).

It is considered, however, that relief of symptoms and signs by sympathetic blockade is of the greatest diagnostic value. The easiest way of doing this is by the intravenous administration of an alpha blocker such as phentolamine. (This is not recommended for treatment as its effects are of too short a duration.) Local perfusion of guanethidine may also be used for diagnostic purposes (see below for details).

Treatment Treatment by physiotherapy and movement is essential. To that purpose the aim is to reduce pain to a level where this can be achieved. If pain cannot be satisfactorily controlled by analgesics alone, regional sympathetic blockade should produce relief. In the upper limb the stellate ganglion may be injected, and in the lower limb, the lumbar sympathetic chain. Alternatively, a regional perfusion technique may be employed. To do this, a cannula is inserted in a superficial vein and a tourniquet is applied to the limb. The limb is exsanguinated with an Esmarch bandage before the cuff is inflated to 250 mmHg. 20 mg of guanethidine sulphate in a 40 mL solution is then injected, and the tourniquet released after 20 minutes. Relief of pain and an improvement in the clinical signs for 1–4 days after the perfusion is regarded as being diagnostic (even although it is recognised that peripheral vasodilatation is the main effect of guanethidine) and of value in permitting intensive physiotherapy. Failure to respond to such a procedure suggests that another cause for the patient's symptoms should be sought.

Additional treatment. Regional perfusion with guanethidine may be repeated (between three and six blocks may be required) with or without the use of oral sympatholytic drugs (such as prazosin or phenoxybenzamine); nifedipine is also sometimes tried, and good results have been claimed following the empirical use of prednisolone. Only rarely are surgical or chemical sympathectomy advised.

Where the knee is involved, a particularly aggressive approach is advocated. This it is said may often lead to rapid and complete resolution. After confirmation of the diagnosis as described above, an epidural blockade is maintained for 4 days, during which time the limb is mobilised vigorously by measures which include continuous passive motion, alternating hot and cold soaks, muscle stimulation and manipulation.

Avascular necrosis   Avascular necrosis is death of bone due to interference with its blood supply. It is an important and serious complication of certain fractures.

There is no doubt that in many comminuted fractures, fragments of bone are often completely detached from their surrounding tissues and deprived of their blood supply. If the fragments are small, healing is usually uneventful. If the fragments are larger, healing may be delayed, but it is often difficult to attribute the relative effects of avascularity and the poorer immobilisation associated with comminution. It is not, however, with the shafts of long bones that this complication is most closely associated. Avascular necrosis is seen in the *femoral head* after some intracapsular fractures of the femoral neck or after dislocation of the hip. It is found in the *scaphoid* after certain fractures of the proximal half of that bone. It sometimes occurs in the *talus* after fractures or dislocations. In the *lunate* it may follow frank dislocations or apparently occur without any obvious previous trauma.

The importance of avascular necrosis is that the affected bone becomes soft and distorted in shape, leading to pain, stiffness, and secondary osteoarthritis. The following points are of some importance:

1. Interference with the blood supply to the bone is a direct result of the fracture: the fracture shears those blood vessels which are travelling within the bone towards its articular surface.
2. As the fracture is responsible for the disruption of the blood supply, it follows that the disruption is attributable to the injury, and dates from the time of injury.
3. There is no treatment that will lead to rapid restoration of the normal bony microcirculation.
4. The greater the displacement of the fracture, the greater is the vessel disturbance and the greater the chance of this complication ensuing.
5. When an injury has occurred at one of the high-risk sites, the chances are that any patent circulatory channels are highly vulnerable. Reduction should be carried out with minimal force and delay if there is to be any hope of avoiding this complication.
6. Avascular necrosis is quite distinct from non-union. In the majority of femoral neck and scaphoid fractures with avascular necrosis, *the fracture has united*.
7. Clear-cut radiological evidence of this complication may be quite slow in appearing, especially in the case of the femoral head. (MRI scans are however said to be helpful in early diagnosis, and with this in mind titanium implants (with which MRI scans are compatible) may be used in preference to others.) Symptoms of pain and stiffness usually *precede* the radiological changes. In the case of femoral neck fractures it is common practice to look for avascular necrosis for up to 3 years after the injury.

Treatment   The natural course of avascular necrosis is for the slow revascularisation of necrotic bone from the periphery. This process takes 6–18 months, and it is believed that drilling of the affected bone in some cases may facilitate the ingrowth of a fresh blood supply. In spite of this secondary osteoarthritic changes in the affected joints are inevitable. In the lower limb, deformity of the avascular bone may be minimised by the avoidance of weight bearing, and this is of some value at least in the case of the talus.

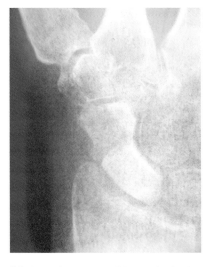

11. Avascular necrosis of the proximal pole of the scaphoid.

If symptoms are commanding, and secondary osteoarthritis is well established, surgery may be required (e.g. hip replacement in the case of femoral neck fractures – see under appropriate sections).

Myositis ossificans (heterotopic ossification) Myositis ossificans is a complication of trauma. In its commonest form, a calcified mass appears in the tissues near a joint, leading generally to considerable restriction of movements because of its mechanical effects.

The commonest site is the elbow. It may, for example, develop some weeks after a supracondylar fracture, especially where there has been difficulty in reduction and manipulation has been repeated. Myositis ossificans is also found in the elbow after dislocations or fractures of the radial head. It is thought that these injuries result in haematoma formation in the brachialis muscle at the front of the joint, and that this is dealt with by the tissues in the same way as a fracture haematoma, i.e. by calcification and ossification.

The ensuing mass may be as large as a plum, and will greatly restrict flexion of the elbow. It is known that myositis ossificans can follow passive stretching of joints and in the past it was frequently seen in cases where, in good faith, this treatment had been carried out to encourage movement after injury. The risks of this complication are so great, however, that passive stretching must never be practised round the elbow.

Myositis ossificans is also seen at other sites, especially the shoulder, knee and hip, e.g. after the open reduction and internal fixation of acetabular fractures or after hip replacement procedures. It is found particularly frequently in patients suffering from head injuries or paraplegia. In some cases, especially where there is limb spasticity, routine passive joint movements may be a causal factor.

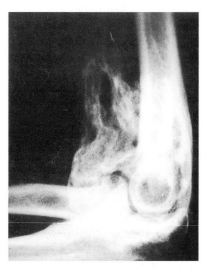

12. Myositis ossificans at the elbow.

Prophylaxis Where the risks of this complication are considered to be especially high, indometacin may be used as a prophylactic. The dose recommended is 2×50 mg daily for either 7 or 14 days.

Treatment of established cases Early excision of the mass gives bad results, being almost always followed by massive recurrence. Late excision (say after 6–12 months) is often successful in removing the mechanical obstruction to movement with less risk of recurrence. The risks of recurrence are reduced with a single dose of irradiation after surgery. The recommended dose is 7 Gy units. Irradiation with the same dose may also be used as a prophylactic in those unable to tolerate indometacin.

Osteitis/osteomyelitis Infection in closed fractures (due to systemic spread of organisms) is rare and seldom diagnosed until infection is well established. It is sometimes seen in patients suffering from rheumatoid arthritis who have been treated with anti-inflammatory preparations. Recurrent pyrexia, a raised sedimentation rate and white count, and unduly prolonged pain, local tenderness and swelling should arouse suspicion. Radiological changes may not be diagnostic and are slow in appearing.

Bone infection is a feared complication of open fractures, and is also seen on occasion after the internal fixation of closed (and open) fractures. The symptoms and signs are as detailed above. In addition, when well established, there will usually be a purulent wound discharge with staining of the plaster or dressings, which become foul smelling.

Glycocalyx, a mucopolysaccharide, is secreted by bacteria and may be deposited on large surfaces of metal including plates and screws, rendering the organisms less susceptible to macrophage attack, so that once an infection takes hold in the presence of retained implants, it may be very difficult to eliminate it.

Treatment

1. The risk of this complication should always be kept in mind in the handling of open fractures or when internal fixation is planned, so that the techniques practised may be above criticism. In addition, the prophylactic administration of antibiotics should be considered.
2. Once firmly established, bone infections are peculiarly resistant to treatment, and may become virtually incurable. Delay must therefore be avoided at all costs.
3. Any doubtful wound should be swabbed so that the bacteriology and antibiotic sensitivity may be firmly established. In patients being treated in plaster casts, access to the wound may be obtained by windowing of the plaster. The appropriate antibiotic must then be administered in adequate dose for an adequate time (usually 4 weeks as a minimum). If a choice is available, preference should be given to an antibiotic which may achieve high concentration levels in bone. In those cases where infection has been established, appropriate monitoring by a bacteriologist/ infectious diseases physician should be sought.
4. If, after an internal fixation procedure, there is evidence of any systemic manifestation such as elevation of temperature, consideration should be given to the removal of any infected material including a wound haematoma before pus formation becomes established. This may be done by opening the wound and irrigating it copiously, preferably with a pulsatile lavage system; the aim is to avoid the bacteriological seeding of, for example, a large plate and screws. The wound may then be left open and closed at 48 hours or later depending on the post-debridement situation and bacteriology.
5. If infection has not been discovered and controlled at an early stage, drainage should be established, and regular dressings performed with aseptic precautions in an attempt to allow healing by granulation tissue.
6. Although discharge from the wound may persist until any internal fixation device is removed, this should be delayed until fracture healing is well advanced unless a satisfactory alternative method of the holding the fracture can be provided (e.g. by using an external fixator).
7. When infection is well established and unresponsive, more radical measures may be called for. These include:

(i) Saucerisation of the area, with radical excision of all infected bone and open packing of the wound.

(ii) Raising the local concentrate of antibiotics by the implantation of irrigation tubes or acrylic beads impregnated with gentamycin or other antibiotics.

(iii) Rarely, amputation may have to be considered where there is profound toxaemia with deterioration of the patient's general condition, uninfluenced by treatment, or where there is widespread bone destruction or avascularity, poor control of the infection, and certain continued infection and non-union.

Acute arterial arrest The arterial blood flow distal to a fracture is occasionally interrupted, and assessment of the circulation in a fractured limb is an essential part of the examination. Arterial arrest results in loss of the distal pulses, pallor and coldness of the skin, loss of the capillary responses, severe pain in the limb, paraesthesiae and eventually muscle paralysis. The commonest cause is kinking of the main arterial trunks by the displacement of a fracture or dislocation. In these cases, the circulation is immediately restored by correction of the deformity, and this should always be carried out as expeditiously as possible. In closed fractures other arterial disturbances are found, but these are relatively uncommon. A ragged bone edge may cause arterial rupture, leading to the rapid formation of a large haematoma. A fracture may also give rise to profound arterial spasm, aneurysm, or intimal stripping. In open fractures, arterial rupture often declares itself by the nature and the extent of the accompanying haemorrhage.

Diagnosis If the pulses distal to the injury site cannot be palpated, the patient should be resuscitated and reassessed within an hour. The most reliable guide to the situation is the Doppler pressure. To take this, a sphygmomanometer cuff should be positioned above the injury site and the Doppler signal located. The cuff is then inflated; the pressure at which the signal disappears is the Doppler pressure. Repeat the examination on the good side. If the pressures are not equal, the advice of a vascular surgeon should be sought *immediately*. If no Doppler equipment is available, then advice should be sought, again without delay, should the peripheral pulses on the injured side be reduced or absent. Angiography may be required.

Treatment It is obvious that the survival of a useful limb is dependent on restoration of the circulation. Where this is not achieved by reduction of the fracture, exploration of the affected vessel is mandatory. Treatment is then dependent on the findings. If the artery is cleanly divided, an end-to-end anastomosis may be performed. In the presence of a deficit, an in-line reversed vein graft is often used. In either case, to prevent damage to the suture line, internal fixation of the fracture is an essential part of the procedure and is often performed first.

Most of the cases which appear to be due to arterial spasm are in fact associated with intimal damage. Opening of the vessel is necessary to elucidate this, although preliminary irrigation with papaverine is sometimes tried. If intimal damage is confirmed, resection of the affected segment with grafting may be required.

Arterial obstruction leading to muscle death and nerve palsy may also result from swelling within the muscle compartments of a limb (see below).

Compartment syndromes Post-traumatic swelling may gradually compromise the circulation within a closed fascial compartment in a limb. If unchecked, there may be necrosis of the muscles and loss of function in the nerves contained in the compartment. The effects depend on the speed of onset of the increased pressure, its duration, and degree. (For example, in the anterior compartment of the leg, local haemorrhage or oedema of muscles following trauma or overactivity may lead to an inexorable rise of pressure beyond the systolic blood pressure. This will result in necrosis of the anterior compartment muscles, loss of conduction in the deep peroneal nerve, sensory disturbance in the foot and foot drop.)

The clinical findings most commonly found include:

- *Pain* out of proportion to the injury.
- Pain on *passive movements* of the fingers or toes (where the muscles being stretched lie within the confines of the suspect compartment).
- Diffuse *tenderness* over the muscles of the compartment (and not just over a fracture).
- Distal *pallor*.
- *Progressive paralysis* of the muscles within the compartment.
- *Paraesthesia* and *loss of vibration sense* in the territory supplied by the nerves passing through the compartment.
- Loss of any *pulse* which is dependent on any vessel passing through the compartment (but beware of false negatives from retrograde flow).

Confirmation may be obtained by measuring the pressure within a suspect compartment, and this should be done as close to any fracture as possible for the most accurate results. This may be done using a simple needle technique, a slit catheter, a side ported needle, or an electronic transducer-tipped catheter. The last would seem to give the most accurate results, and is good for continuous monitoring (which is particularly desirable in cases complicated by head injury). It is considered that when the intracompartmental pressure exceeds 30 mmHg then operative intervention is indicated. However, the measurement of differential pressure (the diastolic blood pressure minus the intracompartmental pressure) is to be preferred, and if this falls below 30 mmHg fasciotomy is indicated. In the case of the fascial compartments of the hand, threshold pressures for intervention are lower, being in the order of 15–20 mmHg.

Treatment This is by means of a fasciotomy which is extensive enough to completely relieve pressure build-up within the compartment concerned. In some cases it is advisable to extend fasciotomy to any adjacent compartments which are also at risk of being compromised. *Prophylactic fasciotomies* should be considered in all open fractures of Grade II and above and in any severe crushing injury. (For further details see under the appropriate regional sections.)

Immediate neurological disturbance   Neurological complications occurring immediately after fractures and dislocations are comparatively uncommon. Nevertheless, in certain situations a nerve may be stretched over a bone edge in a displaced fracture, or over a bone end in a dislocation. If prolonged this will lead to local ischaemia and interruption of nerve conduction. If stretching is more severe there may be rupture of axons or of neural tubes. Actual nerve division is rare, being seen mainly in association with compound injuries (especially gunshot wounds). The commoner fractures and dislocations associated with nerve palsies include the following:

Injury	Nerve palsy
Dislocation of the shoulder	Axillary nerve palsy; rarely, other brachial plexus lesions
Fracture of the shaft of the humerus	Radial nerve palsy
Dislocation of the elbow	Ulnar nerve palsy; sometimes median nerve affected
Fractures around the elbow	Median nerve palsy; less commonly, ulnar nerve or posterior interosseous nerve
Dislocation of the hip	Sciatic nerve palsy
Dislocation of the knee or rupture of lateral ligament of the knee and fracture of medial tibial table	Common peroneal nerve palsy

Treatment   The majority of nerve lesions are in continuity. Assuming that the fracture or dislocation has been reduced, recovery often begins after 6 weeks, progressing quite rapidly thereafter. *The skin* must be protected during the recovery period against friction, burns and other trauma so long as sensation remains materially impaired. *The joints* should be exercised passively to avoid stiffness. *Deformity* due to overactivity of unaffected muscles should be prevented: this applies particularly to the drop wrist of radial palsy, and the drop foot where the sciatic or common peroneal nerves are involved. Lively splintage may be particularly helpful in these circumstances.

   Where there is a nerve palsy accompanying a fracture which is going to be treated surgically, opportunity may be taken to inspect the affected nerve. This will often help in establishing a prognosis, and may also permit definitive treatment of the injury (e.g. by removing any local pressure on the nerve). In the case of fractures of the humeral shaft accompanied by radial nerve palsy, primary open reduction, inspection of the nerve, and compression plating has been advocated in preference to conservative management of the fracture and expectant treatment of the palsy.

   When an expected recovery does not occur, electromyography (EMG) and nerve conduction studies may be of occasional diagnostic value, but exploration is often required. Some also advocate a more aggressive approach in dealing with nerve palsies accompanying fracture, advising an EMG at three weeks, with exploration at 6 weeks if there is no change in a second EMG performed at that time.

In the case of nerve injury complicating a fresh injury, primary suture should be undertaken if the risks of infection are judged to be slight and facilities are good. Otherwise the nerve ends should be approximated with radio-opaque sutures or markers, and elective repair delayed until sound wound healing has been obtained. If nerve repair is not possible, reconstructive surgery or orthotic support of the paralysed part may be required.

Delayed neurological disturbance Sometimes a nerve palsy gradually develops long after a fracture has healed.

Tardy ulnar nerve palsy This is the most striking example of this process. In a typical case, the patient gradually develops, over a period of a few months, an ulnar nerve palsy which may become complete. The injury responsible is usually a supracondylar fracture or a Monteggia fracture–dislocation. The striking feature is the interval between the fracture and the nerve palsy. It is usually in the order of several years, and indeed may be as much as 60.

In a number of these cases there is a cubitus valgus deformity, and the resultant stretching of the nerve is usually regarded as being responsible for the onset of the palsy. Nevertheless, tardy ulnar nerve palsy also occurs in the presence of cubitus varus, so that progressive ischaemia of the nerve has come to be considered as another possible factor.

Treatment Tardy ulnar nerve palsy is usually treated by early transposition of the ulnar nerve. (The nerve is mobilised from its exposed position behind the medial epicondyle, brought round to the front of the elbow, and buried in the flexor muscles of the forearm just beyond their point of origin.)

Median nerve palsy Signs of median nerve compression may gradually develop a few months after a Colles fracture of the wrist. This is generally akin to the partial nerve lesions seen in the carpal tunnel syndrome. Some residual displacement of the fracture may reduce the space available in the carpal tunnel leading to pressure on the nerve and an incomplete palsy.

Treatment Symptoms are usually relieved by carpal tunnel decompression (by dividing the flexor retinaculum).

Delayed tendon rupture This uncommon fracture complication is seen most frequently at the wrist, when after a Colles fracture a patient loses the ability to extend the terminal joint of the thumb. This is due to rupture of the extensor pollicis longus tendon some weeks or months after the fracture. The rupture may result from the gradual fraying of the tendon as it rubs against the healing fracture, or it may be caused by traumatic or fibrotic interference with its arterial blood supply, resulting in local sloughing of the tendon.

Treatment In the case of the thumb, the best results are obtained by transposition and suture of the tendon of extensor indicis to the distal segment of extensor pollicis longus (but see page 197).

Visceral complications

1. Rupture of the urethra or bladder and perforation of the rectal wall may complicate fractures of the pelvis.
2. Rupture of the spleen, kidney or liver may follow severe local trauma, abdominal compression or crushing (such as, for example, run-over injuries).
3. Rupture of the intestines or tearing of the mesenteric attachments may also follow abdominal compression.
4. **Paralytic ileus**: Paralytic ileus is occasionally seen following fractures of the pelvis and lumbar spine, the most likely cause being disturbance of the autonomic control of the bowel from retroperitoneal haematoma. Distension of the abdomen, absent or faintly tympanitic bowel sounds and vomiting are the usual features. It is, of course, imperative to exclude the possibility of perforation, especially when there is a history of a run-over injury. The diagnosis may be made on the basis of the history and clinical findings, but plain radiographs of the abdomen, abdominal paracentesis, an ultrasound examination, laparoscopy or laparotomy may be necessary where there is a history of direct injury. Treatment is by:

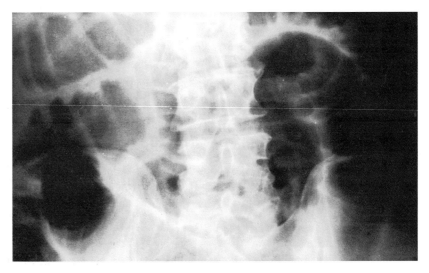

13. Paralytic ileus secondary to pelvic fracture: note the air distension of bowel loops in this plain abdominal film.

    (i)   Nasogastric suction.
    (ii) Intravenous fluids – the quantity and proportions being determined by the amount of aspirate and other losses, and serum electrolyte estimations. In the majority of cases, bowel sounds return within 36 hours, and intravenous fluids and suction may be discontinued shortly afterwards.

5. **The cast syndrome**: Abdominal distension and vomiting sometimes occur in patients being treated in plaster jackets, hip spicas, or plaster beds, especially if the spine is hyperextended. When the onset is extremely rapid leading to shock and prostration, the superior mesenteric artery or cast syndrome may be suspected (i.e. there is a high intestinal obstruction due to duodenal compression by the superior mesenteric artery). Treatment is as follows:
    (i)   If a plaster jacket has been applied, it should be removed. A patient being nursed in a plaster bed should be transferred to an ordinary bed or a Stryker frame.

(ii) A large-bore gastric tube should be inserted.

(iii) Fluid replacement therapy may be required.

Fat embolism This condition is usually thought to be due to microglobules of marrow fat escaping into the circulation from the region of the fracture, and lodging primarily in the lung parenchyma. It occurs most frequently after fractures of the femoral shaft and pelvis, and excessive mobility at the fracture site may be a contributory factor.

The finding of fat globules in the lungs is extremely common, and only a small percentage of cases progress to the more serious fat embolism syndrome (FES), where the fulminating form may often be fatal. The pathology is by no means clear cut, and disturbance of lipid metabolism may account for certain features of the condition. The frequently observed effects on the brain, kidneys and skin are less easy to explain unless cardiac septal defects are more common than supposed.

The *major features* are:

1. Respiratory insufficiency: there is increased frequency of respiration; there may be dyspnoea and use of the accessory muscles of respiration. Radiographs of the chest often show mottling of the lung fields, and there are changes in the blood gases.
2. Cerebral involvement, with the patient becoming confused, aggressive or comatose.
3. The occurrence of petechial haemorrhages in the skin. These appear most frequently in the axilla, anterior chest wall and the conjunctiva.

The *minor features* are pyrexia, tachycardia, jaundice, retinal changes and renal insufficiency.

Diagnosis Fat embolism syndrome should be suspected when there is an unexplained deterioration in the condition of a patient a few days after sustaining a femoral, pelvic or other major fracture. Any one of the following is considered to be diagnostic (Lindeque, B.G.P. et al):

1. A respiratory rate of more than 35, sustained after sedation.
2. A PaO_2 of less than 60 mmHg.
3. A $PaCO_2$ of more than 55 mmHg, or a pH of less than 7.3.
4. Increased work of breathing, with use of the accessory muscles and tachycardia.

The development of FES may be anticipated by routine examination of the blood gases, and some advocate that this be carried out on admission in the case of any long bone fracture.

Prevention The risks of this complication are reduced when:

1. Fluid replacement during and after surgery is impeccable.
2. In cases of multiple injury, any femoral fracture is rigidly fixed: in practice this generally implies intramedullary nailing, but to avoid excessive intramedullary reaming in a patient with known pulmonary contusion an external fixator may be used.
3. All efforts are made to reduce the occurrence of infection in any open injury.

Treatment

1. Aggressively carry out all routine resuscitative measures such as the administration of oxygen and intravenous fluids. If indicated by the blood gas levels, proceed to endotracheal intubation and the use of a ventilator. (In rare cases a cardiopulmonary by-pass pump may be required.) Where possible, active physiotherapy is advised.
2. If there is progressive deterioration in blood gas levels, surgical stabilisation of any femoral fracture is advocated. After such a procedure the patient should be left on a ventilator for not less than 24 hours; this may be discontinued when the blood gases improve, and there is an improvement in the tidal volume and the patient's level of consciousness.
3. The administration of methylprednisolone in cases where the PaO_2 is less than 60 mmHg, whether discovered before the onset of frank symptoms or later, has been shown to have a beneficial effect. (A dose of 30 mg per kg body weight on admission, and repeated after 4 hours has been recommended.)

Osteoarthritis   See under causes of joint stiffness (p. 91).

Implant complications

Mechanical effects Plates and intramedullary nails reduce the natural elasticity of the bone in the area where they lie. As a result, the loads to which a bone is subjected are not absorbed evenly throughout its length; stress concentrations tend to occur at the ends of internal fixation devices. In some cases this may lead to susceptibility to fracture, which may occur with less violence than is needed in a normal bone. It is well known that after a plated fracture of the tibia has united, comparatively minor violence may result in a further fracture of the limb at either end of the plate. Similarly, after a minor fall on the side, the forces which would be absorbed by a normal femur may result in a fracture of the femoral neck in someone who has had an intramedullary nailing.

Corrosion No metal implant is completely inert, and the long-term risks of retention of implants within the body have not been fully evaluated. It is not uncommon for the tissues surrounding a stainless steel implant to become discoloured, with the formation of substantial masses of fibrous tissue. This is especially likely to occur if there has been fretting between components (e.g. between a plate and screw). There may be local aching pain, and this is an indication for removal of the device, assuming that the fracture is soundly healed.

The individual elements in the alloy that has been used for the fabrication of the implant may separate, giving rise to local toxic effects, and having the potential, once they enter the transport systems, of causing problems elsewhere. Stainless steel contains in the order of 13% chromium, and this element is well known for its local irritant effect and its potential for inducing sensitisation. Neoplasia has been reported in bone at the site of plates, and the implants have been considered as being responsible. It is possible that freed metal elements, after transportation, may be capable of causing neoplasia in the liver and elsewhere. Aluminium is used in certain other alloys used for implants; this is neurotoxic, competing with magnesium in the formation of tubulin, a primary structural protein in the nervous system: this mechanism has been linked with Alzheimer's disease.

Treatment While it must be stressed that problems of the above nature are rare, the risks of any long-term effects should be avoided where possible by the routine removal of implants once they have served their purpose; this is the general advice in patients under the age of 40. Over that age the indications are less powerful, but as a general rule intramedullary nails should be removed, as should any other device where there is evidence of local tissue reaction.

PATHOLOGICAL FRACTURES

A pathological fracture is one which has occurred in a bone which is abnormal or diseased.

In some cases the pathological process leads to progressive weakness of the bone so that fracture may occur spontaneously or after slight injury only. Fracture may occur as an inevitable event in some disease process, e.g. a fracture in the course of a destructive, chronic osteitis: always unwelcome, but causing no surprise. On the other hand, the disease process may be unknown to the patient and his practitioner, the trivial nature of the trauma giving concern to both.

Where bone strength is not materially impaired, the causal violence producing the fracture may not cause comment; in these circumstances the radiographs taken after the incident may give the first indication to anyone that something else is amiss. It follows that virtually any condition capable of being detected by radiographs of the skeleton may fall into this category – a limitless range of congenital, metabolic and neoplastic disease. Diagnosis as a result may be difficult, but fortunately there is one important point to take into consideration: where fracture is the presenting feature, the number of conditions commonly responsible is small. These include the conditions described in the following pages.

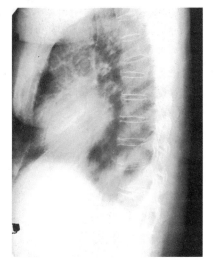

14. Osteoporosis: This is the commonest cause of pathological fracture, being especially important in the spine, the wrist and the femoral neck. It is most frequently due to lowering of hormone levels in association with age or the menopause: less frequently it follows disuse, rheumatoid arthritis or vitamin C deficiency, which lead to a failure of osteoid tissue formation and the translucent appearance of bone on the radiographs. (Illus.: fracture of D6.)

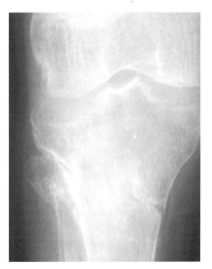

15. Osteomalacia (a): This is due to a failure in osteoid mineralisation and the radiographic appearances may be difficult to differentiate from osteoporosis. (Illus.: fracture of tibia and fibula.) It is usually secondary to an inability to utilise vitamin D (adult rickets) but is also seen where calcium is deficient in the diet (or excreted in renal acidosis), where phosphate is excreted in excess (Fanconi syndrome) or where vitamin D is not absorbed (e.g. steatorrhoea).

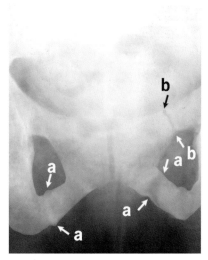

16. Osteomalacia (b): Stress fractures are common. Areas of bone translucency (Looser's zones) in the pelvis and long bones are characteristic. (Illus.: note changes in ischium (a) and pubic ramus fracture (b).) There are disturbances in the blood chemistry: the serum PO_4 is reduced, while the serum calcium is normal or reduced. If the product of the serum calcium and phosphate (in SI units) is lower than 2.25, the diagnosis is confirmed.

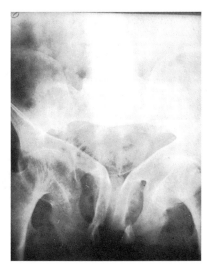

17. Osteomalacia (c): Occasionally a triradiate pelvis may be present and also be diagnostic. Osteomalacia may be treated with calciferol 1.25 mg per day, and calcium gluconate 1–2 g per day. The serum calcium, phosphate and urea should be monitored at regular intervals. Fracture healing is not materially impaired in either osteomalacia or osteoporosis.

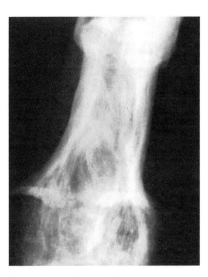

18. Paget's disease (a): This common condition is frequently seen in association with fracture, particularly in the tibia and the femur. (Illus.: two healing fractures of the femur.) The radiological picture is complex with, frequently, cyst formation, bone thickening, increased bone density and disturbances of bone texture. Stress fractures are common, and complete fractures are usually transverse.

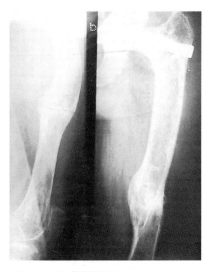

19. Paget's disease (b): Increased bone density and deformity may in many situations make the use of internal fixation devices difficult. (Illus.: femoral neck fracture pinned in coxa vara; healing fracture of shaft.) The rate of healing and the soundness of bone union are not, however, usually greatly affected. In many situations conservative methods may be employed with success.

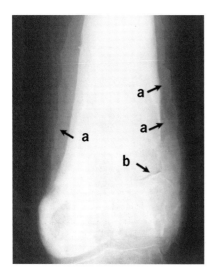

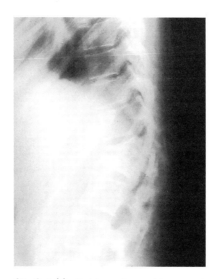

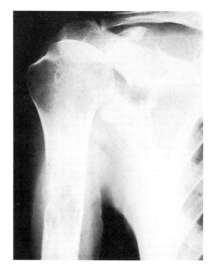

20. Paget's disease (c): Note that sarcomatous change (a) in this condition may be followed by fracture (b) as the cortical bone is eroded. Note, too, that the bone changes found in hyperparathyroidism and sometimes in metastatic disease may mimic Paget's disease.

21. Osteitis: Sudden collapse of bone secondary to infection is comparatively uncommon as a presenting feature, but is seen where the destructive processes are comparatively low grade. Thorough investigation and appropriate treatment is mandatory. (Illus.: Tuberculosis at the thoracolumbar level.)

22. Malignant bone tumours (a): The commonest malignant bone tumour is the metastatic deposit. Secondaries in bone occur most frequently from primary growths in lung or bronchus, breast, prostate or kidney. Any bone may be affected, but the spine, subtrochanteric region of the femur and the humeral shaft are amongst the commonest sites. (Illus.: metastatic deposit in humerus, primary in lung.)

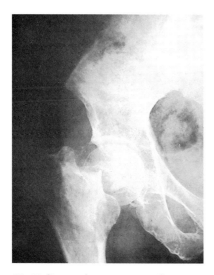

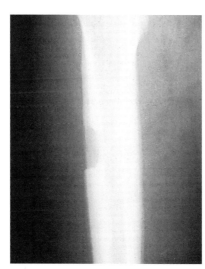

25. Malignant bone tumours (d):
Treatment: Note the following points:
(1) Without treatment, union of a fracture occurring at the site of a malignant bone tumour seldom occurs.

(2) If the tumour is responsive to local radiotherapy or to chemotherapy, healing may occur with appropriate splintage, but will be slow.

(3) In the case of metastatic disease, internal fixation has much to recommend it unless the patient is moribund. Acrylic cement is sometimes used to reinforce a bone defect.

(4) In the case of primary malignant bone tumours, the occurrence of fracture may be a factor in some circumstances in the advocation of amputation.

23. Malignant bone tumours (b):
Multiple myeloma in the pelvis (Illus.: with fracture of the femoral neck and a destructive lesion of the ilium) may sometimes be confused with secondary deposits from carcinoma of the prostate or other organs; full investigation is essential.

24. Malignant bone tumours (c):
Primary malignant tumours of bone generally present with pain and swelling rather than fracture, but this is not always the case, especially perhaps in Ewing's tumour (Illus.: radiograph prior to fracture) and osteosarcoma. The aggressive, locally malignant osteoclastoma again usually presents with pain and swelling rather than fracture.

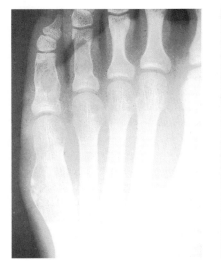

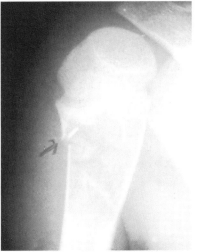

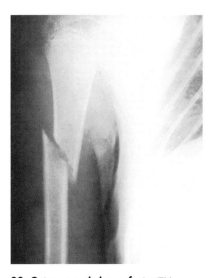

26. Simple bone tumours and cysts (a): In the metacarpals, metatarsals (Illus.) and phalanges (Illus.), enchondromata are frequently encountered as a cause of pathological fracture. These are generally best treated by exploration, curettage and the packing of the resultant cavity in the bone with cancellous bone grafts.

27. Simple bone tumours and cysts (b): In children between 5–15 years, unicameral bone cyst is one of the most frequent causes of pathological fracture, especially in the proximal humeral shaft. The bone cortex may be thinned, but expansion is rare. The fracture should be treated conservatively. (If the fracture fails to heal and the cyst disappears, curette and pack with bone grafts.)

28. Osteogenesis imperfecta: This hereditary disorder (dominant transmission) is characterised by bone fragility leading to bowing of the long bones, deformities of modelling, pathological fractures and stunting of growth. (Illus.: fracture of humerus with deformities of ribs.) Deafness and blue sclerotics are commonly associated. The condition generally declares itself in

infancy or childhood, but occasionally may not be diagnosed until skeletal demineralisation is noted later in life. Fracture healing is usually quite rapid, and most fractures may be treated successfully by conservative methods. Occasionally in the more severe forms of this condition, which present in childhood, internal fixation of the long bones by intramedullary nailing may be advocated as a prophylaxis against further fracture and to lessen bowing and other deformities of the legs.

Investigation of pathological fractures

Investigation of a pathological fracture may require some or all of the following:
1. A full personal and family history.
2. Full clinical examination, including pelvic examination.
3. Radiographs of the chest.
4. Radiographs of the pelvis.
5. Radiographs of the skull and skeletal survey.
6. Estimation of the sedimentation rate.
7. A full blood count, including a differential cell count.
8. Estimation of the serum calcium, phosphate, alkaline phosphatase and, where appropriate, the acid phosphatase.
9. Estimation of the serum proteins.
10. Serum electrophoresis.
11. Examination of the urine for Bence-Jones proteose.
12. A bone scan.
13. Marrow biopsy.
14. Bone biopsy.
15. Occasionally, radiographs of parents or sibs.

RECORDING AND COMMUNICATING: SOME SUGGESTED GUIDELINES

RECORDS

Careful note-taking in good patient management should already be recognised and practised, but in a field of medicine where evidence for insurance claims and litigation is commonly required, it is of particular importance. There are a number of areas where inadequacy is commonly found: these include the following:

1. Not infrequently, when the handling of a case is being studied some time after the event, problems arise because entries or letters have been *undated*; and if, as is often the case, they are on separate sheets, the time that they have been made cannot be determined by their context. It is vital that any entry is clearly dated, and in the seriously ill patient whose condition is rapidly changing during the first few hours after admission, the *time* should be clearly stated as well.
2. Illegible handwriting is always a problem, but there should be no excuse for numerals and capital letters which are so badly formed that they cannot be read by others or even by the originator. When contractions are used (and these can be helpful in providing oases of upper case meaningful clarity) only those in common use should be employed.
3. Paucity of notes (often very unfairly) suggests a similarly brief and, by implication, incomplete examination. In the heat of dealing with a seriously ill patient there is no time for detailed note-taking, but as soon as pressure eases, a full record should be made, and certainly this should be done *on the day of the admission*.
4. The interpretation of radiographs should be included in the notes, giving negative as well as positive findings. With the growing tendency to practise a degree of defensive medicine, radiographs should certainly be taken if there is any doubt about the nature or severity of an injury, and if radiographs are not taken, it is perhaps wise to say at the time why this has not been thought to be necessary.
5. If there is something that you are not sure of, indicate what this is (so that it cannot be claimed later that you had not considered it), and state the course you tend to take (with, if appropriate, the reasons for doing so).

TELEPHONING

Be clear whether the purpose of your call is to inform, to ask for advice, or to seek assistance, and have all the appropriate information at your finger tips. It is necessary to be able to describe a fracture patient in an unequivocal fashion, so that an unconfused picture of the problem is conveyed. There are undeniably different styles of doing this, but the following method is suggested:

1. Preamble.
2. Precise fracture details.
3. Particular qualifiers.
4. Reason for call.

Preamble After any niceties, including if necessary stating exactly who you are, give the age and sex of the patient along with any special attributes which bear directly on the reason for the call:

*'I have just admitted a 35-year-old man who is
a professional ice skater. He has been in a road
traffic accident and his main problem is ....'
(Note that it is probably best to avoid
contractions such as 'RTA' as they have to be
translated, and may grate when used over the
telephone.)*

Precise fracture details The description of the fracture should always
start with whether it is open or closed, and be followed by the bone involved
and at what level; then the pattern of the fracture, and any displacement or
angulation should be given:

*'... an open fracture of his right tibia in
midshaft. It's a transverse fracture, but it's
displaced medially and there's some lateral
angulation. There's some shortening, and
there's no bony contact.'*

Particular qualifiers Where relevant these would include the
following:
1. Complications of the local injury: this would include a description of the
   size, nature, location and potential contamination of a wound. It would
   also include details of any vascular or neurological problem.
2. Details of any other injuries sustained, e.g. other fractures, head injury,
   chest or abdominal injuries.
3. General condition of the patient, with, if appropriate, the time when they
   would be considered fit enough for anaesthesia and surgery.
4. Details of any treatment already carried out, e.g. fluid replacement,
   splintage etc:

*'... The fracture is from within out, and the
wound is 1 cm in length. It looks pretty clean,
and there's no neurological or circulatory
problem, and he has had no other injury. His
general condition's fine; he seems to have had
very little blood loss and his pulse and BP are
OK. I've set up an i.v. line and put him in a
back splint. He's not had anything by mouth for
the last 6 hours. He's been seen by the
anaesthetist who is happy to do him any time.'*

Reason for call

1. When this is to inform only, the details of the treatment carried out and
   what is further proposed could, with profit, be expanded:

   *'I am planning to take him to theatre to
   debride the wound. I think I'll be able to get a
   good stable reduction under vision and I'll put
   the limb in plaster afterwards.'*

2. When advice is sought, the nature of the problem should be clearly stated:

   *'I think this fracture might do best if internally
   fixed, but I'm wondering whether this should*

be done right away, or whether I should just reduce it and splint it, and add it to the beginning of tomorrow's list.' (Not generally the best solution!)

3. When help is required, this should be clearly stated:

'I think this is one you would want to treat by closed intramedullary nailing, and I've laid on theatre for seven thirty.'

For suggestions on the making of follow-up notes, see Chapter 16, The Fracture Clinic.

SECTION

B

REGIONAL INJURIES

CHAPTER

6

The shoulder girdle and humerus

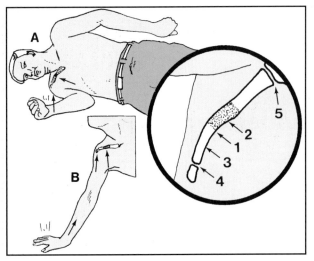

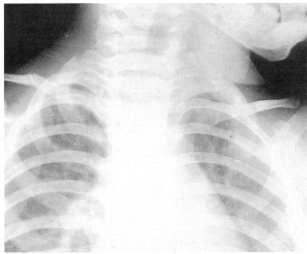

1. Clavicular injuries – Mechanism of injury: Most (94%) clavicular injuries result from a direct blow on the point of the shoulder, generally from a fall on the side (A). Less commonly, force may be transmitted up the arm from a fall on the outstretched hand (B). Under the age of 30 road traffic and sporting injuries are the commonest causes.

Fracture is commonest at the junction of the middle and outer thirds (1) but is also common throughout the middle third (2) and, to a lesser extent, the outer third where the incidence is 18% (3). *Subluxations* and *dislocations* may involve the acromioclavicular joint (4) and the sternoclavicular joint (5). Fractures of the clavicle involving the acromioclavicular joint are uncommon (2.8% of cases).

2. Common patterns of fracture (a): Greenstick fractures are common, particularly at the junction between the middle and outer thirds. Fractures may not be particularly obvious on the radiographs and it is often helpful in children to have both shoulders included for comparison. The only abnormality visible in many cases is local kinking of the clavicular contours. (Illus.: Fracture of right clavicle.) Healing of this type of fracture is rapid, and *reduction is not required*.

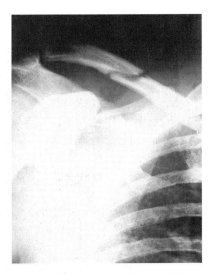

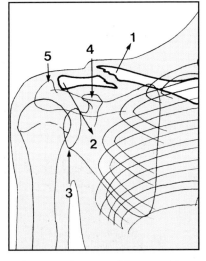

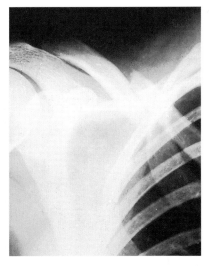

3. Common patterns of fracture (b): In the adult, undisplaced fractures are also common, and are comparatively stable injuries. Late slipping is rare. Symptoms settle rapidly and minimal treatment is required.

4. Common patterns of fracture (c): With greater violence, there is separation of the bone ends. The proximal end, under the pull of sternomastoid, often becomes elevated (1). The shoulder loses the prop-like effect of the clavicle, so that it tends to sag downwards and forwards (2). Note (3) the glenoid, (4) the coracoid, (5) the acromion.

5. Common patterns of fracture (d): With greater displacement there is overlapping and shortening. In spite of this, union is usually rapid, and remodelling, even in the adult, is so effective that strenuous attempts at reduction are unnecessary. Rare non-union is nevertheless seen most often in highly displaced fractures and those of the outer third. Pathological fracture may result from radionecrosis (following radiotherapy for breast carcinoma) and may be mistaken for a local recurrence.

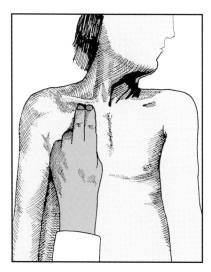

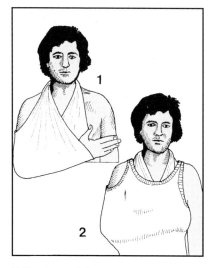

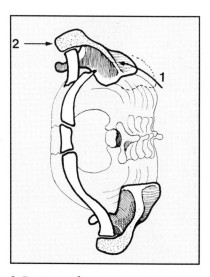

6. Diagnosis: Clinically there is tenderness at the fracture site; sometimes there is obvious deformity with local swelling, and the patient may support the injured limb with the other hand. In cases seen some days after injury, local bruising is often a striking feature. Diagnosis is confirmed by appropriate radiographs; a single AP projection of the shoulder is usually adequate in the adult.

7. Treatment (a): The most important aspect of treatment is to provide support for the weight of the arm which has lost its clavicular tie. As a rule this is best achieved with a broad arm sling (1). Additional fixation may be obtained by wearing the sling under the clothes (2). No other treatment is needed in greenstick or undisplaced fractures.

8. Treatment (b): Where there is marked displacement of a clavicular fracture it is usual practice to attempt to correct the anterior drift of the scapula round the chest wall (1). There is no simple way of achieving this. All methods attempt to apply pressure on the front of the shoulder (2) and, although they are comparatively ineffective in terms of reduction, are helpful in reducing pain.

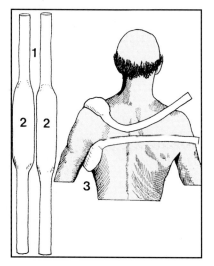

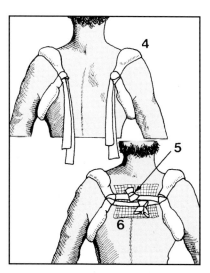

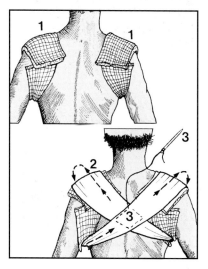

9. Treatment (c) – Ring or Quoit method: Narrow gauge stockinet is cut into two lengths of about a metre each (1). The central portions are stuffed with cotton wool (2). One of the strips is taken and the padded area positioned over the front of the shoulder and tied firmly behind (3).

10. Treatment (d): The second strip is applied in a similar manner to the other shoulder (4). The patient is then advised to brace the shoulders back and the free ends of the ring pads are tied together (5). A pad of gamgee (sandwich gauze/cotton wool) may be placed as a cushion beneath the knots (6).

11. Treatment (e) – Figure-of-eight bandage: Pads of gamgee or cotton wool alone are carefully positioned round both shoulders (1). The patient, who should be sitting on a stool, is asked to brace back the shoulders; a wool roll bandage is then applied in a figure-of-eight fashion (2). For added security the layers may be lightly stitched together at the crossover (3).

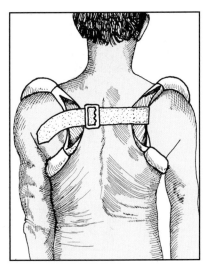

12. Treatment (f): Commercially available clavicle rings, covered with chamois leather, may be applied and secured with a strap. Many other patterns of off-the-shelf clavicular supports are available. With all of these care must be taken to avoid pressure on the axillary structures and the additional support of a sling is desirable for the first 2 weeks or so. Note also that elderly patients tolerate clavicular bracing methods poorly, and sling support only may be advisable. (For internal fixation see Frame 25.)

13. Aftercare: 1. Clavicular braces of all types require careful supervision and, at least initially, may require inspection and possible tightening every 2–4 days. 2. Where braces are used in conjunction with a sling, the sling may usually be discarded after 2 weeks. 3. All supports may be removed as soon as tenderness disappears from the fracture site. 4. Physiotherapy is seldom required except in the elderly patient who has developed shoulder stiffness. 5. A child's mother should always be advised that the prominent callus round the fracture is a normal occurrence, and that it will disappear in a few months with remodelling.

Note: If there is evidence of *torticollis* accompanying a clavicular fracture, further investigation of the cervical spine is indicated, as this finding may indicate a coincidental injury at the C1–2 level (locked facet joints). If plain radiographs are insufficient to clarify the situation, a CAT scan should if possible be carried out.

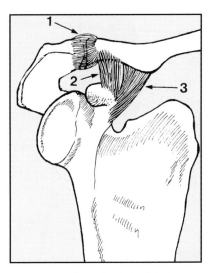

14. Acromioclavicular joint injuries: Injury to the acromioclavicular joint usually results from a fall in which the patient rolls on the shoulder. Note that the clavicle is normally attached to the scapula by (1) acromioclavicular, (2) conoid and (3) trapezoid ligaments. The scapular component of shoulder abduction requires free acromioclavicular movement.

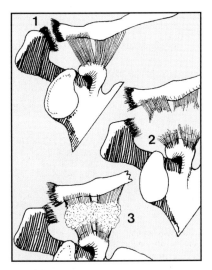

15. Pathology: Note that: (1) in subluxations and sprains, damage is confined to the acromioclavicular ligaments, and the clavicle preserves some contact with the acromion. In dislocations (2) the clavicle loses all connection with the scapula, the conoid and trapezoid ligaments tearing away from the inferior border of the clavicle. The displacement may be severe, and the ensuing haematoma may ossify (3).

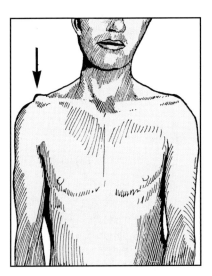

16. Diagnosis (a): The patient should be standing and the shoulders compared. The outer end of the clavicle will be prominent, and in cases of damage to the conoid and trapezoid ligaments the prominence may be quite striking. Local tenderness is always present.

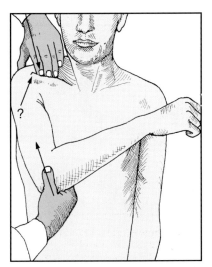

17. Diagnosis (b): Confirm any subluxation by supporting the elbow with one hand, gently pushing the clavicle down with the other. Improvement in the contour of the outer end of the clavicle will confirm the diagnosis of subluxation or dislocation.

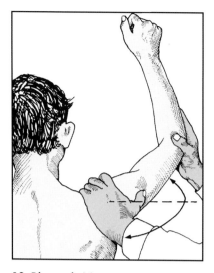

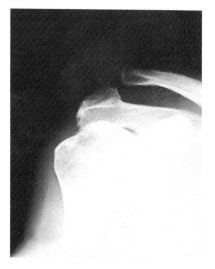

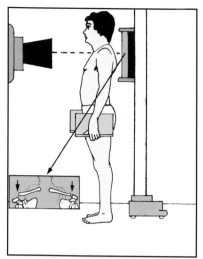

18. Diagnosis (c): Now stand behind the patient and abduct the arm to 90°. Flex and extend the shoulder while gently palpating the acromioclavicular joint. *Failure of the outer end of the clavicle to accompany the acromion indicates rupture of the conoid and trapezoid ligaments.*

19. Radiographs (a): Displacement of the clavicle by a diameter or more relative to the acromion (Illus.) suggests rupture of the conoid and trapezoid ligaments. The radiographs however are often fallacious in indicating the severity of the injury (and indeed may not show it). The reason is that spontaneous reduction tends to occur in recumbency – the position in which AP radiographs are normally taken.

20. Radiographs (b): It must be clearly indicated on the radiograph request form that the acromioclavicular joint is suspect. The radiographs should then be taken with the patient standing. The weight of the limb is often sufficient to show up the dislocation, but it is common practice to have the patient hold weights in both hands, and to include both shoulders for comparison.

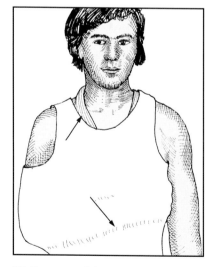

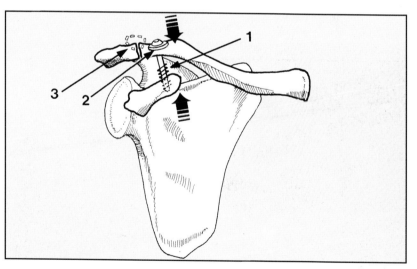

21. Treatment (a): If there is no gross instability, treat by the use of a broad arm sling under the clothes for 4–6 weeks. Physiotherapy is seldom required and an excellent result is the rule.
NB: Subluxations are easily reduced and held by adhesive strapping, but this treatment should *not* be employed as early skin reactions will always force abandonment.

22. Treatment (b): In cases of gross instability, good results usually follow conservative management. Complications are common after surgery, but this should be considered in patients who are engaged in work which is heavy or involves prolonged elevation of the arms. A common method is to hold the clavicle in alignment with the acromion, using a lag screw (1) run into the coracoid. A washer (2) is used to spread local stresses, and some advise reinforcement of the fixation with absorbable transarticular sutures (3) in the acromioclavicular joint. Any tears in the deltoid or trapezius should also be repaired.
Treatment (c): Other methods of internal fixation include figure-of-eight acromioclavicular wiring; PDS (polydioxanone) sutures or polyester tape may be used in the form of slings passed round the clavicle and under the coracoid. Kirschner wires passed across the joint tend to migrate, and their use is not recommended. In all cases there is a strong tendency for the devices to cut out, and it is imperative that there is the additional support of a broad arm sling (under the clothes or with a body bandage) for 8 weeks. *Internal fixation screws must be removed at 6–8 weeks before mobilisation.*

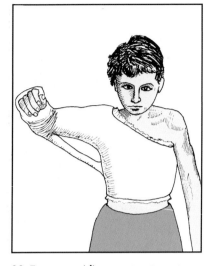

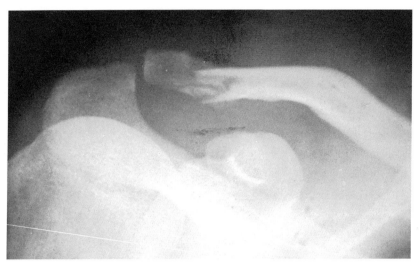

23. Treatment (d): If a dislocation reduces with the arm in abduction, a shoulder spica (for 6–8 weeks) may be used as an alternative to surgery. Complications: Symptoms from acromioclavicular osteoarthritis may be relieved by acromionectomy or excision of the outer 2 cm of the clavicle. Fascial reconstruction of the coracoclavicular ligaments can be used for persistent instability.

24. Fractures of the outer third of the clavicle: Displacement is generally minimal as the coracoclavicular ligaments are not usually torn. When these ligaments are damaged, however, displacement may be marked and give rise (rarely) to non-union. (It should be noted however in this context that non-unions in outer third fractures of the clavicle are often symptom free.)

There are two approaches to the treatment of outer third fractures of the clavicle. Good results are generally the rule with conservative management, which should follow the lines previously described for acromioclavicular injuries. Clavicular bracing is valueless and a sling under the clothes for 4–5 weeks is usually quite adequate.

Alternatively, to lessen the risks of non-union, some prefer to treat all outer third fractures by reduction and plating of the clavicle. If the ligaments are torn these should also be dealt with; PDS sutures or polyester tape in the form of slings passed round the clavicle and coracoid are particularly useful in this situation.

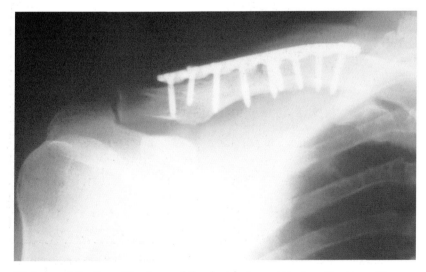

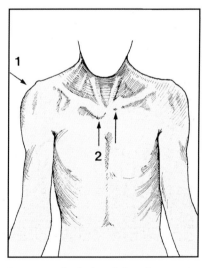

25. Internal fixation of fractures of the clavicle: Internal fixation of fractures of the clavicle in the acute situation may be considered in cases of so-called 'floating shoulder', where there is a fracture of the clavicle associated with a fracture of the proximal humerus or of the glenoid. Good fixation reduces pain, improves patient mobility, and may facilitate union at each site. Some also advise internal fixation routinely in all outer third fractures. In a large male, two 3.5 mm stainless steel plates or small fragment reconstruction plates may be used; alternatively a low profile titanium plate may be preferred.

Complications of clavicular fractures: 1. Glenohumeral joint stiffness in the elderly may require physiotherapy. 2. Even after normal remodelling (which continues for many months) a persistent sharp clavicular spike may cause discomfort against the clothes and require excision. 3. Non-union is rare, but if causing symptoms is treated by bone grafting and internal fixation.

26. Sternoclavicular dislocation: This is sometimes seen without any history of trauma, but generally the commonest lesion, a minor subluxation, follows a fall or blow on the front of the shoulder (1) or fall on the outstretched hand. *There is asymmetry of the inner ends of the clavicles* (2) due to the clavicle on the affected side subluxating downwards and forwards. There is local tenderness. *The diagnosis is essentially a clinical one.*

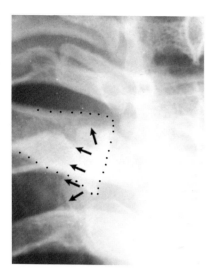

27. Radiographs: AP and oblique radiographs are difficult to interpret but are nevertheless usually performed; they may confirm the diagnosis when there is a major dislocation and the inner end of the clavicle is displaced onto the sternum. Note that in rare cases (illustrated) the clavicle passes *behind* the sternum where it may endanger the great vessels. As a rule tomographs or CAT scans may be more useful in elucidating these injuries.
(Clavicle: dotted line; sternal edge: arrows.)

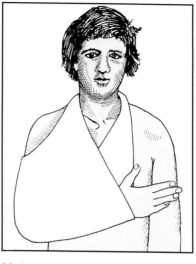

28. Treatment (a): Minor subluxations should be accepted. The clavicle stabilises in the subluxated position; some prominence of the inner end of the clavicle may persist with some asymmetry of the suprasternal notch, but a pain-free result is usual. The arm should be rested in a sling for 2–3 weeks until acute pain has settled.

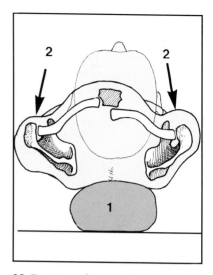

29. Treatment (b): Gross displacements should be reduced under general anaesthesia. A sandbag (1) is placed between the shoulders which are firmly pressed backwards (2). Clavicular braces are then applied (see Frame 9), along with a broad arm sling for 4–5 weeks. Should the reduction be extremely unstable, surgical repair with fascia lata slings should be considered. The rare irreducible dislocation may require open reduction, which may be hazardous.

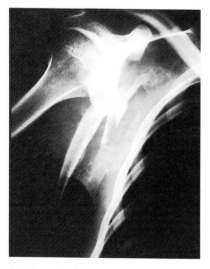

30. Scapular fractures (a): Fractures of the *blade* of the scapula are usually caused by direct violence. Even when comminuted and angled (Illus.) healing is usually extremely rapid and an excellent outcome is the rule. Treatment is by use of a broad arm sling and analgesics. Mobilisation is commenced as soon as acute symptoms have settled, and is usually possible after 2 weeks.

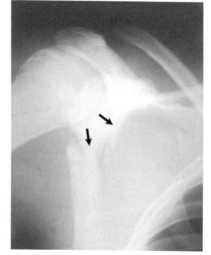

31. Scapular fractures (b): Fractures of the *scapular neck* lead to much bruising and swelling. Comminution is common. If involvement of the glenohumeral joint is suspected, check the position of the humeral head and any steps in the articular surface of the glenoid by CAT scan, with a view to possible open reduction. In spite of frequently daunting radiographs, a good outcome usually follows conservative management with early mobilisation. Fractures of the scapular spine or coracoid may usually be treated conservatively.

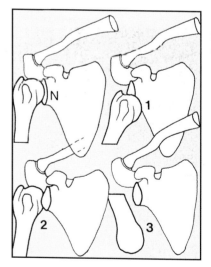

32. Dislocation of the shoulder: When the shoulder dislocates, the head of the humerus may come to lie *mainly* (1) in front of the glenoid (anterior dislocation of the shoulder), (2) behind the glenoid (posterior dislocation of the shoulder) or (3) beneath the glenoid (luxatio erecta). Anterior dislocation is *by far* the commonest of these.

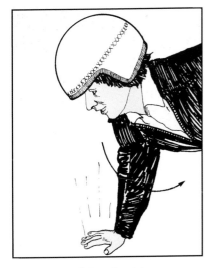

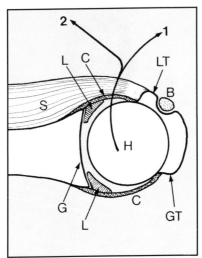

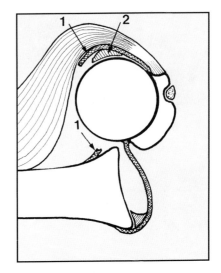

33. Anterior dislocation (a): This most commonly results from a fall leading to external rotation of the shoulder (e.g. the trunk internally rotating over a fixed hand). It is rare in children, common in the 18–25 years age group (from motorcycle and athletic injuries) and comparatively common in the elderly, where the stability of the shoulder may be impaired by muscle degeneration and where falls are common.

34. Anterior dislocation (b): The head of the humerus externally rotates out of the glenoid (1) and, having become free, comes to lie medially in front of the scapula (2). B = biceps tendons; C = capsule; G = glenoid; GT = greater tuberosity; H = head of humerus; L = glenoid labrum; LT = lesser tuberosity; S = subscapularis.

35. Anterior dislocation (c): Anterior dislocation is inevitably associated with damage to the anterior structures. Commonly, the capsule is torn away from its attachment to the glenoid (1). This is the so-called Bankart lesion, although the frequent simultaneous displacement of the glenoid labrum (2) usually attracts this term. The humeral head may be damaged, and it is said may even show a Hill-Sachs type lesion (see later) on an apparently first dislocation. (This abnormality is usually associated with recurrent dislocations.)

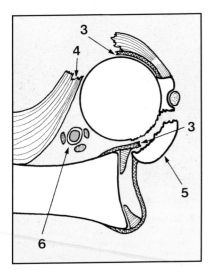

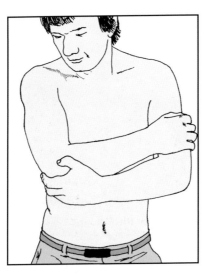

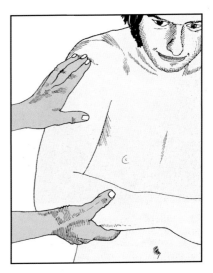

36. Anterior dislocation (d): In the older patient, especially, there may be tearing or stretching of the anterior capsule (3), sometimes with associated damage to the shoulder cuff, especially subscapularis (4). The greater tuberosity may fracture (5) and occasionally there is damage to the axillary artery or brachial plexus (6).

37. Diagnosis (a): The shoulder is very painful: the patient resents movement, and to prevent this often holds the injured limb at the elbow with the other hand. The arm does not always lie into the side, appearing to be in slight abduction. The outer contour of the shoulder may appear to be slightly kinked due to the displacement of the humeral head.

38. Diagnosis (b): Palpate under the edge of the acromion. The usual resistance offered by the humeral head will be absent. If in doubt, compare the two sides. The displaced humeral head may be palpable lying anteriorly.

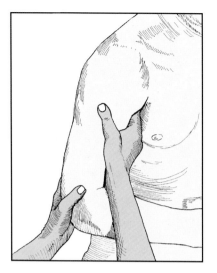

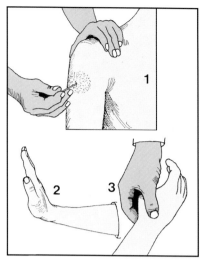

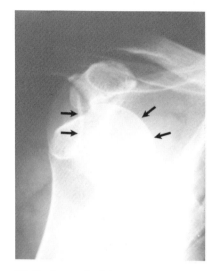

39. Diagnosis (c): Nevertheless, the acromion and clavicle make examination difficult. In the doubtful case, it may be helpful to try to assess the relative positions of the humeral head and glenoid by palpation in the axilla.

40. Diagnosis (d): Axillary (circumflex) nerve palsy is the commonest neurological complication. Test for integrity of the nerve by assessing sensation to pin prick (1) in its distribution over the 'regimental badge' area. (The shoulder is usually too painful to assess deltoid activity with certainty.) Look for other (rare) involvement of the radial portion of the posterior cord (2) and involvement of the axillary artery (3).

41. Radiographs (a): The majority of anterior dislocations of the shoulder show quite clearly on the standard AP radiographs of the shoulder. The humeral head is displaced anteriorly and medially; in its final position it may be described as lying (i) preglenoid (ii) subcoracoid, (iii) subclavicular. This classification is of little practical importance; the important diagnostic feature is the loss of congruity between the humeral head and the glenoid, as illustrated.

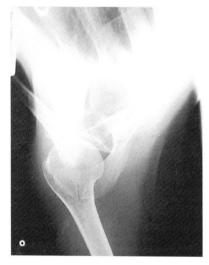

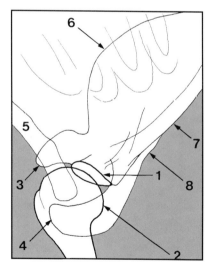

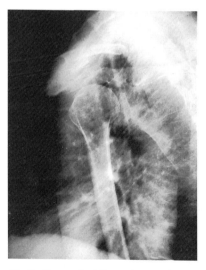

42. Radiographs (b): *A second radiographic projection is essential if the diagnosis is in doubt.* Note that if the humeral head has minimal medial displacement the AP view may appear *normal*. (This is especially the case in posterior shoulder dislocations.) The most useful additional projection is the axial lateral (sometimes called the tangential lateral). (Illus.: the *normal* appearances in such films.) In recurrent dislocation this view may show a defect in the posterior aspect of the humeral head (see Frame 69).

43. Radiographs (c): The axial lateral is usually taken with the patient lying on their back with the arm abducted to 90°. The X-ray tube is adjusted so that it lies roughly parallel to the trunk; the central ray passes through the axilla to the plate which is placed above the shoulder. The bony features are easy to identify. 1 = glenoid; 2 = humeral head; 3 = coracoid; 4 = acromion; 5 = clavicle; 6 = vertebral body of the scapula; 7 = lateral border of scapula; 8 = spine of scapula.

44. Radiographs (d): If the shoulder is too painful to allow an axial lateral, *obtain an apical oblique projection*; the landmarks are similar to those seen in the AP, but may be easier to interpret. Alternatively, if the patient is not overweight, a *translateral* projection, at right angles to the plane of the AP, may be helpful. This view is often difficult to interpret, but note that in the *normal* shoulder (Illus.) the posterior border of the humerus and the axillary border of the scapula form a shallow parabolic curve (see also Frame 61),

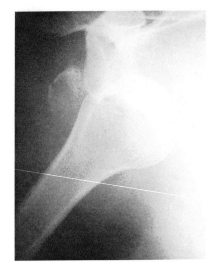

45. Radiographs (e): An associated fracture of the greater tuberosity is not uncommon. This does not influence the initial treatment of the dislocation by reduction, but may require subsequent attention (see Frames 57, 107). The radiographs of an acute dislocation may show evidence of previous episodes (for description see Frame 71).

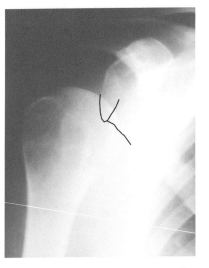

46. Radiographs (f) – Subluxation of the glenohumeral joint: Note that if any painful lesion of the arm is treated in a sling for several weeks wasting in the shoulder girdle will commonly result in a minor subluxation; this is most obvious if the AP radiograph is taken with the patient erect. No active treatment is required, but frank dislocation should be excluded by a lateral projection.

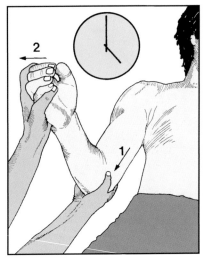

47. Treatment – Reduction by Kocher's method (a): This, one of the most popular of reduction methods, may often be successfully carried out in the older patient after the administration of intravenous diazepam, or in the younger patient after a substantial dose of intramuscular pethidine. Severe pain, or if the patient is of muscular build, are indications for general anaesthesia. Apply traction (1) and begin to rotate the arm externally (2).

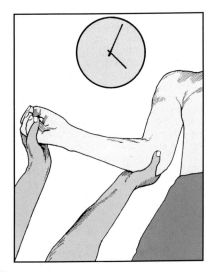

48. Kocher's method (b): Take plenty of time over external rotation. In the conscious patient, if muscle resistance is felt, stop for a moment and then continue, distracting the patient's attention with conversation. It should be possible to reach 90° of external rotation. (If severe pain and muscle spasm prevent rotation, general anaesthesia will be required.) *Excessive force must be avoided* in order to prevent fracture of the humeral shaft.

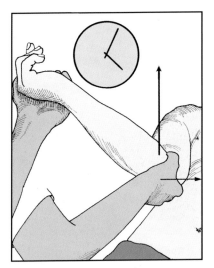

49. Kocher's method (c): The shoulder frequently reduces with a clear 'clunking' sensation during the external rotation procedure, but if this does not happen, flex the shoulder (by lifting up the point of the elbow) and then adduct it, bringing the elbow across the chest. (These and the following movements may be carried out rapidly.)

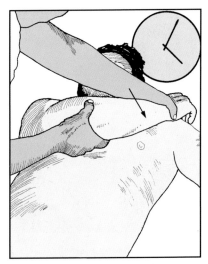

50. Kocher's method (d): Now internally rotate the shoulder, bringing the patient's hand towards the opposite shoulder. If reduction has not occurred, repeat all stages, attempting to get more external rotation in stage b. If doubt remains, repeat radiographs should be taken. Complete failure is rare under general anaesthesia. In the sedated patient, failure is an indication for general anaesthesia.

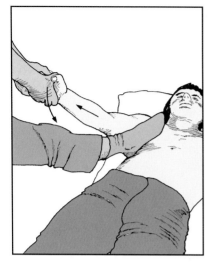

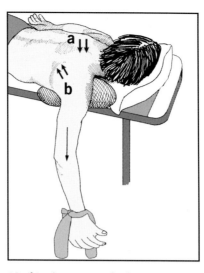

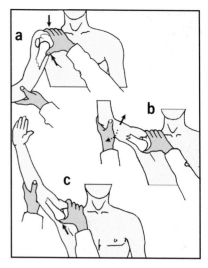

51. Alternative methods of reduction: In this common and generally easy to reduce dislocation there is no shortage of alternative procedures. These include the following.
(a) Hippocratic method: The principle is that traction is applied to the arm and the head of the humerus is levered back into position. The stockinged heel is placed against the chest (without being pressed hard into the axilla) to act as a fulcrum, while the arm is adducted.

52. (b) Stimson's method: The patient is given a powerful analgesic (e.g. 200 mg of pethidine in a fit athletic male) with resuscitation facilities available. The patient should be prone, with the arm dependent, a sandbag under the clavicle and a weight of about 4 kg tied to the wrist. The joint normally reduces spontaneously within six minutes: if not, with one hand fix the superomedial angle of the scapula (a), and with the other push the inferior angle medially (b).

53. (c) Milch's method: This method is based on neutralising the power of the shoulder muscles by abducting the joint. Place the fingers over the shoulder and steady the displaced humeral head with the thumb (a). Now gently abduct and externally rotate the arm (b). When full abduction is reached, increase thumb pressure to slide the humeral head over the glenoid margin (c). Variations of this method include the use of traction and an erect posture. Sedation or anaesthesia may or may not be required.

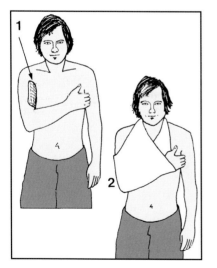

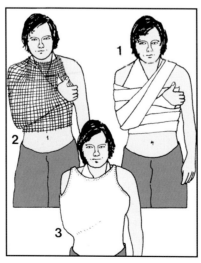

54. Aftercare (a): Check radiographs should be taken. This should be done before any anaesthetic is discontinued if there is doubt about the reduction. The arm should be supported after reduction to lessen the risks of immediate redislocation and to help relieve pain. Begin by placing a gamgee or wool pad in the axilla (for perspiration) (1) and apply a broad arm sling (2).

55. Aftercare (a) cntd: External rotation should be prevented by a body bandage (1), stretchable net (Netelast®) (2) or, less securely, by the outside clothes (3). The supports may require changing for the sake of hygiene from time to time until they are discarded. If there is some residual pain, an outside sling may be worn for a further week. Mobilisation is usually rapid without physiotherapy being required.

56. Aftercare (b): In patients under 40 there is a comparatively high incidence (said to be as high as 50%) of recurrence within 2 years, and some advocate aspiration of the haematoma and a primary arthroscopic stabilisation procedure. The common practice is to continue supporting the limb as described for a *4 week period*, the rationale being that this gives the torn tissues time to heal. The efficacy of prolonged fixation in this respect is in doubt, and where early mobilisation is particularly desirable it would seem reasonable to curtail the period of post-reduction support. If the shoulder has been dislocated four times or more the patient should be assessed for reconstructive surgery.
Aftercare (c): In the elderly patient the risks of recurrent dislocation are minimal, but the risks of stiffness are great. A sling support under the clothes should be applied initially and discarded as soon as pain will permit. Mobilisation of both the shoulder and the elbow may usually be started after 1–2 weeks and the patient referred for physiotherapy. In some elderly patients there may be joint instability problems due to damage to the shoulder cuff. If this is suspected it may be confirmed by arthroscopy, and good results have been claimed for subsequent secondary repairs.

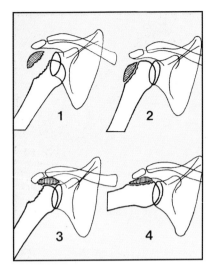

57. Aftercare (d): If there has been an associated fracture of the greater tuberosity (1) this generally reduces adequately with the dislocation (2). Again, mobilisation should be commenced as soon as pain will permit (usually after 3–4 weeks). If the tuberosity remains seriously displaced, e.g. under the acromion (3), and cannot be reduced by placing the arm in abduction (4) it should be openly replaced and fixed with a screw (see Frame 107).

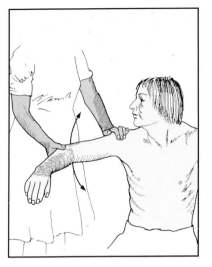

58. Aftercare (e): Where there has been an axillary nerve palsy with loss of deltoid function, physiotherapy will be required. Although the lesion is usually in continuity and full recovery may occur, this may take several months and is not invariable. Assisted movements will be required – either normally, with the aid of slings and perhaps weights, or by hydrotherapy. If there is no sign of recovery after 6 weeks, nerve conduction studies should be undertaken.

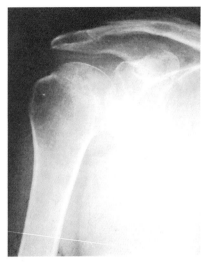

59. Posterior dislocation of the shoulder (a): This may result from a fall on the outstretched, internally rotated hand or from a direct blow on the front of the shoulder. The head of the humerus is displaced directly backwards and, because of this, a single AP projection may show little or no abnormality as illustrated here. Nevertheless, clinically there is pain, deformity and local tenderness. *Note:* Posterior dislocation may accompany (and be missed) in obstetrical and Erb's palsies.

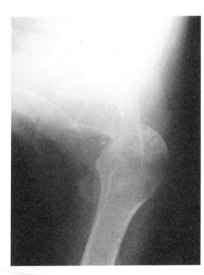

60. Posterior dislocation (b): The frequently apparently normal AP projection makes it essential for an additional lateral view to be obtained when there is any suspicion of posterior dislocation. Where pain is not severe (as, for example, if the dislocation occurs as a complication of a neurological disorder) a tangential lateral may show the humeral head lying clearly behind the glenoid.

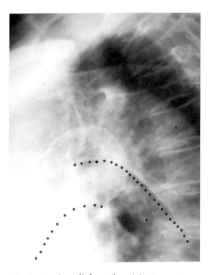

61. Posterior dislocation (c): Generally, however, pain will permit a translateral projection only. The parabolic curve, shaped like the path of a comet, formed by the shaft of the humerus and the edge of the scapula will be broken and further study will show the humeral head to lie behind the glenoid shadow (compare with Frame 44).

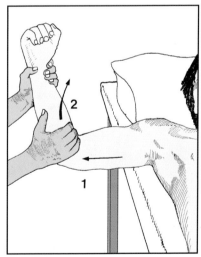

62. Treatment (a): Reduction is usually easily accomplished by applying traction to the arm in a position of 90° abduction (1) and then externally rotating the limb (2). If the reduction appears quite stable the arm should be rested in a sling as described for anterior dislocation of the shoulder.

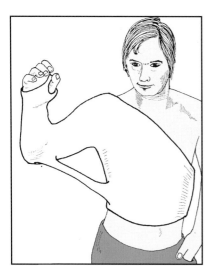

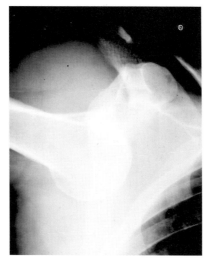

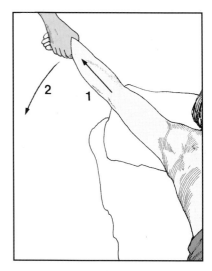

63. Treatment (b): If the reduction is unstable, it is essential that the arm be kept in 60° lateral rotation for 4 weeks to give the torn capsule and labrum a reasonable chance of healing. This can only be reasonably achieved by the application of a shoulder spica, with the shoulder abducted to about 40°, externally rotated 60° and fully extended.

64. Luxatio erecta (a): In this comparatively rare type of shoulder dislocation, there is obvious deformity, with the arm being held in abduction. The radiographs pose no difficulty in interpretation. The patient should be carefully examined for evidence of neurological or vascular involvement, and reduction carried out without undue delay.

65. Luxatio erecta (b): Reduction is usually easily obtained by applying traction in abduction (the position in which the limb is lying) (1) and swinging the arm into adduction (2). The shoulder should be supported after reduction as for anterior dislocation.

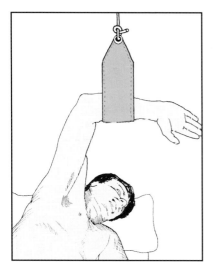

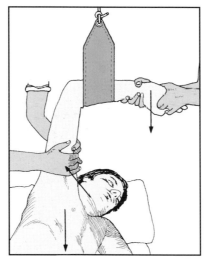

66. Late diagnosed anterior dislocation (a): The diagnosis may have been overlooked, the dislocation not being discovered until some weeks after the injury. Up until about 6 weeks or so, closed reduction (which is often successful) should be attempted. The forearm should be suspended by a canvas sling or bandage from a ceiling hook or improvised fixture above the table. A general anaesthetic is required, and at the time of the actual manipulation a muscle relaxant may be helpful.

67. Late diagnosed anterior dislocation (b): The patient should be on their side and the sling adjusted so that, by using the arm as a lever, an assistant can exert considerable traction through the patient's body weight. The humeral head is then manipulated over the glenoid lip. An image intensifier may give considerable assistance. Mobilisation should be commenced at an early stage (say 1 week).

68. Late diagnosed anterior dislocation (c): If closed reduction fails, open reduction may have to be considered. This is seldom an easy procedure, and a substantial blood replacement may well be required. An anterior approach is usually employed; it the reduction is unstable, temporary pin fixation may be required. If reduction cannot be achieved, resection of the humeral head with or without replacement (excisional arthroplasty, hemi- or total replacement arthroplasty) may have to be considered.

If the dislocation is not discovered until some months after the injury, in the older patient the dislocation should generally be left until the results of a prolonged period of physiotherapy have been assessed. (Many become pain-free, albeit with a marked restriction in shoulder movements.) In the younger patient, exploration and open reduction or arthroplasty should be considered.

Late diagnosed posterior dislocation: Manipulative reduction should be attempted as late as a year from the time of the dislocation. The same technique as that described for late diagnosed anterior dislocation may be employed, with, in the case of posterior dislocation, pressure being applied from behind the shoulder on the posteriorly displaced head. Failure of reduction should be managed in the same way as anterior dislocation, but using a posterior approach for any operative procedure.

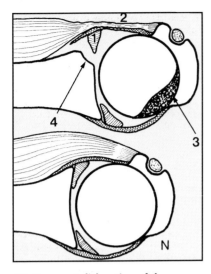

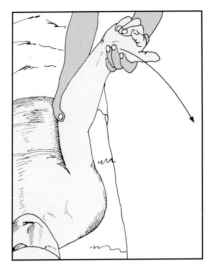

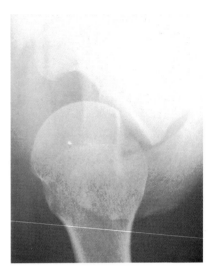

69. Recurrent dislocation of the shoulder: Even after early adequate treatment, redislocation of the shoulder may occur. Progressively less trauma is required on each occasion: eventually the patient may be able to reduce the dislocation voluntarily. Pathological features may include (1) a Bankart lesion, (2) attrition of the anterior shoulder cuff, (3) a defect with flattening of the posterolateral aspect of the head (Hill-Sachs lesion), (4) rounding of the glenoid margin and decreased retroversion of the head. N = normal.

70. Diagnosis (a): The history is usually clear, and clinically, external rotation of the shoulder may cause apprehension. Distinguish between *recurrent* and *habitual* dislocation. In children, this has a good prognosis; in adults, the patients are often psychotic or suffer from joint laxity. They can often voluntarily dislocate and reduce the joint without pain. Arthroscopy shows a lax capsule and capacious joint. Treat by biofeedback re-education of the shoulder muscles and avoid surgery.

71. Diagnosis (b): An axial view may clinch the diagnosis. Posterolateral defects in the humeral head (Hill-Sachs lesion, illustrated) are often striking in recurrent dislocation, but do not occur in habitual dislocation. *Other investigations:* 1. Arthroscopy; or 2. An air contrast CAT or MRI scan may show bony defects or Bankart lesions; 3. Look for abnormal excursion of the humeral head by intensifier examination (or taking stress films) with the shoulder in 90° abduction.

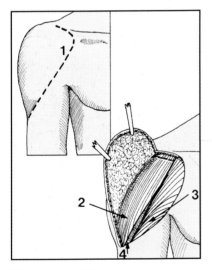

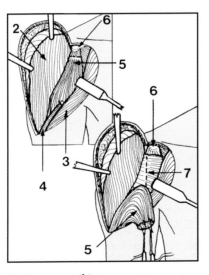

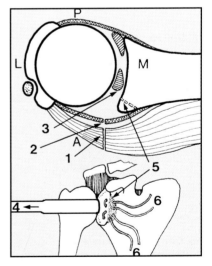

72. Treatment (a): Arthroscopic repair with re-attachment and repair of the damaged structures has a failure rate in the order of 20%, and many prefer an open Bankart procedure. An anterior approach to the shoulder is usually used: an incision is made along the line of the medial border of the deltoid, turning laterally along the clavicle (1) or over the crest of the shoulder. The groove between the deltoid (2) and pectoralis major (3) is identified and opened up; the cephalic vein (4) may need to be ligated.

73. Treatment (b): The deltoid is turned back (2) by incising some of its fibres close to the clavicle. The common tendon of the coracobrachialis and the short head of biceps (5) is divided close to the coracoid (6) and turned down, taking care to avoid the musculocutaneous nerve. This reveals the subscapularis (7).

74. Treatment (c) – Bankart repair: The shoulder joint is opened by dividing the subscapularis (1) and the capsule (2). If the glenoid labrum is loose and displaced into the joint (3) it is excised; if not, it is ignored. Access is improved by lateral retraction of the humeral head (4). The glenoid edge is rawed (5) and drilled obliquely to take anchoring sutures (6). (Alternatively, soft tissue anchors may be used.)

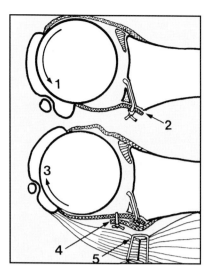

75. Bankart repair cntd: Now the shoulder is internally rotated (1) and the sutures which have been passed through bone are used to anchor the lateral part of the capsule to the raw edge of the glenoid (2). With the shoulder in neutral rotation (3) the medial part of the capsule is sewn over the lateral (4). The subscapularis is repaired (5) followed by layer closure. The arm is bandaged to the side for 4 weeks before mobilisation is commenced.

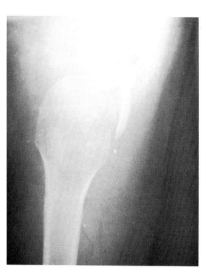

76. Bone-block repair: A bone graft may be used to buttress the joint in both anterior or posterior dislocations (Illus.) where there is a substantial bony defect. In recurrent anterior dislocation the joint may be reinforced anteriorly by a coracoid transfer procedure. **Putti–Platt repair:** Here there is no formal repair of any Bankart lesion; the divided subscapularis is sewn in double breasted fashion across the front of the joint, forming a soft tissue buttress and temporarily restricting external rotation.

77. Recurrent posterior dislocation of the shoulder: Surgical repair of the shoulder (using Bankart or Putti–Platt-like procedures through a posterior approach) may be considered, using criteria similar to those for recurrent anterior dislocation. Recurrent dislocation of the shoulder may also be treated by arthroscopic surgery: there is an appreciable failure rate, and the long term results are not known.

Fracture–dislocations of the shoulder, with fracture of the greater tuberosity or the neck of humerus: see Frame 111.

Neurological complications of shoulder dislocations. Any type of brachial plexus lesion may be seen, and most make a reasonable functional recovery spontaneously. Isolated axillary nerve lesions are the commonest, and have the poorest prognosis in terms of motor recovery. Suprascapular nerve palsies have an excellent recovery rate. No recovery after 6 weeks or so is an indication for nerve conduction studies. Where there is a diffuse plexus lesion, if joint stiffness is not overcome before neurological resolution occurs, function may be permanently impaired: the lesson is that every effort must be made to mobilise the shoulder as quickly as possible where there is *any* neurological complication. If no recovery has occurred after 3–5 months in major plexus lesions, exploration is indicated: a wide exposure is generally required to allow, if indicated, nerve resection and free nerve grafting.

78. Shoulder cuff tears: With advancing years degenerative changes occur in the shoulder cuff. Minor trauma may then produce small tears which, through impingement on the acromion, give rise to a painful area of movement centred at 90° abduction. Physiotherapy in the form of local heat and exercises and local infiltrations of hydrocortisone are usually helpful in relieving symptoms. More extensive tears may follow the sudden application of traction to the arm, and may give rise to difficulty in abducting the shoulder. There is initial tenderness under the acromion and the shoulder is hunched when the patient tries to abduct the arm; at a later stage they may be able to abduct the joint by trick movements. The diagnosis and the extent of the lesion may be confirmed by arthroscopy, air contrast CAT scan, or MRI scan. These injuries are usually treated by prolonged physiotherapy once the acute symptoms have settled. If pain remains a problem, surgery may be advised; good results have been obtained as long as 2 years from the onset of symptoms. (Surgery involves an attempt at repairing the rent in the cuff, using plastic surgical techniques if necessary; partial acromionectomy may be performed if the soft tissues are seen to impinge against the acromion. Certain arthroscopic repair techniques are also

used.) Surgery may be advised at an earlier stage should the problem arise (as it does only rarely) in the younger patient.

79. Fractures of the proximal humerus: There are many different patterns of fracture which occur in this area; although some are of considerable rarity, they can be important because of the complications which may follow them.
A number of attempts have been made to classify fractures in this region, but in order to accommodate the bewildering array of injuries which occur, simplicity has not been one of the results. (The same outcome is to be seen in the classification of ankle fractures.) Two general classifications are of importance: one by Neer, and the other by the AO Group. (The latter is placed at the end of this Chapter.) It is suggested that these are used for reference, and that only the bare facts in Frame 80 be committed to memory.

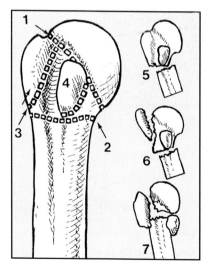

80. Fractures of the proximal humerus: Fractures in this region may involve the anatomical neck (rare) (1), the surgical neck (2), the greater tuberosity (3) or the lesser tuberosity (4). Combinations of these injuries are common, and it is customary to describe fractures in this region by the number of fragments involved, e.g. two-part (5), three-part (6) and four-part fractures (7).

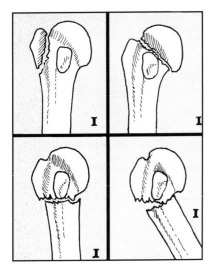

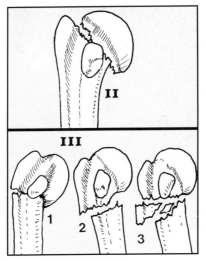

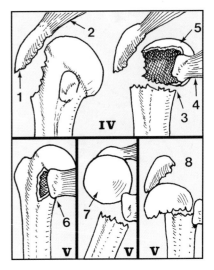

81. Classification of proximal humeral fractures: In the commonly accepted Neer's classification, proximal humeral fractures are divided into 6 groups. **Group I:** This group includes *all* fractures in this region (irrespective of the degree of comminution) where there is minimal displacement or angulation. (Minimal displacement is defined as being less than 1 cm; minimal angulation is (surprisingly) defined as being < 45°.)

82. Neer's classification – Group II: This includes all fractures of the anatomical neck displaced by more than 1 cm. These rare injuries may be complicated by avascular necrosis of the humeral head.
Group III: This includes all appreciably displaced or severely angled fractures of the surgical neck; there are no problems with avascular necrosis. They may be impacted (1), displaced (2) or comminuted (3). Angulation is often anterior, and may give an erroneous impression of abduction or adduction.

83. Group IV: This includes all fractures of the greater tuberosity (1), displaced by the pull of supraspinatus (2). In three-part fractures, a fracture of the surgical neck (3) allows the subscapularis (4) to rotate the head internally so that its articular surface (5) faces mainly posteriorly. **Group V** injuries involve the lesser tuberosity (6). In three-part injuries the humeral head may be abducted and externally rotated so that its articular surface faces anteriorly (7). Four-part injuries (8), identical with four-part injuries of Group IV, may render the head avascular.

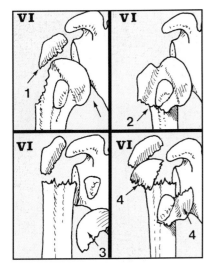

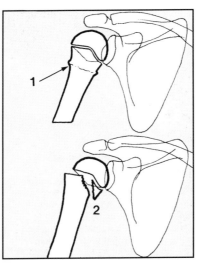

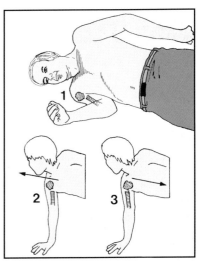

84. Group VI: This comprises the fracture–dislocations. Dislocation of the shoulder with an associated greater tuberosity fracture (1) is included in the two-part injuries in Group VI (see also Frame 57). More serious are the dislocations where the two-part fracture of the proximal humerus is through the surgical neck (2). Most difficult of all are the three- and four-part injuries, especially when the humeral head is completely detached and displaced (3), or worse still, split (4).

85. Children's injuries: Note that in children the commonest injury is a greenstick fracture of the surgical neck (1); this may be classified as a Neer Group I, two-part fracture. Also common is a slight or moderately displaced proximal humeral epiphyseal injury with an associated juxta-epiphyseal fracture (2) (Salter–Harris Type 2 injury). This would fit into Group I or II, depending on the displacement and angulation.

86. Mechanism of injury: These fractures may be caused by a fall on the side (often leading to impacted, minimally displaced fractures) (1), by direct violence or by a fall on the outstretched hand. The pattern of injury following the latter may be influenced by the direction of motion of the trunk over the fixed arm (2, 3).

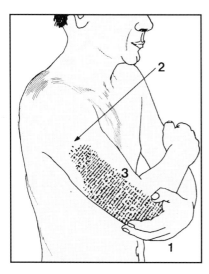

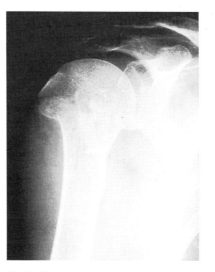

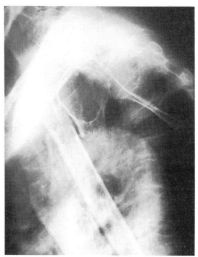

87. Diagnosis: The patient tends to support the arm with the other hand (1). There is tenderness over the proximal humerus (2) and in severely angled or displaced fractures there may be obvious deformity. Later, gross bruising gravitating down the arm is an outstanding feature (3). (This may worry the patient unless this possibility has been previously mentioned to him by the surgeon.)

88. Radiographs (a): The diagnosis is established firmly by the radiographs. In a fair number of cases two features may be clear: namely that the fracture involves the cancellous bone of the head and neck and that there is impaction of the fragments. Both these factors contribute to the rapid healing associated with most fractures of proximal humerus. (Illus.: three-part Group I fracture.)

89. Radiographs (b): Note that a second radiographic projection of the shoulder is desirable for a clear assessment of these injuries. An apical oblique or a good translateral will generally be able to clarify the relationships of the major elements. The illustration, a translateral, shows complete loss of bony contact between the main elements of a two part fracture.

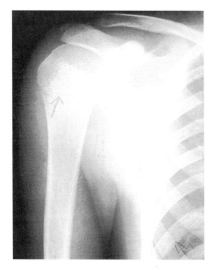

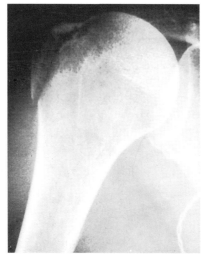

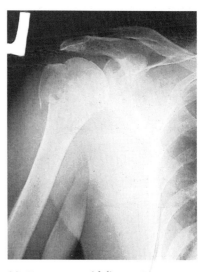

90. Radiographs (c): Note that in children the epiphyseal line is frequently mistaken for a fracture. In many radiographic projections the epiphyseal plate lies obliquely so that instead of appearing as a line it is seen as an oval; as one part of this will be less distinct than the other (see arrow) it may be misinterpreted. (Illus.: normal shoulder.)

91. Treatment guidelines – Group I injuries (a): The following classical examples are arranged in order of severity. *Undisplaced fracture of the greater tuberosity.* This type of injury may occur in isolation or accompany a spontaneously reduced dislocation of the shoulder. The arm should be supported in a collar and cuff sling until the acute symptoms have resolved (1–2 weeks), when mobilisation may be commenced. Watch carefully in case of late displacement.

92. Treatment guidelines – Group I injuries (b): *Impacted fracture of the surgical neck.* (Illus.: three-part fracture involving the greater tuberosity as well as the neck.) There is minimal displacement and angulation showing in this single projection. Prolonged immobilisation is not necessary. Again, a collar and cuff sling should be worn until pain has settled (2–3 weeks usually); shoulder mobilisation may then be commenced. If initial symptoms are severe, proceed as described in Frame 94.

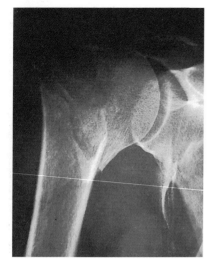

93. Treatment guidelines – Group I injuries (c): Unimpacted fracture of the surgical neck. (Illus.: two-part fracture involving the surgical neck.) In spite of not being impacted, an appreciable area of cancellous bone is in contact, generally assuring rapid healing. Secondary displacement is unlikely provided the limb has some initial protection (required anyway to relieve the severe pain, aggravated by movement, which often accompanies these injuries). Treat along the lines indicated in the following frames.

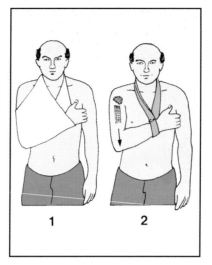

94. Treatment guidelines – Group I injuries (d): Slightly displaced and moderately angled humeral neck fractures may be treated satisfactorily by external support alone; many other fractures may be managed along similar lines. Firstly, the arm should be supported in a sling. Where disimpaction is undesirable (e.g. Frame 92) a broad arm sling is preferable (1). Where the fracture is disimpacted (e.g. Frame 93), then a collar and cuff sling (2) has some potential for gravitational correction of any angulation.

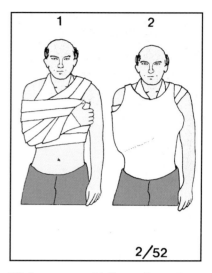

95. Treatment guidelines – Group I injuries (e): In addition, the arm should be protected from rotational stresses by a body bandage (e.g. of crepe bandages) (1) under the clothes (2). Alternatively, an expanding net support may be used (e.g. Netelast®) and this is certainly more comfortable in hot weather. Pain is often severe, and analgesics will be required in the first 1–2 weeks.

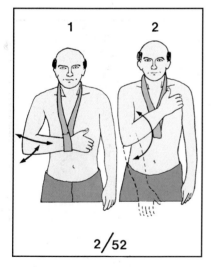

96. Treatment guidelines – Group I injuries (f): After 2 weeks the body bandage may be discarded unless pain is commanding. The sling should be worn under the outer clothes. The patient is advised to commence rocking movements of the shoulder (abduction, flexion (1)) and to remove the arm from the sling three or four times per day to flex and extend the elbow (2).

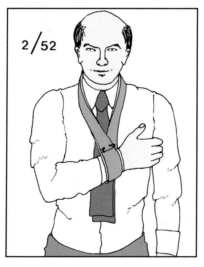

97. Treatment guidelines – Group I injuries (g): At 4 weeks the sling can be placed outside the clothes. Gentle active movements should be practised throughout the day. Over the next 2 weeks the patient should be encouraged to discard the use of the sling in gradual stages.

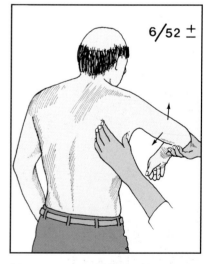

98. Treatment guidelines – Group I injuries (h): At 6 weeks the patient should be referred for physiotherapy if, as is usual, there is considerable restriction of movement. The range of movements (particularly glenohumeral, Illus.) should be recorded at fortnightly intervals, and physiotherapy discontinued when gains cease. Some permanent restriction of glenohumeral movement is common, but seldom incapacitating.

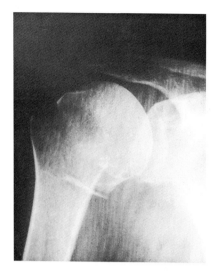

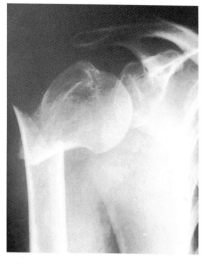

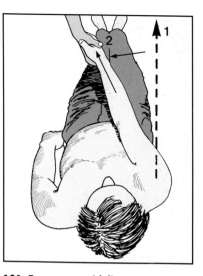

99. Treatment guidelines – Group II injuries (displaced fractures of the anatomical neck): These fractures are often complicated by avascular necrosis of the humeral head. Unless the displacement is very severe (e.g. with off-ending), or there is some complication (such as vascular obstruction in the arm) avoid manipulation or open reduction, and treat as in Frames 94–98. If manipulative reduction is required see Frames 101–103. If avascular necrosis ensues, joint replacement may have to be considered.

100. Treatment guidelines – Group III injuries (severely displaced or angled fractures of the surgical neck): In the elderly patient a good result can be expected in injuries of this pattern where the deformity is accepted and conservative management is pursued along previously indicated lines (Frames 94–98). Nevertheless, there will be some restriction of abduction, so where the deformity is particularly severe or the patient very active, manipulative reduction should be attempted.

101. Treatment guidelines – Group III injuries; Manipulative reduction (a): The patient is anaesthetised; if an image intensifier is available it should be employed and positioned in such a way that the surgeon has adequate access to the shoulder. Apply traction in the line of the limb (1) and swing the arm into *adduction* (2).

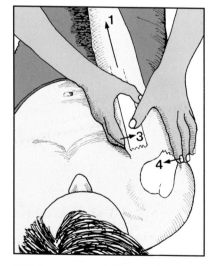

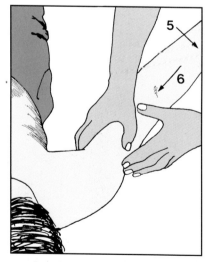

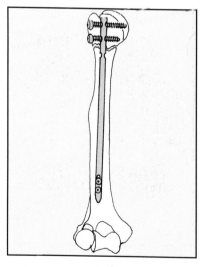

102. Treatment guidelines – Group III injuries; Manipulative reduction (b): An assistant maintains traction in adduction (1). Now apply pressure on the humeral shaft, pushing it laterally (3). At the same time, attempt to control the proximal fragment with the other hand, applying firm pressure beneath the acromion (4).

103. Treatment guidelines – Group III injuries; Manipulative reduction (3): If the medial edges of the fracture can be opposed, reduction may be completed by the assistant abducting the arm gently (5) and gradually releasing the traction (6). After reduction of the fracture, the limb should be supported in a broad arm sling and body bandage.

104. Treatment guidelines – Group III injuries cntd: If closed methods fail, consider open reduction and internal fixation, using for example an intramedullary nail with proximal and distal cross-bolting. Rush pins are sometimes used in this situation: these are solid intramedullary nails with hooked ends. They can preserve alignment, but offer poor control of axial rotation unless used in pairs.

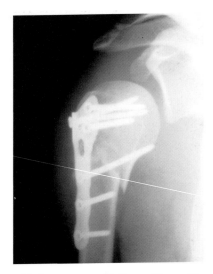

105. Treatment guidelines – Group III injuries cntd: The fracture may instead be held with a plate and screws. (Illus: titanium plate.) A good hold in the soft cancellous bone of the proximal humerus may be obtained with a T-plate and multiple cortical bone screws; alternatively cancellous bone screws may be employed, with cortical screws to fix the plate to the shaft. If there is a problem with a T-plate encroaching on the biceps tendon in the bicipital groove, an L-plate may be used.

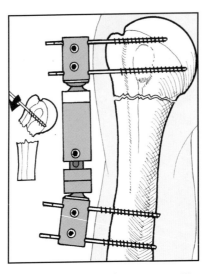

106. Treatment guidelines – Group III injuries cntd: Good results may also be obtained in this class of fracture using an external fixator system. Under image intensifier control a Steinmann pin is inserted into the humeral head and the fracture reduced. Two half pins with continuous threads are inserted into the humeral head, and 2–3 pins into the shaft. After connecting the external neutralising bar the Steinmann pin is removed.

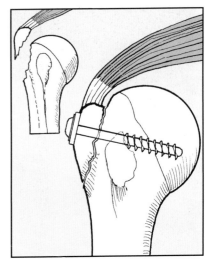

107. Treatment guidelines – Group IV injuries (displaced fracture of the greater tuberosity): Two-part injuries may be reduced by closed methods, but are liable to displace as the result of the unopposed action of the supraspinatus. It is probably best to internally fix these fractures, and this may be done with a single cancellous screw (with a washer under the head). This is also indicated in Group I injuries where there is late displacement.

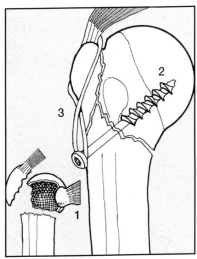

108. Treatment guidelines – Group IV injuries cntd: In three-part injuries the articular surface (1) is directed posteriorly by subscapularis. The viability of the head is usually preserved. In the young and active, consider open reduction and internal fixation. This may be technically difficult, but it may be possible to reduce the fracture using a cancellous screw to oppose the head and shaft (2) and a tension band (3) anchored to the screw head for the tuberosity. (For treatment in the elderly, see Frame 110.)

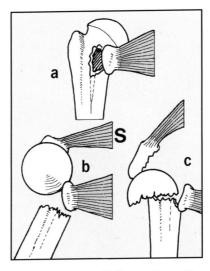

109. Treatment guidelines – Group V injuries (displaced fractures of the lesser tuberosity): Two-part injuries (a) are rare and should be treated conservatively. In three part injuries, supraspinatus (S) is unopposed and the humeral head points forwards (b). Treat as three-part Group IV injuries. Group V four-part injuries (c) are identical with four-part injuries in Group IV; there is a high incidence of avascular necrosis of the detached head. These injuries may also be managed conservatively, and complications dealt with as they arise.

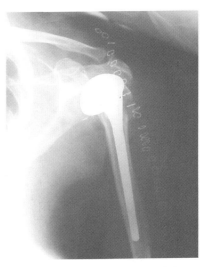

110. Treatment guidelines – Group IV and V injuries in the elderly: If the patient is fit, a joint replacement procedure may offer the best chances of a good functional result. Alternatively, where there is no gross osteoporosis, it may be possible to realign the fragments under intensifier control using Steinmann pins, and subsequently hold them with cannulated screws inserted through small stab incisions. Otherwise treat conservatively (see Frames 94–98). A stiff shoulder is inevitable, but overall function is often surprisingly good.

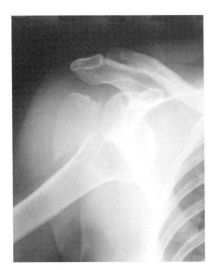

111. Treatment guidelines – Group VI injuries (fracture–dislocations): Two-part injuries in which there is a dislocation of the shoulder and a fracture of the greater tuberosity are dealt with as though they were uncomplicated dislocations, i.e. by manipulative reduction. The greater tuberosity usually returns to its normal location, but if it remains severely displaced reduction should be undertaken (see Frames 57 & 107).

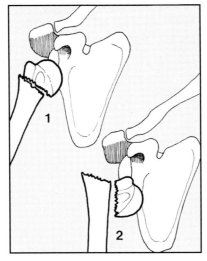

112. Treatment guidelines – Group VI injuries (fracture–dislocations) cntd: If a two-part injury involves the surgical neck, the degree of separation of the fragments affects the chances of a satisfactory closed reduction. Where there is little separation (1) an intact periosteal sleeve will generally permit manipulative reduction. Where there is wide separation of the elements (2) closed reduction is difficult. If a CAT scan shows the head is fractured, a joint replacement should be considered.

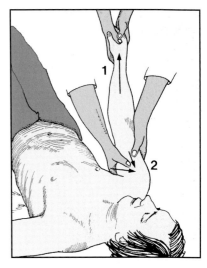

113. Treatment guidelines – Group VI injuries cntd: Unless the patient is too frail, reduction should be carried out. Where there is severe separation, the risks of failure are high, necessitating an open procedure and appreciable blood loss should be anticipated. *Closed reduction technique:* Apply strong traction in the neutral position or slight abduction (1) and manual pressure to the head via the axilla and front of the shoulder (2). Avoid hyperabduction.

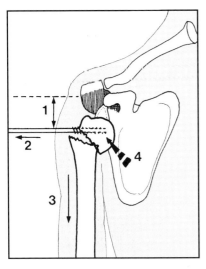

114. Treatment guidelines – Group VI injuries cntd: If the previous technique fails, pass a threaded pin into the humeral head (under intensifier control); introduce the pin on the lateral aspect of the arm 3 cm below the acromial arch (1). Apply lateral traction to the pin (2) with slight traction to the arm (3) and manual pressure over the humeral head (4). *Aftercare* is as for Group III injuries.

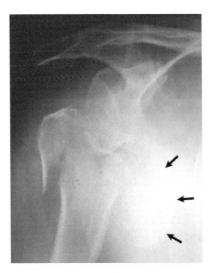

115. Treatment guidelines – Group VI injuries cntd: If closed methods fail or are thought unlikely to succeed, open reduction should be considered. In *three- and four-part injuries*, especially where there is splitting of the head fragment, the risks of avascular necrosis with persistent pain and stiffness are high. Under these circumstances, excisional arthroplasty, hemiarthroplasty or total joint replacement should be considered. (Illus.: four-part fracture–dislocation with arrows pointing to the humeral head.)

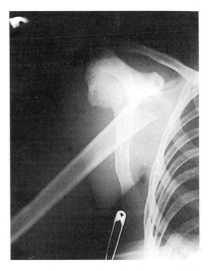

116. Treatment: In children, unimpacted fractures may be of adult pattern (Illus.) or Group 2 epiphyseal injuries, and open reduction is best avoided. Manipulate as described: thereafter the fracture may be held with K-wires inserted percutaneously from the shoulder down, or from the humeral shaft proximally across the growth plate into the head. The wires should be retained for 4–6 weeks. Alternatively, a shoulder spica may be used. Angulation of up to 30° can be accepted.

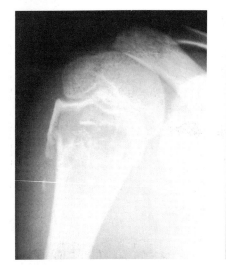

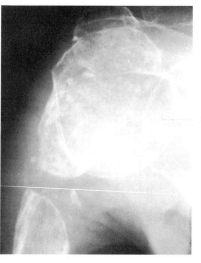

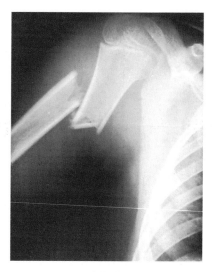

117. Complications (a): Pathological fracture from simple bone cyst is common in the proximal humeral shaft in children. The injury should be treated as an uncomplicated fracture. Healing usually proceeds normally, often with spontaneous disappearance of the cyst. Only rarely (following repeated fracture or cyst expansion) is curettage and packing with bone chips indicated.

118. Complications (b): Radionecrosis may follow radiation therapy for breast carcinoma, leading to pathological fracture. Active treatment is difficult due to local fibrosis and vascular change, but joint replacement might be considered in the selected case. **(c)** Arterial obstruction generally responds to reduction of the fracture; if exploration is required, preliminary exposure and taping of the subclavian trunk at the root of the neck must be anticipated.

119. Fractures of the humeral shaft – Pathology (a): 1. Fractures of the humeral shaft may result from indirect violence (e.g. a fall on the outstretched hand) or from direct violence (e.g. a fall on the side or blow on the arm). 2. In fractures involving the upper third (Illus.) the proximal fragment tends to be pulled into adduction by the unopposed action of pectoralis major.

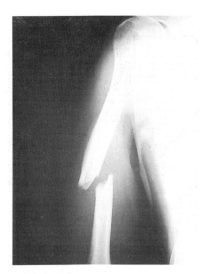

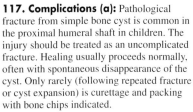

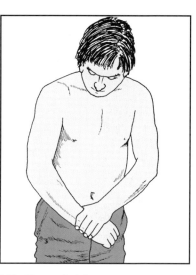

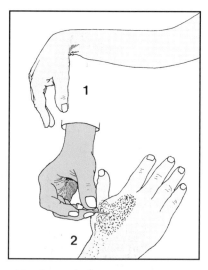

120. Pathology (b): 3. In fractures involving the mid third, the proximal fragment tends to be abducted due to deltoid pull. 4. Radial nerve palsy, and non-union are commonest in *middle third* fractures, and open fractures of the humerus are seen most often at this level.

121. Diagnosis (a): The arm is flail and the patient usually supports it with the other hand. Obvious mobility at the fracture site leaves little doubt regarding the diagnosis. Confirmation is obtained by radiographs, which seldom give difficulty in interpretation.

122. Diagnosis (b): In all cases, look for evidence of radial nerve palsy – drop wrist (1) and sensory impairment on the dorsum of hand (2). This is, in fact, an uncommon complication, as a slip of brachialis lies beneath the nerve – this generally prevents it from coming in contact with the musculospiral groove or the fractured bone ends. If, however, radial nerve palsy accompanies an open fracture, exploration is mandatory.

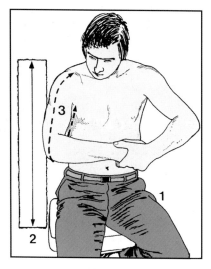

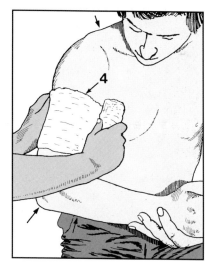

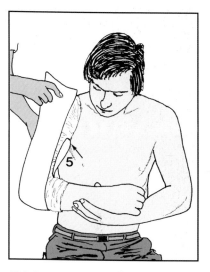

123. Treatment (a) – U-slab method: Simple, single fractures may be treated by the application of a U-plaster. If angulation is slight, no anaesthetic is required. The patient should be seated (1) and a plaster slab prepared of about eight thicknesses of 15 cm (6″) plaster bandage (2). The length should be such as to allow it to stretch from the inside of the arm round the elbow and over the point of the shoulder (3).

124. Treatment (b): Wool roll is then applied to the arm (4). Particular attention is paid to the elbow. The padding should extend from the shoulder to a third of the way down the forearm.

125. Treatment (c): The slab is now wetted and applied to the arm, starting on the medial side at the axillary fold (5) and then bringing it round the elbow up to the shoulder. The slab should be carefully smoothed down. Overlapping of the edges of the slab anteriorly or posteriorly is of little consequence.

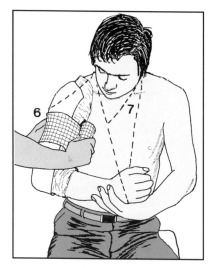

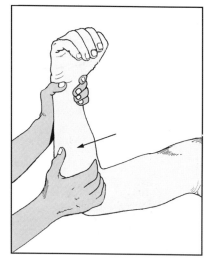

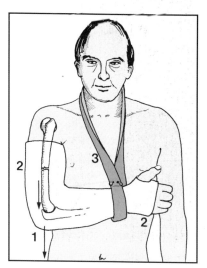

126. Treatment (d): The plaster is secured with a wet open weave cotton bandage (6). During the setting of the slab, the fracture may be gently moulded and slight angulation corrected. Thereafter the arm should be supported in a sling (7), which should be worn under the clothes.

127. Treatment (e): If the fracture is badly displaced, heavy sedation or general anaesthesia is desirable. An assistant should apply light traction to the arm. A U-slab is applied as before, with careful moulding of the fracture as the plaster sets. A sling is worn under the clothes for additional support.

128. Treatment (f) – Hanging cast method: The principle of this form of treatment is that the weight of the limb plus the plaster reduce the fracture and maintain reduction (1). A long arm plaster (2) is applied along with a collar and cuff sling (3). The patient must be ambulant for this line of treatment to succeed, and it is claimed that there may be a higher rate of non-union from occasional distraction.

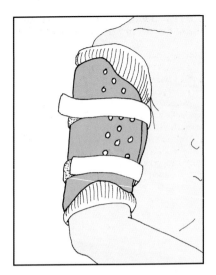

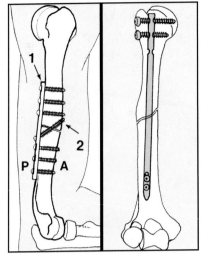

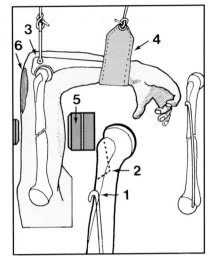

129. Treatment (g): After the initial pain has settled (say 2–3 weeks) the hanging cast may be replaced by a Sarmiento splint (which some use from the outset). Where the fracture is distally placed, a hinged pattern brace should be used; this is retained until union (often at about 9 weeks). Thereafter a sling may be worn as an additional precaution for 2 weeks, but mobilisation of the elbow should be commenced. Depending on progress, the patient should be considered for physiotherapy.

130. Treatment (h): Consider internal fixation if there is a segmental fracture, two fractures in the same limb; multiple injuries, fractures of both arms, a significant head injury, pathological fracture, a radial nerve palsy in an open and otherwise suitable fracture, or after failed manipulation. The most reliable method is to use a plate (1) applied to the posterior surface with an interfragmental screw (2). Alternatively, an intramedullary nail with interlocking screws may be used.

131. Treatment (i): Intramedullary nails may also be introduced retrogradely. The Rush pin (Illus.) is able to correct alignment and apposition, but not rotation, and the quality of fixation is less good than a locked nail. It is inserted just proximal (1) to the olecranon fossa (2). The patient lies supine; traction is applied with an olecranon pin (3) and the hand and forearm supported (4) from an overhead bar. The fracture is reduced using an image intensifier (5) and the fixation device is then introduced through a small triceps splitting incision (6).

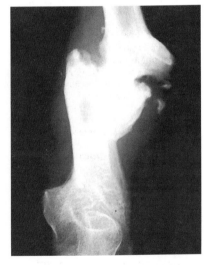

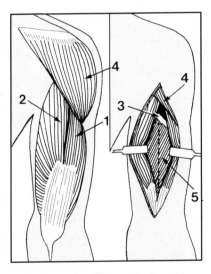

134. Complications (b) – Radial nerve palsy: This is generally a lesion in continuity, and recovery often commences 6–8 weeks after the initial injury. If there is no indication for initial exploration, then the patient may be treated expectantly. A radial palsy in the presence of an open fracture of the humerus is, however, an absolute indication for exploration.

The patient should be provided with a drop-wrist splint, preferably of lively type, as soon as possible, and should attend the physiotherapy department so that they can be encouraged in active and passive movements of the fingers, thumb and wrist. If there is no evidence of recovery in 8 weeks, further investigation by electromyography should be carried out. If this shows no sign of recovery, exploration of the radial nerve should be undertaken.

132. Complications (a) – Non-union (i): This is seen most frequently in middle third fractures, especially in the obese patient where support of the fracture may be difficult or where gravitational distraction of the fracture occurs. Rigid internal fixation with a locked intramedullary nail or compression plating are advised; in the case of the latter, a whole length plate is required in the elderly. Supplementary bone grafting is usually advised, with postoperative support with a Sarmiento brace.

133. Non-union (ii): Visualisation of the radial nerve is essential to avoid damage, and a posterior approach is frequently used. A midline posterior incision gives access to the lateral (1) and long heads (2) of triceps, which are separated. The nerve (3) lies close to the deltoid margin (4) and should be identified. The medial head of triceps (5) is split to give access to the humeral shaft.

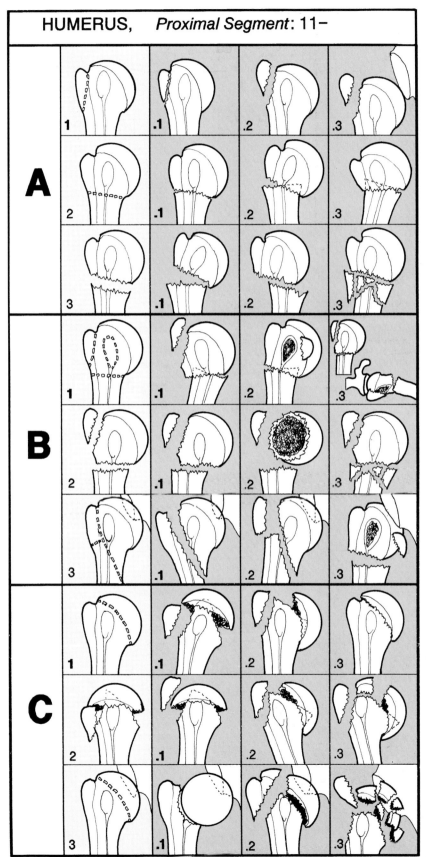

HUMERUS, *Proximal Segment*: 11–

135. AO classification of fractures of the humerus, proximal segment (11–)

Type A fractures are extra-articular and unifocal, involving either the surgical neck *or* the greater tuberosity *or* the lesser tuberosity.
A1 = Fracture of the greater tuberosity: .1 undisplaced; .2 displaced; .3 with an associated dislocation.
A2 = Impacted fracture of the surgical neck: .1 undisplaced; .2 with varus deformity; .3 with valgus deformity.
A3 = Non-impacted fracture of the surgical neck: .1 with angulation; .2 with displacement; .3 multifragmentary.

Type B fractures involve the surgical neck and a tuberosity.
B1 = Impacted fracture of the surgical neck of the humerus with a fracture of the greater or lesser tuberosity: .1 with valgus deformity and a fracture of the greater tuberosity; .2 with varus deformity and a fracture of the lesser tuberosity; .3 with anterior angulation and a fracture of the greater tuberosity.
B2 = Unimpacted fracture of the surgical neck with a fracture of a tuberosity:
.1 without rotation (torsional deformity); .2 with rotation; .3 with a multifragmentary fracture of the metaphysis.
B3 = Bifocal fracture with glenohumeral dislocation (fracture–dislocation of the shoulder): .1 with a vertical fracture line and greater tuberosity intact (classified atypically here as a bifocal fracture because of the obliquity of the fracture line); .2 vertical fracture line and an associated fracture of the greater tuberosity; .3 posterior dislocation and a fracture of the lesser tuberosity.

Type C fractures are articular, with involvement of the anatomical neck and the articular surface.
C1 = Slightly displaced articular fracture: .1 with involvement of the anatomical neck and the greater tuberosity, with some valgus deformity; .2 involvement of the anatomical neck and the greater tuberosity, with some varus; .3 solely of the anatomical neck.
C2 = Markedly displaced but impacted articular fracture: .1 with involvement of the anatomical neck and the greater tuberosity, and valgus deformity; .2 with involvement of the anatomical neck and the greater tuberosity and varus deformity; .3 with the fracture involving the head and the greater tuberosity and varus angulation.
C3 = Dislocated articular fracture (anatomical neck fracture–dislocation): .1 unifocal; .2 with tuberosity fracture; .3 multifragmentary fracture of the head.

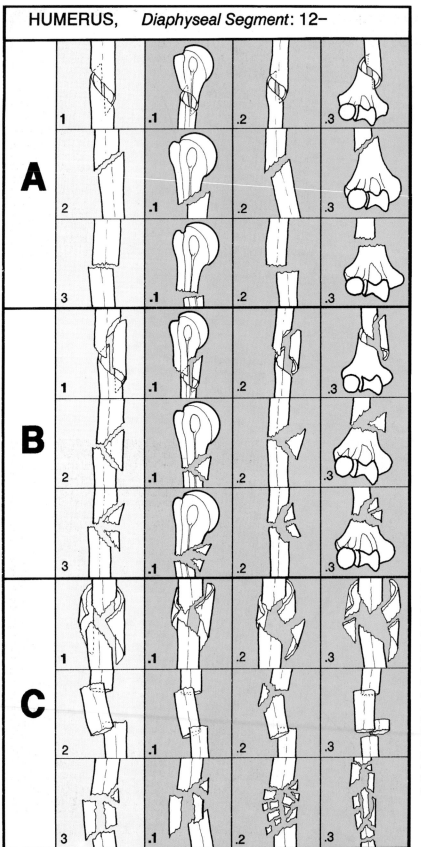

HUMERUS, *Diaphyseal Segment*: 12–

136. AO classification of fractures of the humerus, diaphyseal segment (shaft) (12–)

Type A are simple (i.e. there is a circumferential disruption of the bone).
A1 = Spiral fracture; .1 in the proximal zone; .2 in the middle or central zone; .3 in the distal zone.
A2 = Oblique fracture (i.e. fractures where the fracture lies at 30° or more to a line drawn at right angles to the shaft); the subgroups are the same as in **A1**.
A3 = Transverse fractures (i.e. the fracture line lies at less than 30° to a line drawn at right angles to the shaft); the subgroups are the same as in **A1**.

Type B fractures are wedge fractures (i.e. there is a separate (butterfly) segment, but after reduction there is contact between the main fragments (a so-called hitch)).
B1 = Spiral wedge fracture (usually as the result of twisting stresses): .1 in the proximal zone; .2 in the central zone; .3 in the distal zone.
B2 = Bending wedge fracture (usually as the result of bending stresses): the subgroups are as in B1 above.
B3 = Bending wedge fracture: here the wedge is fragmented. The subgroups are as in B1 above.

Type C fractures are complex (i.e. they have more than two fragments, and even after reduction the pattern is such that there is no contact between the main proximal and distal fragments).
C1 = Complex spiral: .1 with two intermediate fragments; .2 with three intermediate fragments; .3 with more than three intermediate fragments.
C2 = Complex segmental: .1 with one intermediate segment ('double fracture'); .2 with one intermediate segment and an additional wedge fragment; .3 with two intermediate segments.
C3 = Complex, irregular fracture: .1 with two or three intermediate fragments; .2 with shattering of the bone over a length of less than 4 cm; .3 with shattering of the bone over a length of 4 cm or more.

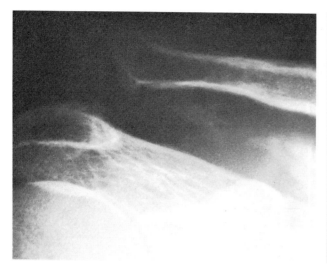

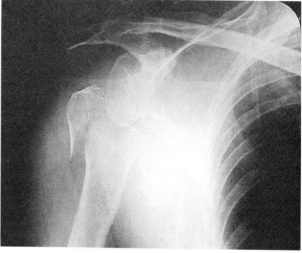

137. What injury and what sequel to injury is shown in this localised radiograph of the shoulder?

138. What is your analysis of this injury?

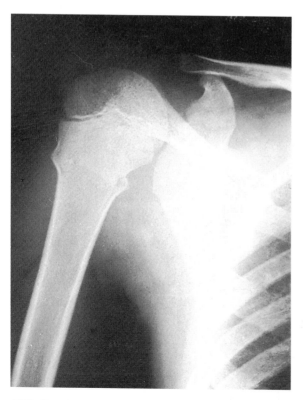

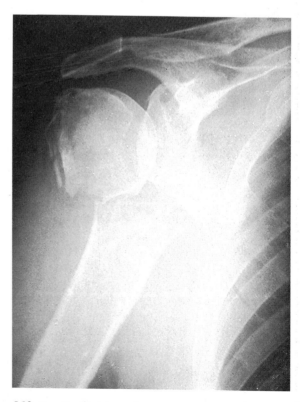

139. Classify this injury and comment on the position.

140. Describe this injury: what complication might you suspect?

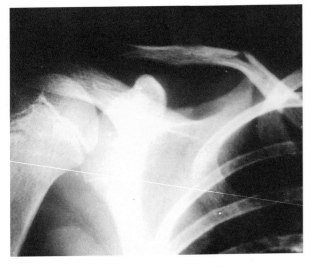

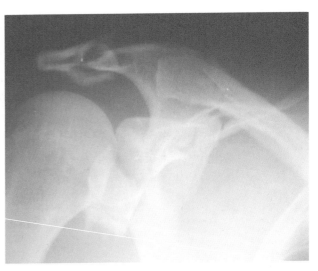

141. What injury is present? Is reduction required?

142. What is this injury? What treatment would normally be advised?

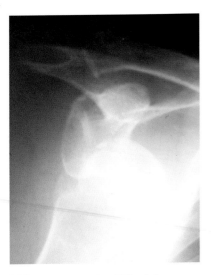

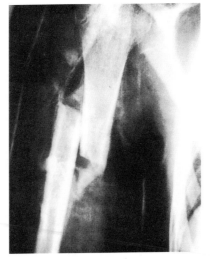

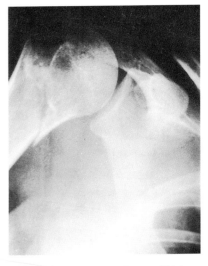

143. What is this injury? What is its commonest neurological complication?

144. What does this radiograph show? What is the prognosis, assuming there is no additional deformity present in the second view? What neurological complication might accompany this injury?

145. Classify this injury. How would it be treated?

ANSWERS TO SELF-TEST

137. Acromioclavicular dislocation with massive calcification in the acromioclavicular ligaments (no active treatment is likely to be required apart from physiotherapy).

138. There is a fracture–dislocation of the shoulder (Neer Group VI, three-part injury). The faint shadow of the humeral head is in the medial wall of the axilla, and there is a separate fracture of the greater tuberosity. (AO = 11–C3.2.)

139. This is a greenstick fracture of the proximal humerus. There is no apparent angulation, but a second projection would be necessary to make certain of this. It is probably a Neer Group I, two-part injury. (AO = 11–A2.1.)

140. Fracture of the surgical neck of the humerus; the fracture is of the unstable type, and the shaft is displaced medially so that it has lost contact with the head. The axillary artery and the brachial plexus are at risk. There is a comminuted fracture of the greater tuberosity (Neer Group IV, three-part injury). (AO = 11–B2.1.)

141. This is a greenstick fracture of the clavicle. No reduction is required.

142. Fracture of the glenoid. There is in addition an undisplaced fracture of the acromion. This injury may be treated by resting the arm in a sling followed by mobilisation as soon as the acute symptoms have settled, although some would consider internal fixation.

143. Anterior dislocation of the shoulder (an additional lateral projection would be required to confirm). An axillary nerve palsy might be associated.

144. The radiograph shows a fracture of the humerus in a child with complete loss of bony contact (off-ending). Callus is plentiful, and union is far advanced with considerable shortening. The late result would normally be excellent, with the length discrepancy being made good. Radial nerve palsy is a possible complication in this type of injury. (AO = 12–A1.1; the fracture is slightly spiral in pattern.)

145. Undisplaced fracture of the surgical neck of the humerus in an adult (Neer Group I, two-part fracture). It may be treated conservatively by resting the arm in a sling, but some would prefer to stabilise the fracture by a plate and screws, or a locked intramedullary nail. (AO = 11–A2.1.)

CHAPTER
7
Injuries about the elbow

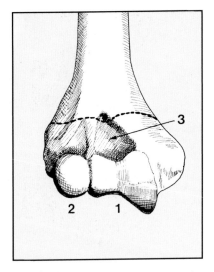

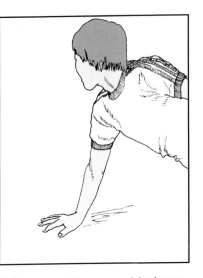

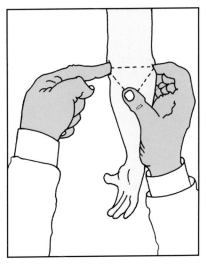

1. Definition: A supracondylar fracture of the humerus is a fracture which occurs in the distal third of the bone. The fracture line lies just proximal to the bone masses of the trochlea (1) and capitulum (capitellum) (2) and often runs through the apices of the coronoid (3) and olecranon fossae. The fracture line is generally transverse.

2. Occurrence: The supracondylar fracture is a common fracture of childhood; its incidence reaches a peak about the age of 8 years. It generally results from a fall on the outstretched hand, and should always be suspected when a child complains of pain in the elbow after such an injury.

3. Diagnosis: The olecranon and medial and lateral epicondyles preserve their normal equilateral triangular relationship (unlike dislocation of the elbow, also common in children). There is tenderness over the distal humerus, there may be marked swelling and deformity, and the child generally resists examination. Radiography is mandatory, but interpretation requires care.

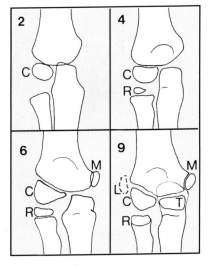

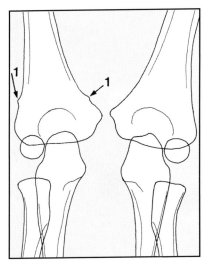

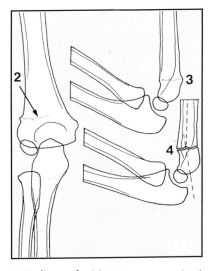

4. Radiographs (a): The interpretation of radiographs is made difficult by the changing complexities of the epiphyses. Typical appearances at ages 2, 4, 6 and 9 years are shown.
Note: C = capitulum – present usually within the first year of life;
R = radial head – appears 3–5 years;
M = medial epicondyle – present by 6;
T = trochlea – appears 7–9;
L = lateral epicondyle – 11–14; (Olecranon – 8–11 years.)

5. Radiographs (b): Variations in appearances occur, and if there is any difficulty in interpreting the radiographs, there should be no hesitation in having films taken of the other side for direct comparison. These may for example, draw attention to (1) the slight cortical irregularity of a minor greenstick fracture.

6. Radiographs (c): In fractures associated with more violence, the next detectable sign may be a hairline crack, visible on the AP view only (2). With more violence, the fracture line will be detectable in the lateral projection as well (3). Next, the distal fragment is tilted in a backward direction (4).

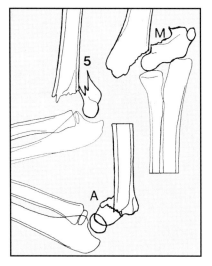

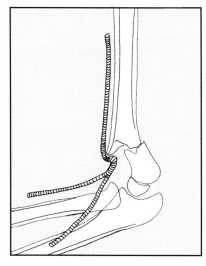

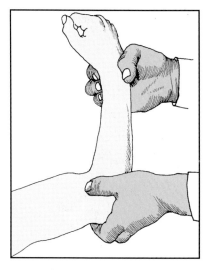

7. Radiographs (d): With still greater violence there is backward displacement (5), often leading to loss of bony contact. In the AP view there is often medial or lateral shift of the epiphyseal complex (M). The complex may also be rotated relative to the humeral shaft (generally lateral rotation). Rarely, as a result of other mechanisms the distal fragment is displaced and titled anteriorly (A). Occult fractures may be suggested by the posterior fat pad becoming apparent in the lateral projections.

8. Vascular complications (a): Where there is appreciable displacement of the fracture, the brachial artery may be affected by the proximal fragment. In the majority of cases this is no more than a kinking of the vessel, but occasionally structural damage to the wall may occur, with the risk of Volkmann's ischaemic contracture. (Rarely, the neurovascular bundle is trapped between the fracture and the biceps tendon, with tethering of the overlying skin; this is an indication for exploration.)

9. Vascular complications (b): In every case check and record the circulation prior to any manipulation. Seek the radial pulse, and note any evidence of arterial obstruction (pallor and coldness of the limb, pain and paraesthesia in the forearm, and progressive weakness of the forearm muscles). Look for excessive swelling and bruising round the elbow. **Neurological complications:** Note any evidence of impaired function in the ulnar, median or radial nerves, said to occur in 6–16% of cases.

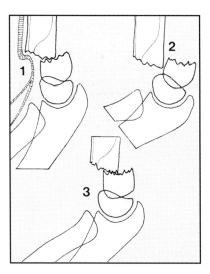

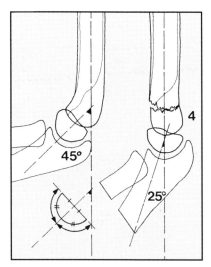

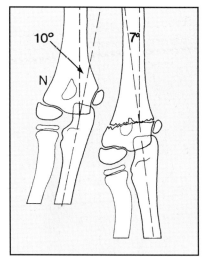

10. Interpretation of radiographs (a): Certain *displacements* showing in the lateral give a clear guide to the necessity for reduction.
(1) Displacement with accompanying evidence of arterial obstruction. (This absolute also applies to angled fractures with vascular complications.)
(2) Displacements with complete loss of bony contact.
(3) Ideally, where the displacement is such that there is less than 50% of bony contact.

11. Interpretation of radiographs (b): (4) If there is *backward tilting* (anterior angulation) of the distal fragment by 15° or more, then correction should be attempted. Note that in the normal elbow the articular surfaces of the distal humerus lie at 45° to the axis of the humerus. (The construction is shown and the actual deformity is 20° (45–25°).) Remodelling of persistent angulation is slow and may be poor, leading to loss of flexion.

12. Interpretation of radiographs (c): Reduction is required if there is significant *lateral or medial tilting*. Note that the normal 'carrying angle' of the elbow is about 10°. (Illus.: a cubitus varus deformity of 17° (10° + 7°).) Cubitus varus and cubitus valgus do not remodel well, and may ultimately be associated with tardy ulnar nerve palsy. Some regard any degree of tilting as significant and meriting correction, and certainly a deformity of 10° and above is unacceptable.

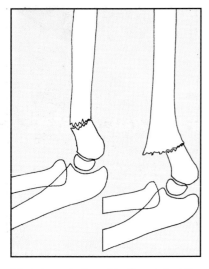

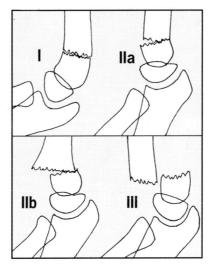

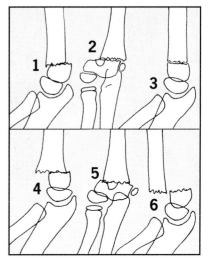

13. Interpretation of radiographs (d):
Reduction is required if there is any significant *rotational* deformity. This is generally most obvious in the lateral projection. (Left above: no rotational (torsional) deformity present; Right: rotational deformity present.) Rotation, like cubitus valgus and varus, does not remodel well. In this context 'significant' is in effect any degree of rotation that is obvious in the plain films.

14. Classification of supracondylar fractures: Simple and useful is the Wilkins modification of the Gartland system. **Type I:** Undisplaced fracture. **Type IIa:** Greenstick fracture with anterior angulation (posterior tilting of the distal fragment); **Type IIb:** Greenstick fracture with anterior angulation and rotation; **Type III:** Completely displaced fracture. Types I and IIa do well, almost irrespective of treatment. Results are poorer in Type IIb and Type III, and internal fixation is preferred by many for injuries in these categories.

15. Summary of indications for reduction: Assuming no vascular complication, pure posterior displacement (1), lateral or medial displacement (2) of 50% or less, and angulation of less than 15° (3) may be accepted, as remodelling is generally rapid and effective. Rotation (4), valgus or varus (5), or loss of bony contact (6) require correction. In the next frames the techniques for closed reduction and cast fixation for any supracondylar fracture are followed by alternative methods using internal fixation.

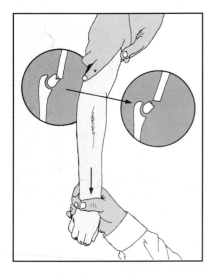

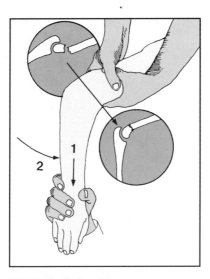

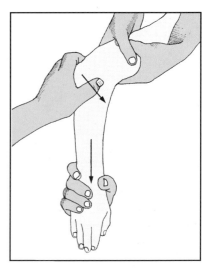

16. Manipulation techniques (a): The arm should be manipulated under general anaesthesia. Gentle/moderate traction is applied at about 20° of flexion while an assistant applies counter-traction. This leads to disimpaction of the fracture. Some surgeons advise that this and the following stages should be carried out with the arm in supination.

17. Manipulation (b): Now, maintaining traction and counter-traction (1), flex the elbow to 80° (2). This lifts the distal fragment, thereby reducing any posterior displacement and correcting any backward tilting (anterior angulation).

18. Manipulation (c): During this manoeuvre, the epiphyseal complex may be further coaxed into position by grasping it in the free hand. The thumb can be used to steady the proximal humeral shaft. Lateral displacement and torsional deformity (axial rotation) may also be corrected in this way.

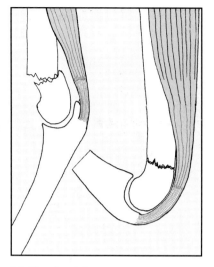

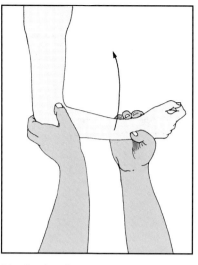

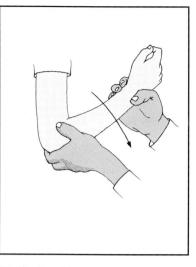

19. Fixation (a): After reduction, the fracture must be maintained in a stable position. Flexion of the elbow stretches the triceps over the fracture, often splinting it most efficiently. *The aim should be to flex the elbow as far as the state of the circulation at the time will permit, while making an allowance in anticipation of further swelling.*

20. Fixation (b): Assuming that at 80° a pulse is present (if present before the manipulation it should still be there, and if absent it will have hopefully been restored) continue flexion of the elbow until the pulse disappears (due to the elbow flexure crease along with the swelling compressing the brachial artery).

21. Fixation (c): Now extend the elbow slowly for about 10° beyond the point when the pulse returns. *This is the position in which the arm should be maintained.* If 110–20° or more of flexion can be preserved, a sling and body bandage, well secured with adhesive strapping, may suffice for fixation.

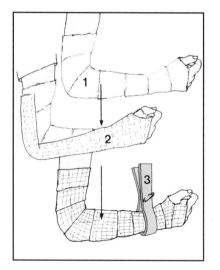

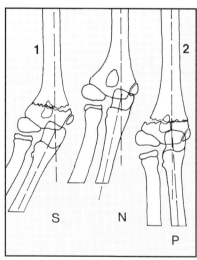

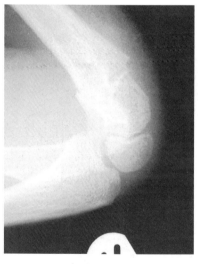

22. Fixation (d): Unfortunately further extension of the elbow may be required to restore the circulation. In such cases, apply a generous layer of wool (1), followed by a long arm plaster slab (2) secured with bandages and a sling (3). *Many surgeons favour this in every case.* **Warning:** Never apply a *complete* plaster because of the risks of swelling, and avoid applying any pressure with encircling bandages at the front of the elbow – some skirt this area, only bandaging the cast into position above and below the joint.

23. Fixation (e): While the slab is being applied, the risks of recurrence of valgus or varus deformity may be reduced by careful positioning of the forearm: if there has been valgus deformity (lateral tilting, medial angulation) (1) place the arm in supination (S). With varus (2) place the arm in pronation (P). With insignificant angulation the neutral (N) position may be employed.

24. Check radiographs: Check radiographs must now be taken in two planes. (For interpretation of AP radiographs, see later.) In the lateral projection illustrated there has been a good reduction: note how all posterior displacement has been corrected and the normal angulation of the epiphyseal complex has been largely restored. (For key see following frame.)

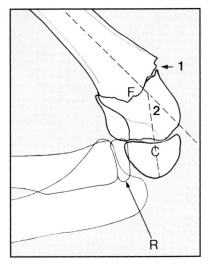

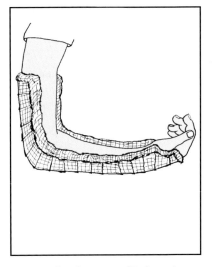

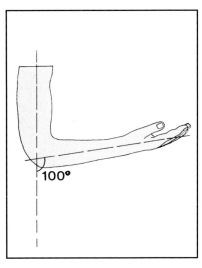

25. Check radiographs cntd: This diagram is based on the previous radiograph, and shows correction of all posterior displacement (1), and restoration of the normal angulation of the epiphyseal complex (2). (F = fracture line; C = capitellum; R = radial head.) If a good reduction has been achieved: 1. discontinue the anaesthetic; 2. admit the child for overnight observation; 3. elevate the arm in a roller towel or similar device; 4. leave access in the dressings for observation of the pulse and finger circulation.

26. Late development of ischaemia: If while under observation the pulse disappears, and especially if there are other signs of ischaemia, *all* encircling bandages should be cut, and *all* wool in front of the elbow teased out. If this does not lead to improvement, the elbow should be placed in a more extended position (e.g. by cracking the slab and slackening the sling).

27. Absent pulse after manipulation: Returning to Frame 20 – If after manipulation the pulse is *not* palpable, the elbow should be flexed to *not more than 100°* and maintained in that position with a sling and a back slab (applied over wool and held with a lightly applied bandage). The anaesthetic should be continued while check radiographs are taken.

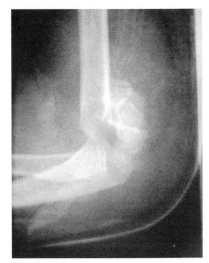

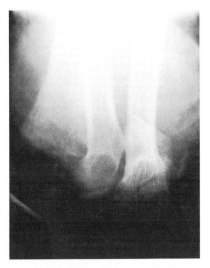

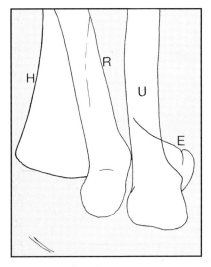

28. Radiographs (a): If the radiographs show a poor reduction, then no more than two further attempts at manipulation may be permitted under the same anaesthetic. The illustration shows a typical unsatisfactory lateral projection where there is complete loss of contact between the distal fragment and the humeral shaft, with proximal displacement of the distal fragment (compare with Frame 24).

29. Radiographs (b): An AP projection should also be taken and the position checked in every case, even although faults in reduction demonstrated in the lateral projection are the ones more usually associated with circulatory impairment. As the AP view cannot be obtained with the elbow straight, superimposition of the radius, ulna and humerus make interpretation difficult (but see following frame). Be careful to avoid disturbing the reduction during the taking of these radiographs.

30. Radiographs (c): The epiphyseal complex preserves its relationship with the radius and ulna. In turn, with a good reduction, the radius and ulna regain their alignment with the humerus. Note in this unsatisfactory reduction the radius (R), ulna (U) and epiphyseal complex (E) are displaced medially in relationship to the humerus (H).

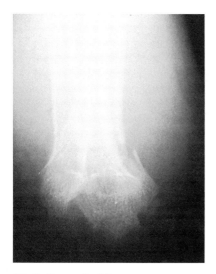

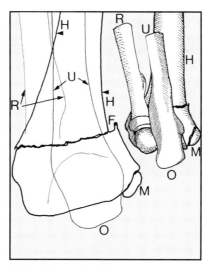

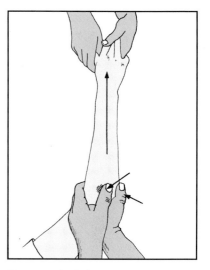

31. Radiographs (d): The preceding case with vascular impairment was remanipulated and the above correction obtained. This is a good reduction, and was accompanied by restoration of the pulse at the wrist.

32. Radiographs (e): A line drawing of the preceding radiograph is shown along with a sketch of the forearm bones drawn in roughly the same position (compare also with Frame 29). R = radius, U = ulna, H = humerus, F = fracture, O = olecranon, M = medial epicondyle.

33. Remanipulation: If a poor reduction has been obtained and remanipulation is necessary, the preceding technique may be repeated; alternatively, while an assistant applies light traction to the forearm, the distal fragment is pushed forwards with the thumb while the fingers control the proximal fragment. Plaster fixation may be applied as described before.

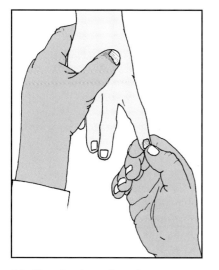

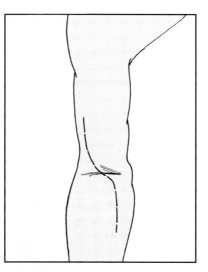

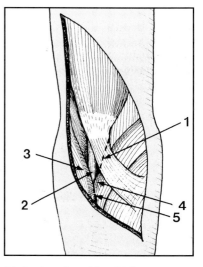

34. Absent pulse, adequate circulation: If a good reduction has been obtained and the pulse remains absent (this occurs in 3% of cases) the circulation should be checked more critically. The use of a pulse oximeter before and after manipulation is often helpful. If the hand is warm and pink, with good capillary return in the nails, there is no immediate indication for further intervention. *Admission, elevation and close observation for 24 hours* are essential. (Generally the pulse returns spontaneously over 2–3 days.)

35. Absent pulse, ischaemia: If there are incontrovertible signs of gross ischaemia, either in the face of a good reduction or a failed reduction, *exploration of the brachial artery* must now be undertaken. (Volkmann's ischaemic contracture occurs in roughly once in every thousand cases of supracondylar fracture, and is generally avoidable.) Exposure of the artery is straightforward. (i) A lazy S incision may be used, following the lateral edge of biceps and crossing the elbow near the fold.

36. Exploration of brachial artery cntd: (ii) The skin edges are reflected and the bicipital aponeurosis (1) divided close to the tendon (2). (iii) The arm is put in full pronation and the space (5) between brachioradialis laterally (3) and pronator teres medially (4) opened up with the finger tips.

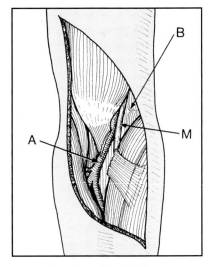

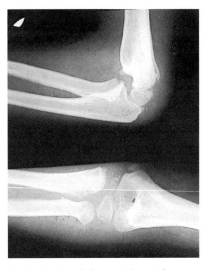

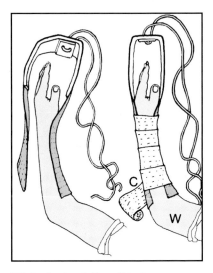

37. Exploration of brachial artery cntd: (iv) The brachial artery (A) is found lying close to the biceps tendon. The median nerve (M) lies on its medial side. The fracture lies deep to the brachialis (B) in the floor of the wound. In some cases relief of local pressure on the vessel (e.g. from the fracture) may restore the circulation, but other measures, requiring experience in vascular surgery, may be necessary.

38. Reduction failure with satisfactory circulation (a): It is unwise to repeat manipulation beyond the third attempt owing to the risks of increasing swelling. In these circumstances, marked displacement (but not angulation, valgus or varus) may be accepted, relying on later remodelling. The fracture illustrated had no bony contact (completely off-ended) in the lateral: after a year, considerable remodelling has occurred, with loss of 15° only of flexion.

39. Reduction failure (b): If displacement and angulation are outside acceptable limits, open reduction is not generally recommended. Instead, continuous traction may be employed. This is especially indicated where there is minimal circulatory impairment, brachial artery exploration is not indicated, and the elbow cannot be flexed. In *Dunlop traction,* traction tapes are applied to the limb. W = wool; C = lightly applied crepe bandage.

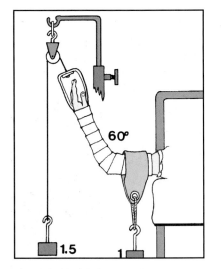

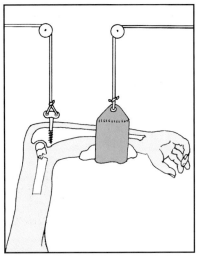

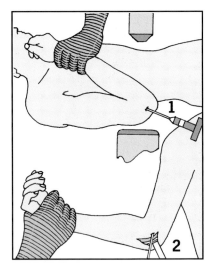

40. Reduction failure (c): The arm is abducted at the shoulder and traction of 1.5 kg applied with the elbow at 60° flexion. Counter-traction of 1 kg is applied directly with a canvas sling applied well above the elbow to avoid compression in this vulnerable area. After swelling subsides the situation may be re-appraised, or the traction discontinued and a plaster slab substituted at 2–3 weeks.

41. Reduction failure (d): Alternatively, skeletal traction may be employed: this may be achieved with a butterfly screw or similar device in the ulna. Traction is applied with weights, and the forearm supported with a sling. Elbow flexion may be controlled with the sling which may be elevated or lowered as thought necessary – this avoids any direct pressure in the antecubital fossa.

42. Alternative fixation technique: This is recommended (where image intensification is available) for all fractures where it is difficult to maintain a reduction. Many advise it for *all* Type IIa and Type III fractures. Begin by reducing the fracture by traction and elbow flexion as described; with the elbow flexed, correct any rotation. Now flex the elbow fully and insert a K-wire laterally, aiming for the axilla (1). Extend the elbow to 90°, locate the ulnar nerve by a small incision over it, and insert a second medial K-wire above it (2).

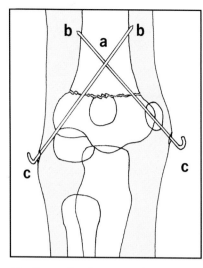

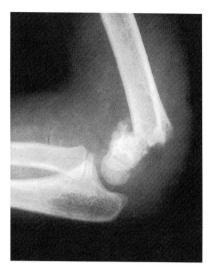

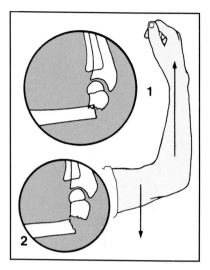

43. Alternative fixation technique cntd:
The K-wires (a) should not be less than 1.6 mm in diameter, and should engage the opposite supracondylar ridge (b). They may cross the growth plate without causing any obvious growth problem. They should remain proud of the skin (c). Single wire fixation is less secure and is not recommended. Additional support with a cast and sling is recommended. The wires may be removed as an out-patient procedure, without anaesthetic, after 3–4 weeks.

44. The anterior (reversed) supracondylar fracture (a):
Supracondylar fractures in which the distal fragment is displaced anteriorly are comparatively uncommon. The normal angle (45°) between the epiphyseal complex and the shaft is increased. *This deformity is aggravated by flexion of the elbow.*

45. Anterior supracondylar fracture (b): An uncommon but related injury is the more distally situated traumatic separation of the epiphyseal complex (Salter–Harris Type 1 or 2) in which the displacement is identical. To reduce either of these injuries, light traction is applied to the elbow in the flexed position (1). This disimpacts the fracture (2).

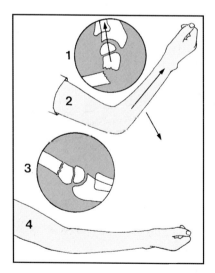

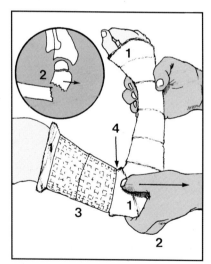

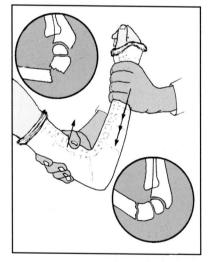

46. Anterior supracondylar fracture (c): Continuing the traction (1) the elbow is slowly extended (2), reducing the angulation (3). The arm is put in a plaster back slab in a position of 10° flexion (4). *This position should not be maintained for more than 3 weeks.* At that stage the elbow should be gently flexed (usually about 70–80° can be achieved) and supported either with a sling or further slab until union.

47. Anterior supracondylar fracture (d): An alternative technique is to apply wool to the limb (1) and disimpact the distal fragment by direct traction on the epiphyseal complex (2). A plaster cuff (3) is then applied by an assistant and allowed to set. Care must be taken to avoid ridging at the distal end (4) which has the potential for causing circulatory impairment.

48. Anterior supracondylar fracture (e): The rest of the plaster is quickly applied, and while it is still soft flex to 110° or less and exert pressure on the distal fragment through the forearm; the position is held till the plaster has set. Check radiographs are taken and fixation continued as for a normal supracondylar fracture. Note that many prefer to fix anterior displaced supracondylar fractures by K-wires (in the manner described for (posterior) supracondylar fractures).

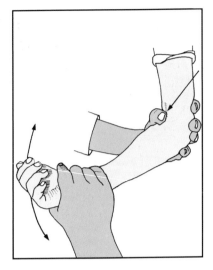

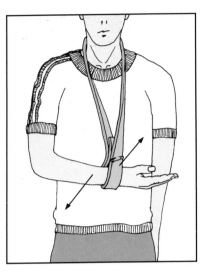

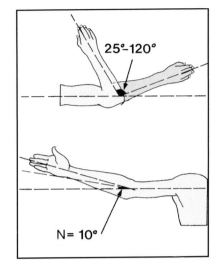

49. Supracondylar fractures – Aftercare (a): Assess union at about 3–4 weeks for a child of 4 years, and about 4–5 weeks for a child of 8 by radiographs and fracture site tenderness. A further useful test is to place your thumb over the biceps tendon, and then flex and extend the elbow through a total range of 20°. Spasm of the biceps indicates that union is not advanced. Mobilisation may be commenced when there is evidence of union, and often earlier in cases treated by K-wires.

50. Supracondylar fractures – Aftercare (b): Mobilisation may be commenced from a sling (i.e. the arm is removed from the sling for 10 minutes' active exercises three to four times per day). The sling is discarded as soon as any discomfort has settled. This procedure may also be used where there is a little residual fracture tenderness and biceps spasm. Physiotherapy is indicated if, after 2 weeks' mobilisation, there is still gross restriction of

51. Supracondylar fractures – Aftercare (c): Physiotherapy can be safely stopped when a range of 25–120° is reached (normal 0–145°). The parents should be cautioned against using passive movements, and advised that some loss of elbow movements may be expected for up to a year after this injury. If any cubitus varus or valgus is present it should be recorded and the child assessed yearly regarding deterioration and the need for corrective osteotomy.

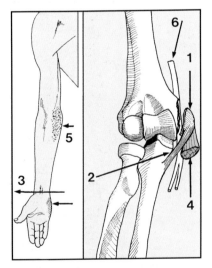

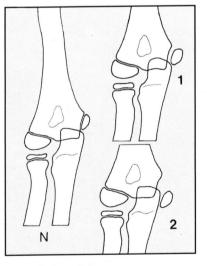

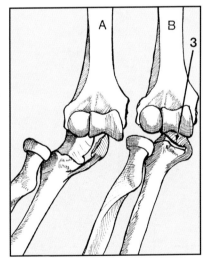

52. Medial epicondylar injuries: Pathology (a): The medial epicondyle (1) may be pulled off by the ulnar collateral ligament (2) when the elbow is forcibly abducted (3). It may be injured by direct violence, and possibly avulsed by sudden contraction of the forearm flexors which are attached to it (4). Suspect if there is medial bruising (5) and always test the integrity of the ulnar nerve (6).

53. Pathology (b): The most minor degrees of violence result in slight separation of the medial epicondylar epiphysis (1). Comparison films may be helpful in diagnosis. Injuries of these types may be treated by immobilisation in a long arm padded plaster for 2–3 weeks. In some cases tardy ulnar nerve palsy may occur. With greater violence the epiphysis is separated and displaced in a distal direction (2). Fixation with K-wires is often advised for separations of 5 mm and greater.

54. Pathology (c): *The potentially most serious injury is when the medial epicondyle is trapped in the elbow joint.* This may follow dislocation of the elbow (A), which must always be accompanied by rupture of the ulnar collateral ligament or avulsion of the medial epicondyle. In the latter case, when the elbow is reduced (B), the epicondyle may be trapped in the joint (3).

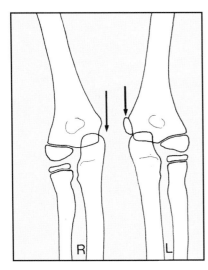

55. Pathology (d): A further hazard in diagnosis is when the medial epicondyle is trapped in an elbow which has been momentarily dislocated but has reduced spontaneously. *Note:* 1. If the child is over 6 years and the medial epicondylar epiphysis cannot be seen in the AP view it is probably in the joint. 2. If there is any doubt comparison films should be taken.

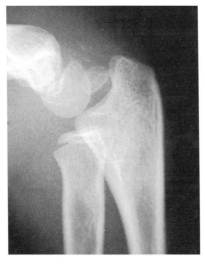

56. Pathology (e): In the normal lateral projection, the medial epicondyle cannot be seen; if it can, as in the case here, it is lying in the joint. The rules are quite clear: 1. Should the medial epicondyle be visible (i.e. what is the child's age)? 2. Does it show in the AP view? 3. Is it visible in the lateral?

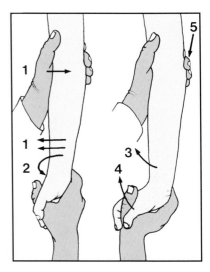

57. Treatment of trapped medial epicondyle (a): Removal by manipulation is often successful. Under general anaesthesia, increase valgus (1), supinate (2), extend elbow (3) and jerk wrist into dorsiflexion (4). A finger placed over the medial side of the elbow (5) may detect the medial epicondyle slipping out of the joint. (Aftercare as described in Frame 53.)

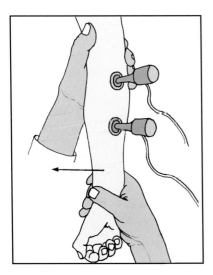

58. Trapped medial epicondyle (b): If the previous method fails, the medial epicondyle may be brought out by electrically stimulating the flexor mass. General anaesthesia is required, the elbow *must* be strongly abducted and a good muscle contraction must be obtained. The necessary equipment and expertise in its use may be available through the physiotherapy department.

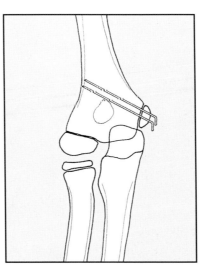

59. Trapped medial epicondyle (c): If both measures fail the medial epicondyle must be extracted through a small anteromedial incision and held in position by K-wires (retained for 3 weeks) (or a screw if over 12).

Ulnar nerve palsies: The majority of palsies found in association with medial epicondylar injuries are lesions in continuity, and recovery usually commences in 3–6 weeks. Some treat these expectantly, while others explore all, with a view to decompression where applicable.

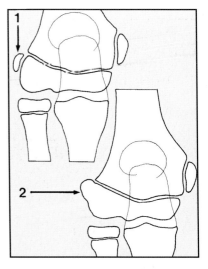

60. Lateral epicondylar injuries in children: The epiphysis for the lateral epicondyle is inconstant, but usually appears about 11 years, fusing with the main epiphysis 2–3 years later (1). It may, however, ossify by direct extension from the capitellum (2). Detachment may follow adduction stress; rarely it may become trapped in the joint after a dislocation. Treat as for medial epicondyle.

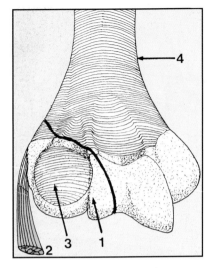

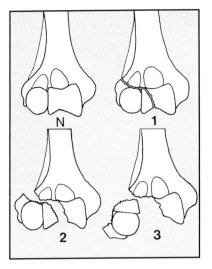

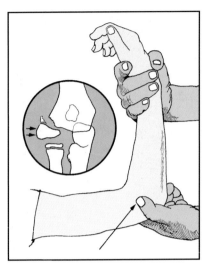

61. Lateral condylar injuries in children – Pathology (a): The common pattern of injury involves the whole of the capitellum and nearly half the trochlea (1). This large fragment may be displaced by the forearm extensors (2) or the lateral ligament. As the capitellar epiphysis (3) and the shaft (4) may be the only structures visible on the radiographs, *their relationship may be the only clue to injury.*

62. Lateral condylar injuries – Pathology (b): Fractures of the lateral condyle may be (1) undisplaced, (2) laterally displaced, (3) rotated. **Treatment (a):** *Undisplaced fractures* should be treated conservatively by a long arm padded back shell and sling for 3–4 weeks. As it is important to make sure no late slip occurs *radiographs should be taken at weekly intervals.*

63. Lateral condylar injuries – Treatment (b): Where there is slight to moderate lateral shift of the complex, closed reduction may be attempted by applying local pressure under general anaesthesia. In many cases this fails, with the deformity recurring as soon as the local pressure is released. If however the reduction is successful, a long arm padded back shell should be applied and retained with a sling for 3–4 weeks. Again it is vital to detect any early slipping by weekly radiographs.

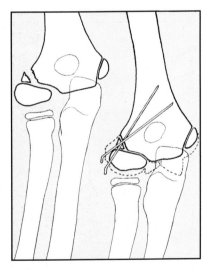

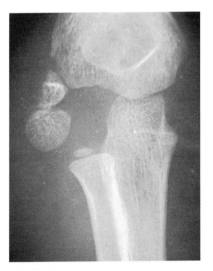

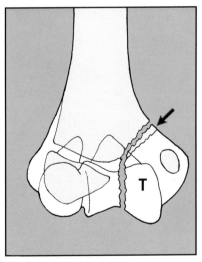

64. Lateral condylar injuries – Treatment (c): Where there is a lateral displacement which is unstable, or late slipping occurs, K-wire fixation is indicated. Where image intensification is available, it may be possible to do this as a closed procedure, but in many cases open operation is required. Two wires must be used, followed by a plaster shell and sling. The wires may be removed after 3–4 weeks and mobilisation commenced at 4 weeks.

65. Lateral condylar injuries – Treatment (d): In injuries where there is rotation of the complex, such as illustrated here, closed methods are unlikely to give a satisfactory reduction, so that there is risk of non-union, growth disturbance and progressive cubitus valgus. Open reduction and K-wire fixation are therefore indicated. (Aftercare as above.) Note that if there is some uncertainty over the position or extent of the epiphyseal fragments, films taken after the injection of a radio-opaque dye into the fracture haematoma may be helpful.

66. Medial condylar injuries in the child: Isolated medial condylar (unicondylar) injuries are uncommon in children, and may be missed as the trochlear centre of ossification does not appear until age 7–9. If the injury is suspected (e.g. by the presence of medial instability of the joint or juxta epiphyseal fractures) further information may be obtained by examination under anaesthesia and arthrography. If the fracture is displaced or unstable it should be opened and fixed with K-wires.

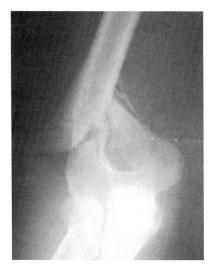

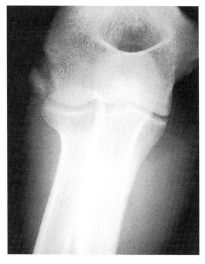

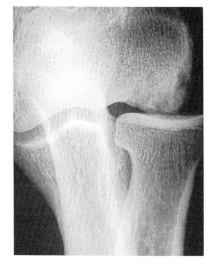

67. Adult fractures – Supracondylar fractures: In adults, the fracture line tends to lie a little more proximal than in children: comminution, obliquity or spiralling and medial or lateral tilting are common. Although undisplaced stable fractures may be treated in a cast, elbow stiffness from delays in mobilisation is a common and serious complication. *Open reduction and internal fixation (e.g. with medial and lateral plates) is the preferred method of treatment for the majority of adult supracondylar fractures.*

68. Medial and lateral epicondylar fractures: Displacement of these fractures is seldom severe and, although potential instability of the joint may be present, symptomatic treatment only is usually required. A crepe bandage applied over wool to limit swelling and a sling for 3–4 weeks is usually adequate. A short period in a long arm plaster is indicated if pain is severe.

69. Fractures of the capitellum (a): The cartilaginous and bony surfaces of the capitellum may be damaged by force transmitted up the radius from a fall on the outstretched hand, often in association with radial head injuries. There may be late osteochondritis dissecans and osteoarthritis.**Treatment:** Initially, symptomatic; later, excise loose bodies and drill the capitellum to encourage revascularisation.

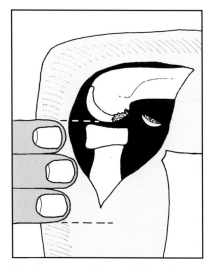

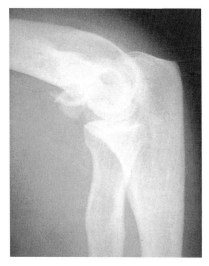

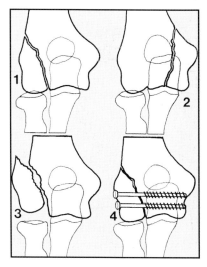

70. Fractures of the capitellum (b): A small flake may be detached from the capitellum as a result of force transmitted up the radius; it may come to lie in the front of the joint. It should be treated as a loose body and excised. This may be carried out safely through a small lateral incision (which must not extend as far as three finger breadths below the joint line to avoid damage to the posterior interosseous nerve).

71. Fractures of the capitellum (c): A more serious fracture involves the major portion of the anterior half of the articular surface of the capitellum. Generally the corresponding part of the trochlea is involved. Severe disability will result if this is not accurately reduced, and generally exposure through an anterior approach will be necessary. Smillie pins or a Herbert screw may be used for fixation.

72. Fracture of a single condyle in the adult (a): Fracture of the lateral (1) or medial (2) condyle (AO = 13–B1 and B2, see p. 167) may be caused by the same mechanisms responsible for the more severe Y-fractures. Displacement may be slight or marked (3). Where there is displacement, best results are obtained by open reduction and internal fixation: this can usually be achieved using one or two cancellous lag screws (4), with an additional plate along the supracondylar ridge if required.

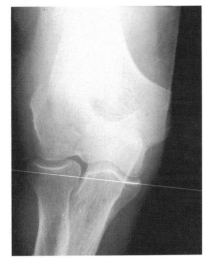

73. Fracture of a single condyle (b): If displacement is minimal, as illustrated, and particularly if the patient is elderly and frail, conservative treatment may be preferred: apply a long arm plaster (over wool) and support the arm in a sling. The plaster may usually be discarded safely after 4–5 weeks, and mobilisation commenced from the sling. Physiotherapy may be started shortly thereafter.

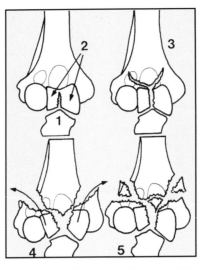

74. Intercondylar Y- or T-fractures (a): This potentially serious injury is caused by the coronoid (1) being driven like a wedge between the two halves of the trochlea (2), often by a fall or blow on the elbow. The vertical split bifurcates (3), and with further violence the two main fragments may separate (4) (AO = 13–C1). Fragmentation (comminution) (5) is often a further problem (AO = 13–C2).

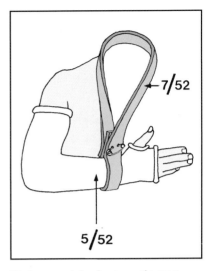

75. Intercondylar fractures (b): While internal fixation is generally the first choice, conservative treatment (as in Frame 73) may be undertaken if the fracture is undisplaced. With gross comminution, primary joint replacement should be considered. In other cases, where operation is thought inadvisable (e.g. because of anticipated technical difficulty), apply a long-arm plaster over wool; before this sets, apply traction, and side-to-side pressure. Remove the plaster and mobilise from a sling at an early date (e.g. 4–5 weeks).

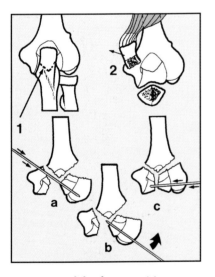

76. Intercondylar fractures (c): In displaced and moderately fragmented fractures, especially in the younger patient, open reduction should be carried out. *Approaches:* (i) through a lateral incision; (ii) through a triceps splitting incision, or (iii) through a chevron osteotomy of the olecranon (1) with its proximal reflection (triceps attached) (2). *Reduction:* The articular fragments should be reduced first using K-wires: it may be helpful to manipulate the lateral element using a wire inserted in the retrograde fashion (a, b, c).

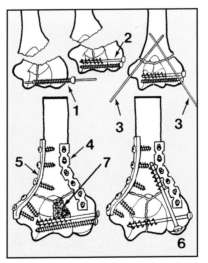

77. Intercondylar fractures (d): After reduction insert a cannulated screw (1) and compress the fragments using a cancellous screw (2). The articular complex may then be lined up with the shaft, and temporarily held with K-wires (3). Then a posterolateral 3.5 mm reconstruction plate (4), and a medial dynamic compression or reconstruction plate (5) may be used to hold the articular complex in alignment with the shaft. Additional compression screws may be used (6) and defects should be packed with bone grafts (7). *Mobilise early.*

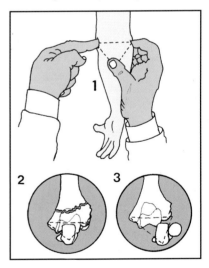

78. Dislocation of the elbow (a): Dislocation of the elbow is common in both children and adults and generally results from a fall on the outstretched hand. It is sometimes confused with a supracondylar fracture. The two may be distinguished clinically by searching for the equilateral triangle formed by the olecranon and epicondyles (1). This is undisturbed in supracondylar fractures (2) but distorted in elbow dislocations (3).

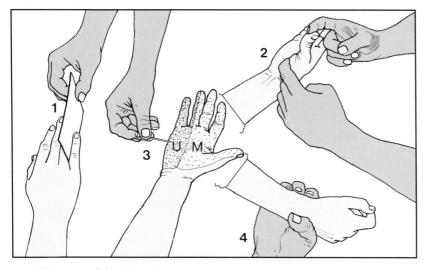

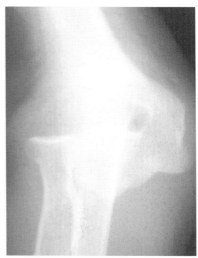

79. Dislocation of the elbow (b): Damage to the ulnar nerve, median nerve or brachial artery is uncommon, but nevertheless should always be sought. A number of motor tests may be used to assess function in both nerves. In the case of the *ulnar nerve*, the ability to grip a sheet of paper between the ring and little finger (1) may be used to assess good interosseous muscle function. It is important that the fingers are not allowed to flex at the MP joints. In the case of the *median nerve*, contraction and power in abductor pollicis may be assessed by feeling the muscle (2) while the patient attempts to resist the thumb being pressed from a vertical position into the plane of the palm. Sensory function in the areas supplied by the median (M) and ulnar (U) nerves should also be quickly tested (3). In the case of the *brachial artery* the quickest assessment is of course by identification of the radial pulse (4).

80. Radiographs: The above frame shows the typical appearances in the AP projection of a dislocation of the elbow. Note how the radius and ulna are displaced laterally and proximally.

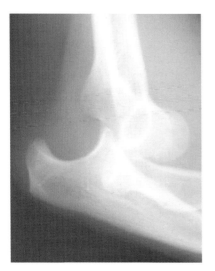

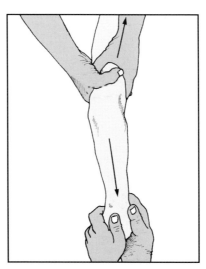

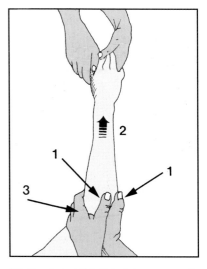

81. Radiographs cntd: The lateral shows posterior and proximal displacement. These combined appearances are those found in the commonest dislocation of the elbow, the posterolateral dislocation. Accompanying fractures are uncommon, but it is wise to assume that there is an associated injury until you have demonstrated otherwise. In particular, post-reduction films should be carefully scrutinised. In adults, look for fractures of the coronoid process and the radial head, and in children, the epicondyles or the lateral condyle.

82. Treatment (a): Reduction should be carried out under general anaesthesia. A fair amount of force is often required, although the use of a muscle relaxant will reduce this. Apply strong traction in the line of the limb, and if necessary slightly flex the elbow while maintaining traction. Success is usually accompanied with a characteristic reduction 'clunk'.

83. Treatment (b): If the last manoeuvre is unsuccessful, clasp the arm and push the olecranon forwards and medially (1), using traction in moderate flexion (2) and counter-traction with the fingers (3).

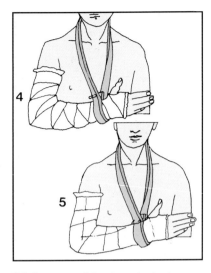

84. Treatment (c): After reduction has been achieved, take check radiographs, and apply a padded crepe bandage; this may be worn with a sling for two weeks (4). Alternatively, apply a plaster back slab and sling with the elbow in 90° flexion (5). Avoid too early or too vigorous mobilisation, and also passive movements which run the risk of myositis ossificans.

85. Late diagnosed posterior dislocation in children: Between 3 weeks and 2 months, open reduction carries an unacceptable risk of myositis ossificans; if the dislocation is discovered within that period the injury should be treated conservatively and the elbow just mobilised. A quarter do well and need no further treatment; in the remainder (and in cases discovered later than 2 months) operative reduction should be attempted.

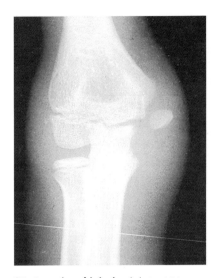

86. Associated injuries (a): In children, the medial epicondylar epiphysis may be detached. On *reduction of the elbow*, it will generally be restored to an acceptable position. A plaster slab and a sling are advised for 4 weeks. **(b)** The medial epicondyle may be retained in the joint: this must always be excluded (see Frame 55 et seq.).

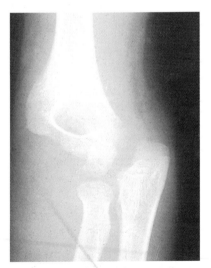

87. Associated injuries (c) – Lateral condylar injury: Note the following points. 1. The capitellar epiphysis (along with half the cartilaginous trochlea) has been carried medially by the radius, and is slightly rotated. 2. The medial epicondylar epiphysis has just appeared and is not displaced. 3. The *medial* dislocation of the elbow is unusual.

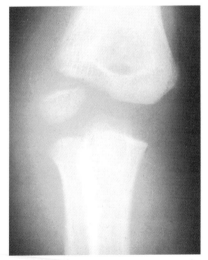

88. Associated injuries – Lateral condylar injuries cntd. The preceding injury was treated by manipulative reduction; the lateral condylar complex remained displaced. (Reduction could be achieved by firm local pressure, but displacement occurred in this unstable injury as soon as pressure was released.)

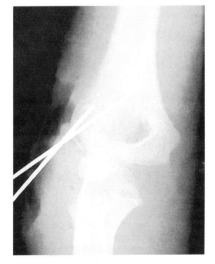

89. Associated injuries – Lateral condylar injuries cntd: Open reduction was therefore carried out and the condylar mass held in position with two K-wires. Note the small bone fragment from the shaft (Salter–Harris Type 2 injury). Fixation was complemented by a long arm plaster back shell for 4 weeks.

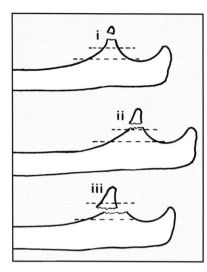

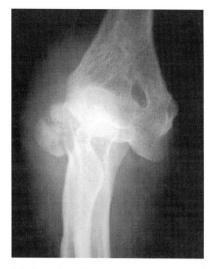

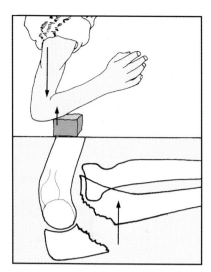

90. Associated injuries (d) – Fracture of the coronoid: Coronoid fractures can be classified into three types: (i) Simple avulsions; (ii) fractures involving half or less; (iii) fractures involving more than half. Groups (i) and (ii) may be treated conservatively, commencing mobilisation before 3 weeks. Group (iii) injuries may be internally fixed to reduce the risk of recurrent dislocation. *Established recurrent dislocation* (rare) may be treated by bone block reconstruction of the coronoid and/or repair of the capsule and medial ligament.

91. Associated injuries (e) – Fracture of the radial head: In general the dislocation should be reduced and if the radial head fracture is found to be of Type I or Type II (see Frame 114), then the treatment appropriate to that type of fracture should be followed without further delay. In highly comminuted Type III fractures of the radial head (as illustrated), primary radial head replacement is normally the treatment of choice.

92. Anterior dislocation of the elbow (a): This is an uncommon injury, but may follow a fall on the elbow which results in the forearm bones being pushed forwards. For dislocation to occur, the olecranon must fracture, and this becomes a potentially very unstable injury (see also p. 180).

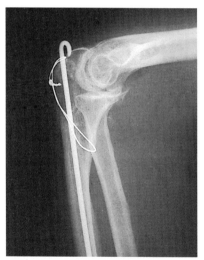

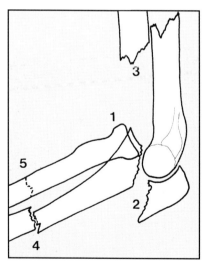

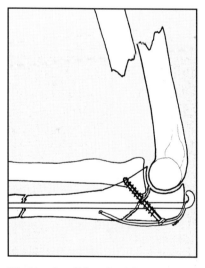

93. Anterior dislocation (b): The elbow may be reduced by applying traction and extending the joint. If the reduction is stable, it may then be treated by plaster fixation for a limited period in extension as in an anterior supracondylar fracture. Nevertheless, there is appreciable risk of late subluxation and difficulty in elbow mobilisation so that, on the whole, internal fixation is recommended for this injury (Illus: a Rush pin with tension band wiring: see Frame 95 for a preferred position for the wire).

94. Anterior dislocation (c): A more complex form of anterior dislocation is seen in the side swipe injury ('baby car fracture'). This occurs when a driver rests the elbow on a car's window ledge, and is struck by a passing vehicle. Typically the elements of this injury include (1) anterior dislocation of the elbow with fractures of (2) the olecranon, (3) the humerus, (4) the ulna and sometimes (5) the radius.

95. Anterior dislocation (d): It is vital to reduce the dislocation immediately, and this may be held by immediate internal fixation. (Illus: tension band wiring with an oblique cancellous bone screw; accompanying humeral and elbow fractures have been dealt with by plating and screwing.) Alternatively, the elbow may be reduced and held in plaster in extension for 2–3 weeks prior to delayed internal fixation. The other injuries may be treated with less urgency, conservatively or surgically.

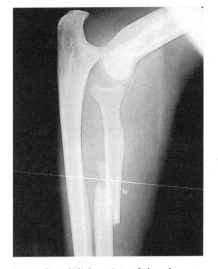

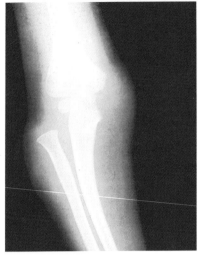

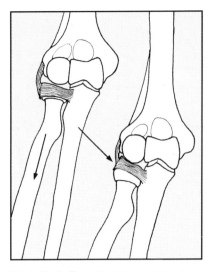

96. Isolated dislocation of the ulna:
Dislocation of the ulna may occur in association with a fracture of the radial shaft. As such fractures may be quite distal, it is important that adequate radiographs of the forearm are taken. This double injury may be treated by manipulative reduction of the elbow followed by a long arm plaster until the radius has united. However, to permit early mobilisation and the avoidance of elbow stiffness, internal fixation of the radius is to be preferred.

97. Isolated dislocation of the radius:
Lateral, anterior or posterior dislocation of the proximal end of the radius is almost invariably part of a Monteggia lesion (see p. 180) which is sometimes concealed because the ulnar fracture is of greenstick pattern (Illus.). Great care must be taken in the assessment and treatment of these injuries which is dealt with in detail later (pp. 180–181).

98. Pulled elbow (a): This condition is due to the radial head stretching the orbicular (annular) ligament and slipping out from under its cover. It occurs in children in the 2–6 age group, and is normally caused by a parent suddenly pulling on the child's arm (e.g. to prevent the child from running on to a road). It is also said to occur in wrestlers.

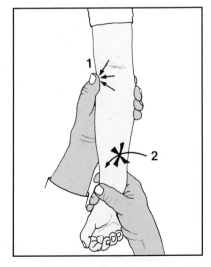

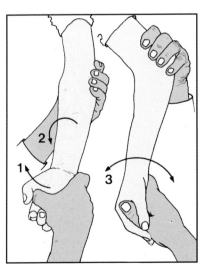

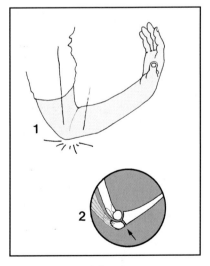

99. Pulled elbow (b) – Diagnosis: In addition to having the appropriate history of sudden traction on the arm, the child will be found to be fretful. There is tenderness over the lateral aspect of the joint (1) and supination is limited (2). Radiographs are usually normal, there being seldom any detectable increase in the radiohumeral joint space even with comparison films.

100. Pulled elbow (c) – Treatment: In most cases reduction can be achieved by either (i) placing the wrist in full radial deviation (1) and forcibly supinating the arm (2) or (ii) rapidly alternately pronating and supinating the forearm (3). If these measures fail, the arm should be rested in a sling, when spontaneous reduction usually occurs within 48 hours.

101. Fractures of the olecranon (a):
The olecranon may be fractured as a result of a fall on the point of the elbow (1). Such fractures may be displaced as a result of triceps contraction (2). The olecranon may also be fractured as a direct result of triceps contraction.

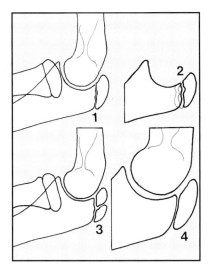

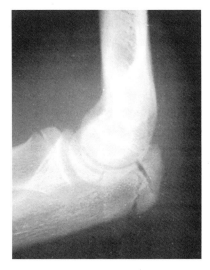

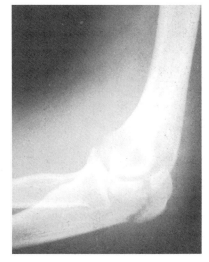

102. Fractures of the olecranon (b):
Diagnosis is usually straightforward, but beware of the following fallacies: (1) the normal epiphyseal line, (2) duplication of the normal line due to obliquity of the projection, (3) normal bifid olecranon epiphysis (the epiphyses appear between the ages of 8–11 and fuse at 14 years), (4) patella cubiti due to ossification in the triceps tendon (note rounded edges).

103. Treatment (a): If the fracture is hairline and undisplaced, it may be treated by immobilisation of the arm in a long arm plaster (3–4 weeks in a child, 6–8 weeks in an adult). Note the three lines running through the olecranon in the radiograph: the most distal is a fracture, the middle the epiphyseal line, the most proximal either a bifid epiphysis or a fracture of the epiphysis (differentiate by looking for tenderness).

104. Treatment (b): If the fracture line is pronounced but still undisplaced, it may be treated in the same way, but radiographs should be taken at weekly intervals during the first 3 weeks in case of (unlikely) late displacement. Minor epiphyseal separations may also be treated conservatively. Slight to moderate displacement may be accepted in the frail elderly.

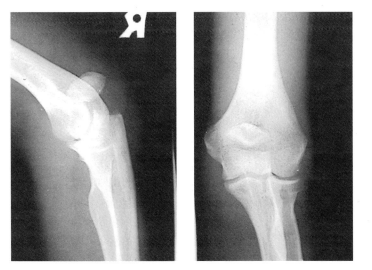

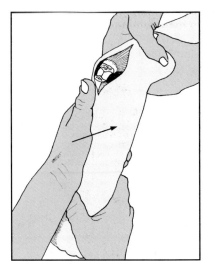

105. Treatment (c): If the olecranon fragment is small (a third or less of the articular surface) and significantly displaced (by triceps pull) surgical excision gives excellent results. This procedure is particularly useful in the elderly where the fragments may be osteoporotic. *Operation*: The operation is performed under a general anaesthetic using a pneumatic tourniquet to obtain a clear bloodless field. The fragment is exposed through a vertical posterior incision and excised. The tear in the triceps insertion is then carefully repaired with horizontal mattress sutures and the wound closed in layers. A pressure bandage (crepe over wool) and a collar and cuff sling are applied (or a plaster back shell and sling may be employed). The elbow may be mobilised after 2 weeks.

106. Treatment (d): If there is any doubt regarding the stability of the elbow (i.e. if the olecranon fragment is fairly substantial) this should be tested on the table by attempting to produce an anterior dislocation with the elbow flexed at 90°. If the elbow can in any way be subluxated, the olecranon must be retained.

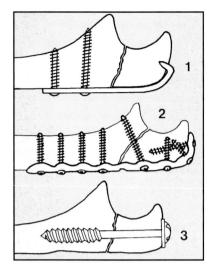

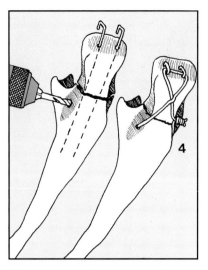

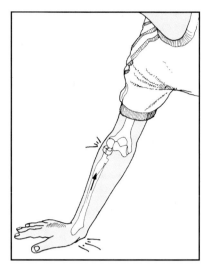

107. Treatment (e): If the olecranon fragment is substantial it must be reduced and held by some form of internal fixation. The many methods available include: (1) a Zuelzer or other hooked plate and screws; (2) a dynamic compression or other plate, contoured to fit round the olecranon; (3) a Croll or other pattern lag screw (e.g. an AO cancellous screw). During the final tightening of such a screw it is important to check that elbow movements are not prevented by the fracture components binding like calliper brakes.

108. Treatment (f): Tension band wiring: K-wires control alignment and rotation and the twisted stainless steel wire compresses the fragments together. The ends of the K-wires are bent over and hammered home. A Rush pin may also be used. The security of fixation dictates the need for any external fixation and when mobilisation may be commenced. Major separations in children may be treated by the insertion of two K-wires and a figure of eight of suture material rather than wire.

109. Fractures of the radial head – Mechanics of injury (a): Although the radial head may be fractured by direct violence, such as a fall or blow on the side of the elbow, injury frequently results from indirect violence (Illus.). A fall on the outstretched hand results in force being transmitted up the radius, with the radial head striking the capitellum (capitulum).

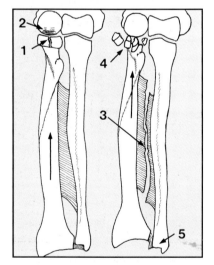

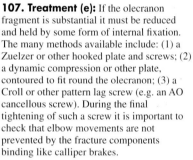

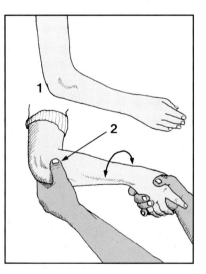

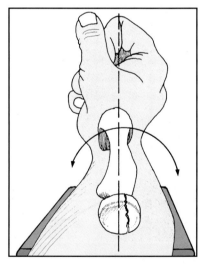

110. Mechanics of injury (b): The radial head fractures (1) but may also damage the articular surface of the capitellum (2), prolonging recovery. In some cases, where violence is severe, the interosseous membrane tears (3), severe comminution of the head occurs (4) and there is *subluxation of* the *distal end of the ulna* (5) due to proximal migration of the radial shaft. (Essex–Lopresti fracture–dislocation.)

111. Diagnosis (a): There is complaint of pain in the elbow and there may be local bruising and swelling (1). In minor fractures, tenderness may not be apparent until the damaged portion of the head is rotated under the examining thumb (gently pronate and supinate while palpating the radial head) (2). Somewhat paradoxically, the range of pronation and supination is often full, although elbow *extension* is usually restricted.

112. Diagnosis (b) – Radiographs: Most radial head fractures will show in the standard lateral and (supination) AP projections, but if there is clinical evidence of fracture and negative radiographs, *additional* AP projections should be taken in the midprone and full pronation position, so that all portions of the radial head will be visualised in profile.

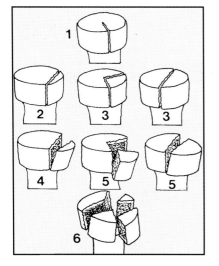

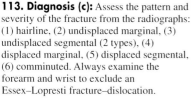

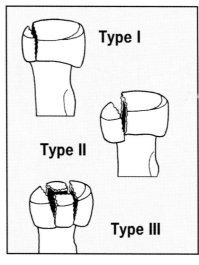

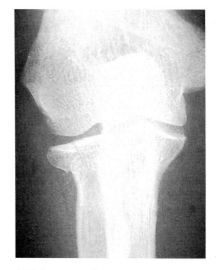

113. Diagnosis (c): Assess the pattern and severity of the fracture from the radiographs: (1) hairline, (2) undisplaced marginal, (3) undisplaced segmental (2 types), (4) displaced marginal, (5) displaced segmental, (6) comminuted. Always examine the forearm and wrist to exclude an Essex–Lopresti fracture–dislocation.

114. Classification of radial head fractures: The Hotchkiss modification of Mason's recognises three types. **Type I:** Small marginal fractures with displacements of less than 2 mm, and which do not appreciably compromise stability or affect rotation. **Type II:** Includes large two part fractures displaced by 2 mm or more, any fracture that restricts rotation, and comminuted fractures amenable to operative fixation. **Type III:** Highly comminuted fractures where operative fixation is not possible.

115. Treatment (a): Type I fractures such as of the pattern illustrated should be treated with a light compression bandage and a sling before mobilisation from the sling is commenced after 2–3 weeks. The sling alone may be worn for a further 2 weeks. If pain is very severe initially, a plaster back slab may be used. An excellent outcome is usual, but note that many months may elapse before full *extension* is regained.

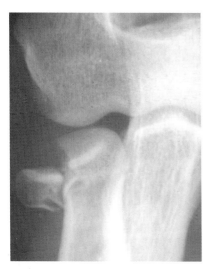

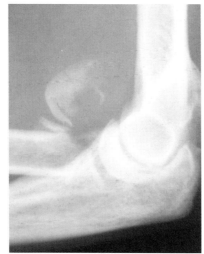

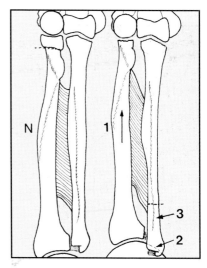

116. Treatment (b): Type II fractures (illustrated is a typical example) are probably best treated by open reduction and internal fixation (but see Frame 117), using, for example, small fragment screws. The procedure may be carried out through a lateral incision, taking care to avoid damaging the posterior interosseous nerve. Postoperatively the elbow should be supported in a sling, and mobilisation commenced as soon as possible, this being dependent on the quality of the fixation.

117. Treatment (c): Type III, severely comminuted fractures should be treated by immediate excision of the radial head. All fragments must be removed. The arm is then rested in a sling for 2–3 weeks before mobilisation. If there is valgus instability of the joint, demonstrable before or during surgery, then prosthetic replacement is advised, using, for example, a titanium implant.

118. Treatment (d): Sometimes excision of the radial head is followed by proximal drift of the radius (1) so that the distal end of the ulna becomes prominent and painful (2). This in turn may be treated by excision of the distal end of the ulna (3), albeit with some weakening of the grip. Proximal drift is a feature of the Essex–Lopresti lesion, and may be minimised by delaying radial head excision for 6 weeks.

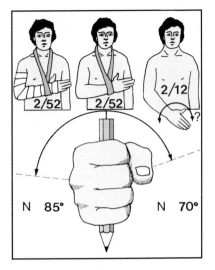

119. Treatment (e): Type II fractures may also be treated conservatively (see Frame 115), often with excellent results. They should be reassessed after 2–3 months. If pronation, supination and extension are severely restricted, *late excision* of the radial head should be considered. *Note*: It is generally advised that excision of the radial head should be performed *either* within the first 48 hours *or* after union (between carries the risk of myositis ossificans). *Late diagnosed injuries should be left until union.*

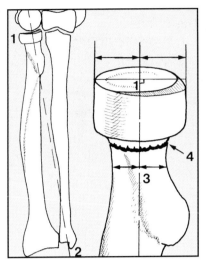

120. Fractures of the radial neck (a): The axis of rotation of the radioulnar joints passes through the centre of the radial head (1) and the attachment of the triangular fibrocartilage (2). The axis passes through the centre of the neck (3) and lies at right angles to the plane of the head. Fractures through the neck (4) have the potential to disturb this relationship between the head and the neck.

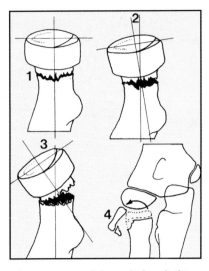

121. Fractures of the radial neck (b): Fractures of the radial neck may result from the same mechanisms as those causing fractures of the radial head, and the diagnostic features are also similar. Patterns: The fractures may be hairline and undisplaced (1) or result in slight (2) or gross tilting (3). In children, the epiphysis of the head may be completely separated and widely displaced (4).

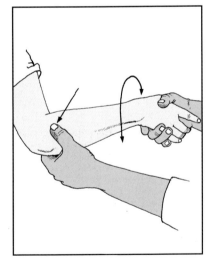

122. Treatment (a): With slight or no tilting (1 and 2) and up to 30° in children treat conservatively (as in Frame 115). With marked tilting (3) (20° or more in adults) manipulate. Do so by applying traction and gently pronate and supinate, feeling for the prominent part of the radial head to present; then apply pressure when the head is at its zenith. (Thereafter treat as in Frame 115.) Open reduction is indicated if closed methods fail.

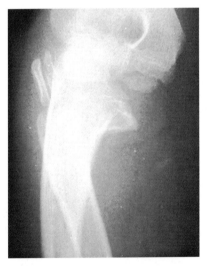

123. Treatment (b): Where there is gross epiphyseal displacement, operative reduction is indicated. On reduction, the fragments may be found to lock in a stable position. If not, a K-wire may be used for 2–3 weeks to achieve stability. *Note*: In some cases of severe tilting it is possible to obtain a reduction by inserting a temporary percutaneous wire into the radial head and levering it back into position under intensifier control.

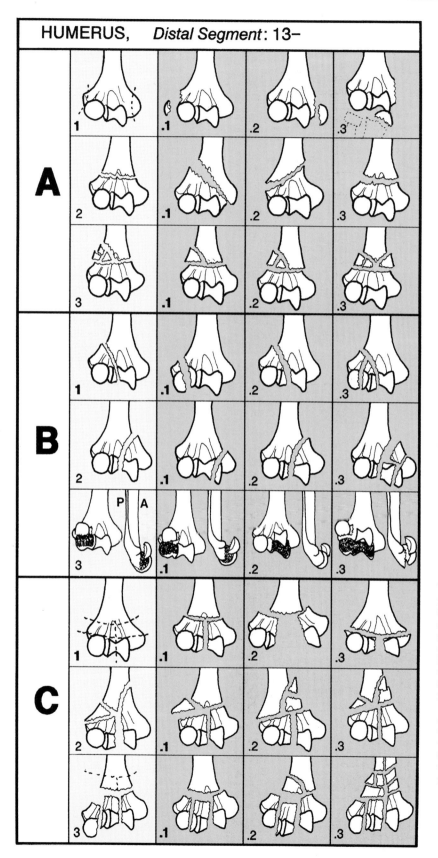

HUMERUS, *Distal Segment*: 13–

124. AO classification of fractures of the humerus, distal segment (13–):

Type A fractures are totally extra-articular.
A1 = Avulsion fracture (of apophysis): .1 lateral; .2 medial; .3 medial, with the fragment trapped in the joint.
A2 = Simple metaphyseal (supracondylar fracture): .1 with the proximal part of the fracture line lying lateral; .2 with proximal part of the fracture line lying medial; .3 with the fracture line lying transverse.
A3 = Multifragmented metaphyseal; .1 with an unbroken wedge; .2 with the wedge fragment fractured; .3 complex.

Type B fractures are partially articular.
B1 = Lateral sagittal (i.e. generally most obvious in the AP radiographic projection): .1 involving the capitellum; .2 simple trochlear; .3 multifragmentary trochlear.
B2 = Medial sagittal: .1 medial side of the trochlea; .2 through the trochlear notch; .3 multifragmentary trochlear.
B3 = Frontal (i.e. generally most obvious in the lateral radiographic projection): .1 of the capitellum; .2 of the trochlea; .3 of both the capitellum and the trochlea.

Type C fractures are complete articular fractures, and are multifragmentary.
C1 = Simple fractures of both the epiphysis and the metaphysis (T- and Y-fractures): .1 slight displacement only; .2 with marked displacement; .3 T-fractures with the horizontal limb distally placed so that it is in the epiphysis.
C2 = Simple fracture of the epiphysis, multifragmentary fracture of the metaphysis: .1 wedge intact; .2 wedge fractured; .3 complex.
C3 = Multifragmentary epiphyseal fracture with a simple or multifragmentary fracture of the metaphysis; .1 metaphysis simple; .2 wedge fracture of the metaphysis; .3 complex metaphyseal fracture.

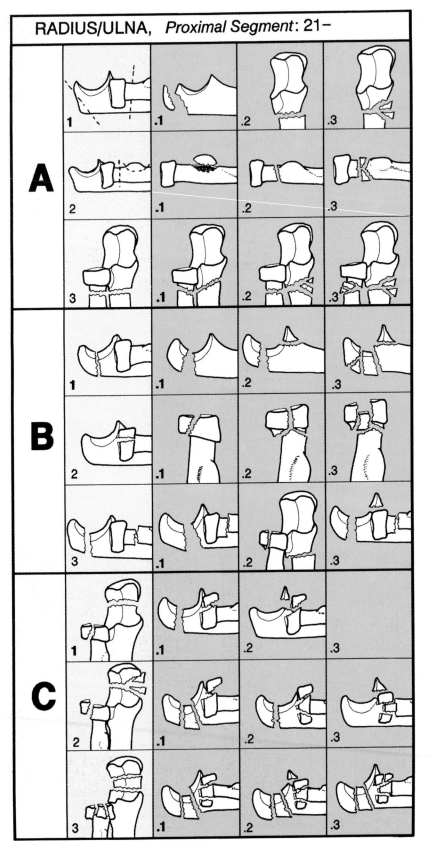

RADIUS/ULNA, *Proximal Segment*: 21-

125. AO classification of fractures of the radius/ulna, proximal segment (21-):

Type A fractures are extra-articular.
A1 = Fracture of the ulna only: .1 avulsion of the triceps insertion (olecranon); .2 simple, of the metaphysis; .3 multifragmentary, of the metaphysis.
A2 = Fracture of the radius only: .1 avulsion of the biceps insertion (radial tuberosity); .2 simple fracture of the neck; .3 multifragmentary of the neck.
A3 = Fracture of both the radius and ulna; .1 both simple; .2 one simple and the other multifragmentary; .3 both multifragmentary.

Type B fractures are partial articular fractures.
B1 = Articular fracture of the ulna with the radius intact: .1 unifocal, of the olecranon or coronoid; .2 bifocal (olecranon and coronoid) – both simple; .3 bifocal multifragmentary.
B2 = Articular fracture of the radius with the ulna intact: .1 simple fracture of the radial head; .2 multifragmentary fracture of the radial head without depression; .3 depressed multifragmentary fracture of the radial head.
B3 = Articular fracture of one bone, with an extra-articular fracture of the other: .1 simple articular fracture of the ulna; .2 simple articular fracture of the radius; .3 multifragmentary articular fracture of either bone.

Type C fractures are complete articular fractures.
C1 = Simple articular fractures of both bones: .1 head of radius and olecranon; .2 head of radius and coronoid. [There is no third subgroup here.]
C2 = Articular fractures of both bones, one simple and the other multifragmentary: .1 radial head simple, olecranon multifragmentary; .2 olecranon simple, radial head multifragmentary; .3 coronoid simple, radial head multifragmentary.
C3 = Both bones multifragmentary; .1 three fragments in each bone; .2 more than three fragments in the ulna; .3 more than three fragments in the radius.

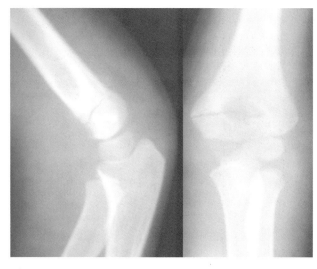

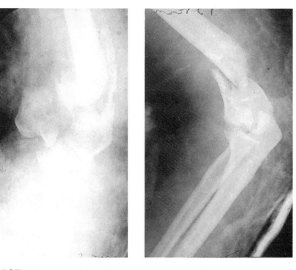

126. Diagnose and suggest treatment.

127. What is this injury? Comment on the position.

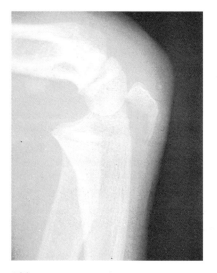

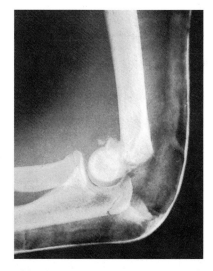

128. Diagnose and suggest treatment.

129. Comment on this AP radiograph of the elbow. What force has been responsible for the injury?

130. Comment on this supracondylar fracture which has been manipulated and put in plaster.

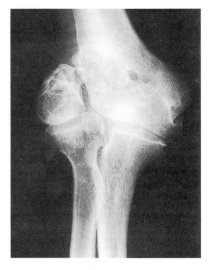

131. What is this fracture? What complication has occurred?

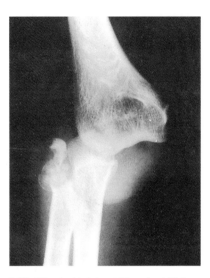

132. What is this injury? How should it be treated?

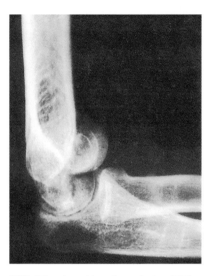

133. What does this radiograph show? What treatment will probably be required?

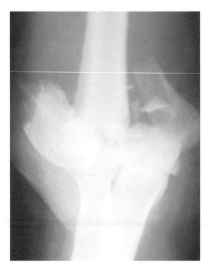

134. What is the nature of this fracture? How might it be treated?

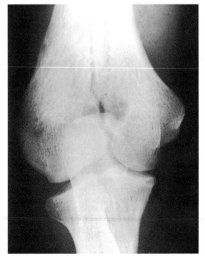

135. What fracture is present? How should this be treated?

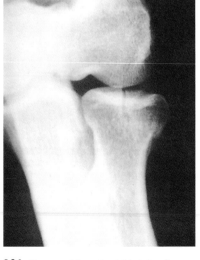

136. How would you treat this injury?

126. The radiographs show an undisplaced supracondylar fracture of the humerus in a child. Assuming there were no circulatory problems, a collar and cuff sling under the clothes should suffice for initial treatment. (AO = 13–A2.3.)

127. Y-fracture of the humerus. There is considerable separation of the two distal components, and open reduction and internal fixation should be considered unless the patient is particularly frail (when repeat manipulation with side-to-side compression may be undertaken). (AO = 13–C2.1.)

128. Dislocation of the elbow with fracture of the olecranon. The elbow should be reduced and check radiographs taken. Moderate residual displacement of the olecranon should be accepted, but if there is marked residual displacement then this should be reduced and fixed (e.g. with K-wires and a figure of eight suture not using wire). Note that the ossification centres for the olecranon have not yet appeared and this really represents a Salter–Harris Type 2 injury. (AO = 21–B1.1.)

129. There is a double injury – avulsion of the medial epicondyle and fracture of the radial neck, almost certainly both due to an abduction (valgus) injury. (Humerus: AO = 13–A1.2; radius: AO = 21–A2.2.)

130. This has been an anterior supracondylar fracture and the reduction is unacceptable. (AO = 13–A2.3.)

131. Fracture of the lateral condyle with non-union. (AO = 13–B1.1.)

132. Dislocation of the elbow with highly comminuted fracture of the radial head. Treat by reduction and immediate excision of the radial head, preferably with prosthetic replacement. (AO = 21–B2.3.)

133. Displaced fracture of the capitellum. Open reduction and internal fixation (e.g. with a Herbert screw) would be advised. (AO = 13–B3.1.)

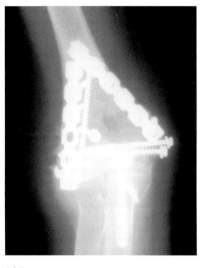

134. This is a comminuted Y-fracture of the distal humerus in an adult. (AO = 13–C1.3.) Here it has been dealt with by reduction and cross-screw stabilisation of the articular elements, which have subsequently been realigned and fixed to the shaft using reconstruction plates.

135. Undisplaced fracture of the distal humerus involving the elbow; more stress would probably have produced a Y-fracture. Treat by rest in a sling and early mobilisation. (AO = 13–B2.2.) Greater separation of the fragments would merit cross-screwing.

136. Undisplaced Type I fracture of the radial head: treat by crepe bandaging and rest in a sling. Mobilise after 2 weeks. (AO = 21–B2.1.)

Note

Fractures of the olecranon –
see Chapter 7, p 162

Fractures of the radial head –
see Chapter 7, p 164

Fractures of the radial neck –
see Chapter 7, p 166

For Colles fracture and other
fractures close to the wrist –
see Chapter 9

CHAPTER

8

Injuries to the forearm bones

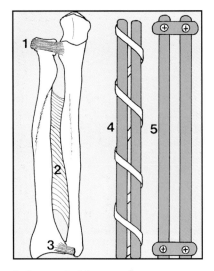

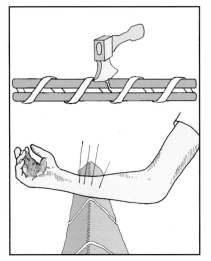

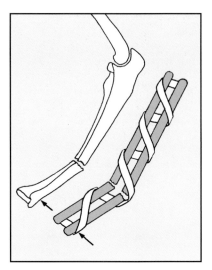

1. Anatomical features: The radius and ulna are bound together by (1) the annular (orbicular) ligament, (2) the interosseous membrane, (3) the radio-ulnar ligaments and the triangular fibrocartilage. This gives the radius and ulna some of the features of (4) a bundle of sticks and (5) a linked parallelogram.

2. Direct violence: With direct violence it is possible to fracture either of the forearm bones in isolation. These injuries are comparatively uncommon, but do occur, especially in the ulna when in a fall the shaft strikes a hard edge. They may also occur when the ulna is struck by a weapon as the victim attempts to protect the head with their arms.

3. Indirect violence: More commonly, the forearm is injured as the result of indirect violence, such as a fall on the back or the front of the outstretched hand. The force of impact on the hand stresses the forearm bones: the most common occurrence is for both to fracture.

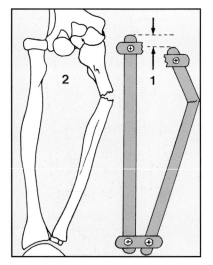

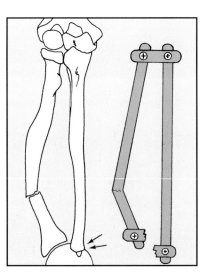

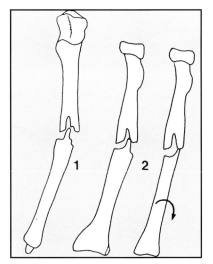

4. Fracture–dislocations (a): If *one* forearm bone is seen to be fractured and angled, it has inevitably become relatively shorter (1). If its attachments to the wrist and humerus are intact, the other forearm bone *must* be dislocated. The commonest fracture–dislocation of this type is a fracture of the ulna with a dislocation of the radial head (Monteggia injury) (2).

5. Fracture–dislocations (b): The same pattern of injury occurs in the Galeazzi fracture–dislocation when a dislocation of the distal ulna accompanies a shaft fracture of the radius. *Never accept a single forearm bone fracture as an entity until a Monteggia or Galeazzi injury has been eliminated.*

6. Axial rotation (a): In any forearm injury, when the ulna fractures it may angulate or displace like any other bone (1). When the radius fractures, however, *in addition* to angulation one fragment may rotate relative to the other (axial rotation) (2).

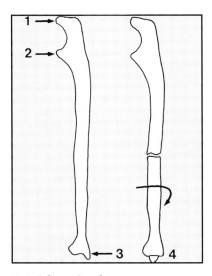

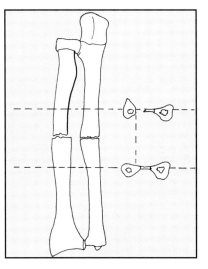

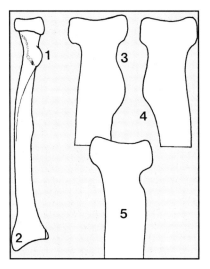

7. Axial rotation (b): Axial rotation of the ulna is rare, but always check to see that it is not present. To do so, note that in the lateral projection the olecranon (1), coronoid (2) and styloid process (3) should be clearly visible. This relationship is lost in the presence of axial rotation (4).

8. Axial rotation (c): In the case of the radius, note any discrepancy in the widths of the fragments at fracture level. A difference as illustrated indicates the presence of axial rotation.

9. Axial rotation (d): Note also the normal relationship between the radial tubercle (1) and the styloid process (2) in this AP view of the radius in full supination. In full supination the radial tubercle lies *medially* (3). In pronation it lies *laterally* (4). In the mid position it is concealed (5). The position of the radial styloid should always correspond.

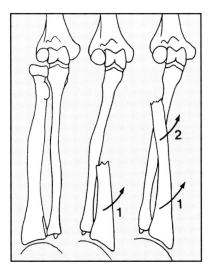

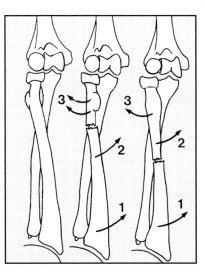

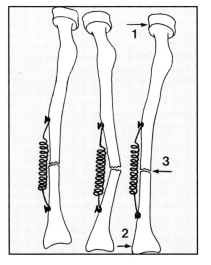

10. Axial rotation (e) – Forces responsible (a): In all radial shaft fractures, pronator quadratus tends to pronate the distal fragment (1). In all upper (proximal) third fractures, pronator teres helps to pronate the distal fragment (2), assisting pronator quadratus in this movement.

11. Axial rotation (f) – Forces responsible (b): In upper third fractures, the proximal fragment is fully supinated by biceps (3) while the distal fragment is fully pronated by pronators teres and quadratus (1 & 2), (i.e. there is a maximal tendency to axial rotation). In fractures distal to the mid third, biceps is opposed, so the proximal fragment tends to lie in the mid position.

12. Fracture slipping (a) – Greenstick fractures: In children's greenstick fractures any intact periosteum on the original concave surface of the fracture exerts a constant, springy force which may cause recurrence of angulation if the plaster slackens, impairing three-point fixation. *Frequent check films may be essential in any conservatively treated fracture.*

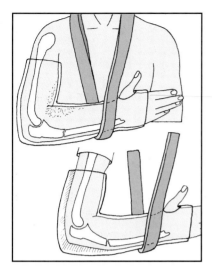

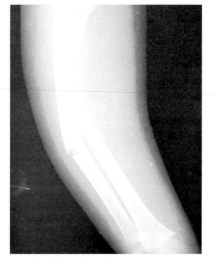

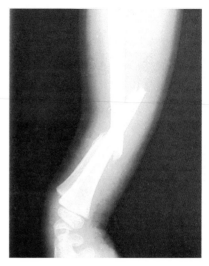

13. Fracture slipping (b): Another contributory cause of fracture slipping is when muscle wasting occurs in a patient in a full arm plaster wearing a collar and cuff sling. Loss of brachialis and brachioradialis bulk leads to plaster slackening and angulatory deformity. (*Note:* soft tissue shadow Frame 26.) *Patients with conservatively treated fractures should be given broad arm slings.*

14. Fracture of both bones of the forearm in children – Patterns (a): Most fractures are greenstick in pattern as illustrated. The radiograph shows fractures of the radius and ulna in the middle thirds. The distal fragments are tilted anteriorly (posterior angulation) but there is no displacement. An extensive, intact periosteal hinge can be assumed and reduction of such a fracture involves correction of the angulation only.

15. Patterns (b): When there is off-ending of one or both bones there is potential instability. Shortening and angulation are more likely, and axial rotation may occur; reduction may therefore be more troublesome. In some difficult cases the use of Nancy flexible intramedullary nails may be considered.

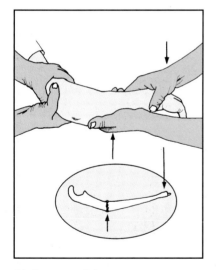

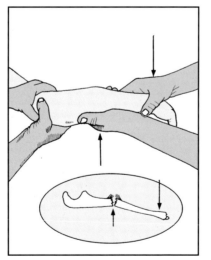

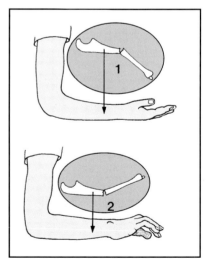

16. Treatment (a): In the undisplaced angulated greenstick fracture, the child should be given a general anaesthetic and the angulation corrected. One hand applies a little traction and the corrective force, while the other acts as a fulcrum, under the fracture.

17. Treatment (b): If the fracture is overcorrected, the periosteum on the initially concave side of the fracture will be felt to snap. This will immediately give the fracture more mobility: this has the advantage of reducing the risks of late angulation, but has the disadvantage of requiring greater care with respect to the initial positioning in plaster.

18. Treatment (c): In the undisplaced greenstick fracture where there is no rotational deformity, the arm should be placed in a stable position while the cast is applied. To prevent re-angulation, fractures with *posterior tilting* (anterior angulation) (1) are generally most stable in full pronation, while the commonest fractures with *anterior tilting* (posterior angulation) (2) are best in full supination. If an extreme position is required, the cast should be changed at four weeks and the arm put in a more neutral position.

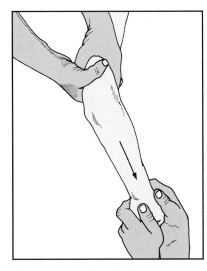

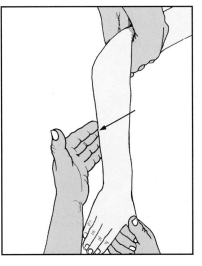

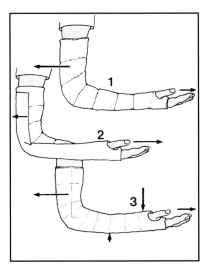

19. Treatment (d) – Displaced fractures: When the fracture is displaced, axial rotation of the fragments should be looked for and the appropriate position in the pronation/supination range evaluated. The forearm is then placed in that position, and strong traction is applied for a quarter of a minute or so, with the patient well relaxed under a general anaesthetic. The elbow is flexed at a right angle for counter-traction.

20. Treatment (e) – Displaced fractures cntd: Assessment of reduction is difficult, but often residual displacement may be detected by feeling the subcutaneous surface of the ulna in the region of the fracture. In the difficult case it is sometimes possible to gain bony apposition by applying traction and *increasing* the deformity before finally correcting it. Only rarely is open reduction and internal fixation indicated.

21. Treatment (f) – Fixation: To lessen the risks of ischaemia apply a back shell only, maintaining traction while this is done. Wool (1) is followed by the shell (2), held by cotton bandages. Just before the plaster sets give a final moulding (e.g. 3 – post-angulation fracture). Review the check radiographs before withdrawing the anaesthetic. (Note that some proximal third fractures in children are only stable with the elbow in extension, and this position can be maintained for 5 weeks with relative safety.)

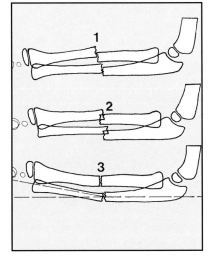

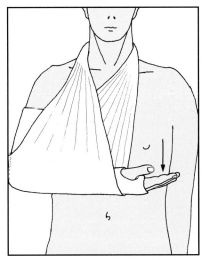

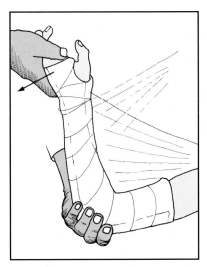

22. Radiographs: (1) Persistent displacement without angulation may be readily accepted. (2) Complete off-ending without angulation: remanipulate but accept if no improvement can be gained. Careful surveillance to detect early angulation is essential. (3) Slight angulation (10° or less), while undesirable, *will* correct with remodelling in the younger child, and should be accepted. Marked angulation requires remanipulation.

23. Treatment (g): A broad arm sling, keeping the arm well elevated, should be employed, and the fingers exposed. If there is much swelling, or the reduction has been difficult, the patient should be admitted for elevation of the arm and circulatory observation: otherwise the child must be seen within 24 hours of the application of the plaster and the parents given the usual warnings.

24. Treatment (h): On review, the fingers should be checked for swelling, colour and active movements. If there is some doubt, slowly and gently extend the fingers – if this produces excessive pain, it is suggestive of ischaemia. If ischaemia is present, the encircling bandages must be split and the situation carefully re-assessed after a short interval. If the circulation is perfect, the plaster may be completed.

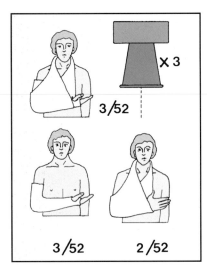

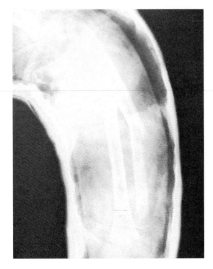

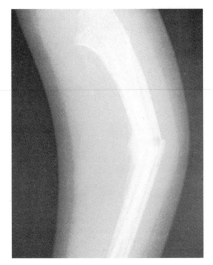

25. Treatment (i): In stable and unstable injuries check the cast and the position of the fracture at fortnightly or weekly intervals respectively for 3–4 weeks; if satisfactory, the sling may then be discarded. Plaster fixation is maintained till union (usually after a further 3–4 weeks in a child of 10 years, and a further 1–2 weeks in a child of 4). The arm may be placed in a neutral position at 4 weeks if an extreme position was initially required. Thereafter mobilisation may be commenced from a sling.

26. Management of late angulation (a): (Detected by progress films.) Slight angulation of up to 10° may be accepted, especially under the age of 10, but a slack plaster must be changed to prevent *further* angulation. Where angulation is more severe and has been detected before callus has appeared (Illus.) the plaster should be changed under general anaesthesia and the angulation corrected by manipulation. (If the fracture is rigid, consider drilling the bone and an osteoclasis.)

27. Management of late angulation (b): In a young child, if callus has appeared, accept any angulation unless gross (20° or more). In the older child, say 10 years or over, if angulation is marked remanipulation (or osteoclasis) should be considered even in the presence of callus (Illus.), as the powers of remodelling are less good. Union after remanipulation is usually rapid.

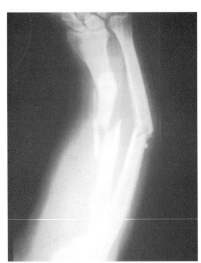

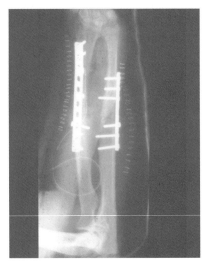

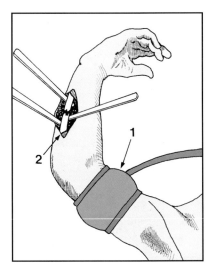

28. Adult fractures: In the adult displacement, angulation, rotation and comminution may be quite marked and closed reduction is often difficult or impossible to achieve. Even if an acceptable position can be obtained, and a cast successfully applied, late slipping of the fracture is extremely common and difficult to treat. The best treatment for displaced fractures of the forearm bones in the fit adult is open reduction and internal fixation, usually by plating both bones through separate incisions.

29. Adult fractures cntd: 3.5 mm AO dynamic compression plates are commonly used, with the radial plate contoured to fit the curve of the shaft. The screws should preferably engage 6 cortices above and below the fracture, using, where possible, additional interfragmentary screws and a bone graft if there is any residual gap. Bone grafting is also advised if there is no sign of callus by six weeks. The aim is to achieve a rigidity of fixation which will permit early mobilisation.

30. Treatment (a): The radius and ulna are exposed separately to minimise the risks of cross union, and a tourniquet is used (1). The ulna is subcutaneous along its posterior border; a longitudinal posterior incision, followed by exposure and cleaning of the bone ends, usually permits easy reduction (2). Plating is usually carried out to stabilise the fracture; intramedullary nailing may not always control any (slight) tendency to axial rotation.

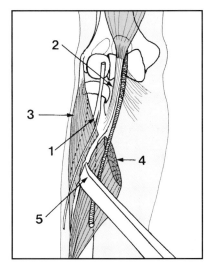

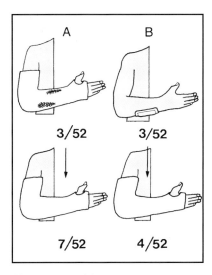

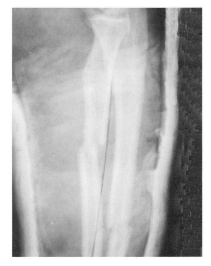

31. Treatment (b): Unless the radial fracture is in the distal third, a formal (Henry) exposure is required to avoid damage to the posterior interosseous nerve (1). The biceps tendon (2) is followed down to the tubercle, and the plane between the supinator (3) and the pronator teres (4) located. The supinator is reflected laterally (5) carrying the nerve away from danger. The rest of the shaft may then be exposed safely for reduction and plating.

32. Treatment (c): *If the internal fixation is rigid, no external support is necessary and the arm can be fully mobilised from the start.* If the fixation is not rigid (A), a cast may be used until there is reasonable callus formation round both fractures (often at about 10 weeks), changing the cast to remove the sutures at 3 weeks. With better fixation (B), after few days with a crepe support the arm may be mobilised fully and then a cast provided for a short period after discharge from hospital.

33. Treatment (d): It is reasonable to treat fractures of the forearm bones in the adult conservatively (Illus.): 1. if the fractures are undisplaced, 2. in the elderly, or in the patient suffering from multiple injuries where the duration of anaesthesia required for open reduction and internal fixation is considered hazardous. If manipulation is required, proceed (as described at Frame 19) with attention to axial rotation.

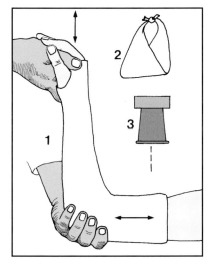

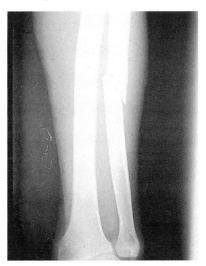

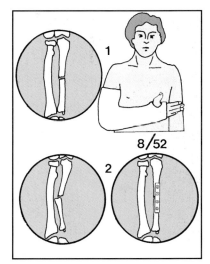

34. Treatment (e): In conservatively treated fractures, the following precautions must be taken. (1) The plaster should be checked weekly for slackness, and changed if necessary. (A complete plaster, applied over wool, should be used in an adult.) (2) A broad arm rather than a collar and cuff sling should be used. (3) Weekly radiographs are necessary to detect and allow the correction of early slipping.

35. Isolated fracture of the ulna (a): This injury may result from direct violence (e.g. in warding off a blow from a stick or falling object, or by striking the arm against the sharp edge of, for example, a machine or a step). In all cases, however, the whole of the radial shaft should be visualised to exclude, in particular, an associated dislocation of the radial head.

36. Isolated fracture of the ulna (b) – Treatment: As there is an appreciable incidence of non-union, some prefer early open reduction and internal fixation for all these fractures. Where displacement is slight, conservative treatment may be used. A long arm plaster should be applied with the hand in mid pronation (1). Beware however of late slipping. The plaster is retained until union is advancing (usually about 8 weeks). If angulation is marked, then open reduction and internal fixation will have to be considered (2).

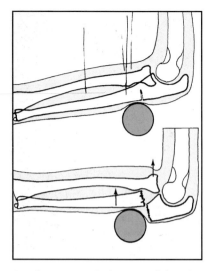

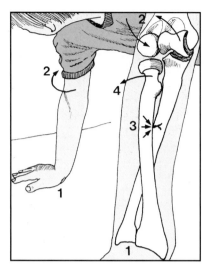

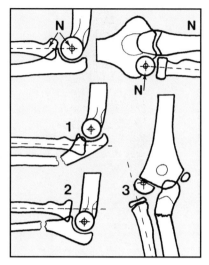

37. The Monteggia fracture–dislocation and related injuries – Mechanisms (a): Severe angulation of a forearm bone is normally accompanied by fracture or dislocation of the other (see Frames 3 and 4). In the Monteggia fracture–dislocation, fracture of the ulna is associated with dislocation of the radial head. The most easily understood mechanism is when a violent fall or blow on the arm fractures the ulna and displaces the radial head anteriorly.

38. Mechanisms (b): More commonly, the injury results from forced pronation. A fall on the outstretched, fully pronated arm (1) is followed by further pronation as the trunk continues to turn over the fixed hand (2). The radius is forced against the ulna, fracturing it (3) and in turn is levered away from the capitellum (4). Rarely, the radial head may dislocate without damage to the ulna; *supination* of the arm is needed for reduction.

39. Patterns (a): (N) In the normal elbow a line through the axis of the radius cuts the centre of the spherical capitellum). (1) The radial head may dislocate backwards with fracture and posterior angulation of the ulna (posterior Monteggia). (2) The radial head may dislocate anteriorly, with anterior angulation of the ulna (anterior Monteggia). Or (3) the radial head may dislocate laterally, with lateral angulation of the ulna (lateral Monteggia).

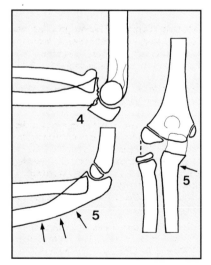

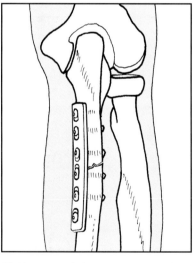

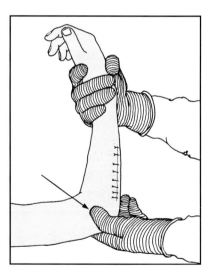

40. Patterns (b): (4) The radial head may dislocate anteriorly and be as associated with a fracture of the olecranon (Hume fracture). (5) Greenstick fracture of the ulna, often difficult to detect, partly accounts for the fact that Monteggia lesions are frequently overlooked in children. *Always* check the position or the radial head in both views, and *always* look for distortion and kinking of the ulna.

41. Treatment (a): The key to successful management of this potentially difficult injury is accurate reduction of the ulnar fracture. In the adult, and in children with displaced fractures, this is best achieved by open reduction and internal fixation. The fracture is easily approached through a posterior incision, and the reduction may be held with a plate applied to the medial aspect of the ulnar shaft with cortical screws.

42. Treatment (b): Thereafter the elbow should be placed in right-angled flexion. The position of the radial head should be checked by palpation and by radiographs. Full supination may be required to maintain reduction, but generally the neutral position will be satisfactory in maintaining stability after the ulna has been fixed. If the radial head will not reduce in full supination, it should be exposed, any loose cartilage fragments removed, and any tear in the orbicular ligament sutured.

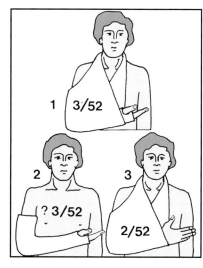

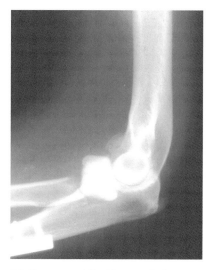

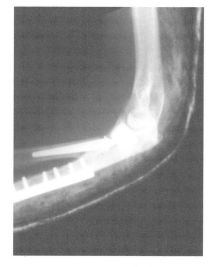

43. Treatment (c) – Aftercare: (1) The plaster is changed at 3 weeks and the stitches removed. (2) Plaster is finally discarded when, on your assessment, there is adequate stability. Your opinion will be based on the type of fixation, its technical adequacy, callus formation, etc. In practice, mobilisation from a sling (3) may often be started about 4 weeks. Physiotherapy is often required.

44. Treatment (d) – Monteggia fracture associated with comminution of the radial head: In this example, the ulnar shaft fracture was reduced and plated. There was an open comminuted fracture of the radial head. A thorough debridement of the wound was carried out and the fragmented radial head was removed. A plug of antibiotic impregnated cement (Palacos™) was then inserted as a temporary spacer.

45. Treatment – Monteggia fracture associated with comminution of the radial head cntd: Once sound wound healing had been obtained, the cement was excised and a bipolar radial head replacement substituted. Immediate mobilisation could then be commenced.

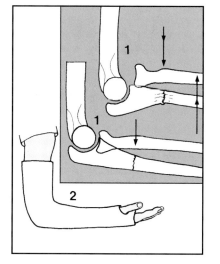

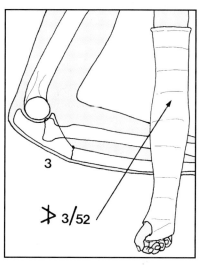

46. Treatment (e) – Monteggia fractures in children (a): Any greenstick angulation of the ulna should be corrected by manipulation (1). Anterior Monteggia fractures should be put up in a position of 90° flexion at the elbow and in supination (2).

47. Treatment – Monteggia fractures in children cntd: Posterior Monteggia fractures (3) are often stable in full extension and may be fixed for not more than 3 weeks in this position: the elbow should be brought into a more flexed position for the remainder of the time in plaster. The position of the radial head must be confirmed by weekly radiographs; if there is any evidence of incongruity, exploration may have to be considered.

48. Late diagnosed Monteggia lesions:
1. In the adult, some restriction of elbow movements may be the only complaint. Excision of the radial head may give temporary relief, but is often followed by proximal drift of the radius and troublesome subluxation of the ulna at the wrist.
2. Tardy ulnar nerve palsy may be the patient's first complaint; transposition of the ulnar nerve is often effective in arresting the progress of this condition.
3. In children, excision of the radial head is contraindicated – it would lead to growth disturbance. In some cases manipulative correction may be possible depending on the delay.

In exceptional circumstances the condition may be very late in being brought to light. In children under the age of 10 good results have been claimed for surgery performed as late as 4 years after the initial injury. (Such late reconstructions involve:
1. Excision of scar tissue in the region of the radiohumeral joint.
2. Proximal ulnar osteotomy.
3. Reduction of the radial head.
4. Reconstruction of the annular ligament using palmaris longus or triceps fascia.)

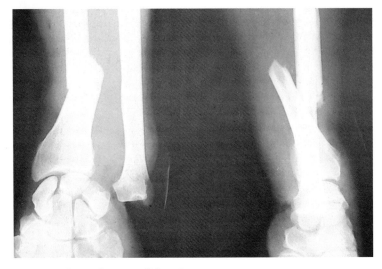

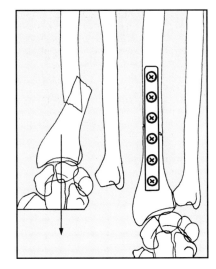

49. The Galeazzi fracture–dislocation: This is a fracture of the radius associated with a dislocation of the inferior radio-ulnar joint. Note that in the normal wrist the distal end of the ulna (excluding the styloid process) lies just proximal to the articular surface of the radius, the space between being occupied by the triangular fibrocartilage. If the radius is fractured, *always* look for subluxation of the ulna.

50. Galeazzi fracture – Treatment (a): In the adult, open reduction and plating of the radius through an anterior incision eliminate the risks of late slipping. Reduction of the radius is followed by spontaneous reduction of the ulnar subluxation, and only in exceptional circumstances does the inferior radio-ulnar joint require opening. With stable internal fixation and an intact ulna, there is less need for additional external fixation.

53. Isolated fracture of the radius (b): *In the adult,* isolated fractures of the radius with no significant angulatory or rotational deformity may be treated in plaster with the arm in supination. Slight axial rotation may be controlled by careful positioning of the forearm; in all cases careful surveillance is vital to detect early slipping, an indication for operative intervention.

In children, isolated fractures of the radius should also be treated conservatively.

Non-union of the radius: This complication may be treated along standard lines by internal fixation and bone grafting.

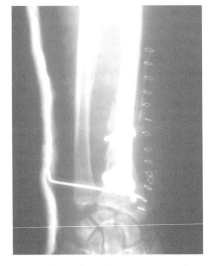

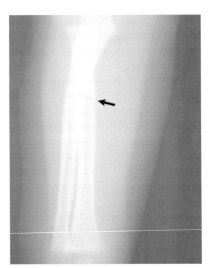

51. Galeazzi fracture – Treatment (b): If displacement of the ulna persists after internal fixation of the radius, a K-wire for 3 weeks may be used to stabilise the inferior radio-ulnar joint.
Galeazzi fracture–dislocations in children: Manipulate and put up in plaster in supination. Open reduction is seldom required.
Late diagnosed Galeazzi lesions: Prominence of the ulna with pain in the wrist is the commonest complaint and excision of the distal ulna may give relief.

52. Isolated fracture of the radius (a): Fracture of the radius can occur without initial involvement of the inferior radio-ulnar joint. This comparatively uncommon situation may follow direct injury to the radius which results in an undisplaced fracture. Nevertheless, late subluxation of the inferior radio-ulnar joint may appear when, as is frequent, late angulation of the fracture occurs.

54. Forearm compartment syndromes:

These occur most frequently after fractures of both the forearm bones, but may follow supracondylar fractures and fractures of the radial head and neck in children. The condition should be suspected if: 1. There is marked pain on passive extension of the fingers; 2. There is reduced sensation or paraesthesia in the hand; 3. There is a significant rise in compartment pressure: this is most useful in the unconscious patient. Both anterior and posterior compartments may be affected, but the anterior is most commonly involved. Release of pressure in the anterior compartment usually results in a fall of pressure in the posterior compartment, but if pressure monitoring shows pressure in the posterior compartment separate decompression (through an additional, linear posterior incision) may be required)

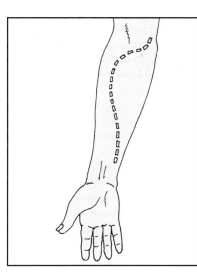

Method: A curvilinear incision is generally advised. (McConnell's approach (Illus.), as described by Henry, not only allows decompression of the anterior compartment, but exposure if required of both the median and ulnar nerves.) The decompression must include:

1. The lacertus fibrosus (bicipital aponeurosis).
2. The fascia over flexor carpi ulnaris.
3. The fascia over the edge of flexor digitorum superficialis.

If injury to the median nerve is suspected, the likely sites of its compression are:

1. At the lacertus.
2. Over the proximal margin of pronator teres.
3. At the proximal margin of flexor digitorum superficialis.

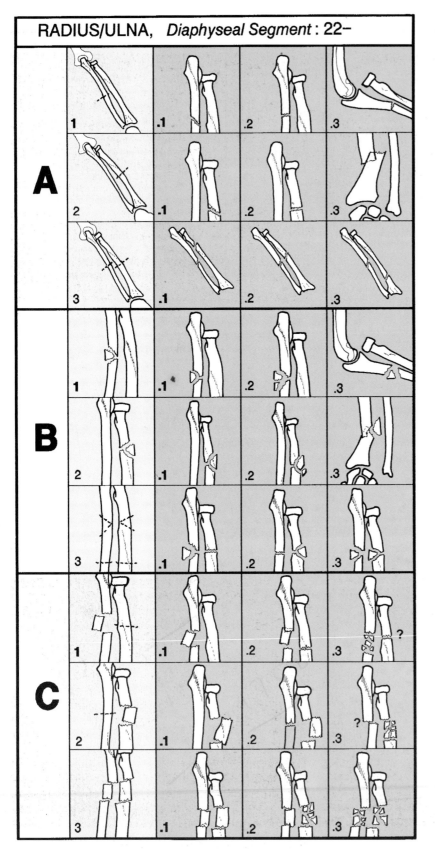

RADIUS/ULNA, *Diaphyseal Segment : 22–*

55. AO classification of fractures of the radius/ulna, diaphyseal segment (22–):

Type A are simple (i.e. there is a circumferential disruption of the bone), involving one or both bones.

A1 = Simple fracture of the ulna with an intact radius: .1 oblique; .2 transverse; .3 with dislocation of the radial head (Monteggia fracture–dislocation).

A2 = Simple fracture of the radius, with the ulna intact: .1 oblique; .2 transverse; .3 with dislocation of the distal radio-ulnar joint (Galeazzi fracture–dislocation).

A3 = Simple fracture of both bones: .1 proximal part of radius involved; .2 middle third of radius fractured; .3 fracture of distal radius.

Type B fractures are wedge fractures (i.e. there is a separate (butterfly) segment, but after reduction there is contact between the main fragments (a so-called hitch)); one or both bones are involved.

B1 = Wedge fracture of the ulna and an intact radius; .1 wedge intact; .2 multifragmentary wedge; .3 with dislocation of the radial head (Monteggia fracture–dislocation).

B2 = Wedge fracture of the radius and an intact ulna: .1 wedge intact; .2 multifragmentary wedge; .3 with dislocation of the distal radio-ulnar joint (Galeazzi fracture–dislocation).

B3 = Wedge fracture of one bone, with a simple or wedge fracture of the other: .1 wedge ulna; .2 wedge radius; .3 wedge fractures of both bones.

Type C fractures are complex (i.e. they have more than two fragments, and even after reduction the pattern is such that there is no contact between the main fragments); one or both bones may be involved.

C1 = Complex fracture of the ulna: .1 bifocal with radius intact ; .2 bifocal with radius fractured; .3 irregular, with or without fracture of radius.

C2 = Complex fracture of the radius: .1 bifocal with ulna intact; .2 bifocal with fracture of ulna; .3 irregular, with or without fracture of ulna.

C3 = Complex fracture of both bones; .1 bifocal of both bones; .2 bifocal of one bone and irregular fracture of the other; .3 irregular fracture of both bones.

SELF-TEST

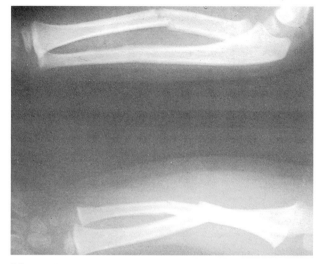

56. Describe this fracture. What treatment would you advocate?

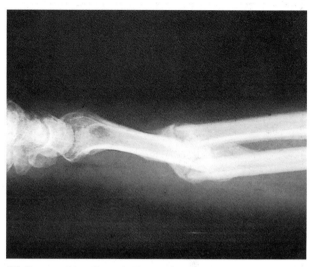

57. Interpret this radiograph. How might this appearance be avoided?

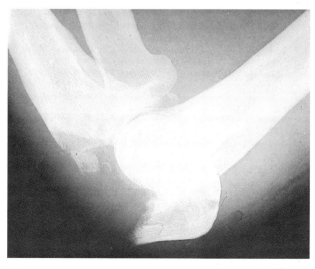

58. What is this injury?

59. Describe this injury. How would you treat it?

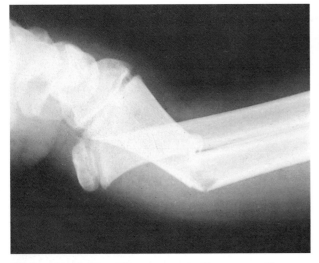

60. Describe this injury. What treatment would you carry out?

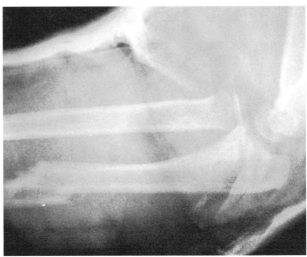

61. Comment on this radiograph.

ANSWERS TO SELF-TEST

56. Greenstick fractures of the radius and ulna, with anterior angulation. Treat by manipulation under general anaesthesia and the application of long arm plaster slab. (AO = 22–A3.3.)

57. Cross-union has occurred in this fracture of the radius and ulna. The distal fragments have rotated 90° relative to the proximal fragments (malunion). No pronation or supination will be possible. This would be avoided by open reduction and internal fixation through separate incisions. (AO = 22–A3.3.)

58. Hume fracture (anterior Monteggia fracture–dislocation where the ulnar fracture involves the olecranon). (In the AO classification this would appear as a special variety of radius/ulnar proximal segment; as there is a small coronoid fracture this would be classified as 21–B1.2.)

59. Adult anterior Monteggia fracture–dislocation, with a fracture of the ulna in the proximal part of its middle third, with anterior angulation; the radial head is dislocated anteriorly. Treatment would be by open reduction and internal fixation of the ulna; reduction of the radial head would then have to be confirmed. (AO = 22–A1.3.)

60. Galeazzi fracture–dislocation in a child; there is a greenstick fracture of the radius with anterior angulation. The distal end of the ulna is dislocated anteriorly. (AO = 22–A2.3.)

61. The radiograph is of an arm in plaster; there is a fracture of the ulna, apparently in reasonable alignment in this single view but the radial head is dislocated anteriorly, i.e. this is an anterior Monteggia fracture–dislocation which has not been satisfactorily reduced. The arm appears to be in the mid-prone position, and reduction of the radial head might have been achieved if the arm had been placed in supination. Further treatment here is imperative (e.g. remanipulation and placing the arm in supination; should this fail to reduce the dislocation of the radial head, exploration of the radiohumeral joint would have to be considered (preferably after plating of the ulna). (AO = 22–A1.3.)

CHAPTER

9

The wrist and hand

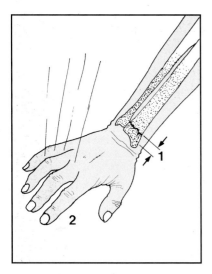

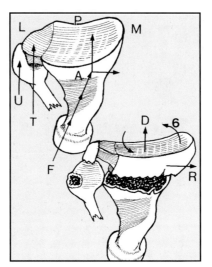

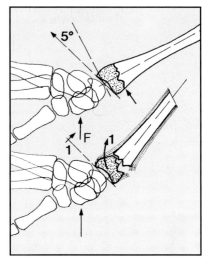

1. Colles fracture: A Colles fracture is a fracture of the radius within 2.5 cm of the wrist (1), with a characteristic deformity if displaced. It is the commonest of all fractures. It is seen mainly in middle-aged and elderly women, and osteoporosis is a frequent contributory factor. It usually results from a fall on the outstretched hand (2), and generally the distal radial fragment remains intact. (See Frame 44 et seq for those other cases where the radiocarpal joint is involved.)

2. Displacements (a): The *six* characteristic features of a displaced Colles fracture (see later for details) are shown in this foreshortened view of the pronated right arm, viewed from below. The slight obliquity of impact (F) produces the two most striking features of *dorsal* and *radial* displacement (D & R) of the distal fragment. (T = triangular fibrocartilage; U = ulnar styloid; M = medial; L = lateral.)

3. Displacements (b): The deformity can be followed by studying the wrist in the two planes in which the radiographs are usually taken. The impact (F) fractures the radius through the cancellous bone of the metaphysis. With greater violence the anterior periosteum tears, and the distal fragment tilts into *anterior angulation* (1) with loss of the 5° anterior tilt of the joint surface.

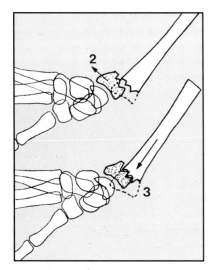

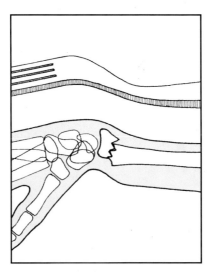

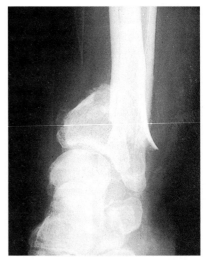

4. Displacements (c): With greater violence there is *dorsal displacement of the distal fragment* (2). The shaft of the radius is driven into the distal fragment leading to impaction (3). (The dotted lines indicate the position of the distal fragment prior to any displacement.)

5. Displacements (d): The altered contour of the wrist in a badly displaced Colles fracture is striking, and is referred to as a 'dinner fork deformity'. When viewed from the side, the wrist has the same curvature as a fork, with the tines resembling the fingers.

6. Displacements (e): This radiograph shows a typical displaced Colles fracture. The anterior angulation, dorsal displacement, and impaction are obvious (deformities 1, 2, 3 in previous frames).

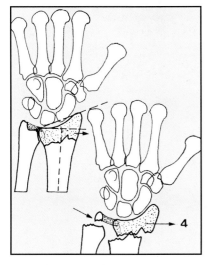

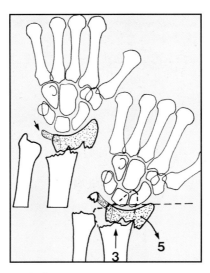

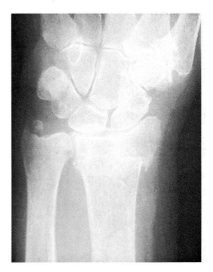

7. Displacements (f): In the AP plane, a small lateral component of the force of impact causes *lateral (radial) displacement of the distal fragment* (4). The distal fragment is attached to the ulnar styloid by the triangular fibrocartilage, and generally this leads to avulsion of the ulnar styloid. Note that in the AP projection of the normal wrist that the joint surface has a tilt of 22°.

8. Displacements (g): Sometimes the triangular fibrocartilage is torn; in either case there is disruption of the inferior radio-ulnar joint. The distal fragment tilts laterally into *ulnar angulation* (5) (reducing the tilt to less than 22°) and impacts (3). The sixth feature is a rotational or torsional deformity (6) (see Frame 2), not obvious in either AP or lateral projections.

9. Displacements (h): In this AP radiograph of a Colles fracture, note the features just mentioned, i.e. radial deviation, ulnar angulation and impaction of the distal fragment.

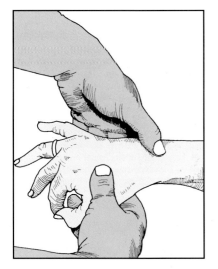

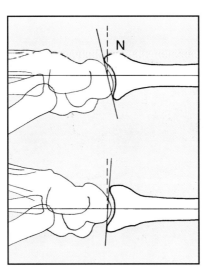

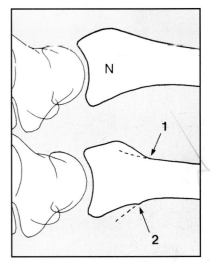

10. Diagnosis: 1. If there is pain in the wrist and tenderness over the distal end of the radius after a fall, radiographs must be taken in every case. The site of maximum tenderness will help to differentiate fracture of the scaphoid (but see scaphoid fractures). 2. Where there is marked displacement the characteristic appearance leaves little diagnostic doubt. Note that in the normal wrist the radial styloid lies 1 cm distal to the ulnar.

11. Radiographs (a): In the majority of cases the fracture is easily identified. Sometimes it may be missed because impaction has rendered the fracture line inconspicuous. If in doubt, look at the angle between the distal end of the radius and the shaft in the lateral radiograph. Decrease to less than 0° is suggestive of fracture (but enquire about previous injury). N = normal.

12. Radiographs (b): The minimally displaced fracture will also reveal itself in the lateral projection by an increase in the posterior radial concavity, often with local kinking (1) or by a separate or accompanying break in the smooth curve of the anterior surface of the radius (2). N = normal.

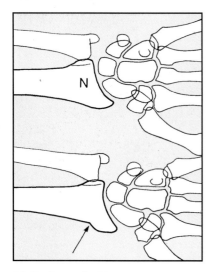

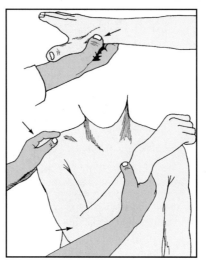

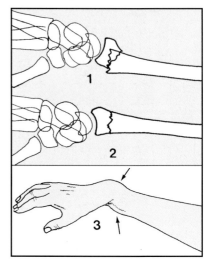

13. Radiographs (c): In the AP view of the wrist, look for any irregularity in the smooth lateral aspect of the radius. If there is any doubtful radiographic feature suggesting fracture, return to the patient *and confirm whether there is any localised tenderness over the suspect area.* N = normal.

14. Diagnosis cntd: As stated, a Colles fracture is generally caused by a fall on the outstretched hand – a mechanism common to many upper limb fractures. Although other injuries in the arm occurring in association with Colles fracture are *uncommon*, clinically the scaphoid, elbow and shoulder should be examined, and on the radiographs the scaphoid should be scrutinised. (Special views are required if an associated scaphoid fracture is strongly suspected.)

15. Treatment – Does the fracture require manipulation? (a): If the fracture is grossly displaced, it obviously should be reduced (1). If undisplaced, no manipulation is needed (2). Between these extremes, the following additional factors may be considered: if there is a readily appreciated naked eye deformity (3) manipulation should be carried out (but distinguish between *swelling* and *deformity*).

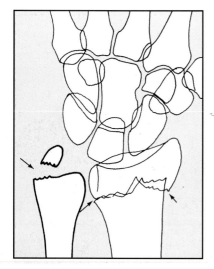

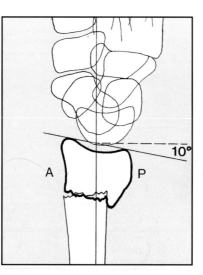

18. Reduction technique (a): Anaesthesia is necessary for the reduction of this fracture, and either a general anaesthetic or intravenous regional anaesthetic (Bier block) may be used with success. Although the latter has a good safety record, it should not be employed unless facilities for resuscitation are freely available. Where there is a preference for general anaesthesia but the patient attends late at night with a history of recent intake of food or drink, it is permissible and often safer to apply a temporary plaster back shell and an arm sling, and delay reduction of the fracture until morning.

16. Does the fracture require manipulation? (b): If there is displacement of the ulnar styloid, this indicates *serious disruption of the inferior radio-ulnar joint.* (Acute ulnar angulation of the distal fragment is also evidence of this.) An attempt at correction should be made *irrespective of other appearances.*

17. Does the fracture require manipulation? (c): If the joint line in the lateral projection is tilted 10° or more posteriorly rather than anteriorly, the fracture should be manipulated: but in the very old, frail patient somewhat greater degrees of deformity may be accepted.

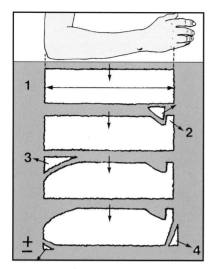

19. Reduction technique (b): Before any manipulation, start by preparing a suitable plaster back slab. The *length* should equal the distance from the olecranon to the metacarpal heads (1). The *width* in an adult should be 15 cm (6″), and it should be about eight layers thick. The slab should be trimmed with a tongue (2) for the first web space, a large radial curve to allow elbow flexion (3) and allowance for ulnar deviation (4).

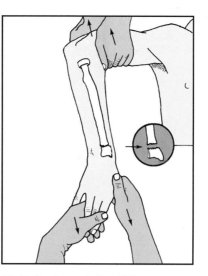

20. Reduction technique (c): The essential first stage in the reduction of a Colles fracture is to disimpact the distal radial fragment. The elbow is flexed to a right angle and the arm held by the interlocked fingers of an assistant (1). Traction is applied in the line of the forearm (2).

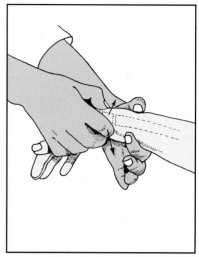

21. Reduction technique (d): Traction need only be applied for a few seconds, and disimpaction may be confirmed by holding the distal fragment between the thumb and index. It should be easy to move anteriorly and posteriorly. When disimpacted the radial styloid should lie 1 cm distal to the ulnar styloid.

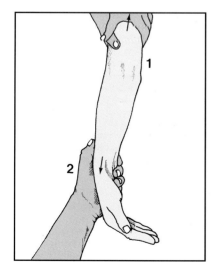

22. Reduction technique (e): The elbow is now extended (1). The heel of one hand should be placed over the dorsal surface of the distal radial fragment, and the fingers curled round the patient's wrist and palm (2). This grip allows traction to be re-applied to the disimpacted fracture.

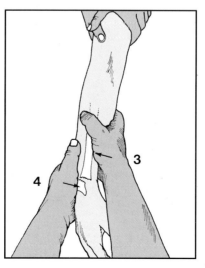

23. Reduction technique (f): Now, by using the heel of the other hand as a fulcrum (3) firm pressure directed anteriorly (4) will correct all the remaining deformities normally visible in lateral radiographs of the wrist (posterior displacement, anterior angulation).

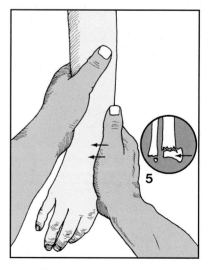

24. Reduction technique (g): Still maintaining traction, alter the position of the grip so that the heel (here of the right hand) is able to push the distal fragment ulnarwards and correct the radial displacement (5). Ulnar angulation, the other deformity seen in the AP radiograph, is corrected by placing the hand in full ulnar deviation at the wrist.

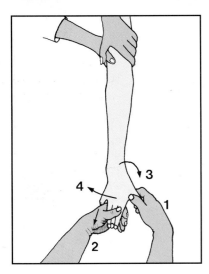

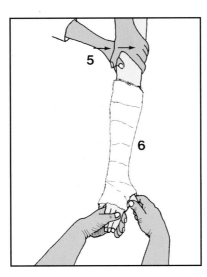

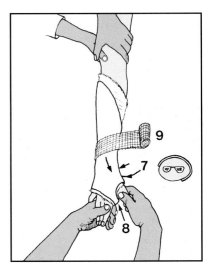

25. Reduction technique (h): Change the grip to allow free application of the plaster (which follows Charnley's principle of three point fixation). Note that one hand holds the thumb fully extended (1). The other holds three fingers (to avoid 'cupping' of the hand) maintaining slight traction (2). The limb should be in full pronation (3), *full* ulnar deviation at the wrist (4) and *slight* palmar flexion.

26. Reduction technique (i): Note that the elbow must be *extended* (either by an assistant (5) or by resting the upper arm against the edge of the table) to maintain this position. The skin may be protected with wool roll (6). If stockinet is preferred, it must be applied prior to reduction.

27. Reduction technique (j): The wetted slab should now be positioned so that it covers the anterior, lateral and posterior aspects of the radius (7). The tongue should be carefully turned into the palm (8). The slab should be held in position with two wetted 10 cm (4″) open weave bandages (cotton, gauze or Kling™ bandages) (9). The end can be secured with a wetted scrap of plaster bandage.

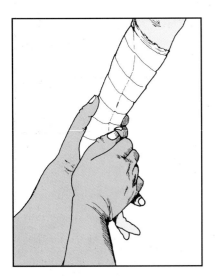

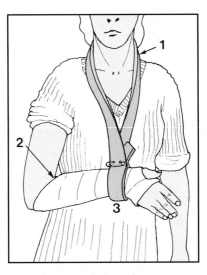

28. Reduction technique (k): Before the plaster sets, many surgeons like to apply further pressure over the posterolateral aspect of the distal fragment, and maintain this until setting occurs ('final moulding'). This precaution ensures maintenance of the reduction, but care should be taken not to dent the plaster.

29. Reduction technique (l): A collar and cuff sling should be applied (1). Make sure that there is no constriction at the elbow (2) or at the wrist (3), and try to flex the elbow beyond a right angle so that the forearm is not dependent.

30. Alternative techniques: It is not unexpected that in this common fracture methods of reduction are legion. As it is generally an easy fracture to reduce, it follows that success can rightly be claimed for many techniques. The method given is logical in so far as it correlates with the pathology as seen on the radiographs. Note, however:
1. A direct, simple and extremely effective procedure is to disimpact the fracture (Frame 20), apply a plaster slab (Frame 27) and correct the deformity before the plaster sets by applying pressure on the posterolateral aspect of the distal fragment (as in Frame 28).
2. In the elderly patient, unfit for general anaesthesia (but preferably after intravenous diazepam), a *marked* dorsal displacement may be corrected by quick application of pressure (without previous disimpaction) over a dorsal slab.
3. In the young adult, if a good reduction cannot be secured and held, so that there is recurrence of severe deformity, the use of an external fixator, K-wires or plating should be considered (see Frame 42).

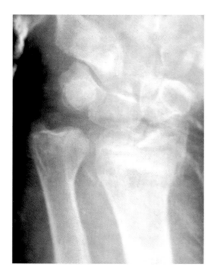

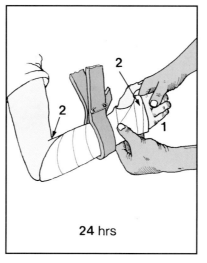

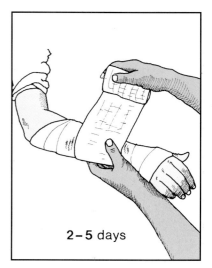

31. Treatment cntd: Check radiographs should be studied. Severe persisting deformity, *especially in the AP projection* (Illus.) should not be accepted, and remanipulation should be undertaken. If difficulty is anticipated, radiographs may be obtained before discontinuing the anaesthetic. If the position is acceptable, the patient is shown finger exercises and advised regarding normal plaster care.

32. Aftercare (a): The patient is seen the next day and the fingers examined for adequacy of the circulation and the degree of swelling (1). The palm, fingers, thumb and elbow are checked for constriction caused by bandaging or elbow flexion, and any adjustments made (2). Thereafter the patient should be seen within the next 2–5 days with a view to completion of the plaster.

33. Aftercare (b): At the next review (usually a fracture clinic) finger swelling is checked: if slight, the plaster is completed (if marked, completion is delayed). *Superficial* layers of cotton bandage are removed, the slab retained, and encircling plaster bandages applied. The patient is instructed in elbow and shoulder exercises, and unless there is still a fair amount of swelling the sling may be discarded.

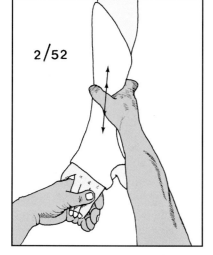

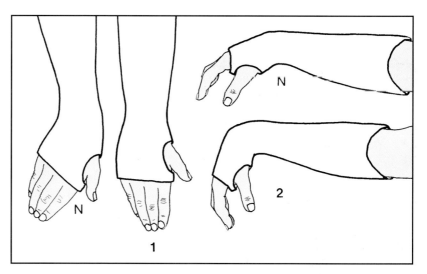

34. Aftercare (c): At 2 weeks the plaster is checked for marked slackening (replace), softening (reinforce) and technical faults (see next two frames). Movements in the fingers, elbow and shoulder are examined and appropriate advice given or physiotherapy started. In some centres radiographs are taken at this stage; slight slipping is inevitable, but marked slipping may be an indication for remanipulation (not usually a profitable procedure). At this stage too, if desired, the plaster may be replaced by a resin cast.

35. Aftercare (d) – Positional errors: (1) The commonest fault is lack of ulnar deviation. This should be sadly accepted if discovered at 2 weeks (but replastered in the correct position if discovered earlier). Lack of ulnar deviation increases the risks of late problems arising from disruption of the inferior radio-ulnar joint; non-union of the ulnar styloid is common, with frequently some restriction of pronation and supination and local pain. (2) Excessive wrist flexion is liable to lead to difficulty in recovering dorsiflexion and a useful grip, and may be associated with compression of the median nerve. If present, the plaster should be re-applied with the wrist in a more extended position. (Full wrist flexion was once advocated in the treatment of Colles fracture – the Cotton–Loder position – but has been abandoned for the reasons given.)

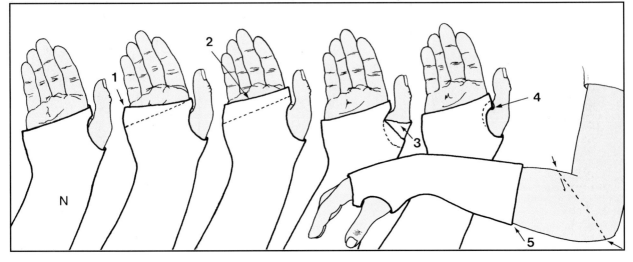

36. Aftercare (e) – Plaster faults: Errors in plastering technique should not occur, but nevertheless are often discovered at this stage. The following faults are common: (1) The distal edge of the plaster does not follow the normal oblique line of the MP joints, and movements of the little and sometimes the ring finger are restricted. The plaster should be trimmed to the dotted line. (2) All the MP joints are restricted by the plaster which has been continued beyond the palmar crease. Trim to the dotted line. (3) The thumb is restricted by a few turns of plaster bandage. Again the plaster should be trimmed to permit free movement. (4) The plaster is digging into the skin of the first web and should be trimmed back to the dotted line. (5) The plaster is too short. Support of the fracture is greatly impaired; the plaster should be extended to the olecranon behind, and as far in front as will still permit elbow flexion.

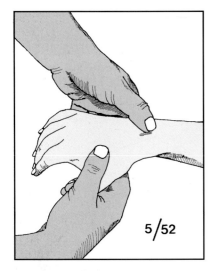

37. Aftercare (f): The plaster should be removed at 5 weeks (or 6 weeks in badly displaced fractures in the elderly) and the fracture assessed for union. (Radiographs are of limited value.) *If there is marked persisting tenderness*, a fresh plaster should be applied and union re-assessed in a further 2 weeks.

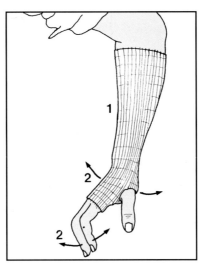

38. Aftercare (g): If tenderness is minimal or absent, (1) a circular woven support (e.g. Tubigrip™ or a crepe bandage) may be applied to limit oedema and to some extent increase the patient's confidence. (2) The patient is instructed in wrist and finger exercises and encouraged to practise these frequently and with vigour. Arrangements are made to review the patient in a further 2 weeks.

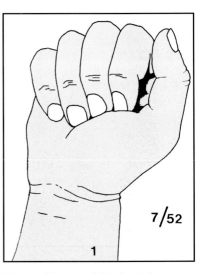

39. Need for rehabilitation (a): At about 7 weeks post injury, you must decide whether to discharge the patient or refer them for rehabilitation. Base your decision on: (i) finger movements, (ii) grip strength, (iii) wrist movements, (iv) the patient's occupation. For example, if finger 'tuck-in' (i.e. the last few degrees of flexion) cannot be carried out (loss of terminal tuck-in is illustrated) physiotherapy should be considered.

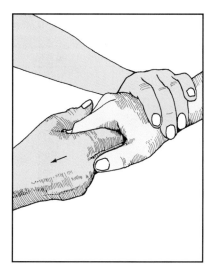

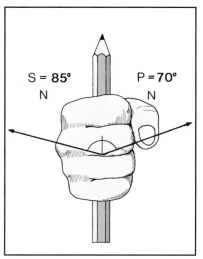

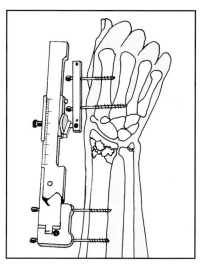

40. Need for rehabilitation (b): Assess the patient's grip strength by first asking them to squeeze two of your fingers as tightly as possible while you try to withdraw them. Compare one hand with the other. Repeat with a single finger. Marked weakness is an indication for physiotherapy.

41. Need for rehabilitation (c): Assess wrist movements. Initially, material restriction of *palmar flexion* is normal and by itself is of little importance. If, however, the total range of *pronation* (P) *and supination* (S) is less than half normal, physiotherapy is advisable. Where there is only slight restriction of movements and power, rehabilitation may still be indicated through the special requirements of the patient's work.

42. Alternative fixation methods (a): These may be indicated where the fracture cannot be satisfactorily reduced or held by closed methods, e.g. where there is severe comminution, or splitting of the radial fragment into two or more substantial fragments. An external fixator (e.g. the Agee–WristJack™ illustrated) allows control of length while avoiding the necessity of having to put the wrist up in marked flexion to maintain the reduction.

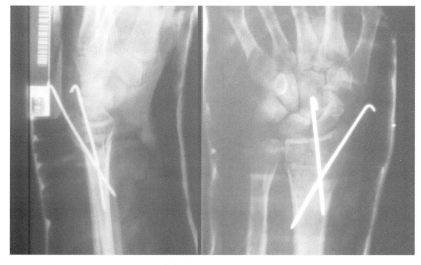

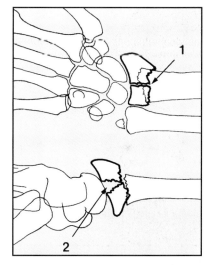

43. Alternative fixation methods (b): Where, during the manipulative procedure, instability is found to be marked, and it is considered that it will be very difficult to maintain any reduction that can be achieved if only a cast is used, then the position may be held with two or more K-wires. An additional plaster cast will be required until union of the fracture is well advanced. The wires may be removed after 3–4 weeks. In similar circumstances, plating of the fracture may also be considered. (For example, see Frame 46.)

44. Splitting of the radial fragment (a): Sometimes there may be a small vertical crack through the radial fragment, showing in the AP view (1). In other cases the fracture may run horizontally, and the scaphoid or lunate may separate the fragments (2). In the young adult, especially where the main fragments are separated and there is no gross fragmentation, some form of internal fixation is indicated.

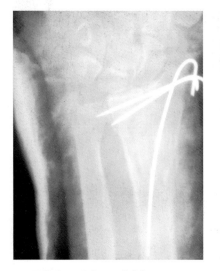

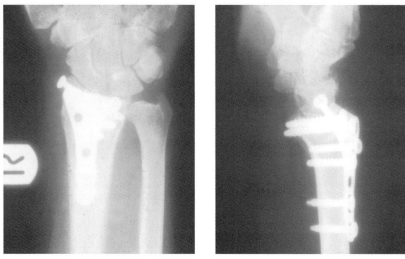

45. Splitting of the radial fragment (b): In a number of cases the fracture may be reduced under intensifier control (or under vision using an arthroscope). K-wires may be used to lever the fragments into position prior to the insertion of the Kirschner fixation wires which are shown in this radiograph. Additional support with a cast will be needed. Some permanent joint stiffness is the rule after injuries of this pattern, and prolonged physiotherapy will usually be required.

46. Splitting of the radial fragment (c): Where comminution is not a problem, fractures of this pattern may also be held by screwing and plating. In this example note the cross-screw which has been used to hold and compress the two radial fragments together, and the plate which holds and aligns the distal complex with the radial shaft.

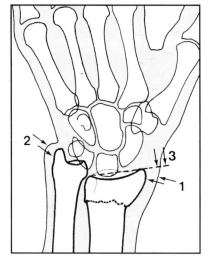

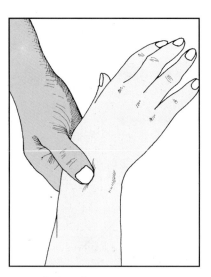

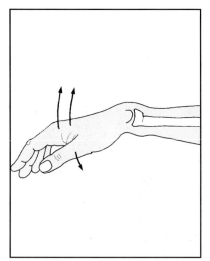

47. Complications (a) – Persistent deformity or malunion (i): Radial drift of the distal fragment results in prominence of the distal radius (1). Radial tilting and bony absorption at the fracture site lead to relative prominence of the distal ulna (2) and tilting of the plane of the wrist as seen in the AP radiographs (3). These deformities may be symptom free, and surgery on purely cosmetic grounds is seldom indicated.

48. Malunion (ii): In some cases there is quite marked pain in the region of the distal radio-ulnar joint, owing to its severe disorganisation. There is generally quite *marked local tenderness* and supination, in particular, is reduced. Physiotherapy in the form of grip strengthening and pronation/supination exercises is indicated. If symptoms remain severe, excision of the distal end of the ulna may be considered.

49. Malunion (iii): Uncomplicated persistence of dinner-fork deformity (i.e. persistent deformity in the lateral but not in the AP radiographs) is accompanied by some loss of palmar flexion, but significant functional disturbance is unusual. This type of residual deformity is generally accepted.

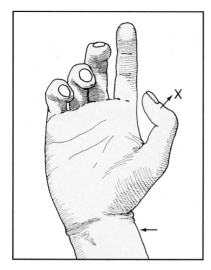

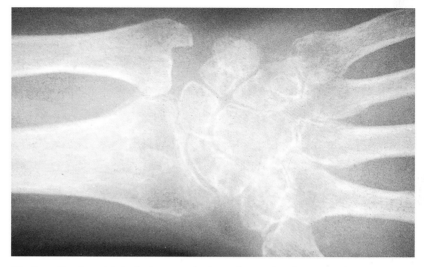

50. Complications (b): *Delayed rupture of extensor pollicis longus* may follow Colles fracture, and be due to attrition of the tendon by roughness at the fracture site, or by sloughing from interference with its blood supply. Disability is often slight, and spontaneous recovery may occur. There is no urgency regarding treatment, and in the elderly this complaint may be accepted or treated expectantly. In the young, extensor indicis proprius tendon transfer is advocated.

51. Complications (c): Sudeck's atrophy/complex regional pain syndrome: This is often detected about the time the patient comes out of plaster. The fingers are swollen and finger flexion is restricted. The hand and wrist are warm, tender and painful. Radiographs show diffuse osteoporosis (Illus.). *Treatment*: The mainstay of treatment is intensive and prolonged physiotherapy and occupational therapy, but if pain is very severe a further 2–3 weeks rest of the *wrist* in plaster may give sufficient relief to allow commencement of effective finger movements. If the MP joints are stiff in extension and making no headway, manipulation under general anaesthesia followed by fixation in plaster (MP joints flexed, IP joints extended) for 3 weeks only may be effective in initiating recovery. In severe cases, a sympathetic block may be attempted by infiltration of the stellate ganglion, or by regional perfusion with guanethidine sulphate. (See Chapter 5 for a fuller discussion.)

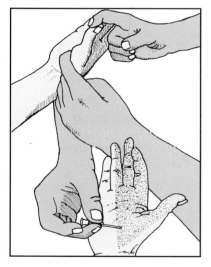

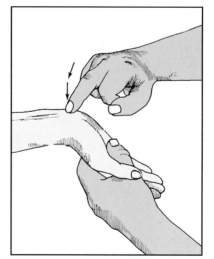

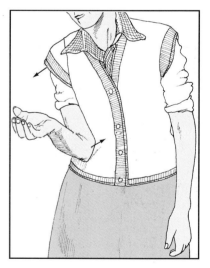

52. Complications (d) – Carpal tunnel (median nerve compression) syndrome: Paraesthesia in the median distribution is the main presenting symptom, but look for sensory and motor involvement. If detected *before reduction:* (i) Complete lesion: reduce, plaster and re-assess. If no improvement, explore, and divide not only the roof of the carpal tunnel but the antebrachial fascia. (ii) Partial lesion: reduce and apply a cast; if motor symptoms remain, or if symptoms persist for a week, decompress.

53. Median nerve compression syndrome cntd: If detected *after reduction,* Release the splints, put the wrist in the neutral position, and use K-wires or an external fixator to hold the reduction; if symptoms persist, explore. If detected *after union,* exploration is generally advised, as symptoms otherwise tend to persist. Note that diagnosis at the late stage may be suggested by the response to tapping over the nerve (Illus.), or by nerve stretching, tourniquet, or nerve conduction tests.

54. Complications (e) – Persisting stiffness: Restriction of movements, even after prolonged physiotherapy, is not uncommon, but is seldom severe enough to impair limb function to a material extent. This is due to compensatory (trick) movements developed by the elbow, shoulder and trunk (e.g. in case of loss of supination).

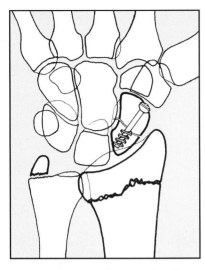

55. Complications (f) – Associated scaphoid fracture: This may be treated by manipulation of the Colles fracture and application of a scaphoid plaster. After the Colles fracture has united, further immobilisation may be required for the scaphoid. Alternatively, the scaphoid fracture may be fixed with an AO lag cancellous screw (Illus.) (or a Herbert screw), the Colles fracture manipulated, and fixation discontinued as soon as the latter has united.

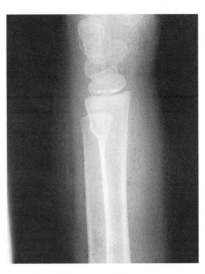

56. Related fractures (a): A number of fractures involving the distal end of the radius, produced by falls on the outstretched hand, have certain similarities to the classical Colles fracture. The commonest of these is the *undisplaced greenstick fracture of the radius*. In its most minor form it may be overlooked; the only sign may be slight local buckling.

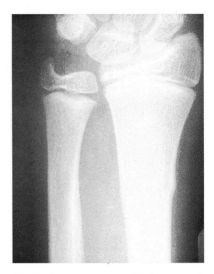

57. Undisplaced greenstick fracture of the radius cntd: The level of the fracture is rather variable, and it may be situated fairly proximally. These fractures may be treated like undisplaced Colles fractures by the application of a plaster slab. This may usually be completed after 1–2 days. Fixation for about 3 weeks only is usually all that is necessary.

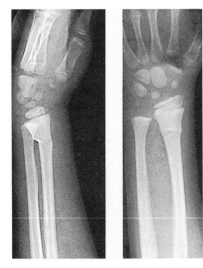

58. Related fractures (b) – Angulated greenstick fracture of the radius: In this type of injury there is both clinical and radiological deformity. Manipulation is required as for a Colles fracture, and the aftercare is similar; the period of plaster fixation may be reduced to 3 or 4 weeks, depending on the age of the child.

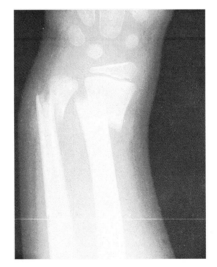

59. Related fractures (c) – Overlapping radial fracture (i): In children the radius often fractures close to the wrist, with off-ending (i.e. complete loss of bony contact). On the ulnar side there may be: 1. Detachment of the triangular fibrocartilage; 2. Separation of the ulnar epiphysis; 3. Fracture and angulation of the distal ulna; 4. Fracture and displacement of the distal ulna (Illus.), in effect a fracture of both bones of the forearm; 5. Dislocation of the ulna (Galeazzi fracture–dislocation).

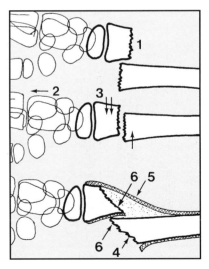

60. Overlapping radial fracture (ii): If the fracture line is transverse (1), reduction is straightforward by traction (2) and local pressure (3). When, however, there is a fracture running obliquely from front to back (4), reduction by traction is often impossible owing to the integrity of the periosteum on the dorsal surface (5) and the overlapping bony spikes (6).

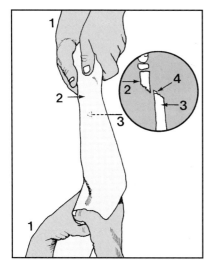

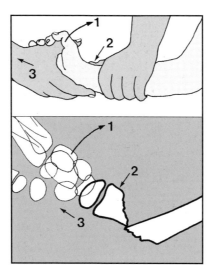

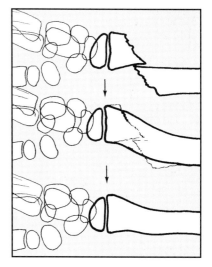

61. Overlapping radial fracture (iii):
Two closed techniques may be tried. For the first, two assistants are essential to apply *maximal* traction to the limb (1). While this is being strongly maintained, the surgeon should press forcibly with the heel of one hand on the distal fragment (2) and use the other to apply counter-pressure (3). Reduction is achieved by shearing off one of the bone spikes (4).

62. Overlapping radial fracture (iv):
Alternatively, by *increasing* the deformity (1) and applying pressure directly over the distal radial fragment (2), whilst maintaining traction (3), reduction may be achieved. After the fragments have interlocked the angulation is corrected. Thereafter plaster fixation is carried out as in other fractures in this region.

63. Overlapping radial fracture (v): If
shortening is marked, and closed methods fail, open reduction may be considered. (Performed through a small dorsal incision under a tourniquet; internal fixation is not required, although a K-wire may be used to hold the fracture temporarily – being withdrawn as soon as the plaster has been applied.) Nevertheless, if persisting overlap is reluctantly accepted, a good result from remodelling is the usual outcome (Illus.) *provided* any angulation is corrected.

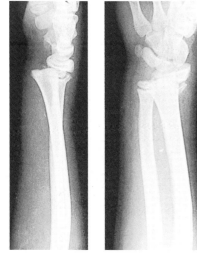

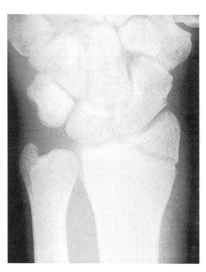

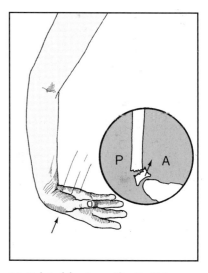

64. Related fractures (d) – Slipped radial epiphysis: This injury is common in
adolescence, and the displaced distal radial epiphysis is usually associated with a small fracture of the metaphysis (Salter–Harris Type 2 injury). Unless displacement is minimal, manipulation followed by plaster fixation (as for a Colles fracture) is indicated. Growth disturbance is rare, but reduction should be carried out promptly (it is often difficult to reduce after 2 days).

65. Related fractures (e) – Fracture of the radial styloid: This fracture is
sometimes caused by an engine starting-handle kickback as well as by a fall on the outstretched hand. Displacement is usually slight, and manipulation is unlikely to be of value. Every case should be checked for scapho-lunate dissociation. A Colles plaster is usually adequate, although some prefer fixation with a lag screw or Kirschner wires. Physiotherapy is usually required, and Sudeck's atrophy a common complication.

66. Related fractures (f) – Smith's fracture (i): This injury frequently results
from a fall on the back of the hand, although a clear history is not always obtainable. The distal radial fragment is tilted anteriorly (posterior angulation) and may be displaced anteriorly. The fracture is usually impacted.

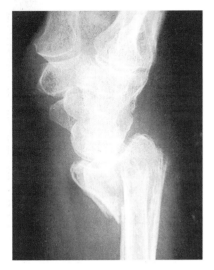

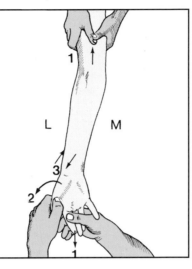

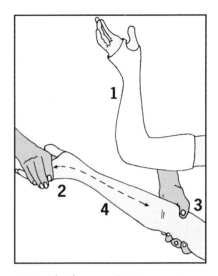

67. Smith's fracture (ii): This fracture is frequently referred to as a 'reversed Colles fracture' because the deformities, when viewed from the side clinically and radiologically, are in the opposite direction to those seen in a Colles fracture. (Note, however, that the two fractures may be identical in AP radiographs.) Comminuted Smith's fractures may involve the articular surface of the radius (Illus.). Greenstick fractures are common.

68. Smith's fracture (iii): To reduce these fractures, traction is applied to the arm (1) in supination (2) until disimpaction is achieved. (This may be confirmed as in a Colles fracture.) Pressure may be applied with the heels of the hands to force the distal fragment dorsally (3).

69. Smith's fracture (iv): The reduction is difficult to hold, and a long arm plaster is required (1). This may be more conveniently applied in two stages, and a complete plaster is better than a simple slab. The arm is held in full supination and dorsiflexion (2). This is easily maintained with the elbow extended (3). The arm is measured for an anterior forearm slab (4) and wool roll applied to the arm.

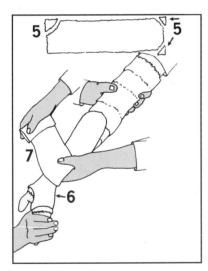

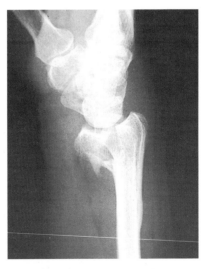

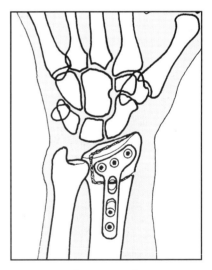

70. Smith's fracture (v): The anterior slab is trimmed (5) and positioned (6) before completion of the forearm part of the cast (7) which may be moulded while setting. The cast is then extended above the elbow. *Aftercare:* Split if necessary; radiographs at weekly intervals for the first 3 weeks (treat any slipping by remanipulation or moulding); change slack plasters with care. Six weeks' fixation is usually required, with physiotherapy after removal of the cast.

71. Related fractures (g) – Barton's fracture: This is a form of Smith's fracture in which the anterior portion only of the radius is involved. Closed reduction may be attempted along thelines indicated for Smith's fracture, but this may fail with the carpus wedging the fragments apart. If this occurs, open reduction and internal fixation are indicated in the younger patient (e.g. by cancellous screw or an Ellis buttress plate).

72. Barton's fracture cntd: In the young patient these potentially unstable and disabling fractures are best treated by open reduction and internal fixation. The most satisfactory procedure is to expose the fracture anteriorly and reduce it under vision; thereafter it is best held with a volar plate (e.g. with an Ellis buttress plate or an AO right-angled or oblique T-plate (Illus.)).

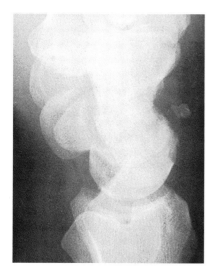

73. Related fractures (h): Forcible palmar flexion may result in a *minor avulsion fracture of the carpus* at a ligament insertion (Illus.). If the wrist is forcibly palmar flexed or dorsiflexed, the carpus impinging on the distal end of the radius may produce a *marginal chip fracture of the radius.* Symptomatic treatment only is required for either of these injuries (e.g. 2–3 weeks in a plaster back slab).

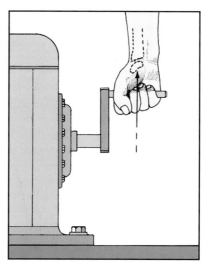

74. Fractures of the scaphoid – Mechanisms of injury: Scaphoid fractures often result from 'kick-back' when using starting handles on internal combustion generators, pumps, compressors and inboard marine engines. (The motorist's avoidance of this fracture is his only dividend from the unfortunate abolition of car starting handles.) Otherwise the fracture may be acquired by falls on the outstretched hand.

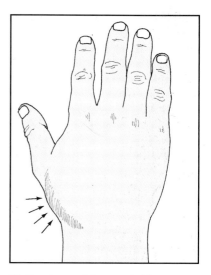

75. Fractures of the scaphoid – Diagnosis (a): Fracture of the scaphoid may be suspected when there is complaint of pain on the lateral aspect of the wrist following any injury (or frequently repeated stress). In those cases which follow starting handle accidents there may be marked and rapid swelling of the hand and wrist.

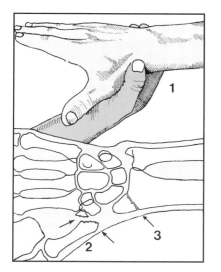

76. Diagnosis (b): Tenderness in the anatomical snuff box (1) is suggestive of this injury, but by no means diagnostic. Many wrist sprains without fracture give rise to tenderness in this site. Beware too of tenderness which may be the result of a Bennett's fracture of the thumb metacarpal (2) or of a fracture of the radial styloid (3).

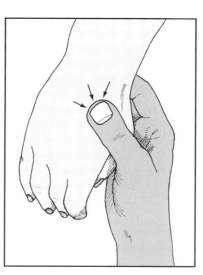

77. Diagnosis (c): In a true scaphoid fracture, tenderness will also be elicited on the application of pressure over the *dorsal aspect of the scaphoid*, and also on pressure over the palmar aspect. Tenderness in these additional sites very seldom occurs in other injuries in this area, no matter how severe.

78. Diagnosis (d) – Radiographs (i): Radiography is required in all suspect cases. Note the following important points:
1. Request cards should be clearly marked 'scaphoid' and not 'wrist'. This is necessary to ensure that the films are properly centred, and that at least three projections of the scaphoid are obtained to improve the chances of the fracture being visualised in the initial radiographic series.
2. The fracture is often hairline, and as a consequence hard to detect.
3. Because of this accepted difficulty – ie that a hairline fracture may not show up on the initial films – it is common practice in all suspected but unconfirmed cases that radiographs should be repeated at 10–14 days. Although there is some controversy about this, the common view is that local decalcification after such an interval may reveal a previously hidden fracture.
4. If doubt remains, a bone scan may be helpful.

Note that there is a 20% rate of false positive reporting of scaphoid radiographs, and *clinical confirmation of the diagnosis is mandatory.*

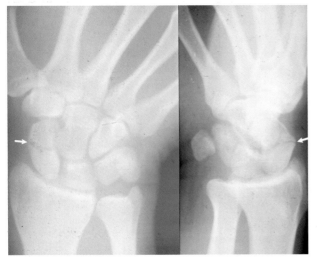

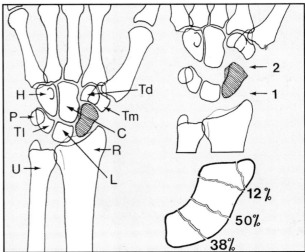

79. Radiographs (ii): This radiograph is typical of a fracture through the waist of the scaphoid. In this example the fracture line is easily seen in both the AP projection and one oblique – but this by no means is always the case.

80. Anatomical features (a): The scaphoid (shaded) plays a key role in wrist and carpal function, taking part in the radiocarpal joint (1) and in the joint between the proximal and distal rows of the carpus (2). It articulates with the radius (R), trapezium (Tm), trapezoid (Td), capitate (C) and lunate (L). The commonest site for fracture is the waist (50%); 38% of fractures occur in the proximal half and 12% in the distal half. (U = ulna, H = hamate, P = pisiform, Tl = triquetral.)

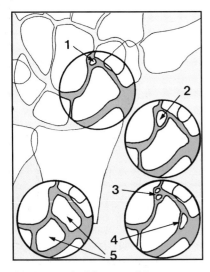

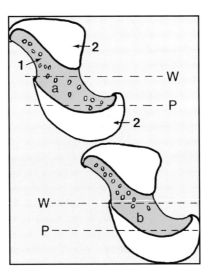

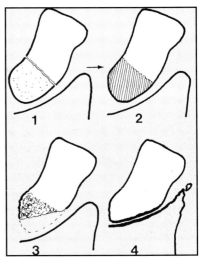

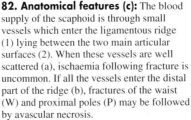

81. Anatomical features (b): A number of abnormalities in ossification may be confused with fractures. The *os centrale* may be small (1), large (2) or double (3). The *os radiale externum* (4) lies in the region of the tubercle and in some cases may represent an old, ununited fracture; certainly the so-called 'bipartite scaphoid' (5) is now generally regarded as being due to this. (Rounded edges differentiate these from fresh fractures.)

82. Anatomical features (c): The blood supply of the scaphoid is through small vessels which enter the ligamentous ridge (1) lying between the two main articular surfaces (2). When these vessels are well scattered (a), ischaemia following fracture is uncommon. If all the vessels enter the distal part of the ridge (b), fractures of the waist (W) and proximal poles (P) may be followed by avascular necrosis.

83. Anatomical features (d): Avascular necrosis is of immediate onset, but 1–2 months may elapse before increased bone density betrays its presence on the radiographs (2). There is usually slow but progressive bony collapse (3) and radiocarpal osteoarthritis (4). This leads to worsening pain and stiffness in the wrist. Avascular necrosis occurs in about 30% of fractures of the proximal pole of the scaphoid.

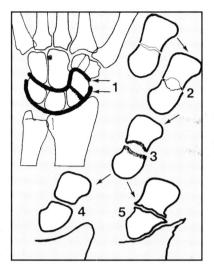

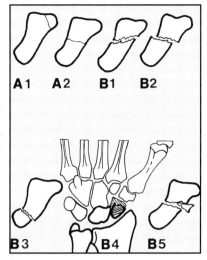

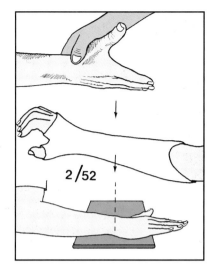

84. Anatomical features (e): Because of its role in two major joints (1), movement of the fragments is difficult to control, and non-union may occur in waist fractures. Cystic changes at the fracture site (2) are followed by marginal sclerosis (3). The edges may round off and form a symptomless pseudarthrosis (4) or osteoarthritis may supervene (5). Note that non-union can occur without avascular necrosis, and that most fractures with avascular necrosis are united.

85. Prognostic features: The prognosis is good in *stable* injuries: these include (Herbert Classification) fractures of the tubercle (A1), and hairline fractures of the waist (A2). The prognosis is poorer in *unstable* injuries which include oblique fractures of the distal third (B1), displaced fractures of the waist (B2), proximal pole fractures (B3), fractures associated with carpal dislocations (B4; Illus.: trans-scapho perilunar dislocation of the carpus – see Frame 102) and comminuted fractures (B5).

86. Treatment of suspected fracture: When there is local tenderness and normal radiographs, apply a scaphoid plaster and sling. Remove the plaster and repeat X-rays at 2 weeks (see also Frame 78). Absorption of bone at the site of any hairline fracture will then usually reveal it. If a fracture is confirmed, apply a fresh cast and treat as for a frank fracture. If the radiographs are negative, the patient is presumed to have suffered a sprain, and is treated accordingly: but if symptoms persist re-examine and X-ray after another 2 weeks.

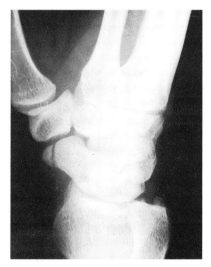

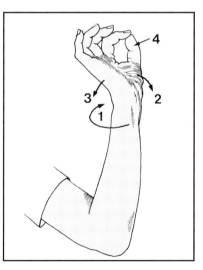

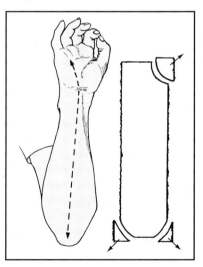

87. Fractures of the tuberosity of the scaphoid: Avascular necrosis never occurs in fractures of this type, and non-union here does not give rise to significant symptoms. Symptomatic treatment only is needed (e.g. a crepe bandage or plaster, depending on pain). Some extend this to include all distal pole fractures, but generally plaster fixation is the mainstay of treatment of all fractures through the body of the scaphoid (but see Frame 98).

88. Treatment of undisplaced fractures of the body of the scaphoid – The classical scaphoid plaster (a): The position of the hand is of some importance and should be made quite clear to the patient prior to the application of the plaster. In the classical scaphoid plaster (a position nevertheless challenged by some) the wrist should be fully pronated (1), radially deviated (2), and moderately dorsiflexed (3). In addition, the thumb should be in mid abduction (4).

89. The scaphoid plaster (b): An anterior plaster slab, although by no means essential, is frequently used. This may be made from 6–8 layers of 10 cm (4″) plaster bandage, or taken from a slab dispenser. The proximal corners should be trimmed and a cut-out made to accommodate the swell of the thenar muscles.

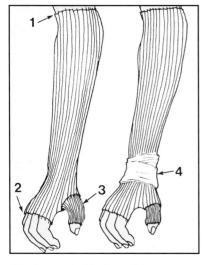

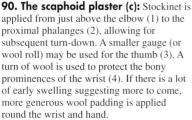

90. The scaphoid plaster (c): Stockinet is applied from just above the elbow (1) to the proximal phalanges (2), allowing for subsequent turn-down. A smaller gauge (or wool roll) may be used for the thumb (3). A turn of wool is used to protect the bony prominences of the wrist (4). If there is a lot of early swelling suggesting more to come, more generous wool padding is applied round the wrist and hand.

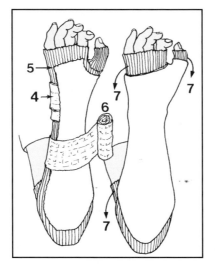

91. The scaphoid plaster (d): The plaster slab may then be wetted and applied to the forearm, taking care not to extend it beyond the proximal palmar crease (5). Encircling plaster bandages are then applied, using 15 cm (6″) bandages for the forearm, 10 cm (4″) for the wrist and 7.5 cm (3″) for the thumb (6). The edges of the stockinet are turned down before completion (7).

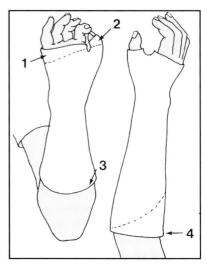

92. The scaphoid plaster (e) – Common faults: Plaster including MP joints of fingers, restricting flexion (1). Terminal phalanx of thumb included, preventing interphalangeal joint flexion (2). Plaster too short (3). Plaster restricting flexion of the elbow (4). (Note that to give the best support to a scaphoid fracture there is some questioning of the position of the wrist and the need to include the thumb. Some use a Colles plaster in neutral or slight flexion, without radial deviation.)

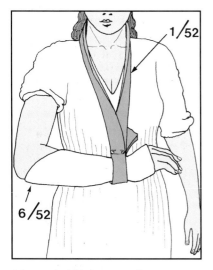

93. Scaphoid fracture – Aftercare (a): A sling should be worn for the first few days until swelling subsides. Analgesics are usually required initially. The patient is reviewed at 2 weeks (assuming the initial plaster check has been satisfactory). If on this visit the plaster is unduly slack, it should be changed. Any softening in the palm should be reinforced.

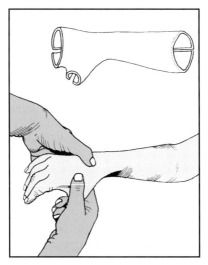

94. Aftercare (b): At 6 weeks the plaster should be removed and the scaphoid assessed clinically and with radiographs. There are several possibilities: (i) If there is no tenderness over the dorsal surface and in the snuff-box, and the fracture appears united on the radiographs, the wrist should be left free and reviewed in 2 weeks (usually for discharge, or further radiographs if pain recurs).

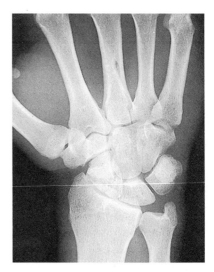

95. Aftercare (c): (ii) The fracture line may still show clearly on the radiographs. (iii) The radiographs may suggest union, but there is marked local tenderness. (iv) There is some uncertainty on either score. These possibilities are all suggestive of delayed union, and a further 6 weeks of plaster fixation is desirable.

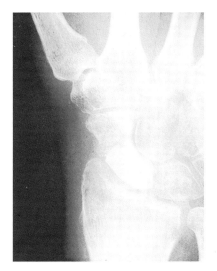

96. Aftercare (d): At 12 weeks, there may be: (i) Evidence of *avascular necrosis* (note density of proximal half in radiograph), (ii) Clear evidence, clinically and radiologically of *union*. In these circumstances, there is no need and no advantage in continuing with plaster fixation.

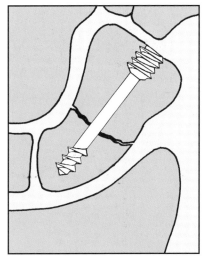

97. Aftercare (e): At 12 weeks, there may be: (iii) No evidence of union, (iv) Evidence of established non-union; internal fixation should be considered (e.g. using a Herbert screw (Illus.) or a cannulated screw inserted percutaneously). In (iv), local bone grafting will also be required. If surgery is refused, or not thought advisable, plaster should be discarded in established non-union. In (iii), a further period of plaster immobilisation may be considered if there is marked persistent pain and local tenderness.

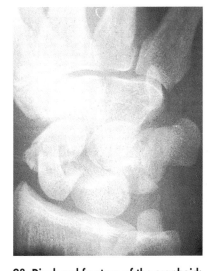

98. Displaced fracture of the scaphoid: If there is marked displacement (Illus.), be sure to exclude a concurrent carpal dislocation. Where displacement or angulation exceed 1 mm or 15° respectively, open reduction and internal fixation (through an anterior approach to avoid impairing the blood supply of the fragments) is indicated; indeed, as the results of internal fixation are so very good, many advocate this for every displaced scaphoid fracture.

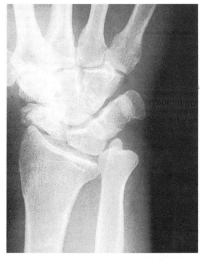

99. Complications (a) – Sudeck's atrophy: Treat as described in Frame 51. **(b) Avascular necrosis:** In the early stages an anterior bone block graft (e.g. Matti–Russe operation) may be considered. In the late stages where there is bony collapse (Illus.) only salvage procedures (such as those detailed in Frame 101) are likely to be of benefit.

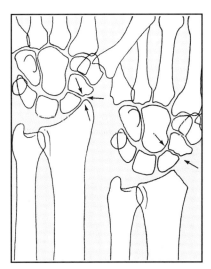

100. Complications (c) – Non-union:
1. Late diagnosed non-union, seen 3–6 months after injury, may still be effectively treated by plaster fixation and pulsed magnetic fields, *provided* that there is no displacement, carpal collapse, or osteoarthritic change.
2. If there is displacement, or if seen later than 6 months, and symptoms are present, internal fixation and bone grafting are advised.

3. If an early impingement osteoarthritis threatens, satisfactory results may be obtained from excision of the radial styloid even although the midcarpal joint is unaffected by this (Illus.).
4. Symptomless non-union of the scaphoid, sometimes discovered by accident, should have the risks of secondary osteoarthritis assessed; if the appearances indicate that these are insignificant, then no treatment is indicated.

101. Complications (d) – Advanced osteoarthritis: This generally occurs as a sequel to avascular necrosis or non-union. The following treatments may be considered:
1. Wrist joint (radiocarpal) fusion: Pronation and supination movements are retained, but all other wrist movements are lost. This is the most reliable procedure and is the only one which should be considered in the patient who undertakes heavy manual labour.
2. Where the retention of some wrist movement is essential, excision of the proximal row of the carpus may be considered. The results are a little unpredictable in terms of final range of movements, strength, and freedom from pain.
3. Where surgery is thought inadvisable, good results in terms of relief from pain with reasonable function may be obtained by the use of a block-leather support, or similar orthotic device.

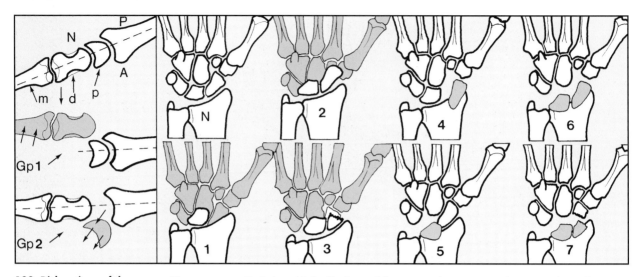

102. Dislocations of the carpus: These may result from a fall on the outstretched hand, and are comparatively uncommon. There are two main groups. In the first, the metacarpals (m), the distal row of the carpus (d) and part of the proximal row (p) dislocate backwards. In classifying injuries within this group, the prefix 'peri' is used to describe undisplaced structures in the proximal row. Occasionally one of the carpal bones fractures, part remaining in alignment and part displacing with the distal row of the carpus. Note in the illustrations that structures drawn in faint lines and shaded in dark grey are *displaced* (N = normal appearance from the side or *volar* aspect):
(1) Perilunar dislocation of the carpus.
(2) Periscapholunar dislocation of the carpus. (3) Trans-scapho perilunar dislocation of the carpus. (Not illustrated are the rare transcapitate, transtriquetral perilunar dislocations and others.)
In the second main group of injuries, the distal row re-aligns with the radius and part of the proximal row is extruded, hence: (4) Dislocation of the scaphoid.
(5) Dislocation of the lunate. (6) Dislocation of the lunate and scaphoid. (7) Dislocation of the lunate and part of the scaphoid. (Note the correspondence between 1 & 5, 2 & 6, 3 & 7.)

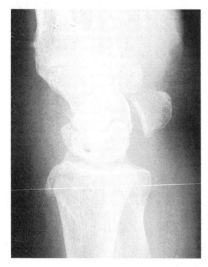

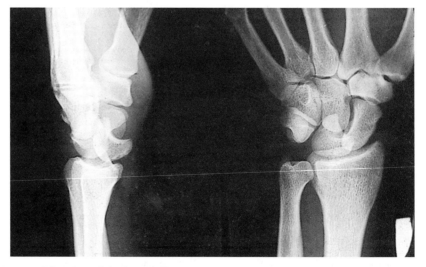

103. Dislocation of the lunate (a): This is the commonest of all the carpal dislocations, and generally results from a fall on the outstretched hand. It is frequently overlooked, and this is nearly always due to failure in interpretation of the radiographs. Note in the normal radiographs of the carpus (Illus.) that the pisiform bone stands out to a varying degree from the rest of the volar surface.

104. Dislocation of the lunate (b): The *shape* of the dislocated lunate is quite different from the ovoid/quadrilateral mass of the pisiform. The concave surface in which the capitate usually sits is *rotated* anteriorly, and the crescent moon shape of the bone (and hence its name) is rendered obvious. The articular surfaces of the scaphoid and triquetral remain aligned with the radius while the lunate is *displaced* anteriorly. In the AP projection, the lunate is sector-shaped (resembling a cheese segment). *Diagnosis:* This is established on the basis of a history of injury, local tenderness and the radiographs. Evidence of median nerve involvement is very suggestive (may result from direct pressure of the displaced bone on the nerve).

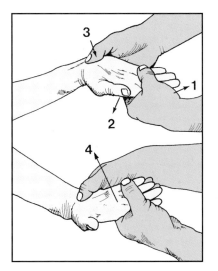

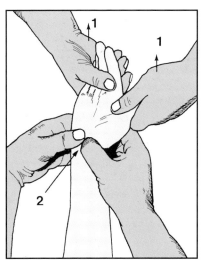

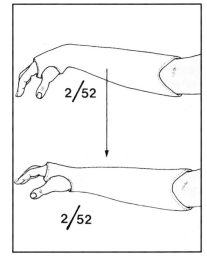

105. Treatment (a): Reduction can generally be achieved by closed methods under general anaesthesia. (1) Apply traction to the supinated wrist. (2) Extend the wrist, maintaining traction, (3) Apply pressure with the thumb over the lunate. (4) Flex the wrist as soon as you feel the lunate slip into position.

106. Treatment (b): Alternatively, if an assistant is available, they should apply traction in supination and extension as before (1) while you use both thumbs to push the lunate posteriorly and distally (2). When it is felt to reduce, the wrist is once again flexed. The reduction should be checked with radiographs before the anaesthetic is discontinued. (Failure is an indication for open reduction.)

107. Treatment (c): (i) The wrist is encased in plaster in a position of moderate flexion for 1–2 weeks. (ii) The plaster is then changed for one with the wrist in the neutral position for a further 2 weeks. (iii) Weekly radiographs should be taken to detect any late subluxation (an indication for K-wire fixation). (iv) Physiotherapy may be required, depending on the degree of residual stiffness. Swelling may be a problem initially, and require generous padding, elevation, and a sling.

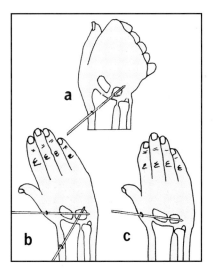

108. Treatment (d): Many prefer K-wire fixation in all cases. To do this the wrist is put in flexion and full ulnar deviation, and the lunate fixed to the radius with a K-wire (a). The wrist is then positioned in dorsiflexion and radial deviation and a second wire passed through the scaphoid into the lunate (b). The wrist is then placed in a more neutral position and the first wire removed (c). A light cast is worn for 5–6 weeks. The wire is retained for 4 weeks.

109. Complications (a) – Late diagnosis: If there is delay in making the diagnosis, manipulative reduction becomes increasingly difficult, and after a week may not be possible. Open reduction is then necessary, and carries with it the greatly increased risk of avascular necrosis. Surgery should be performed through an anterior incision, and every effort made to reduce the bone without disturbing any of its ligamentous attachments (evidence suggests the major blood supply enters anteriorly) or further damaging the median nerve.

(b) Median nerve palsy: Prompt reduction of the dislocation is usually followed by early complete recovery. After late reduction recovery may be incomplete, but seldom requires separate treatment.

(c) Sudeck's atrophy: This is a common complication and is treated along previously described lines (See Frame 51 and Chapter 5).

(d) Avascular necrosis: (Illus.) This leads to collapse of the lunate and secondary osteoarthritis which advances with great rapidity. *All cases of dislocated lunate should have monthly radiographs for 6 months* to allow early detection of this complication. If detected early, excision may prevent progressive osteoarthritis. In many cases, and certainly at the later stages, arthrodesis of the wrist is preferable.

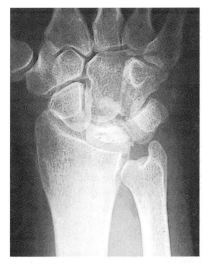

Note that repeated trauma to the wrist without frank dislocation of the lunate may lead to similar radiographic appearances (Kienbock's disease); this condition is found in manual workers such as carpenters, cobblers and jack hammer operators.

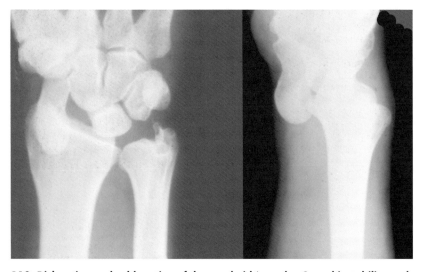

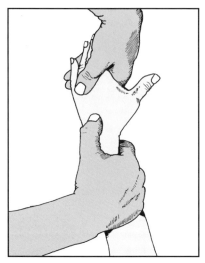

110. Dislocation and subluxation of the scaphoid (see also Carpal instability and Scapholunate dissociation) (a): These uncommon injuries are diagnosed radiologically and, if suspected, AP projections in both radial and ulnar deviation may be helpful. The most striking feature is the widening of the space between the scaphoid and lunate.
Treatment: 1. If the displacement is anterior and complete as shown, manipulate as for dislocation of the lunate. 2. In many cases, dislocation is incomplete, with the proximal pole being tilted posteriorly and the distal pole anteriorly. Such injuries have often a toggle-like instability within the dorsiflexion/palmar flexion range (and the stable position within this phase must be found by trial and error during reduction).

111. (b) cntd: Reduction may be achieved by pressure over the proximal pole. If possible, an image intensifier should be used to check the reduction and stability. If a stable position is found, the wrist should be put up in plaster in that position, with some radial deviation; the plaster should be retained for 6 weeks, with frequent radiographs to check the position. If instability is not easily controlled, then the scaphoid should certainly be fixed with K-wires, a procedure many advocate for all cases.

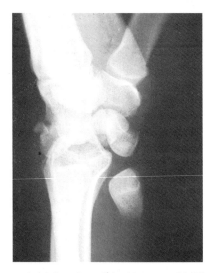

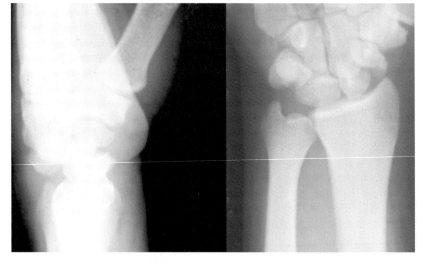

112. Dislocation of the lunate and half the scaphoid: This combination of injuries may be treated by manipulative reduction as described for dislocation of the lunate. Thereafter it is probably best to internally fix the scaphoid fracture, e.g. with a Herbert screw. These injuries have a much poorer prognosis than uncomplicated dislocations of the lunate.

113. Trans-scapho perilunar dislocation of the carpus: This injury corresponds to dislocation of the lunate and half the scaphoid just described. It is the commonest of the first group of carpal dislocations. In some cases there may be associated fractures of the styloid process of the radius and the ulna. *Treatment:* Reduction by traction is usually easy. Thereafter the management is that of fracture of the scaphoid. If, however, the scaphoid reduction is poor or if the wrist is very unstable, internal fixation of the scaphoid must be considered.

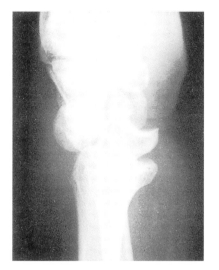

114. Other carpal injuries (a) – Perilunar dislocation of the carpus:
This corresponds to isolated dislocation of the lunate. *Treatment:* 1. Reduce by traction. 2. Apply plaster with the wrist in flexion and retain for 1–2 weeks before 3. Changing the plaster to one with the wrist in the neutral position. This should be retained for a further 2 weeks. 4. Thereafter, physiotherapy may be required to mobilise the wrist.

115. Other carpal injuries cntd:
(b) Dislocation of both the lunate and scaphoid: This should be treated as for dislocation of the lunate.
(c) Periscapholunar dislocation of the carpus: This should be treated in the same way as perilunar dislocation of the carpus.
(d) Dislocation of the trapezium, trapezoid or hamate: These are rare. Closed reduction should always be attempted, but open reduction is frequently required. In the face of instability, transfixion by K-wires may be helpful.
(e) Fractures through the bodies of any of the carpal bones other than the scaphoid: These are rare, and should be treated symptomatically by 6 weeks' fixation in a Colles or scaphoid plaster (depending on the injury). Fractures of the hamate (see also below) and pisiform may be complicated by ulnar nerve palsy, which should generally be treated expectantly.
(f) Small chip fractures of the carpus: These are common and usually result from hyperflexion or hyperextension injuries of the wrist. Direct violence is sometimes responsible. The bone of origin is often in doubt. Rest of the wrist in plaster for 3 weeks is all that is required, and full recovery of function is the rule.

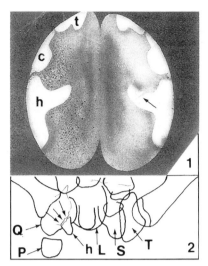

116. Other carpal injuries cntd:
(g) Fracture of the hook of the hamate: This injury is seen most often as a result of a heavy golf or tennis swing, but may follow a fall, or a direct blow in the palm. There is local pain and tenderness. The fracture is best shown by a CAT scan of both wrists in the praying position (1), or by carpal tunnel films (2). The best treatment is to excise the hamate fragment. (h = hamate; c = capitate; t(T) = trapezium; S = scaphoid; P = pisiform; Q = triquetral; L = lunate.)

In the case of scapholunate instability, AP views of the supinated wrist in both radial and ulnar deviation are usually diagnostic. Examination of the wrist in motion using an image intensifier may also be helpful. Other investigations: 1. A radio-isotope bone scan may be carried out. If this is negative, either the diagnosis is incorrect, or local inflammatory changes are of such a minor degree that no more than conservative management should be considered 2. Arthrography may be helpful in detecting the presence and location of (intercarpal) ligament tears. The commonest instability is between the *scaphoid and lunate* (scapholunate dissociation) (Illus.). If untreated this may be followed by osteoarthritis.

Treatment: 1. In the acute case: manipulative reduction using the image intensifier, followed by the insertion of K-wires. The technique is similar to that used for dislocation of the lunate (see Frame 108): in the example shown two K-wires have been used for better carpal fixation. Alternatively an open repair of the torn ligaments may be undertaken. 2. In chronic cases reattachment of the avulsed scapholunate ligament may be carried out, but where there are arthritic changes and subluxation a salvage procedure may have to be considered.

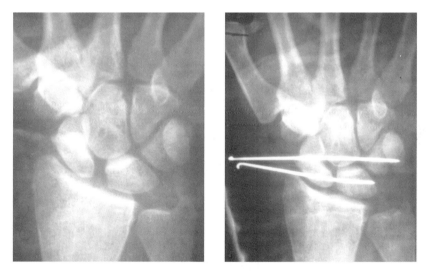

117. Carpal instabilities: A carpal instability is a condition in which there is a loss of normal carpal alignment which develops at an early or late stage after an injury.
In **static carpal instabilities** there is an abnormal carpal alignment which can be seen by careful study of standard AP and lateral radiographs of the wrist. In *dorsiflexion instability* the lunate is rotated into dorsiflexion; in *palmar flexion instability* the lunate is rotated into palmar flexion; in *ulnar translocation* the whole carpus is displaced in an ulnar direction; and in *dorsal subluxation* the carpus in displaced in a dorsal direction.
In **dynamic carpal instabilities** routine radiographs are normal. The patient is usually able to toggle his carpal alignment from normal to abnormal and back, or manipulation of the scaphoid by the examiner may reproduce the sensation of instability of which the patient usually complains. To establish the diagnosis, place lead markers on the skin over points of local tenderness, and take radiographs in both stable and unstable positions.

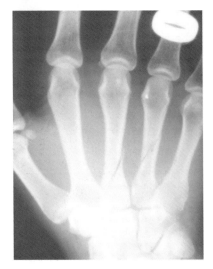

118. Injuries to the metacarpals and phalanges – general principles: In assessing how best to treat a specific injury, begin by making sure there is no significant soft tissue involvement such as nerve or tendon injury, or substantial skin loss (see later for further details). Next, from the radiographs, assess whether the bony alignment can be judged as being acceptable. (Illus: acceptable undisplaced fractures of the shafts of the middle and ring metacarpals.)

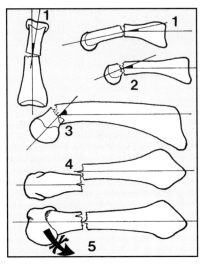

119. Assessing position cntd: Generally speaking, the position of a metacarpal or phalangeal fracture can be considered acceptable (a) if angulation does not exceed 10° in either the lateral or AP projections (1), but in the lateral, 20° may be accepted in the metaphysis (2) and 45° in the neck of the fifth metacarpal (3); (b) if there is at least 50% bony contact (4); (c) if there is no rotational deformity (5).

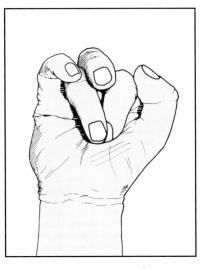

120. Assessing position cntd: Rotational deformity may not always be obvious on the radiographs, or clinically when a finger is in the extended position. Note, however, that when the fingers are individually flexed that they all touch the palm close to the scaphoid. Check that this is the case. (The same precaution should be taken when the quality of a reduction is being assessed or when splintage is being applied.)

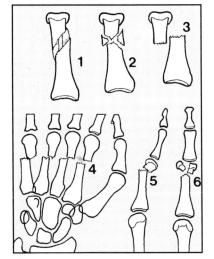

121. Assessing stability: Now go on and make an assessment of the *stability* of the fracture. Undisplaced transverse and longitudinal fractures are generally *stable*, but the following are usually *unstable*: (1) rotated spiral and some oblique fractures; (2) multifragmentary fractures; (3) severely displaced fractures; (4) multiple fractures; (5) fractures through the neck of a proximal phalanx; (6) displaced articular fractures.

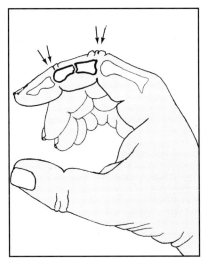

122. Assessing stability cntd: If there is some remaining doubt, assess the *functional stability* of the fracture. This is done by asking the patient to flex the injured finger (without assistance) and assessing the range of movements in the joints on either side of the fracture. If the fracture is functionally stable the range obtained should reach 30% of the normal range. (i.e. MP = 27° (N = 90°); PIP = 30° (N = 100°); DIP = 24° (N = 80°).)

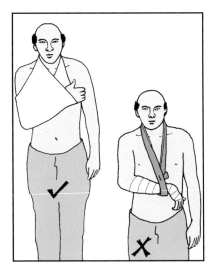

123. Treatment (a): If there is no significant soft tissue injury, if the fracture is in an acceptable position, and if it is clinically and radiologically stable, treatment should be directed at controlling the initial pain and swelling. Elevation of the arm in a sling may be helpful, *provided the sling is applied in such a way that the hand is not dependent.* Any pressure dressing should be applied in such a way that it avoids any local constriction. Mobilise early.

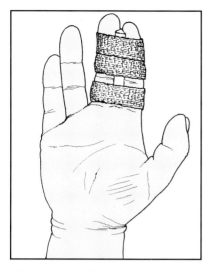

124. Treatment (b): If the position is unsatisfactory, the fracture should be manipulated. If a good stable position can be obtained, treat as above. If the position is acceptable, or an acceptable position has been obtained by manipulation, but the fracture is unstable, splintage will be required. For the less severe injuries buddy (garter) strapping to an adjacent finger with interdigital felt padding provides the ideal combination of stability while retaining movement (Illus.).

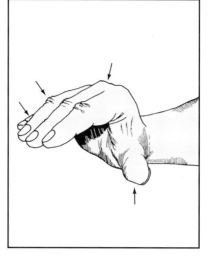

125. Treatment (c): If the injury is more severe, and a more restricting cast or bandaging is necessary, close attention must be paid to the position of the fingers. The MP joints should *never* be splinted in extension. When recovery of movements is hoped for, the MP joints should be flexed to 90°, the IP joints extended, and the thumb abducted. In practice this is often difficult to achieve, but MP joint extension should be studiously avoided.

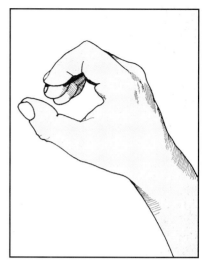

126. Treatment (d): The previously described position, where return of function is expected, reduces the effects of fibrosis in the collateral ligaments, and places the finger joints in a favourable position for mobilisation. It must be carefully differentiated from the position of *fixation* where no return of function is anticipated (e.g. the position a joint is placed in for fusion). In the latter case, the MP and IP joints are put up in midflexion.

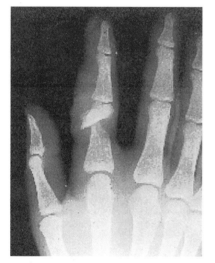

127. Treatment (e): If the fracture cannot be reduced or held with simple splintage in acceptable position, then open reduction and/or stabilisation with some form of internal fixation (or an external fixator) should be considered. Other indications for this approach include: 1. The presence of a significant soft tissue injury; 2. the presence of multiple fractures; 3. fractures involving or disrupting joint surface. (Illus.: open unstable fracture of proximal phalanx in an unacceptable position.)

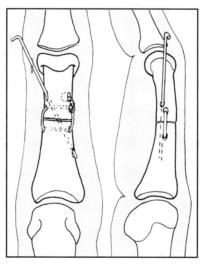

128. Methods of internal fixation: The aim is to achieve a rigidity of fixation that will allow early mobilisation. Unfortunately the bones of the hand are small and soft tissue cover poor. These factors, along with the proximity of the gliding structures, and the risks of tendon and joint adhesions have led to the development of alternative techniques: these include **type A intraosseous wiring.** The latter is suitable for transverse fractures, and employs a single loop of 26G monofilament stainless steel wire and a K-wire.

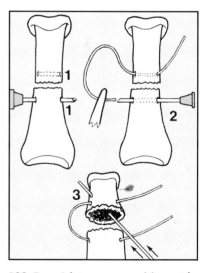

129. Type A intraosseous wiring cntd: *Technique.* The fracture may be approached through a mid-line dorsal incision (except in the case of the distal phalanx, when an H incision is used). Two transverse holes, situated marginally towards the dorsal surfaces and 3–4 mm from the bone ends, are drilled using a trocar pointed 0.035″ (0.89 mm) K-wire (or equivalent drill) (1). Through these holes the wire is threaded using, if required, a 20G needle as a carrier (2). A K-wire is then inserted obliquely through the distal fragment (3).

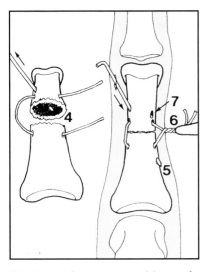

130. Type A intraosseous wiring cntd:
The K-wire is partially withdrawn (4), the
fracture reduced, and the K-wire driven
through the opposite cortex (5). The wire is
twisted (6), and the ends cropped and tucked
into a hole drilled in the cortex (7). External
splintage (e.g. bandages, sling, POP
backshell) may be used for comfort, but this
should be discarded by the seventh day. A
biodegradable bone peg may be used instead
of the K-wire. This form of wiring is not
recommended for metacarpal shaft fractures.

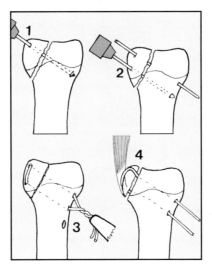

131. Type B intraosseous wiring: This
is suitable for small articular fragments.
Technique: The fracture is reduced, and a
hole drilled at right angles to the fracture
line (1). Leave the drill (0.035″ (0.89 mm)
K-wire) in position, and with a second drill
make a hole parallel to the first (2). Insert the
wire, using a hypodermic needle as a carrier,
tighten, crop and bury as before (3). If the
fragment is too small to drill, it may be
snared by passing the wire next to bone
(e.g. through the collateral ligament
attachment) (4).

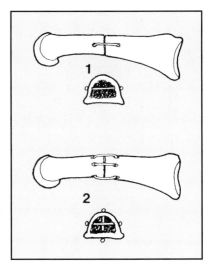

132. 90–90 intraosseous wiring: This
resembles Type A wiring, but instead of a
single wire (1), two wires are used at right
angles to one another (2). It is a strong
method of holding transverse fractures of the
metacarpals and phalanges, and is useful for
fusions and replants. It should not be used if
there is osteoporosis or fragmentation.
Technique: The bone ends are trimmed if
necessary to provide flat contiguous surfaces,
and holes drilled with careful attention to
orientation.

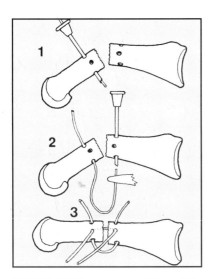

133. 90–90 intraosseous wiring cntd:
A 20G needle may be used as a carrier,
flexing the finger at the fracture site as
required for placing the vertical wire (1 & 2).
When both wires have been inserted (3), the
fracture is reduced and the wires tightened
by twisting. The ends should be buried to
avoid interference with the gliding structures.
After closure, additional external splintage
may be employed for patient comfort; this
should be discarded and mobilisation
commenced within 7 days.

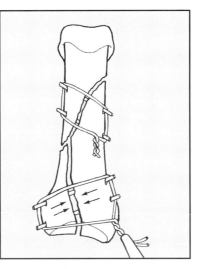

134. Tension band wiring: This can give
very strong fixation, and is useful for
unstable fractures of the phalanges and
metacarpals, especially when there is a
degree of fragmentation. *Technique*: The
fractures are reduced and held with single or
paired K-wires; the wires are cropped so that
the amount protruding from the bone is just
enough to give anchorage for tension band
wires. These are looped round the *dorsal*
surface of the bone before tightening.

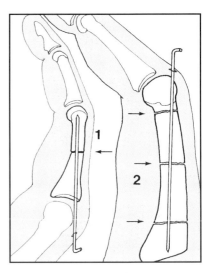

135. Percutaneous K-wires: This is used
most often to stabilise phalangeal (1), and
metacarpal fractures at all levels (2). In many
cases the wires can be inserted without
exposing the fracture. The quality of fixation
is seldom perfect, and additional external
splintage is often required. Although there
can be problems with loosening, migration,
infection, distraction and non-union, it is a
valuable technique. Best results are obtained
when trocar pointed wires are inserted with
slow drilling speeds

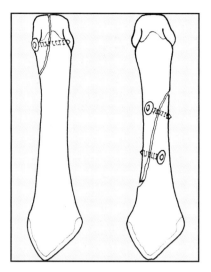

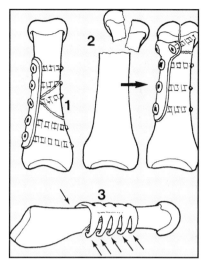

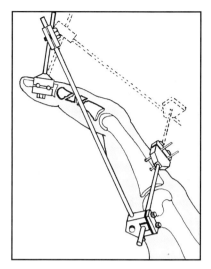

136. Compression screws: These may be used to reconstruct articular fractures, or to hold unstable fractures of the metacarpals or phalanges. The bone fragments are often small and friable, and secure fixation without risk of devascularisation or fragment fracture requires careful case selection. As a general rule, any fragment should be at least three times the diameter of the screw intended to be used. (2.7 mm screws may be used in metacarpal fractures; 2.0 and 1.5 mm screws are used in phalangeal fractures.)

137. Plate fixation: Plates must be carefully placed to avoid interference with the gliding structures. They are of value in fractures which are comminuted (1), have bone loss, or are intra-articular or periarticular (e.g. of T- and Y- (2)) pattern; and as an alternative to that shown in Frames 131–135. Available are $\frac{1}{4}$ tubular, DCP, T-shaped condylar, and Mennen (3). In the latter (used for metacarpal fractures) the prongs are crimped round the bone after the fracture has been reduced.

138. Rigid mini external fixators: Small external fixators may be used for multifragmentary fractures, fractures with bone loss and/or severe soft tissue involvement, infected fractures, and fracture–dislocations of the PIP joint. Traction (e.g. for joint disruptions) or compression techniques may be employed. Unilateral, bilateral, and combination systems (Illus.) can be used. Their application can be difficult, the pin tracks are susceptible to infection, and the pins may interfere with the gliding structures.

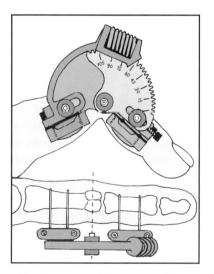

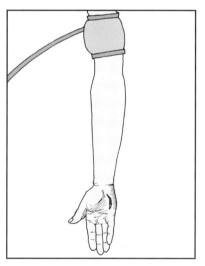

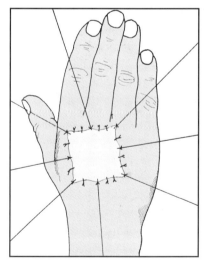

139. Motion-permitting external fixators: The Compass PIP Joint Hinge®, centred over the axis of movement of the joint, is attached to two pins on either side of the fracture, controlling the position of the fragments as in other external fixators, and permitting a degree of distraction to encourage alignment of fragments (particularly intra-articular ones). The worm may be disengaged to permit active movements, or it may be engaged and advanced for passive mobilisation.

140. Soft tissue management (a): Where there is necrotic or foreign material, a thorough debridement should be performed under a tourniquet to minimise the risks of infection. There is little tissue to spare in the hand, and wide excision of wounds is to be avoided. (2) The tourniquet should be released prior to closure to secure bleeding points and reduce wound haematoma.

141. Soft tissue management cntd (b): Where there is skin loss, every attempt should be made to ensure that healing will be achieved as quickly as possible to permit early mobilisation. The exposure of fractures, joints and bones should be avoided, and if the situation permits a primary skin grafting procedure or plastic repair should be carried out.

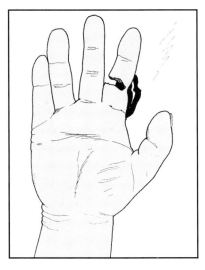

142. Soft tissue management cntd (c):
If there is division of both neurovascular bundles to a finger, amputation should be advised unless facilities for microsurgery are available and the particular circumstances (e.g. employment, hobbies, etc.) make an attempt at preservation particularly desirable. In all cases, the maximum length of thumb must be preserved.

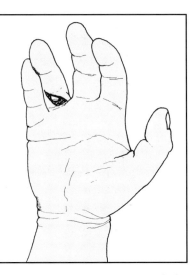

143. Soft tissue management cntd (d):
If there is appreciable risk of infection (e.g. ragged wound, dirty causal instrument) primary suture of nerves and also of tendons in the 'no man's area' of the tendon sheaths should not be undertaken. Where, however, the circumstances are ideal, the experienced surgeon may achieve the best results by primary repair.

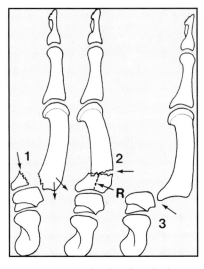

144. Injuries to the thumb – The base:
The commonest injuries involving the base of the thumb are (1) Bennett's fracture (or Bennett's fracture–dislocation as it may be more aptly called); (2) fractures of the base of the thumb metacarpal. When there is a vertical extension into the joint, converting it into a T- or Y-fracture, the prognosis is less good (Rolando fracture, R); (3) carpometacarpal dislocation of the thumb.

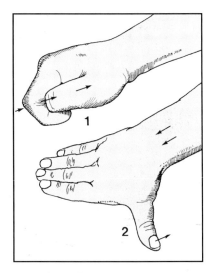

145. Diagnosis: Injuries of the base usually result from force being applied along the long axis of the thumb, e.g. from a fall or blow on the clenched fist (1), or from forced abduction of the thumb (2). Any of these may be mistaken for scaphoid fracture, but tenderness is maximal distal to the snuff box (and deformity may be obvious).

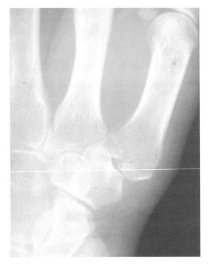

146. Bennett's fracture: Note the distinctive features of this fracture: 1. a small medial fragment of bone which may tilt, but maintains its relationship with the trapezium, 2. the (vertical) fracture line involves the joint between the thumb metacarpal and the trapezium (trapezometacarpal joint), 3. most important, the proximal and lateral subluxation of the thumb metacarpal.

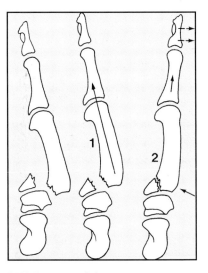

147. Treatment (a): The principle of reduction is straightforward: traction is applied to the thumb (1) and reduction completed by abducting it and applying pressure to the lateral aspect of the base (2). A general anaesthetic or Bier block is usually necessary. Maintaining reduction can be troublesome, and careful attention must be paid to the details of plaster fixation.

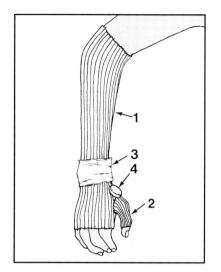

148. Treatment (b): Begin by applying stockinet to the arm (1) and the thumb (2). Bony prominences should be protected as required with wool roll (3). A small felt pad is placed over the base of the thumb metacarpal (4). (*Note:* adhesive felt should not be applied directly to the skin in this situation if a pustular rash is to be avoided.)

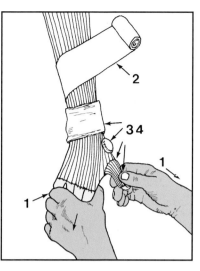

149. Treatment (c): An assistant applies traction to the thumb and steadies the lateral three fingers (1). Two to three 15 cm (6″) POP bandages (with or without an anterior slab) are applied to the *forearm* (2). Two 10 cm (4″) POP bandages are then quickly applied to the wrist and up to the IP joint of the thumb (3).

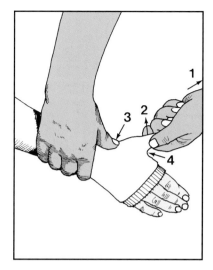

150. Treatment (d): The surgeon now takes the thumb (the plaster being set on the forearm while the distal part remains soft). He must apply traction (1), abduct the thumb (2), maintain pressure over the base of the first metacarpal (3), and mould the plaster well into the MP joint on its flexor aspect (4).

151. Aftercare: 1. Check radiographs are taken to confirm that reduction has been achieved. 2. The arm may require elevating with a sling for the first few days. 3. The patient should be seen at weekly intervals for the first 2–3 weeks and the thumb X-rayed. If the plaster appears slack at any stage it must be changed. If there is evidence of slipping of the fracture a new plaster should also be applied (no anaesthetic is generally required). During the setting of the plaster, light traction should be applied to the thumb while the plaster is well moulded round the base (in the position described for the initial reduction). 4. Plaster fixation should be maintained for 6 weeks.

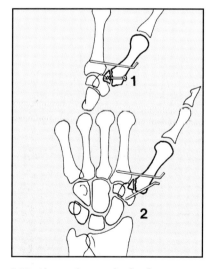

152. Alternative methods of treatment: A good result is the rule following reduction and plaster fixation, but alternative methods of holding this fracture are practised. These include: (1) screw fixation (e.g. using the AO small fragment set, with further stabilisation of the fixation with a K-wire); or (2) the use of two K-wires.

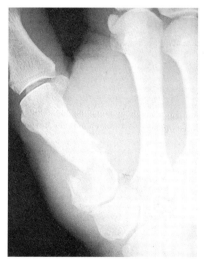

153. Fractures near the base of the thumb metacarpal: Greenstick fractures of this type are common in children. Angulation is usually slight or moderate, and should be accepted; gross angulations should be manipulated, using the technique described for Bennett's fracture. Plaster fixation for about 5 weeks is desirable. **Rolando fractures** require careful reduction, and good results are claimed for stabilisation with an external fixator, the pins being placed in the metacarpal and the trapezium.

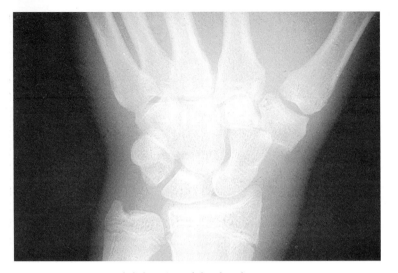

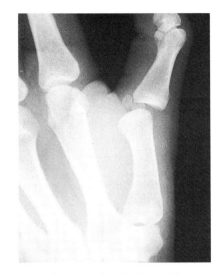

154. Carpometacarpal dislocation of the thumb: The thumb may dislocate at the joint between the metacarpal base and the trapezium, or the whole of the first ray may be involved, the trapezium remaining with the thumb metacarpal, with the dislocation taking place between the trapezium and the scaphoid (Illus.). Both these injuries result from forcible abduction of the thumb. *Treatment*: Reduce by applying traction to thumb and local pressure over the base. Any persisting instability may be controlled with percutaneous K-wires. Thereafter apply a well-padded plaster of scaphoid type for 3 weeks. Elevation of the limb for the first few days is desirable. Physiotherapy is seldom required.

155. Injuries at the MP joint of the thumb – Posterior dislocation (a): This injury generally results from forcible hyperextension of the thumb. It is common in children. In a number of cases there is 'button holing' of the capsule by the metacarpal head and closed methods of reduction will fail. Nevertheless, manipulation should be tried first in all cases.

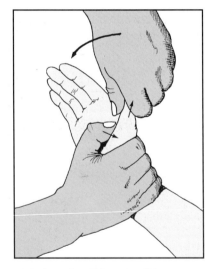

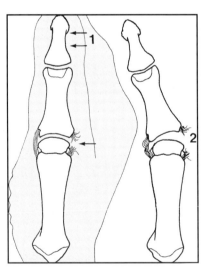

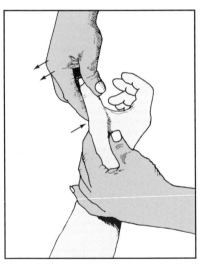

156. Posterior dislocation (b): Manipulative reduction may often be attempted without anaesthesia (by the quick confident application of the traction to the thumb with simultaneous pressure over the metacarpal head). When open reduction is required this should be performed through a lateral incision under a tourniquet. In all cases a light plaster splint should be worn for 2–3 weeks after reduction.

157. Rupture of the ulnar collateral ligament (Gamekeeper's) (a): This injury is caused by forcible abduction (1). If unrecognised and untreated, there may be progressive MP subluxation (2) with interference with grasp, causing significant permanent disability. *Suspect* this injury when there is complaint of pain in this region. *Look for tenderness* on the medial side of the MP joint.

158. Ulnar collateral ligament (b): Extend the MP joint fully and apply stress to the ulnar collateral ligament by abducting the proximal phalanx. Repeat with the thumb flexed at the MP joint. Note the presence of any 'give'. Carefully compare one side with the other. If in doubt, stress radiographs should be taken. Careful palpation may reveal the torn distal portion of the ligament lodged between the adductor pollicis aponeurosis and its normal position (Stener lesion).

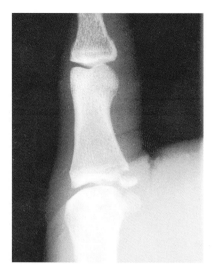

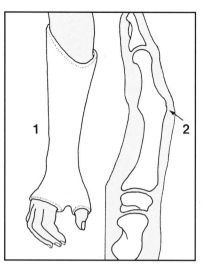

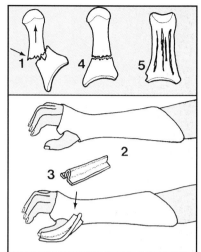

159. Ulnar collateral ligament (c):
Study radiographs of the joint:
1. Subluxation may or may not be apparent in the unstressed films. 2. An avulsion fracture (Illus.) may betray this type of injury (sometimes separately referred to as gamekeeper's fracture). If a fracture is present, note its position. (Marked displacement, or rotation so that its articular surface is pointing distally, and a large fragment are indications for surgery.)

160. Ulnar collateral ligament (d):
Treatment: 1. Slight laxity or minimally displaced avulsion fracture: scaphoid cast for 6 weeks (1). 2. Rotated fragment: reduction and internal fixation. 3. Gross laxity, especially with a palpable Stener lesion: primary surgical repair is usually preferred. (Conservative treatment may give a good result but is less reliable.) 4. Late diagnosed complete tear: repair of the capsulo-ligamentous complex with a palmaris longus free tendon graft; or as a salvage procedure, MP joint fusion (2).

161. Fracture of the proximal phalanx:
The severely angled fracture (1) should be reduced by traction and local pressure. Hold with a dorsal (or volar) slab (2) to which is added a girdered extension (3), held on with bandages. If the position cannot be readily held, internal fixation (e.g. by one of the wiring methods) is indicated. The minimally angled fracture (4) or the splinter fracture (5) may be protected by a local slab (similar to 3) bandaged in position. Elevation may be required.

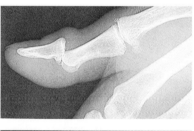

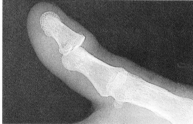

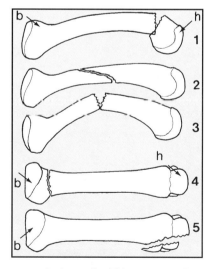

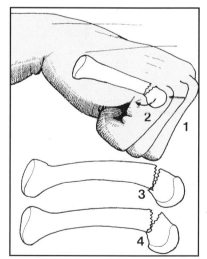

162. IP joint dislocation of the thumb:
Reduce by traction as described for MP joint dislocations. Only occasionally is anaesthesia required (ring or Bier block). Thereafter splint for 2–3 weeks with a local plaster slab. *Fractures of the terminal phalanx:* Crushing injuries are the usual cause, and any soft tissue damage takes priority in management. A light local splint (e.g. of plaster) will prevent pain from stubbing.

163. Injuries to the fifth metacarpal:
The commonest fractures involving the metacarpal of the little finger are:
(1) fractures of the neck; (2) spiral fractures of the shaft, usually undisplaced; (3) transverse fractures of the shaft, often angulated; (4) fractures of the base; (5) fractures of the head. (b = base, h = head.)

164. Fractures of the neck of the fifth metacarpal (a): These are nearly always caused by the clenched fist meeting resistance, e.g. as a result of a fight (1). Angulation and impaction are common (2). When angulation is slight (3) or moderate (4) it should be accepted, and the fracture supported for 3–4 weeks until local pain settles.

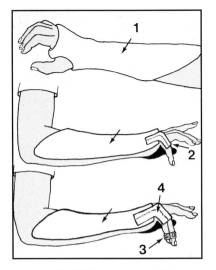

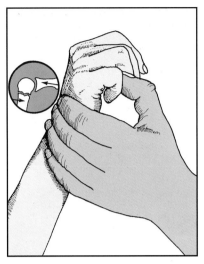

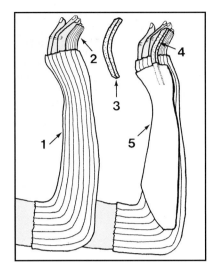

165. Neck of fifth metacarpal (b): A simple dorsal slab (1), completed after a few days, may be quite satisfactory. Better fixation is achieved by the addition of a finger extension (2) to the basic slab. Still more support is provided by the use of buddy (garter) strapping (3) and the inclusion of the ring and little fingers in the extension (4) (securing bandages omitted in Illus. for clarity).

166. Neck of fifth metacarpal (c): If angulation is gross (more than 45°), an attempt may be made to correct it. The MP joint is flexed; pressure is then applied to the head via the proximal phalanx, using the thumb. The fingers apply counter pressure to the shaft. Reduction is generally easy. The position may be maintained using a K-wire or with a plaster cast.

167. Neck of fifth metacarpal (d): The following technique may be employed. Stockinet is applied to the arm (1) and to the little finger (2). A thin strip of felt (3) is placed over the finger (4). A substantial dorsal slab is applied (5). The finger should be flexed into the palm and the striking point checked (see Frame 120).

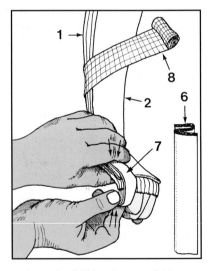

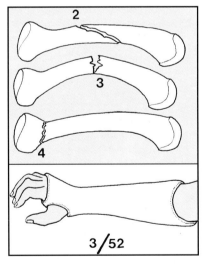

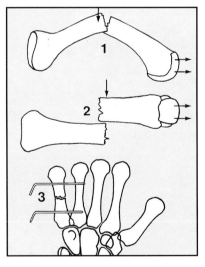

168. Neck of fifth metacarpal (e): A finger slab, made from a thrice-folded slab formed from three layers or so of 10 cm (4″) plaster bandage (6) is applied from wrist to finger tip (7). Pressure is maintained while the slab is setting. Meanwhile an assistant can be securing the slabs with a wet gauze bandage (8). Complete in 2–3 days and retain for 3–4 weeks only.

169. Injuries of the fifth metacarpal cntd: Spiral fractures of the shaft (2), transverse fractures of the shaft with slight or moderate angulation or displacement (3) and fractures of the base (4) may be treated quite adequately by the application of a Colles plaster for 3–4 weeks.

170. Injuries of the fifth metacarpal cntd: Marked angulation of a shaft fracture should be treated by traction and local pressure prior to plaster fixation (1). Displaced fractures may be similarly reduced (2); if unstable they may be held with 1–2 intramedullary K-wires inserted through the neck of the metacarpal. Soft tissue between the bone ends may necessitate open reduction, when the position may be maintained by percutaneous (3) or intramedullary K-wiring, 90–90 intraosseous wiring, or plating.

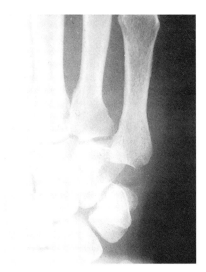

171. Injuries of the fifth metacarpal contd: Fractures of the *head* of the fifth metacarpal (Frame 163(5)) may be treated by buddy strapping and early mobilisation; if symptoms are marked a dorsal slab may also be used for the first 1–2 weeks. If the fragment is substantial and displaced, internal fixation using a screw or Type B intraosseous wiring may be considered. *Dislocation of the base* of the metacarpal (Illus.) is usually easily reduced with traction, but may need K-wire stabilisation.

172 . Injuries to the middle and ring metacarpals: The so-called *inboard fractures* involving the third and fourth metacarpals are inherently stable as they are attached by muscle and ligament to one another and to the stable pillars formed by second and fifth metacarpals. The commonest fracture is a spiral or transverse fractures of the shaft, especially the 4th metacarpal, but fractures involving both or of the base and neck are frequent. Undisplaced fractures may be supported by a Colles type slab, but be on guard for swelling which can be severe, especially in multiple fractures.

When the AP radiographs show the presence of an isolated off-ended fracture (i.e. where there is complete loss of bony apposition) affecting the middle or ring metacarpals, or where there is moderate angulation or shortening, the position can generally be accepted. The striking point of the finger however should be checked, a dorsal slab applied and the limb elevated to counteract swelling. If off-ending or angulation is conspicuous in the *lateral projection*, reduction should be carried out, either by manipulation or by an open procedure.

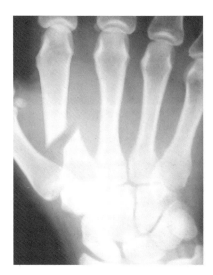

173. Injuries to the index metacarpal: The so-called *outboard fractures* involve the second and fifth metacarpals. Fractures of the fifth metacarpal have already been dealt with and severely displaced fractures of the index should be managed along similar lines. In particular, badly displaced fractures should be reduced, and if necessary secured by some form of internal fixation. If K-wires are used they should be retained for 3 weeks; plaster fixation may be needed for a further 2 weeks.

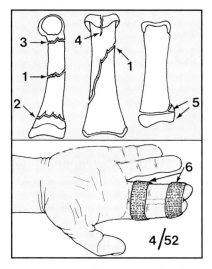

174. Fractures of the proximal and middle phalanges: Undisplaced, simple fractures, e.g. of the shaft (1), base (2), neck (3), intercondylar region (4) or epiphyseal injuries (5), seldom present any problem. Buddy strapping (6) for 3–4 weeks may give adequate support, but if symptoms are marked this may be supplemented by the use of a volar or dorsal slab, with finger extension. Displaced fractures should be assessed and treated as previously indicated (Frame 118 et seq).

175. Aftercare: In all cases:
1. Uninjured fingers should be left free and exercised. 2. Rigid fixation should be discarded as soon as possible. In many situations where a cast support has been used initially, buddy (garter) strapping may be substituted after 2 weeks, and often all support after 4. *In no instance should the MP joints be fixed in extension.*

Complications: *Finger stiffness* is the commonest and most disabling complication, and is due to joint adhesions, fibrosis in the adjacent flexor tendon sheaths and collateral ligament shortening. Infection in open fractures may be a major contributory factor. Stiffness may be minimised by the procedures described (e.g. elevation, correct splinting, early mobilisation) and by intensive physiotherapy and occupational therapy. Physiotherapy and occupational therapy should be continued with vigour until the range of movements and finger power become static. This implies careful recording, at frequent intervals, of these parameters. In this respect it is helpful to note the *total active range of motion* (TAM) in each digit; this overall movement can be assessed by a single goniometer measurement; it is a little less than the sum of the normal maxima of flexion of the individual joints, the normal value of TAM being taken to be 250°.

Early return to work should be encouraged to foster re-adaptation. Inability to work and a static response to physiotherapy require a most careful assessment of the following: 1. possibility of redeployment, 2. Possibility of improvement from further surgery (e.g. tenolysis), 3. amputation.

Amputation as primary treatment must be raised in open phalangeal fractures when they are associated with flexor tendon division. Division of one or both neurovascular bundles, skin loss or severe crushing are additional factors weighing in favour of this procedure (in contrast to attempted repair where treatment is likely to be prolonged and the final result uncertain). With these factors must be considered the patient's age, sex and occupation.

Malunion. Problems may arise from:
1. Recurrence of deformity.
2. Failure to correct initial deformity.
3. Torsional deformity. In some cases epiphyseal displacement may have escaped attention.
In the latter case remodelling may lead to correction, and in the others trick movements and postural adaptations may remove the patient's initial strong desire for corrective surgery. It is wise not to offer surgical correction until at least 6 months have passed since the injury.

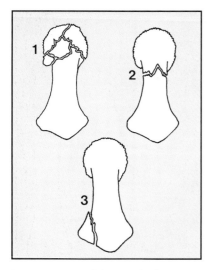

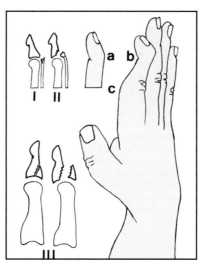

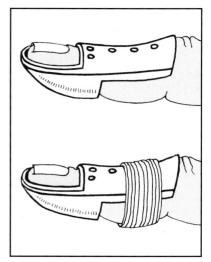

176. Fractures of the terminal phalanx: Fractures of the terminal tuft (often comminuted) (1), of the neck (2), and the base (3) are painful but relatively unimportant injuries. Treatment of any associated soft tissue injury takes precedence (e.g. debridement and suture of pulp lacerations). Nevertheless, strapping the finger to a spatula or use of a plastic finger splint may relieve pain and prevent any painful stubbing incidents.

177. Mallet finger (a): This is caused by forcible flexion of an extended finger. The distal extensor tendon slip is torn at its attachment to bone (Type I injury) or avulses a fragment of bone (Type II). The patient is unable to extend the DIP joint fully; drooping of the finger tip may be slight (a) or severe (b). In late cases there may be hyperextension of the PIP joint (c). In Type III injuries, more than 20% of the articular surface of the distal phalanx is involved, sometimes with anterior subluxation of the phalanx.

178. Mallet finger (b): *Treatment*: All these injuries excepting Type III with subluxation may be treated by splinting the distal joint in extension. A Stack or Abuna splint (Illus.) may be used. Choose the size with care to lessen the risks of skin ulceration. It is strapped to the finger and worn for 6 weeks constantly, and then for a further two at night only. It may be removed for skin hygiene if extension is preserved. Alternatively, support the distal joint with a short length of padded spatula strapped to the volar surface.

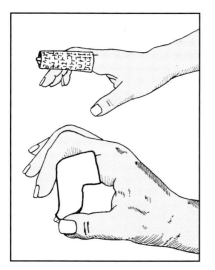

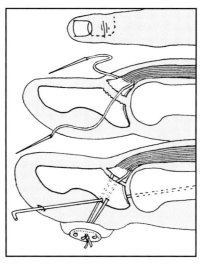

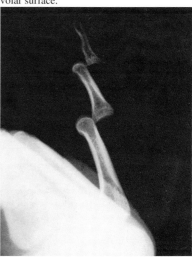

179. Mallet finger (c): Where the patient's cooperation is in doubt, a Smillie plaster may be used for 6–8 weeks, although it can cause some stiffness. Form a 4-layer tube of 7.5 cm (3″) dry POP bandage round the finger. Dip the hand momentarily in water, asking the patient to flex the PIP joint and extend the DIP joint against the thumb while the POP is smoothed. *Note:* In any case there may be some recurrence on removal of splintage, but disability is seldom more than slight, and spontaneous improvement may occur up to a year after the injury.

180. Mallet finger (d): If there is subluxation, splint in flexion or extension if reduction can be achieved in that position: otherwise repair is advised through a C-shaped incision. A pull-out wire may be used with a stabilising K-wire as illustrated, but a suture anchor (such as the Mitek® Micro QuickAnchor®) may be preferred. *Late diagnosed*: Extension splintage may be successful even as late as 6 months. If there is a swan-neck deformity, an oblique retinacular ligament reconstruction has been advocated.

181. MP and interphalangeal joint dislocations: These may be simple or multiple (Illus.) and as they result from hyperextension are almost always posterior dislocations. Reduce as described for the thumb (Frame 156). Thereafter buddy strapping should be applied for 2 weeks unless there is any evidence of instability – when POP splintage may be required for a slightly longer period.

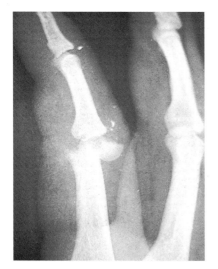

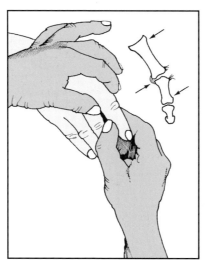

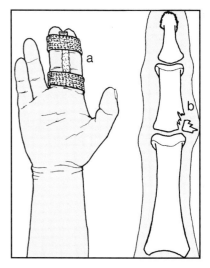

182. Fracture–dislocation: It is essential that the joint surface is correctly relocated, and important that mobilisation is commenced as soon as possible. Open reduction is usually required, and fixation may be achieved with intraosseous wiring, small fragment set screws, or plating. Mobilisation should be commenced immediately with the added support of buddy strapping.

183. 'Sprains' and lateral subluxations (a): These are usually caused by falls in which the side of a finger strikes some resistant object. There is avulsion or tearing of a collateral ligament. Spontaneous reduction is the rule. *Diagnosis:* The injury should be suspected on the basis of the history and the presence of local tenderness. Confirmation is obtained by noting instability on stressing the collateral ligament.

184. Sprains and lateral subluxations (b): Radiographs may show a tell-tale avulsion fracture. If doubt remains, stress films may be taken. *Treatment:* (a) Buddy strapping for 5 weeks should be adequate. (b) If an avulsion fracture is present and has rotated, it should be replaced and fixed. *Complications:* Fusiform swellings of the finger may persist for many months even in the treated injury. If a flexion deformity starts to develop, use an extension assisting lively splint.

185. Compartment syndromes in the hand: There are no less than 10 osteofascial compartments in the hand (7 for the interossei, 1 thenar, 1 hypothenar, and 1 containing adductor pollicis). Increased compartment pressure may follow severe crushing injuries, multiple fractures, and the erroneous administration of unsuitable intravenous infusions. The onset may be heralded by severe pain, loss of finger movements, and increased swelling. The fingers are usually held in a position of extension at the MP joints, and flexion at the proximal IP joints. Sensory disturbance is not a feature. The increased tissue pressure required to produce this condition is about 10 mm lower than that found at other sites.

Treatment: The transverse carpal ligament must be divided. If a midline incision is used then access to the three anterior compartments may be readily obtained through it. The interosseous compartments may be opened through two longitudinal dorsal incisions (over the second and fourth metacarpals). The dorsal incisions may be closed primarily, but secondary closure is usually advised for the volar incision.

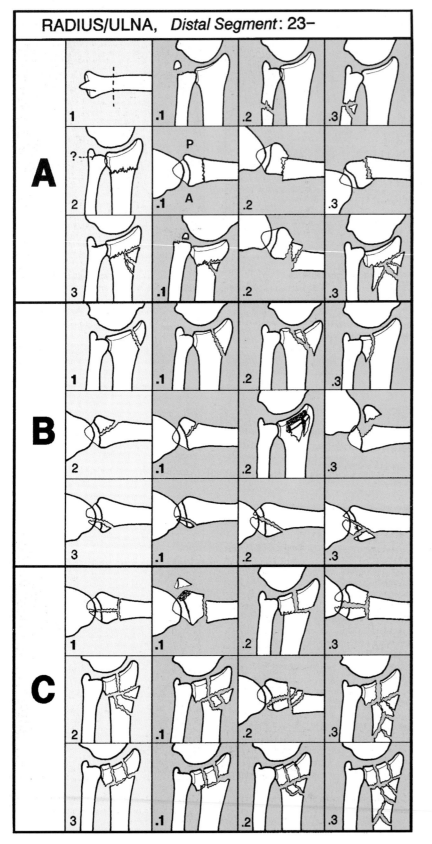

RADIUS/ULNA, *Distal Segment*: 23–

186. AO classification of fractures of the radius/ulna, distal segment (23–):

Type A fractures are extra-articular.
A1 = Fracture of the ulna only: .1 styloid process; .2 simple, of the metaphysis; .3 multifragmentary of the metaphysis.
A2 = Simple impacted fracture of the radius: .1 undisplaced; .2 with dorsal tilting (Colles pattern); .3 with anterior tilting (Smith pattern).
A3 = Multifragmentary fracture of the radius: .1 with axial impaction and shortening; .2 with a wedge; .3 complex.

Type B fractures are partial articular fractures of the radius.
B1 = Partial articular fracture of radius in the sagittal plane: .1 simple lateral; .2 multifragmentary lateral; .3 medial.
B2 = Partial articular fracture of the radius with involvement of the posterior lip (dorsal rim) (Barton's fracture): .1 simple; .2 with an additional lateral sagittal fracture; .3 with dorsal dislocation of the carpus (fracture dislocation of the wrist).
B3 = Partial articular fracture of the radius with involvement of the anterior lip (volar rim) (Reverse Barton's fracture): .1 simple with a small fragment; .2 simple with a large fragment; .3 multifragmentary.

Type C fractures are complete articular fractures.
C1 = Both the metaphyseal and articular elements are simple; .1 with a posteromedial articular fragment; .2 with the articular fracture line in the sagittal plane; .3 with articular fracture line in the frontal plane.
C2 = The articular fracture is simple, but the metaphyseal fracture is multifragmentary: .1 the articular fracture line is in the sagittal plane; .2 the articular fracture line is in the frontal plane; .3 the metaphyseal fracture extends into the diaphysis.
C3 = The articular fracture is multifragmentary: .1 metaphyseal simple; .2 the metaphyseal fracture is also multifragmentary; .3 multifragmentary metaphyseal fracture extending into the diaphysis.

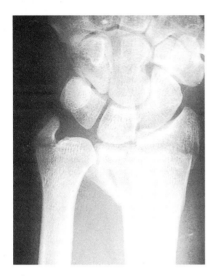

187. Describe this AP radiograph of the wrist; the history is of pain and marked swelling following a fall on the outstretched hand.

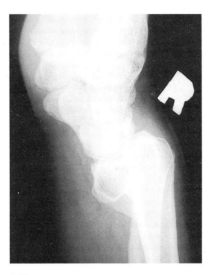

188. There is a history of deformity of the wrist persisting after an injury some years previously. What is the diagnosis?

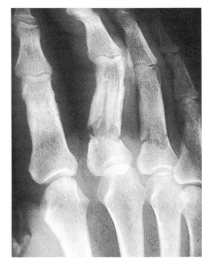

189. The history is of a crushing injury of the hand and fingers. Describe the radiograph.

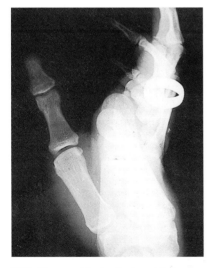

190. The complaint is of pain and deformity of the hand following an injury in which the fingers were forced backwards. What does the radiograph show?

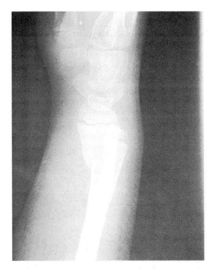

191. Describe this injury sustained by a child in a fall.

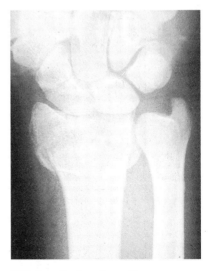

192. Describe the radiographic appearances. The history is of a fall on the outstretched hand.

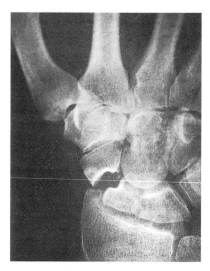

193. What does this radiograph show?

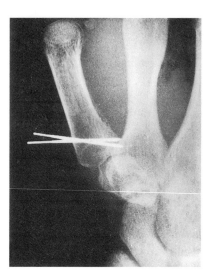

194. What injury is being treated here?

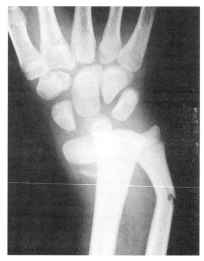

195. What is the injury? How would you treat it?

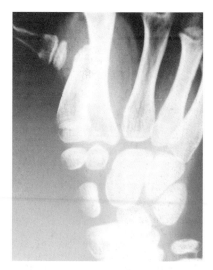

196. What is this injury? What special precaution would you take if attempting treatment by closed methods?

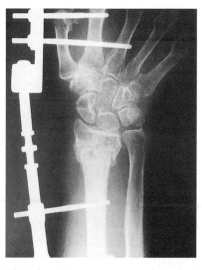

197. What is this injury, and how is it being treated?

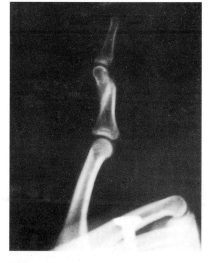

198. What does this radiograph show? What functional restriction would you expect?

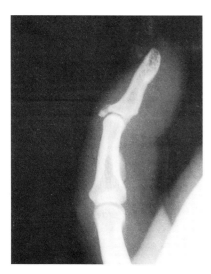

199. What is this injury? How would you treat it?

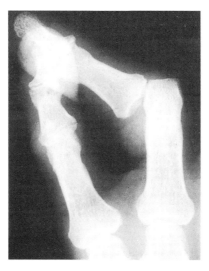

200. What is this injury? How would you treat it?

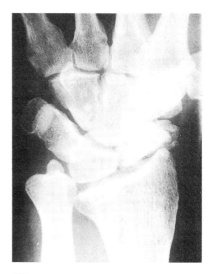

201. What fracture complication is shown on this radiograph?

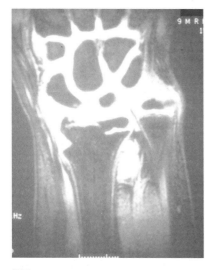

202. What does this scan show?

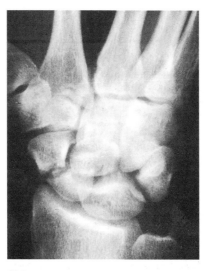

203. What type of fracture is present? What is the prognosis? How might it be treated?

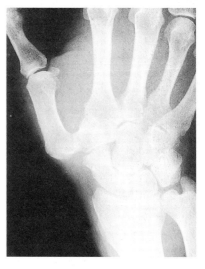

204. What is this injury? How would you treat it?

ANSWERS TO SELF-TEST

187. Fracture of the distal radius; the distal fragment is fragmented, with the fracture line involving the radiocarpal joint; fracture of the ulnar styloid. (AO = 23–C1.2.)

188. Malunion of a Smith's fracture. (AO = 23–C1.2.)

189. There is a transverse fracture of the base of the proximal phalanx of the ring finger; the single film suggests that there is no significant angulation or displacement. There is a fracture of the base of the proximal phalanx of the middle finger, with vertical splinter fractures running into the proximal IP joint. There is angulation of the fracture. The single oblique view suggests that this is mainly anterior angulation.

190. Posterior dislocation of all the fingers at the MP joints. The thumb is not affected.

191. Greenstick fractures of the radius and ulna just proximal to the epiphyseal lines. There is slight subluxation of the distal ulna whose angulation is less than that of the radius. The deformity corresponds to that found in a Smith's fracture, and the combination of fracture of the radius with ulnar subluxation has some of the feature of the Galeazzi lesion.

192. 1. There is a highly comminuted fracture of the distal radius with the radial displacement, ulnar angulation and impaction usually associated with a comminuted Colles fracture with involvement of the radiocarpal joint. A lateral projection would be required to differentiate it with certainty from a Smith's fracture. 2. There is a fracture through the waist of the scaphoid. (AO = 23–C3.1.)

193. Long-standing non-union of the scaphoid, with early secondary osteoarthritic changes in the wrist joint.

194. Bennett's fracture of the thumb being held with fine K-wires.

195. This is a slipped distal radial epiphysis, uncommonly associated with a greenstick fracture of the ulna in its distal third. This should reduce easily by manipulation; subsequent treatment would be by plaster fixation.

196. MP dislocation of the thumb in a child; theatre facilities should be available (for an open reduction) should manipulation under general anaesthesia fail.

197. Unstable, slightly comminuted fracture of the distal radius with an associated injury to the ulnar styloid (Colles type fracture); this is being treated by an external fixator. Stable injuries of this pattern would normally be treated conservatively; the use of an external fixator is generally reserved for open injuries, unstable fractures which are difficult to control, and highly comminuted fractures involving the radiocarpal joint.

198. Malunion of a fracture of a middle phalanx. There would be inevitable loss of flexion in the distal IP joint.

199. Mallet finger, with a small avulsion fracture of the base of the distal phalanx; there is no joint subluxation, and the injury should respond well to 6 weeks' splintage in extension.

200. Dislocation of the proximal IP joint of the ring finger. Treat by manipulative reduction followed by buddy strapping splintage.

201. Avascular necrosis of the scaphoid.

202. The distal end of the ulna extends well beyond the distal radial epiphysis, disturbing the mechanics of the wrist joint. The relative increased length of the ulna is due to a traumatic epiphyseal arrest involving the distal radius; this has followed a previous slipped distal radial epiphysis. The bone block responsible for the growth disturbance can be clearly seen to involve about 50% of the epiphyseal plate.

203. Displaced and possibly slightly comminuted fracture of the waist of the scaphoid. This injury has a bad prognosis, and primary internal fixation is desirable.

204. Carpometacarpal dislocation of the thumb, with a small associated fracture, possibly of the metacarpal base. Manipulative reduction followed by plaster fixation, with K-wire fixation if unstable.

CHAPTER

10

The spine

1. General principles:
1. The **main concern** in any spinal injury is less with the spine itself than with the closely related neurological elements (the spinal cord, issuing nerve roots and cauda equina).
2. If there is no **neurological complication** the chances of later neurological involvement must be assessed; if there is some risk of this, *precautions must be taken to see that this is avoided at all stages.*
3. If there is an **incomplete paraplegia** or other major neurological problem complicating the injury *great care must be taken to see that no deterioration is allowed to occur.*
4. If **paraplegia** is present and complete, the prognosis regarding potential recovery must be firmly established as early as possible. Only if this is pronounced, *total and permanent* can vigilance in the handling of the spinal injury be relaxed.

In summary, the key to the management of spinal injuries is a thorough understanding of the nature of any damage to the bony elements, the supportive ligamentous structures, and the related neurological structures.

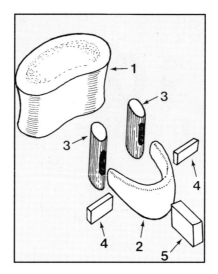

2. Anatomical features (after Kapandji) (a):
The components of a typical vertebra have a complex relationship, and can be illustrated with an exploded diagram. The elements comprise the vertebral body (1) composed of cancellous bone covered with an outer shell of cortical bone, the horseshoe-shaped neural arch (2), two articular masses or processes which take part in the facet (interarticular) joints (3) and the transverse (4) and spinous (5) processes.

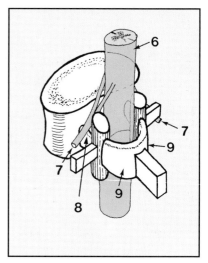

3. Anatomical features (b):
When these components are brought together they form a protective bony covering for the cord (6) and the issuing nerve roots (7) The neural arch (2) is divided by the articular processes (3) into pedicles (8) and laminae (9).

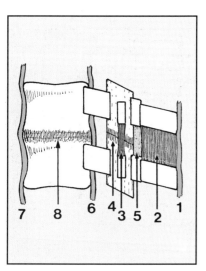

4. Anatomical features (c):
The vertebrae are bound together by the following structures: the supraspinous (1), interspinous (2), intertransverse (3) and capsular (4) ligaments, and the ligamentum flavum (5). Together, these form the so-called posterior ligament complex. Playing a less powerful but nevertheless important role are the posterior (6) and anterior (7) longitudinal ligaments and the annular ligaments (8). Trauma may result in damage to any of the bony or ligamentous structures of the spine, in isolation or in combination.

5. Assessment of spinal injuries (a):
In managing any case of spinal injury it is important to determine which structures have been involved and the extent of the damage they have suffered; with this information an assessment may be made of the risks of complication. *Note:* 1. The history may direct you to the type of injury to suspect; 2. The clinical examination may be a valuable guide to the extent of bony and ligamentous injury (and any neurological complication); 3. Investigation by X-ray and CAT scan is likely to provide the most information; MRI scans, if available, may help clarify the extent of any associated soft tissue damage, especially the intervertebral discs and the posterior ligament complex.

It is important to make an early assessment of the stability of the spine, i.e. to assess whether it is able to withstand stress without progressive deformity or further neurological damage. Instability may be *purely mechanical* (e.g. in some compression fractures where further kyphotic deformity may occur); or *neurological* (e.g. where shifting or further extrusion of bone fragments within the spinal canal may lead to neurological deterioration). Combined *mechanical and neurological* instability may be present. In assessing instability it may be helpful to regard the spine as having three main elements or columns.

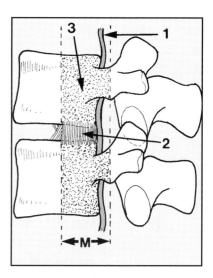

6. Assessment of spinal injuries (b):
The *middle column* (M) consists of the posterior longitudinal ligament (1), the posterior part of the annular ligament (2), and the posterior wall of the vertebral column (3). Unstable injuries occur when damage to the middle column is combined with damage to either the anterior column or to the posterior column.

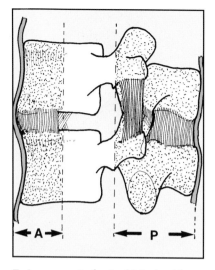

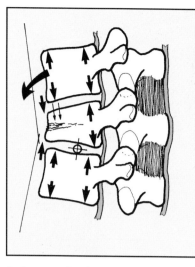

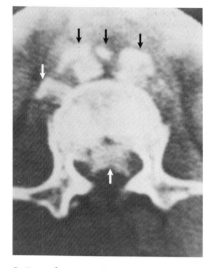

7. Assessment of spinal injuries (c):
The *posterior column* (P), vital for stability, comprises the neural arch, the pedicles, the spinous process, and the posterior ligamentous complex. The *anterior column* (A) is formed by the anterior longitudinal ligament, and the anterior parts of the annular ligament and vertebral body. Note that failure of these columns in their role as supports can be due to bony or ligament involvement. Four categories are recognised in the Denis classification of spinal injury:

8. Compression fractures (a): Simple compression fractures are common stable injuries involving the anterior column only. Hyperflexion of the spine round an axis passing through the disc space leads to mechanical failure of bone with either *anterior* (Illus.) or *lateral* wedging. The height of the posterior part of the vertebral body is maintained. (Note that *severe* wedging – e.g. more than 15–20° – often indicates damage to the other columns and a burst fracture or fracture–dislocation.)

9. Burst fractures (b): Axial loading of the spine may cause failure of the anterior and middle columns. One or both end plates may be involved, and bone fragments may be extruded into the spinal canal, compromising the neurological structures and, more controversially, causing neurological instability. Radiographs may show the vertebral body fracture, loss of vertebral height, and, in the AP, laminar fractures and separation of the pedicles. (Illus: CAT scan showing displacement of bony fragments both anteriorly and posteriorly.)

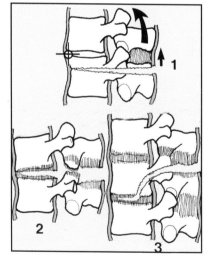

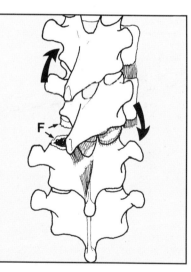

10. Seat-belt type injuries (c): Rapid deceleration causes the spine to jack-knife round an axis brought forward by a lap type seat-belt, and *tension* forces lead to failure of the posterior and middle columns. The spine is unstable in flexion. Failure may occur entirely through bone (Chance fracture) (1), or ligaments (2), or a combination (3), involving either one (1 & 2) or two (3) levels of the spine. Injuries of this pattern may be seen in situations outside road traffic accidents, but the essential element is tension failure.

11. Fracture–dislocations (d): All 3 columns fail in these unstable injuries. Suspect if: 1. there are multiple rib or transverse process fractures (as from D1 to D8 the ribs and sternum give additional support to the spine); 2. there is a slight increase in the height of a disc or a fracture of an articular process. Types: *Flexion–rotation fracture–dislocation*. There is often a fracture of an articular process on one side (F), or a slicing fracture through a vertebral body, leading to rotation and subluxation of the spine.

12. (d cntd): (b) *Shear types of fracture–dislocation:* In the *posteroanterior type* (1) the upper segment shears forwards, often with fracture of the posterior arch at 1 or 2 levels. In the *anteroposterior type* (2) there is complete ligamentous disruption, but often no fracture. In the *flexion–distraction* type (3) there is an anterior annular tear with stripping of the anterior longitudinal ligament allowing anterior subluxation: this is a tension type of injury, as in the seat-belt lesion.

13. Neurological examination – Basic principles:
Where there is evidence of a deficit, a thorough neurological examination is required on admission; this must include as a minimum:

1. Testing for evidence of muscle activity and power in all muscle groups below the level of injury.
2. Testing sensation of pin prick and light touch over the entire area affected.
3. Testing proprioception.
4. Testing the reflexes – the tendon reflexes, the plantar responses, the anal reflex (stimulation of the perineum leading to contraction of the external anal sphincter) and the glansbulbar reflex (compression of the glans leading to perineal muscle contraction).

Note also the following points:
1. Where the spinal cord is involved, the neurological level should be determined.
2. The neurological level and the level of any bony injury should be correlated. Absence of any obvious bony injury at the neurological level should lead to further local investigation (e.g. by MRI scan).
3. The severity of any deficit should be assessed.
4). If the findings indicate a *complete* spinal lesion, the examination should be repeated after 6 hours, 12 hours and 24 hours.

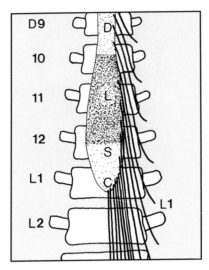

14. Anatomical features (a): *Note:*
1. The spinal cord ends at L1; any injury distal to this can involve the cauda but not the cord. 2. All the lumbar and sacral segments of the cord lie between D10 and L1 only. 3. Injuries at the thoracolumbar junction produce a great variety of neurological disturbances as: (a) the cord may or may not be transected; (b) the nerve roots may be undamaged, partly divided or completely divided.

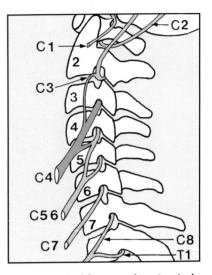

15. Anatomical features (b) – Cervical cord: *Note:*
1. The phrenic nerve arises from C4, with minor contributions from C3 and C5. Cord section proximal to the phrenic nerve will lead to rapid death from respiratory paralysis. Those with lesions at C4–5, and more distal, are capable of respiration without external support.
2. C2 and C3 supply the vertex and occiput (accounting for pain here in upper cervical lesions). C5–T1 contribute to the brachial plexus. (Illustration is diagrammatic.)

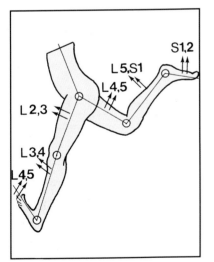

16. Assessing the neurological level of cord or nerve root injury:
Cord or root damage is reflected in disturbance of myotomes or dermatomes. **Myotomes (a):** As a rule, motion in each joint is logically controlled by four myotomes in sequence: viz. *Hip flexion* L2, 3; *extension* L4, 5. *Knee extension* L3, 4 (including knee jerk); *flexion* L5, S1. *Ankle dorsiflexion* L4, 5; *plantar flexion* S1, S2 (including ankle jerk). (In addition, inversion is controlled by L4 and eversion by L5, S1.)

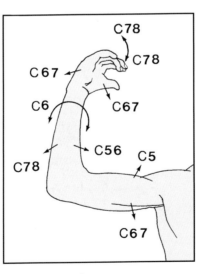

17. Myotomes (b):
In the upper limb, the arrangement is less regular: *Shoulder abduction* C5; *adduction* C6, 7. *Elbow flexion* C5, 6 (including biceps jerk); *extension* C7, 8 (including triceps jerk). *Wrist flexion and extension*, both C6, 7. *Finger flexion and extension* C7, 8. *Pronation and supination* C6 (including supinator jerk). *Hand intrinsic muscles* T1.

18. MRC grading:
Muscle activity should be assessed using the MRC scale:

M0 – No active contraction
M1 – A flicker of movement can be seen or palpated, but this is not enough to produce movement
M2 – Weak contraction which can produce movement if gravity is eliminated
M3 – Contraction weak, but can produce movement against gravity
M4 – Strength not full, but can produce movement against gravity and some resistance
M5 – Full strength

Motor index score: This is useful for assessing the extent of motor loss, and for gauging any improvement or deterioration. In the upper limb, biceps, the wrist extensors, triceps, flexor digitorum profundus and the hand intrinsics are each assessed using the MRC grading system and added together. The totals for the right upper extremity and left upper extremity (RUE and LUE) are noted (25 in each normal limb). The procedure is repeated in the lower limb, using the hip flexors, quadriceps, tibialis anterior, extensor hallucis longus, and gastrocnemius.

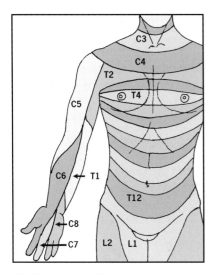

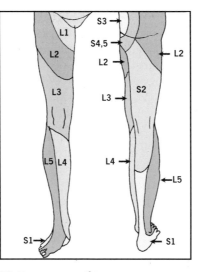

19. Dermatomes (a): In the upper limb, the anterior axial line follows the lie of the second rib from the angle of Louis, and continues down the anterior aspect of the arm, splitting near the middle finger, which is supplied by C7. The other dermatomes are arranged in a regular fashion on either side of the axial line.

If indicated, a **sensory index score** may be made for each limb (0 = absent sensation, 1 = impaired, 2 = normal).

20. Dermatomes (b): The lumbar and sacral dermatomes have a complex arrangement which is difficult to commit to memory. Remember by the facts that: 1. The outer border of the foot is supplied by S1; 2. The medial part of the foot and the lateral part of the leg by L5; 3. The 'stocking top' area by L2; 4. The saddle area by S3. 'We kneel on L3, stand on S1, and sit on S3.'

21. DETERMINING THE SEVERITY OF NEUROLOGICAL INVOLVEMENT

It is helpful to record the extent of any neurological impairment, and the Frankel scale is a simple and direct method of doing so:

Frankel A: Complete paralysis
Frankel B: Only sensory function below the injury level
Frankel C: Incomplete motor function below the injury level
Frankel D: Fair to good motor function below the injury level
Frankel E: Normal function.

TYPES OF INCOMPLETE CORD INJURY

A number of cord syndromes are recognised. These include the following:

Anterior column syndrome The damage is to the anterior two thirds of the cord and commonly occurs in burst fractures of the spine where there is compression of the cord and interruption of its blood supply by fragments of bone which have been forced into the spinal canal. There is complete motor paralysis and loss of sensation to pin prick and light touch, but proprioception and perception of deep pressure are retained. There is greater muscle loss in the legs than in the arms. This has the worst prognosis of all cord syndromes, with only 10–15% having any functional recovery. No return of sensation to pin prick or temperature in the sacral area after 24 hours is a very poor prognostic indicator.

Central cord syndrome This is the commonest incomplete cord syndrome, and generally follows a hyperextension injury. It is particularly common in the older patient who has a degree of cervical spondylosis (see also Frame 69). The cord may be affected over several segments, with involvement of both grey and white matter. The effects are curiously greater in the arms than in the legs. In the upper limbs, lower motor neurone lesions predominate, with a partial flaccid paralysis of the fingers and arms, and loss of pain and temperature sensation. In the lower limbs the lesion is an upper motor one, resulting in a spastic paralysis, usually with sparing of sensation, but sometimes with bladder and bowel involvement.

Brown Séquard syndrome This most commonly results from a unilateral facet joint fracture or dislocation and is due to hemitransection or similar damage to the cord. There is muscle paralysis and loss of discriminatory and joint sensation on the side of the injury, and loss of pain and temperature sensation on the other. The syndrome has a good prognosis, with more than 90% regaining bowel and bladder control and the ability to walk.

Posterior cord syndrome Injuries to the posterior cord are rare, but may follow injuries associated with rupture of the posterior ligament complex or penetrating wounds. There is loss of vibration and position sense, but motor function and pain and temperature sensation are retained.

Cauda equina syndrome Urinary retention is the most consistent finding (see p. 257) and partial injuries often have a good prognosis. In any suspected lesion examine for saddle anaesthesia, rectal tone, the bulbocavernosus reflex and sacral sparing.

THE COMMON LESIONS

1. Spinal concussion causes a temporary arrest of conduction within the cord; its effects are patchy and recovery is rapid. If, for example, there is a *complete* spinal lesion on first examination, spinal concussion is an unlikely but possible cause. If after 12 hours the lesion remains complete, spinal concussion is *not* the cause.
2. If there is any evidence of voluntary motor activity, skin sensation or proprioception below the level of the lesion, the cord has not been transected (and further recovery is possible).
3. After an injury to the cord, the reflexes generally disappear for at least some hours, and sometimes for as long 2 weeks. Return of reflex activity with continued absence of all sensation and voluntary muscle contraction confirms a *transection of the cord*.
4. Where the injury is at a level where there is potential damage to lumbar nerve roots or the cauda equina (e.g. injuries at the thoracolumbar junction) persistent absence of reflexes would confirm such damage.
5. Note that cord transection is irrecoverable, but there is potential recovery where there is involvement of nerve roots and the cauda equina.

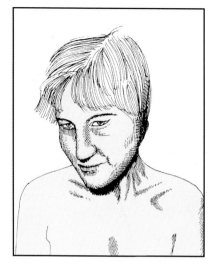

22. Injuries to the cervical spine – Diagnosis: Suspect involvement of the cervical spine where the patient: 1. Complains of neck, occipital or shoulder pain after trauma; 2. Has a torticollis (Illus.), complains of restriction of neck movements or supports the head with the hands; or 3. Is found unconscious after a head injury, especially in road traffic accidents. In all cases, further investigation by radiographs is essential.

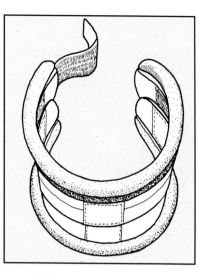

23. Initial management (a): If you suspect that the cervical spine has been injured, your first move should be to safeguard the cord by controlling neck movements. The simplest and best way of doing this is by applying a cervical collar. (Illus.: commercially available collar adjustable in depth and girth.) At the roadside, an adequate collar may be fashioned from rolled newspapers pushed into a nylon stocking and wrapped round the neck. (But see later regarding use of a collar in so-called whiplash injuries.)

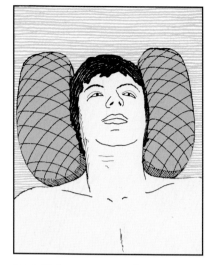

24. Initial management (b): Alternatively, if the patient is on a trolley, the head may be supported by sandbags. *Do not allow the head to flex forwards, and do not hyperextend.* Keep the head in a neutral position wherever possible, and in the conscious patient quickly check that there is active movement in all limbs.

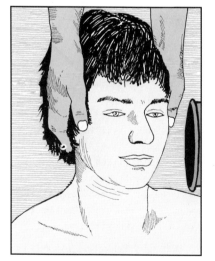

25. Initial management (c): Especially if there is some evidence of neurological involvement, *do not* check the range of movements in the cervical spine. Accompany the patient to the X-ray department, supporting the head during the positioning of the tube and making sure that the spine is not forced into flexion. For initial screening an AP, lateral and a through-the-mouth projection of C1 and C2 should be taken.

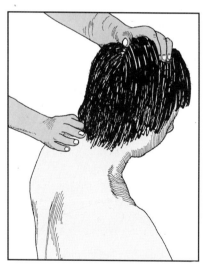

26. Initial management (d): If these films appear normal, you may proceed in reasonable safety to: 1. Further examination of the neck for localising tenderness, restriction of active movements and protective spasm, and 2. A more thorough neurological examination. If these show no departure from normal, the patient may be treated with a cervical collar, with a follow-up review in 1 week.

27. Initial management (e): Investigate further if there is persistent limitation of movements or evidence of neurological disturbance. CAT and MRI scans are likely to provide the best additional information. *CAT scans* may help show hard-to-see fractures, especially of the neural arches and facet joints, and define any neural canal encroachment in burst fractures.

MRI scans may be able to show the state of the posterior ligament complex and the intervertebral discs. Alternatively, the following additional radiographs should be taken: 1. Two more lateral projections, one in flexion and one in extension; these again should be supervised; 2. Right and left oblique projections of the cervical spine.

The commonest difficulty is the technical one of visualising the lower cervical vertebrae in the stocky patient. The upper border of T1 *must* be seen. Accept that detail may be poor. *Do not accept* that the spine cannot be shown in sufficient detail to exclude dislocation of one vertebra over another. If necessary, assist the radiographer by arranging for traction to be applied to the arms – one in adduction and the other in abduction; slight angulation of the tube and increase in exposure may be helpful. In some cases screening of the cervical spine movements may be useful.

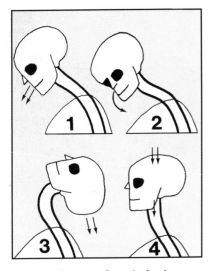

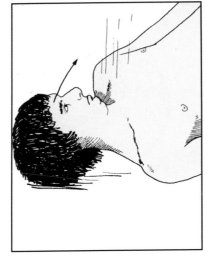

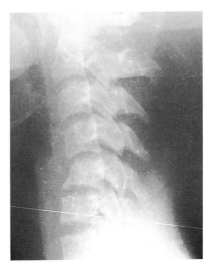

28. Classification of cervical spine injuries: Injuries of the cervical spine may be grouped according to the mechanism of injury:
(1) Flexion (anterior compression) injuries
(2) Flexion and rotation injuries
(3) Extension injuries
(4) Burst (vertical compression) fractures.
(Note that injuries involving the *proximal* cervical spine are dealt with separately at the end of the following section.)

29. Causes of flexion and flexion/ rotation injuries: These may result from: 1. Falls on the back of the head leading to flexion of the neck, e.g. in motor cycle spills, diving in shallow water, pole vaulting and rugby football; 2. Blows on the back of the head from falling objects (e.g. in the building and mining industries); 3. Rapid deceleration in head-on car accidents.

30. Flexion injuries: Stable anterior wedge (compression) fracture (a): The vertebral body is wedged anteriorly, while the posterior part is generally intact. Instability *must* be excluded: there must be no evidence of injury to the posterior ligament complex, with no separation of the vertebral spines (which the radiograph here suggests may possibly be present). Check if possible with an MRI scan. Eliminate damage to the neural arches or facets. Flexion and extension laterals may be carried out to exclude instability.

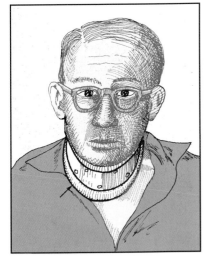

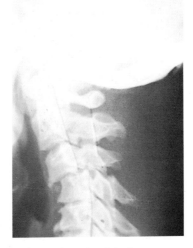

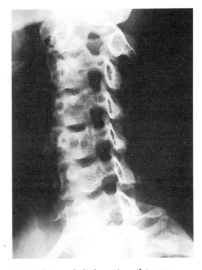

31. Stable anterior wedge fracture (b): Assuming these criteria are satisfied, neurological disturbance is rare and the prognosis excellent. Treat with a cervical collar for 6 weeks. Rarely, when there is a degree of lateral wedging there may be troublesome nerve root involvement usually with (mainly) sensory disturbance in the corresponding dermatome. *If instability is at all suspected, treat as a cervical dislocation.*

32. Flexion/rotation injuries – Unilateral dislocation with a locked facet joint (a): One facet joint dislocates, so that in the lateral projection of the cervical spine one vertebral body is seen to overlap the one below (i.e. there is anterior translation of the upper vertebra with regard to the vertebra below) by about a third. The AP view may not be helpful, or it may show malalignment of spinous processes. There is often little difference between laterals taken in flexion and extension.

33. Unilateral dislocation (b): Oblique projections will, however, confirm the diagnosis. On one side the columnar arrangement of bodies, foramina and facet joints will be regular (Illus.), while on the other (see next frame) it will be broken. Damage to the posterior ligament complex is variable, and *after reduction* these injuries may be quite stable but **note:** if there is an associated fracture involving a facet joint the injury is **most certainly unstable** and fusion will be required after reduction.

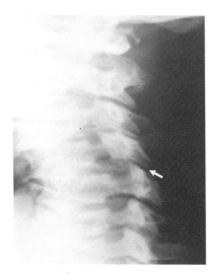

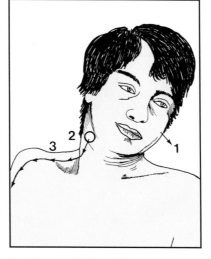

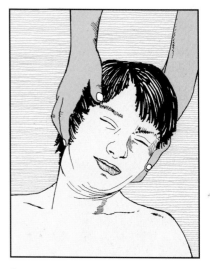

34. Unilateral dislocation (c): The oblique radiograph shows a dislocated facet joint. In all cases requiring reduction a preoperative MRI scan should be carried out to exclude a disc rupture: a significant prolapse may merit an anterior discectomy and interbody fusion in case manipulation precipitates a further disc protrusion and a catastrophic neurological problem. In the elderly, especially, manipulative reduction also carries a risk of causing a central cord syndrome, so that an open procedure may then be preferred.

35. Unilateral dislocation (d): On clinical examination of the patient with a unilateral dislocation, the head is slightly rotated and inclined to the side (1) away from the locked facet (2). There is often great pain with radiation (3) due to pressure on the nerve root at the level of the affected joint, and (rarely) there may be cord involvement. Proceed to treatment if there is no neurological defect or significant disc prolapse, *otherwise see* Frame 68.

36. Treatment (a): The initial aim in treatment is to reduce the dislocation, and the secret of this is well-controlled traction. 1. The patient is given a general anaesthetic; the head must be well supported during induction, the administration of any muscle relaxant and intubation (which must be carried out without undue extension of the neck). 2. X-ray facilities should be available (preferably an image intensifier).

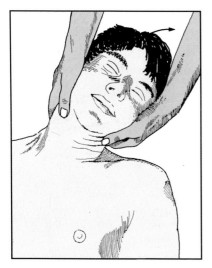

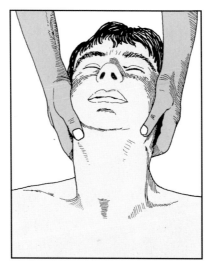

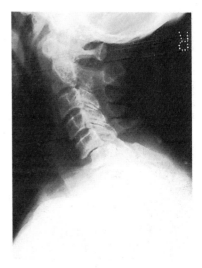

37. Treatment (b): 3. The surgeon must have freedom to manipulate the head, and may do this with the patient fully on the table, or pulled up until the head is supported in the lap of the surgeon seated at the top end of the table. Place the thumbs under the jaw, clasp the fingers behind the occiput, and apply firm traction in *lateral flexion* away from the side of the locked facet, i.e. in the direction the head is usually inclined.

38. Treatment (c): 4. Maintaining traction, bring the head into the midline position, correcting the rotation element *before* lateral flexion. Release the traction, support the head (e.g. with foam plastic blocks) and confirm reduction with the image intensifier or by check radiographs. If however, reduction has not been achieved, repeat the manoeuvre with greater anaesthetic relaxation. If reduction fails (rare), or if preferred, apply traction using skull tongs or a halo as for a bilateral facet dislocation.

39. Treatment (d): 5. Once reduction has been achieved, a cervical collar should be applied, and worn continuously for 6 weeks. 6. Fortnightly radiographs of the neck should be taken, and flexion and extension laterals at the end of the 6 weeks' fixation. *If there is any evidence of late subluxation* (Illus.) the patient should be admitted for local (posterior) cervical fusion. Some also advocate fusion if the initial displacement is more than 25% or 3.5 mm.

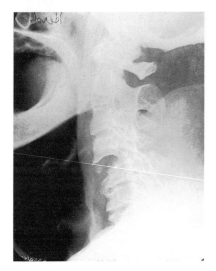

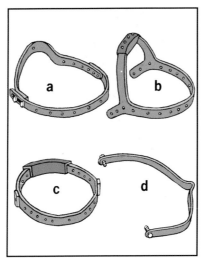

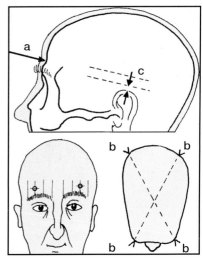

40. Flexion/rotation injuries – Unstable injuries (a): The commonest injury is a *cervical dislocation without fracture.* Displacement may be severe, and there is frequently locking of both facets. Damage to the posterior ligament complex is always present. (This may be associated with an avulsion fracture of a spinous process, widening of the gap between two spinous processes or *evidence of forward slip on a flexion lateral.*) An MRI scan is advised to exclude a significant disc prolapse. (See Frame 68).

41. Unstable injuries (b): Skull traction will be required to achieve and maintain reduction and should be applied without delay. This may be carried out using a halo (which at a later stage may be attached to a vest or plaster jacket for continued support). The Bremer range includes: (a) Adjustable rings; (b) Halo-crown devices; (c) Small, large and custom built paediatric rings; (d) Traction hoops. (Note that where there is no fracture, fusion will be required.)

42. Halo traction pin sites: Palpate the groove between the superciliary ridge and the frontal prominence (a). The anterior pins should lie on this line, caudal to the maximal circumference of the skull, and about 1 cm above the orbital margin. Each should lie in the line of the outer half of the eyebrow (e.g at the junction of the middle and outer thirds). The posterior pins should be sited diagonally opposite (b), at such a level that the halo band clears the ear by about a half centimetre (c).

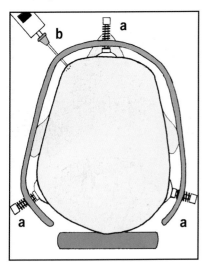

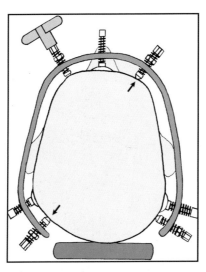

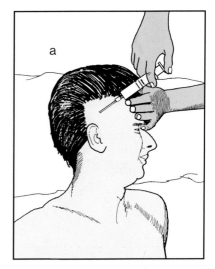

43. Halo application cntd: Support the head manually throughout the procedure. The head of the supine patient should be just clear of the bed, with a board between the shoulder blades extending up to the occiput. Shave and prep the skin round the areas of the proposed pin sites. Slide the halo into position, and hold it with 3–4 suction cups screwed into the halo (a), positioned away from the skull pin sites. These may then be infiltrated (through the holes in the halo) with local anaesthetic (b).

44. Halo application cntd: Adjust the suction cups to ensure the halo is centred. Using the fingers at first, screw in opposite pairs of skull pins, before repeating this with the other pair. (At this stage some make small skin incisions to avoid indentation of the skin.) Now tighten them in stages – again in a diametrically opposed sequence – to a maximum torque of 8 inch/pounds (0.90 Newton/metre) using a torque wrench or torque-limiting caps. Then attach a traction hoop. (See Frame 58 for aftercare.)

45. Applying skull tongs (a): Alternatively, skull tongs may be used when no later need for a halo-vest is anticipated. Several types of calliper are available, and the following description applies to those of Cone's pattern. Shave the skin round the proposed insertion points (approximately 6–7 cm above the external auditory meati) and infiltrate the areas deeply on both sides with local anaesthetic (a).

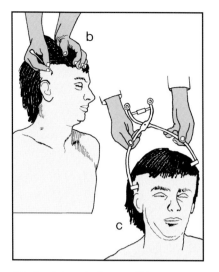

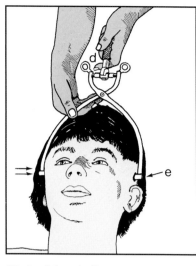

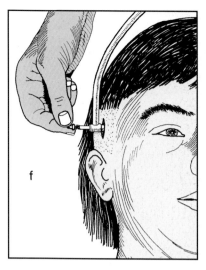

46. Applying skull tongs (b): Make a small incision (about 1 cm in length) on each side down to bone (b). Bleeding is usually brisk, but generally controllable by firm local pressure applied for a few moments; if not, secure and tie off any remaining bleeding points. Now insinuate one point holder through the temporalis muscle fibres until it is in contact with the skull (c).

47. Applying skull tongs (c): Keep the point holder pressed firmly against the skull; straighten out the calliper, and close it with the turnbuckle spanner (d). Guide the second point holder through the skin wound; oscillate the calliper slightly to allow its tapered end to part the temporalis fibres on the second side (e). Close the calliper until both point holders are in firm but not hard contact with the skull.

48. Applying skull tongs (d): Now screw the points in (you should check that their protrusion is limited to about 3 mm) to penetrate the outer cortex only; tighten them with a key (f). If the points fail to enter, either they are blunt or the bone unduly hard. In these circumstances, a small awl may be used as a starter, taking great care to avoid penetration of the inner cortex. Now seal the wound with strips of gauze soaked in Nobecutane™ or a similar preparation.

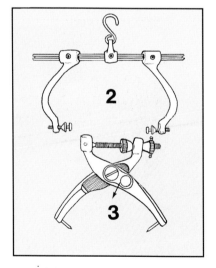

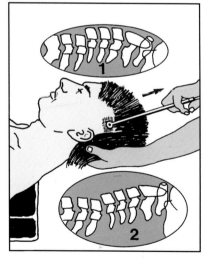

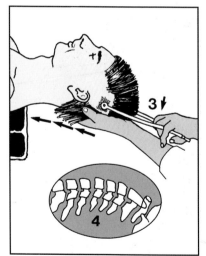

49. Other traction devices: *Blackburn callipers* (2) are designed to hook into the diplöe of the skull, and a trephine is used to remove a tiny lid of outer cortex. Occasionally no diplöe is present, and the points must hook under the full thickness of the skull, and come in contact with the dura. *Crutchfield traction tongs* (3) are inserted nearer the vertex than the other two devices.

50. Reduction (a): Assuming there is no disc prolapse (which might precipitate a neurological problem – see Frame 68), many surgeons prefer to carry out a manual reduction. General anaesthesia with good relaxation and X-ray facilities are essential. Great care must be taken during induction and throughout to avoid uncontrolled movements of the head. When all is ready, the head is supported and the end of the table dropped; firm traction is applied in the neutral position or slight flexion (1) to unlock the facets (2).

51. Reduction (b): Maintaining firm traction, the neck is slowly extended (3). The hand supporting the occiput may be moved in anticipation down the neck to act as a fulcrum (4). The traction is then slowly reduced, the table end raised and, whilst maintaining a little controlling traction, the position is checked with radiographs.

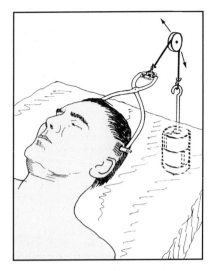

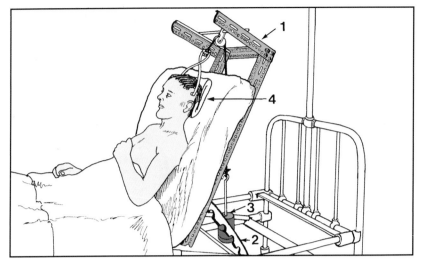

52. Reduction (c) – Alternative techniques: Continuous (weight) traction may be used to overcome muscle tension and unlock overriding facets. Control the *direction* of traction with the position of the traction pulley, or by pads under the head or shoulders. The *amount* of traction can be adjusted by the weights: allow 10 lb (4.5 kg) for the head + 5 lb (2.3 kg) for each interspace: e.g. 35 lb (16 kg) for C5 on C6. The *duration* of maximal traction is monitored by radiographic progress.

53. Reduction (d): A better arrangement is for traction to be applied with the patient in a sitting-up position. Traction is more efficient, being countered by the body weight; the patient can see what is going on, and if paraplegic, breathing is easier as the diaphragm is unobstructed. A framework of slotted angle (e.g. Dexion™) (1) may be attached to the mattress frame if the hospital bed has not this facility, and the frame may be racked up and down (2) while pressure points are being attended to. The weight required (3) should be in the order of that detailed in the previous frame. The line of traction should start in the neutral position or slight flexion (4). The patient should be sedated, *and in the recently injured patient radiographs to check progress should be taken every 15 minutes*. Failure to reduce after several hours is often regarded as an indication for an open procedure.

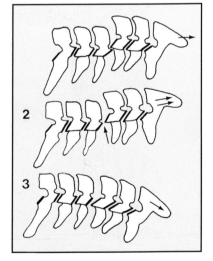

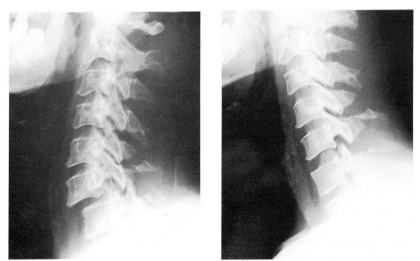

54. Reduction (e): As soon as the neck has been stretched sufficiently to allow the locked facets just to clear one another (2), the neck should be extended to complete the reduction (3) and traction reduced. In longstanding cases (say 1–3 weeks post injury) progress will be much slower, and in extreme cases can extend to days. Generally, if reduction is not achieved after 6 hours, manipulative or open reduction is advised rather than increasing the amount or duration of traction.

55. Reduction (f): The radiograph on the left shows an unstable dislocation of C6 on C7, with locked facets and an associated fracture of the spinous process of C6. On the right the dislocation has been reduced. The C6/7 disc space indicates that a further reduction of traction is required. **Aftercare:** If the original injury was confined to the posterior ligament complex, then to avoid late subluxation a local cervical fusion is necessary. If the instability is due to a *fracture* (as above) and healing of that fracture will restore stability, then it is sufficient to support the neck until union occurs. This may be achieved by continuous traction (in the order of 2.5 kg (6 lb)), taking care that on no account the neck be over distracted. Alternatively, depending on your assessment of the degree of inherent residual instability and local practice, you may use a halo vest, an extensive off the shelf brace, casts, or internal fixation. Note, however, that at the end of any period of conservative treatment *stability must be checked with flexion and extension laterals*.

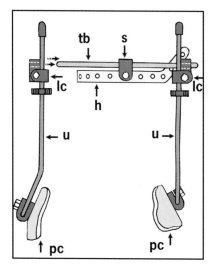

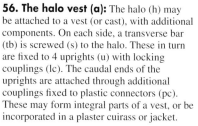

56. The halo vest (a): The halo (h) may be attached to a vest (or cast), with additional components. On each side, a transverse bar (tb) is screwed (s) to the halo. These in turn are fixed to 4 uprights (u) with locking couplings (lc). The caudal ends of the uprights are attached through additional couplings fixed to plastic connectors (pc). These may form integral parts of a vest, or be incorporated in a plaster cuirass or jacket.

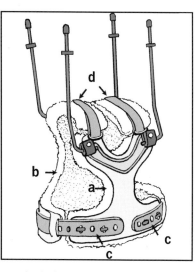

57. The halo vest (b): The Bremer vest has anterior (a) and posterior (b) shells with soft replaceable liners. They are linked inferiorly with thoracic bands (c) secured to locking posts. Above, two shoulder pads which extend from the posterior shell are secured in front with webbing straps (d) which pass through keepers and are fixed superiorly with Velcro fasteners. A range of sizes, including one for paediatric use, is available. A pelvic girdle attachment may be fixed to the vest for additional stability.

58. Attaching the vest: The head is supported and lifted up with the trunk so that the posterior section of the vest (with its paired uprights and transverse bars in place), can be slid into position. The transverse bars are then attached to the halo. The anterior shell is now placed on the chest, and the two parts joined together by tightening the thoracic bands and securing the shoulder straps. The transverse bars are attached to the front uprights and the connectors tightened. After check radiographs, alterations in alignment and traction (using the adjusters on the uprights) may be made. **Aftercare:** 1. Re-tighten the halo pins after 36 hours. Subsequently a loose pin may be tightened if resistance is met – otherwise insert a new pin, tighten it, and remove the old. 2. Clean the areas round the pins daily with soap and water, and remove any crusting with hydrogen peroxide. 3. Treat infected pin tracks with antibiotics and intensified site care. If there is no improvement, introduce a new pin at a fresh site, before removing the old and if necessary carrying out a local debridement. **Other complications:** These include osteomyelitis of the skull; extradural haematoma; extradural, subdural and cerebral abscess. Symptoms include headache, pyrexia, fits, hemiplegia and coma. Treat the complication, abandon skull traction, and use an alternative such as a Minerva plaster.

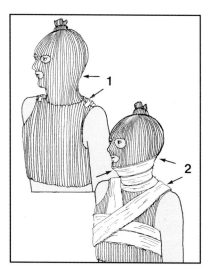

59. Plaster fixation in cervical spine injuries (a): Plaster fixation is occasionally indicated, giving more support than a well-fitting collar. It may be helpful in treating the poorly motivated patient who is tempted to remove a brace. It may also be used in some cases where pin track infections prevent continuation of treatment in a halo vest. Stockinet is applied to the head and trunk (1), and wool padding to pressure areas (2). Felt pads to the chin and occiput are advisable.

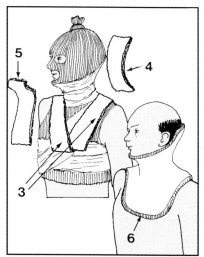

60. Plaster fixation (b): Four plaster slabs are prepared from 15 cm (6″) plaster bandages; two are applied over the shoulders (3), one from midscapular region to the occiput (4) and one over the point of the chin on to the chest (5). The slabs are joined with circular bandages; the stockinet and wool are turned down and trimmed (6). This plaster is best applied with the patient seated on a stool.

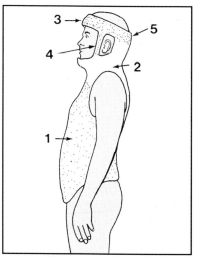

61. The Minerva plaster: This extensive plaster, although perhaps not giving quite as much support as a well fitting halo vest with a pelvic attachment, is sometimes used as an alternative, especially in children. It may also be used where pin track infections prevent further use of a halo. *Method:* A plaster jacket is applied first (1); this is extended with slabs to form a collar (2); additional support is provided with a head band (3) and side struts (4). If to be worn for any length of time, the head should be cropped or shaved (5).

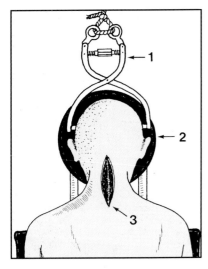

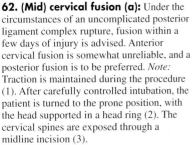

62. (Mid) cervical fusion (a): Under the circumstances of an uncomplicated posterior ligament complex rupture, fusion within a few days of injury is advised. Anterior cervical fusion is somewhat unreliable, and a posterior fusion is to be preferred. *Note:* Traction is maintained during the procedure (1). After carefully controlled intubation, the patient is turned to the prone position, with the head supported in a head ring (2). The cervical spines are exposed through a midline incision (3).

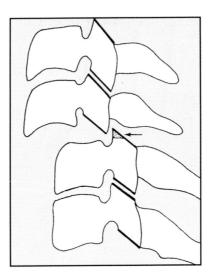

63. Cervical fusion (b): If preliminary traction has failed to obtain a reduction, this may generally be achieved by local trimming of those parts of the facets which are blocking reduction (facetectomy). Failure to obtain reduction is unusual in recent injuries, but there may be difficulty after 3–4 weeks. Note that in very longstanding dislocations, spinal stability is more important than accurate reduction, and the spine may be fused in the dislocated position if reduction cannot readily be obtained.

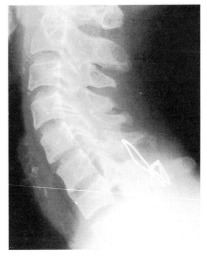

64. Cervical fusion (c): The ruptured posterior ligament is identified and the adjacent spinous processes, laminae and facet joints rawed. The safest and easiest way to perform fixation technique is wiring of adjacent spinous processes, either by plain wire (Illus.) or Songer cables. Two iliac bone grafts are placed (and sometimes wired together) on either side of the spines, bridging them. Cancellous bone chips are packed into the area before closure. The AO Group favour H-shaped cortical bone grafts.

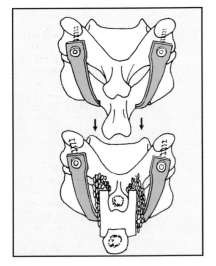

65. Cervical fusion (d): There are a number of other fixation techniques along with bone grafting for cervical spine fusions: 1. Hook plates, similar in concept to Zuelzer plates, may be used, one on each side of the spinous processes. In practice each is bent so that its hook portion can slip under the inferior edge of a lamina, suitably notched to receive it and to prevent it from drifting; its upper end is held with a single screw into the articular mass. A Bosworth H-graft (Illus.) with cancellous bone chips may then be applied.

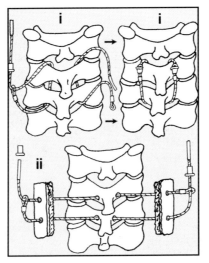

66. Cervical fusion (e): 2. Songer multifilament cables, of stainless steel or titanium, are easier to handle and less prone to failure than plain wires. They may be passed round adjacent laminae, tensioned, and then held with crimps (i); They may be passed through holes drilled through the spinous process bases and incorporate cortical bone grafts (ii); Where fixation of more than two vertebrae is required the repair may be reinforced with rods, moulded to lie snugly and held with sublaminar cables.

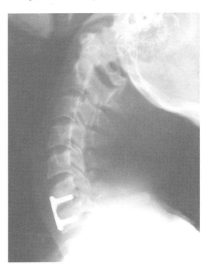

67. Cervical fusion (f): 3. If an anterior approach is required (for example to carry out an anterior decompression) then the spine may be stabilised anteriorly using, for example, a plate with locking screws, or plates on either side of the vertebral bodies. Anterior fusion is sometimes insufficient to stabilise the spine when there has been a massive associated posterior complex disruption, and may require an additional posterior fusion. In all cases supplementary external splintage (e.g. with a neck brace) is advised until union.

68. Treatment of fracture–dislocations where there is a neurological defect on admission: In about 10% of cervical spine dislocations posterior extrusion of intervertebral disc material can compromise the cord, and there is a risk that the situation may be aggravated if reduction is undertaken without prior decompression. A thorough neurological examination should of course be carried out on admission, and if there is evidence of neurological involvement (particularly of the cord) then further investigation of the state of the relevant intervertebral disc should be undertaken. This is best done by a carefully supervised MRI scan; failing this myelography with a postmyelography CAT scan should be carried out. If there is evidence of cord compression, then a decompression by the anterior route *before* reduction is generally advocated. Where there is no indication for decompression, and in the presence of a partial or complete cord lesion, fusion may be delayed for 1–2 weeks, but is still advocated to facilitate nursing and rehabilitation.

69. Extension injuries: Mechanisms: Commonly: 1. From a fall downstairs, the forehead striking the ground; 2. In front-impact car accidents where the forehead strikes the car roof, fascia or bonnet (3rd, 4th and 5th phases of injury); 3. In rear-impact car accidents in which the neck forcibly extends.

Pathology: These injuries are particularly common in the middle aged and elderly who suffer from cervical spondylosis. Osteoarthritic rigidity in the spine may lead to excessive stress concentrations at any area of the spine retaining mobility. A similar predisposition is found in those suffering from ankylosing spondylitis, severe rheumatoid arthritis, or congenital deformities of the spine with localised areas of fusion (e.g. Klippel–Feil syndrome). The neck hyperextends (1) leading to tearing or avulsion of the anterior longitudinal ligament (2). During the period of extension the cord may be stretched at the level of the vertebral lesion (3). At the same time, or when the vertebrae snap together again, the cord may be nipped by backward projecting osteophytes (4) (in the patient with advanced spondylosis). Stretching and kinking of spinal vessels may lead to extensive spreading thrombosis (5). The cord damage is often diffuse and may not correspond exactly with the level of injury (6). Spread of thrombosis may lead to a deteriorating neurological picture (central cord syndrome).

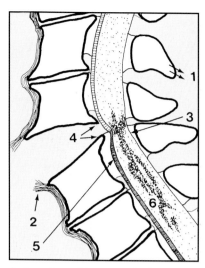

As far as the cord is concerned sole involvement of the central area is rare, but when it occurs the effect is: (a) Motor loss tends to be greater in the arms than in the legs. (b) Temperature and pain conduction are more likely to be affected than proprioception and light touch, which are frequently spared.

Diagnosis: 1. The history of injury, pain in the neck and complaint of weakness in the arms are suggestive. 2. Where the causal force is anterior, bruising or laceration of the forehead is an invaluable sign.

72. Treatment: Extension injuries of the spine are generally stable, but there may be instability when there is profound disruption of the anterior structures including the disc and anterior longitudinal ligament. *Local treatment* consists of the judicious use of a collar until local pain and cervical muscle spasm settle. The *general treatment* is that of the accompanying neurological problem which may be minor or profound.

73. Burst fractures of the cervical spine: *Mechanisms:* These injuries may be caused by: 1. Heavy objects falling on the head; 2. The vertex striking the ground as in falls, diving and other athletic accidents; 3. The head striking the roof in head-on car accidents (phase 2).

Diagnosis: 1. The history of injury may be suggestive. 2. There may be tell-tale lacerations on the crown of the head. 3. Complaint of pain in the neck should lead to the taking of the radiographs which will clarify the diagnosis.

These injuries are often clinically and radiologically similar to certain anterior wedge (compression) fractures, but have generally a better prognosis than the latter, with neurological deficits often being transitory. Nevertheless in the more severe cases there may be damage to the anterior (and sometimes the posterior) column, with instability and gross neurological damage.

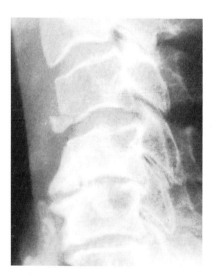

70. Radiographs (a): Spontaneous reduction is the rule, so that the radiographs *may be quite normal.* Nevertheless, plain films may show: 1. Avulsion of the anterior longitudinal ligament from its attachment to the vertebral body (Illus.) or an osteophyte; 2. Anterior displacement of the pharyngeal shadow secondary to haemorrhage; 3. Rarely, there may be fractures of the laminae or spinous processes, or 4. Tearing open of a vertebral body.

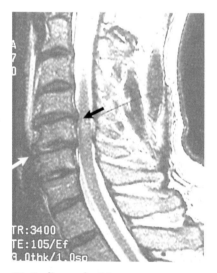

71. Radiographs (b): MRI imaging is often of considerable value in showing any involvement of the related anterior longitudinal ligament and the intervertebral disc, as demonstrated above. It may clarify the nature of the pathology in this and other cases of so-called SCIWORA syndrome – Spinal Cord Injury Without Radiological Abnormality.

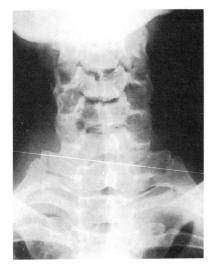

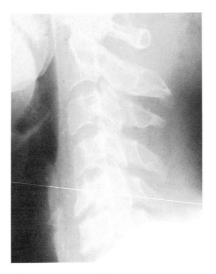

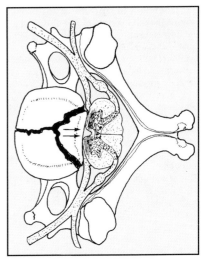

74. Radiographs (a): The appearances are dependent on the degree of causal violence. When the forces are moderate, a fissure fracture of the vertebral body may be produced, most obvious in the AP projection (Illus.: Vertical fracture through the body of C5, with a similar but less marked fracture of C6). Where the deformity is greater, lateral displacement of the pedicles may be obvious.

75. Radiographs (b): In more severe injuries the vertebral body may be comminuted and flattened. Fragments of the vertebral body may be extruded in any direction; when this occurs the cord may be endangered. (Illus.: Compression fracture of C5; note the encroachment on the neural canal by the posterior part of the body.) *CAT scanning is of particular value in clarifying the extent of fractures of this type.*

76. Neurological involvement: The most vulnerable part of the cord lies anteriorly, and bone fragments pushed backwards into the spinal canal tend to result in an anterior cord syndrome (see also Frame 21). The motor supply of the upper limbs tends to be affected *before* the motor pathways to the lower limbs: hence paralysis tends to be maximal in the upper limbs. Next to be involved are the spinothalamic tracts carrying pain and temperature, and lastly the posterior columns (proprioception and light touch).

77. Neurological assessment: On admission, a complete neurological examination should be carried out as previously described. If the paralysis is bilateral, symmetrical and complete, testing should be repeated meticulously at 6 hours, 12 hours, and 24 hours post-injury. No recovery after 24 hours in injuries at cervical level almost certainly indicates a hopeless prognosis. *Be careful to note, however, that a profound neurological loss cannot be declared complete unless proprioception and light touch have been most carefully assessed.* Many apparent recoveries in lesions first described as complete may well have been due to failure in carrying out a careful examination of these modalities of sensation.

Treatment:
1. The posterior ligament complex is generally intact, so that once these fractures have healed there is little tendency to subsequent displacement. The aim should be to protect the spine from movement, and in the ambulant patient this may be achieved with a halo orthosis. Cervical traction for 6 weeks until union has occurred may also be used.
2. Removal of backward projecting bone fragments which are interfering with cord function may be carried out through an anterior approach. Although the value of this is to some extent controversial, it has been advocated in the face of the following criteria:
    (i) an incomplete cord lesion;
    (ii) a deteriorating neurological picture;
    (iii) a local block on myelography;
    (iv) confirmatory evidence on CAT or MRI scan of spinal encroachment. The indications are less clear when the neurological condition is static, and even less so when it is complete. At surgery the fragments of the vertebral body are excised and replaced with three cortical bone struts and an anterior plate bridging the vertebrae above and below.

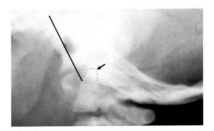

78. The upper two cervical vertebrae: (a) Atlanto-occipital subluxations and dislocations: Traumatic lesions at this level are usually caused by severe hyperextension. They are especially common in children, due to their flatter occipital condyles. Death from respiratory arrest is usual, but a few survive. Subluxations of slow onset from rheumatoid arthritis and spinal and pharyngeal infections are seen more frequently. The radiographs are often difficult to interpret. Subluxation may be detected by means of Wachenheim's basilar line: this is drawn tangent to the posterior surface of the clivus and extended; it should *normally* just touch the posterosuperior aspect of the odontoid process at the point indicated by the arrow. *Treatment:* Traction and flexion are contraindicated. Apply a halo vest and obtain reduction by adjustment of this prior to fusion (occiput to C1 and C2).

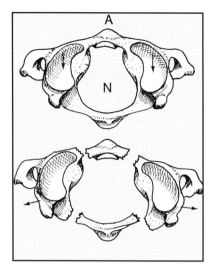

79. (b) Fractures of the atlas (i): The usual pattern of fracture is *quadripartite* (Jefferson fracture), and is produced as a result of severe downward pressure of the occipital condyles on the atlas. Such force may result from: 1. A weight falling on the head (e.g. in the construction industry); 2. The head striking the roof of a car in a road traffic accident; 3. A fall from a height on to the heels.

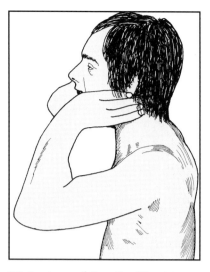

80. Fractures of the atlas (ii): Clinically, if the patient is conscious he may resent sitting up and may support the head with the hands. There may be complaint of severe occipital pain due to local pressure on the great occipital nerve. About 50% of patients survive this injury without significant neurological involvement; but note a third are associated with a fracture of the axis, and half with another cervical spine injury. Most fractures are stable, with an intact transverse ligament.

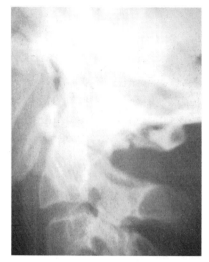

81. Radiographs (a): The *lateral* radiograph may show the fracture of the posterior arch (Illus.). The plain AP view is usually unhelpful. A through-the-mouth projection is generally more valuable and should reveal the lateral displacement of the lateral masses. Nevertheless, pain and resistance to all movement may lead to failure; if this is so, an oblique centred on C3, AP and lateral tomography and CAT scanning may be useful. In children the latter is of particular value.

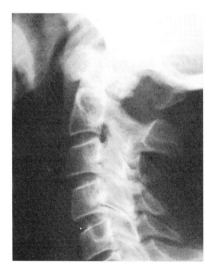

82. Radiographs (b): Congenital absence of part of the posterior arch may cause confusion, but in itself is of no significance, being a stable condition. *Treatment of arch fractures:* These cannot be reduced; with *slight* displacement a well-fitting collar for 6 weeks should suffice. With more severe displacements, 12 weeks in a halo vest is advised. Late subluxation of C1 is rare, but should be looked for at the end of the period of fixation.

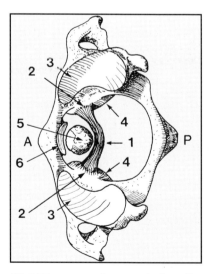

83. (c) Transverse ligament lesions (i): The transverse ligament (1) runs between two bony tubercles (2) which lie between the joint surfaces (3) which articulate with the occiput and those which articulate below with the axis (4). The odontoid process (5) articulates with the anterior arch (6) and the transverse ligament restrains its backward travel.

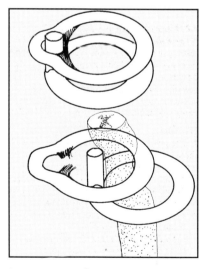

84. Transverse ligament (ii): The ligament may be torn in sudden flexion injuries: it may become attenuated or rupture in rheumatoid arthritis (or in pharyngeal infections in children – Grisel's syndrome). In either case the risk to the cord is great as it becomes pinched between the posterior arch of the atlas and the odontoid peg (as shown here diagrammatically).

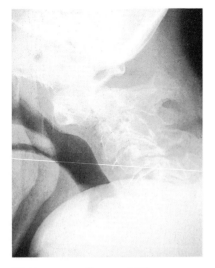

**85. Transverse ligament (iii) –
Diagnosis:** The condition may be suspected from the history, by pain in the neck *and the head*, and by the presence of marked cervical spasm, often with an associated torticollis. Vertebro-basilar insufficiency is occasionally present.

Radiographs: The diagnosis is established by radiographs:

1. Plain lateral films should be examined and the gap between the posterior face of the anterior arch and the odontoid carefully measured (the atlas–dens interval or ADI). With the spine in flexion (which in acute cases should only be permitted under the closest supervision) this should be less than 3 mm in adults and 3.5 mm in children. (Illus.: gross shift in an arthritic spine.)
2. There is generally a degree of rotational deformity, and a through-the-mouth view may show an asymmetrical location of the odontoid peg relative to the lateral masses of the atlas.
3. If there is remaining doubt, flexion and extension laterals should be taken under close supervision. An abnormal excursion of the odontoid peg in relation to the anterior arch of the atlas is diagnostic.
4. If available, CAT scanning may also be used to clarify the relationship between the odontoid peg and the anterior arch of the atlas.

Treatment:

Children:
1. In Grisel's syndrome the majority of cases resolve spontaneously. Where this does not occur, the dislocation should be reduced by skull traction (e.g. using a halo) followed by a period of 3 months in a halo vest.
2. In acute traumatic dislocations, reduction by traction followed by a halo vest for 3 months are also indicated. At the end of this period stability should be checked by flexion and extension laterals. If instability is still present, an atlantoaxial fusion is indicated. Fusion is also advised in late diagnosed cases (over 3 weeks) or where there is neurological involvement.

Adults:
1. Acute traumatic dislocations: As the potential for ligament healing is poor in the adult, fusion is the treatment of choice. This should be preceded by a 2–3 week period of traction with reduction of the deformity. After fusion a halo vest is usually advised for 8–12 weeks.
2. Chronic subluxation: Reduction is inadvisable, and an in situ fusion of C1 and C2 is recommended.

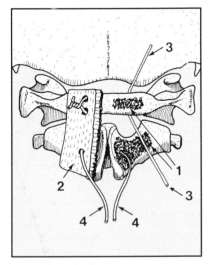

86. Treatment cntd – Atlantoaxial fusion (a): There are many methods used in cervical fusions at this level. A common method is to begin by rawing the posterior arches of C1 and C2 (1). Two stout grafts (from tibia or iliac crest) are wired in position (one side only shown) (2). The upper wires (3) pass round the arch while the lower (4) is passed through a hole drilled in the spine of C2. The area is packed with bone chips.

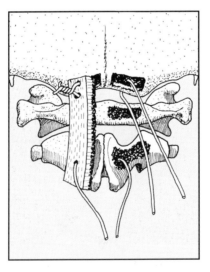

87. Atlantoaxial fusion (b): If the posterior arch of C1 is very frail, it may be necessary to include the occiput in the grafted region; great care must be taken in passing the fixing wires through holes drilled in the edge of the foramen magnum. After surgery, a halo vest is usually worn for 8–12 weeks.

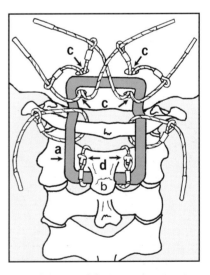

88. Atlantoaxial fusion (c): As an alternative, after cleaning and decortication of the posterior elements (including the facet joints) with a high speed burr, a rectangular bar (a) is bent to fit snugly between the occiput and the spinous process of C2 (b). Songer cables are passed through burr holes made in the occiput (c) and under the laminae of C1 and C2. These are tightened and secured with crimps (as shown at d). Bone grafts are then placed on each side, lateral to the vertical elements of the bar.

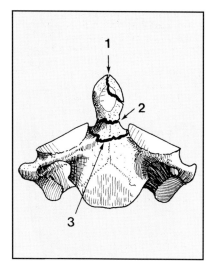

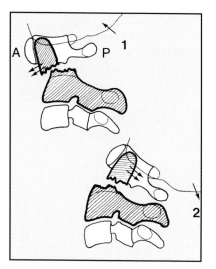

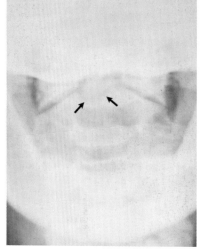

89. Odontoid fractures (a):

Classification: Type I injuries (1) involve the tip of the peg, are generally stable and require symptomatic treatment only with a collar (but exclude an unstable associated atlanto-occipital dislocation). Type II injuries (2), the commonest, involve the junction of odontoid peg with the body. Although Type III fractures (3) run deeply into the body of C2, union fails to occur in about a quarter of cases, so they must be handled as carefully as Type II fractures.

90. Odontoid fractures (b):
Fracture may result from sudden severe flexion (1) or extension (2) of the neck (flexion and extension fractures). *Diagnosis:* This injury may be suspected from the history and the site of pain and protective muscle spasm. Occasionally the original injury may be ignored, and discovered only on investigation of an advancing ataxia or other neurological disturbance.

91. Odontoid fractures (c):
The diagnosis may be readily confirmed by routine radiography; the fracture may show clearly in the through-the-mouth AP projection (Illus.: Fracture of the base) and/or in the standard lateral view. Only if there is doubt need carefully supervised flexion and extension laterals be taken, or CAT scans carried out. Confusion can sometimes arise, however, from certain congenital abnormalities.

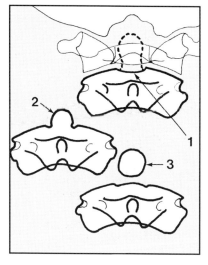

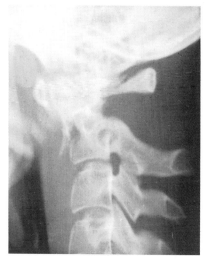

92. Congenital odontoid abnormalities:
These include: (1) Complete absence (predisposing to dislocation); (2) Hypoplasia: (3) Non-fusion of the odontoid process (persistent os odontoideum) (the ossification centre for the apex normally appears at 2 years with fusion occurring by 12). Rounded edges and a separate articulation with the atlas may help to distinguish it from a fracture (even though it may behave as such).

93. Flexion injuries of the dens:
The atlas and dens displace anteriorly in relation to C2. (Illus.: Flexion injury revealed by a flexion lateral.) There may be an associated rotational injury. If the fracture is junctional, the incidence of non-union is about 60%, with risk of progressive subluxation and neurological involvement.

Treatment: In spite of the risks of complications these injuries are frequently treated conservatively, especially in children.

good reduction should be aimed for, in order to lessen the risks of non-union. In the younger patient, persistent displacement can in fact re-model well.

2. After 1–2 weeks in traction, it may be possible to mobilise the patient; this is especially desirable in the elderly patient who will not tolerate prolonged traction and confinement to bed. Continuous external support for the neck is required for 8 weeks, and this may be provided with a halo vest (which is convenient if a halo has been used initially for traction) or a Minerva plaster; in some cases a cervical brace may suffice.

3. Stability should then be assessed with flexion and extension laterals. Surgical treatment (generally a posterior fusion of C1 and C2) is indicated (a) if conservative treatment fails, (b) the case presents late, (c) a good reduction cannot be obtained, or (d) where the delays and complications of conservative management are thought to present a greater hazard than the risks of primary surgery.

In most cases displacement of the os odontoideum may be treated conservatively unless the forward slip is extensive or there are severe or progressive neurological signs. The experienced surgeon may advise internal fixation in certain adult odontoid fractures, using two screws running from the antero-inferior edge of C2 into the odontoid process. An antero-median approach is used, and high resolution two-plane imaging is essential.

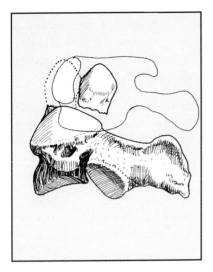

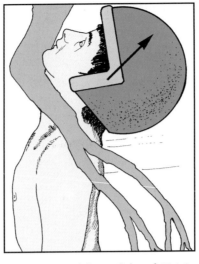

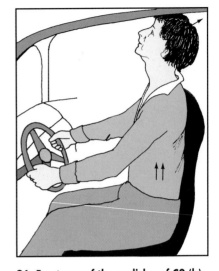

94. Extension injuries of the dens:
Fracture with backward displacement of the odontoid fragment is commoner in the elderly, and is a relatively stable lesion. *Treatment:* 1. If the shift is slight, a collar for 8 weeks should suffice. 2. If marked, apply traction in slight flexion with skull tongs, but slacken off the weight as soon as reduction has been achieved to avoid distraction. After 2–4 weeks a collar may be substituted.

95. Fractures of the pedicles of C2 (a):
Fractures of the pedicles of the axis may occur in two distinct ways: 1. Fracture may follow simultaneous extension and distraction of the neck. This is the mechanism of death by hanging. Similar, and not always fatal, injuries occur in cyclists who are caught under the chin by a tree branch or a rope; nevertheless, neurological disturbance is usually profound.

96. Fractures of the pedicles of C2 (b):
2. Radiologically identical fractures may be produced by forcible extension of the neck accompanied by compression; this may occur in road traffic accidents if the head strikes the vehicle roof and ricochets into extension. Neurological involvement here is rare. These two types of injury may be distinguished by the history, site of bruising (neck or forehead) and neurological disturbance.

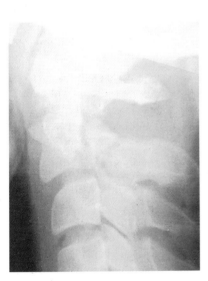

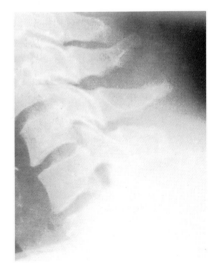

maximum of 2 kg (5 lb). If radiographs suggest distraction, or if there is deterioration in the neurological picture, traction must be abandoned. Fusion would then be indicated.

2. *Extension injuries with compression:*
(i) If the injury appears to be stable and there is no neurological disturbance, a well-fitting collar should be worn for 6 weeks.
(ii) If there is neurological involvement with evidence of deterioration, decompression and fusion are normally advocated.
(iii) If there is any evidence of instability, fusion is also advisable. Posterior and anterior fusion have both been advocated for C2 fractures.

7. Fractures of the pedicles of C2 (c):
The fracture normally shows clearly in lateral radiographs of the cervical spine. Occasionally there is spondylolisthesis of C2 on C3.

Treatment:
1. *Extension injuries with distraction:* Skull traction for a period of 4–6 weeks may be used to maintain position only. There is always the risk in this type of injury of further distraction, and it is therefore important to limit traction to a

98. Isolated spinous process fractures:
Fracture of the spinous process of C7 or T1 (clay shoveller's fracture) may result from sudden muscular contraction (avulsion fracture). This is a stable injury (unless there is evidence of extension into the lamina). Symptomatic treatment only is required (e.g. a cervical collar for 2–3 weeks). It must be carefully distinguished from a cervical dislocation with associated fracture. (If in doubt, flexion and extension laterals should be taken.)

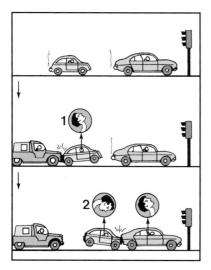

99. WHIPLASH INJURIES

Whiplash occurs most frequently in road traffic accidents. In the classical incident the spine is hyperextended following a rear impact collision (1) and then rapidly flexed as the vehicle in which the patient is travelling hits an object in front – usually another car (2). It is usually agreed that the extension element is the more important in producing disability: amongst the reasons for this include the observation that flexion is generally limited by the chin contacting the chest, while there is no equivalent restriction placed on extension. As distinct from this mechanism, 'whiplash injury' is a somewhat emotive term and has been considerably abused, being at times chosen with regrettable imprecision to describe virtually any injury to the neck.

The Quebec Task Force, an international body of experts interested in all aspects of these injuries, reported in 1995. They defined whiplash as

'an acceleration–deceleration mechanism of energy transfer to the neck. It may result from rear-end or side impact motor vehicle collisions, but can also occur during diving or other mishaps. The impact may result in bony or soft tissue injuries (whiplash injury) which may lead to a variety of clinical manifestations (Whiplash-associated Disorders).'

They went on to classify Whiplash Associated Disorders in the following manner:

Grade I: Complaint of neck pain, stiffness or tenderness only, with no abnormal physical signs.
Grade II: Neck complaint, with musculoskeletal signs (e.g. decreased range of movements or point tenderness).
Grade III: Neck complaint, with positive neurological signs (e.g. reflex disturbance, muscle weakness, or sensory defects).

Other symptoms which may be found in all grades include deafness, dizziness, tinnitus, headache, temporary memory loss, dysphagia and temporomandibular pain. The Task Force gave a fourth grade where there is a neck complaint associated with a fracture or dislocation. Many consider that the inclusion of fractures confuses the issue, and that the term should be reserved exclusively for soft tissue injuries.

Since 1995 publications from other sources have revealed further complexities surrounding this issue. While it has been recognised that there is little clarity regarding the exact nature of the physical basis for the complaints associated with these disorders, it is now apparent that in very many cases there is a non-organic element. It has been noted that the condition is twice as common in women than men, that it is increasing in frequency in spite of the introduction of head restraints and other protective measures, and curiously that it is virtually unknown in Lithuania – where there appears to be little knowledge amongst motorists of the condition and where there is not a climate of litigation. While there seems little doubt that malingering does occasionally occur, this is considered to be rare. It is thought that in many cases a significant component of late disability is psychological, even if this is not at conscious level, and that psychological elements and sometimes illness-related behaviour are often established within three months of injury.

The prognosis for recovery is adversely affected by the severity of the collision (which may sometimes be assessed by reports of the damage to the vehicle), the Quebec Task Force grading of the injury, the age of the patient (the prognosis is poorer in the old), and the position of the passenger in the vehicle (the prognosis being worse for front seat passengers than those in the rear). A high proportion of patients make a full recovery (one series quotes 60% recovered at three months and 90% at six months), but in about 10% of cases disability may continue for years or become permanent, sometimes interfering with or preventing return to previous employment. There is uncertainty as to whether a whiplash injury may precipitate arthritic changes in the neck, although some evidence has been presented to show that joint space narrowing and other spondylotic changes may appear 1–2 years after the incident and be related to it.

DIAGNOSIS

The main symptoms are of pain and stiffness in the neck. In addition there may be radiation of pain and numbness into the shoulder, arm and hand, or to the interscapular region or occiput. In an appreciable number of cases there may be an additional complaint of low back pain, the mechanism of which is uncertain.

Clinically, neck movements are generally restricted, and asymmetrical restriction is considered by some to be of particular significance. Widespread cervical tenderness is usual, often with involvement of the anterior cervical muscles, but localisation should be looked for. Objective neurological signs are rare, but should always be sought.

NEED FOR FURTHER INVESTIGATION

Hoffman considers that further investigation (e.g. by X-ray) is indicated if the patient does not satisfy *all* of the following criteria:

1. No posterior midline tenderness.
2. No intoxication (which may mask the complaints and findings).
3. Normal level of alertness.
4. No focal neurological signs.
5. No painful, distracting injuries.

This is generally very reliable, but is not infallible: if in doubt, there should be no hesitation in commencing further investigation by obtaining X-rays of the neck.

Radiographs If these are taken they may show the following: 1. There may be loss of the usual cervical curvature or localised kinking (of greater significance). 2. Occasionally, there may be evidence of hyperextension (anterior osteophytic avulsion) or hyperflexion (flake fracture of a spinous process). 3. The presence of pre-existing osteoarthritic changes in the cervical spine which predispose to injury (by concentrating local stresses).

MRI scans These are frequently performed, and may show evidence of disc prolapse or nerve root compression. The results however can be unreliable, as abnormalities have been reported in symptomless patients, and vice versa.

TREATMENT

Treatment is primarily conservative, and to minimise the risks of the superimposition of a non-organic element, a positive approach in the handling of these cases, with emphasis of the likelihood of a complete recovery, is strongly advised. It has been suggested that the content of any medico-legal report in the early stages (and which the patient is likely to see) should reflect this.

The Quebec study strongly advised against the prolonged use of cervical collars, which they considered to be associated with cases with poorer outcomes. They advocate:

Grade I: Immediate return to normal activities, with no work restrictions and no medication.

Grade II: To return to normal activities as soon as possible, and preferably within a week. Temporary alteration of work patterns may be required, but the need for these should be reassessed after two weeks unless the clinical circumstances or the working environment are unusual. Non-narcotic analgesics and/or NSAIDs may be prescribed for up to one week only.

Grade III: As in Grade II, but narcotic analgesics may be required for short periods initially. Manipulation may be of transient benefit, but not more than two sessions are recommended. Treatment started by a physiotherapist and continued at home by the patient himself is generally very helpful, with emphasis again being placed on the likelihood of a good recovery. McKenzie exercises are considered to be of particular value.

Cases persisting over three months Carefully reassess and, if necessary, consider the prescription of minor tranquillisers or antidepressants. Grade III patients with progressive neurological deterioration or persisting radicular arm pain may be considered for surgery provided a disc protrusion at the relevant level has been confirmed: then discectomy and anterior cervical fusion generally give a good result.

Barré–Lieou syndrome This may follow a whiplash incident. There is complaint of headache, vertigo, tinnitus, ocular problems and facial pain. It is thought that it may be due to a sympathetic nerve disturbance at the C3–4 level, and in 75% of the cases there is impairment of sensation in the C4 dermatome, with weakness of shoulder and scapular movements. Myelography may show nerve root sleeve disturbances. Good results have been claimed for anterior discectomy combined with local cervical fusion.

100. Fractures of the thoracic and lumbar spine

Mechanism of injury:
Fractures of the thoracic and lumbar spine occur most frequently as a result of forces which tend to produce flexion of the spine. A rotational element is often present.

Causes: The many possible causes of this type of injury include:
1. Falls from a height on to the heels, where the direction of the forces acting on the spine are offset by the normal thoracic convexity, leading to anterior stress concentrations.
2. Blows across the back and shoulders which cause the spine to jack-knife at the thoracolumbar junction, e.g. injuries in the mining and construction industries.
3. Flexion and rotational forces transmitted to the spine from road or vehicle impact in car and motor cycle accidents.
4. Heavy lifting, especially in the middle aged and elderly, where there is often the pathological element of osteoporosis or osteomalacia. Less commonly, malignancy (especially metastatic deposits) may be a factor, when the causal force may be slight or not even remembered.

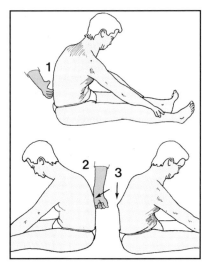

101. Diagnosis: Suspect on a history of back pain after trauma, particularly if there is local spinal tenderness (1), pain on spinal percussion (2), or especially if there is an angular kyphosis (3). Thoracic or abdominal radicular pain may wrongly divert attention to the chest or abdomen, and in the elderly there may be no convincing history of injury; any suspicion merits radiography.

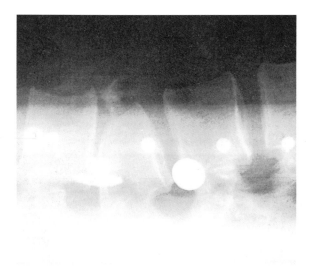

102. Radiographs (a): AP and lateral radiographs only should be taken in the first instance. In the obviously seriously injured patient there may be difficulty in obtaining a lateral because of severe pain, or through fear of causing cord damage. In these circumstances, a shoot-through lateral may be taken using a fixed grid or chest bucky. (Illus.: Shoot-through lateral; note tacks securing canvas to stretcher poles, but detail sufficient to show an anterior wedge compression fracture of L3, with anterior subluxation and obvious instability.)

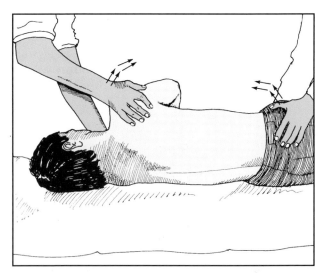

103. Radiographs (b): If these measures are unsatisfactory you should *personally* supervise the turning of the patient on their side in order to obtain a lateral projection; in essence you should see that the patient is turned gently and smoothly in such a way that the upper part of the spine with the shoulders is rotated in pace with the pelvis, and that the patient remains well supported (e.g. by pillows) when on their side. This is often a convenient time to physically inspect the back, looking for bruising, swelling and deformity, and palpating to detect tenderness, local oedema and any palpable gap between the spinous processes (signifying a posterior complex injury with implied instability).

104. Note:
1. The most important decision to make in any spinal injury is whether it is stable. This obviously profoundly influences the approach to treatment.
2. Most *stable fractures* are uncomplicated by damage to the cord or cauda equina (although certain *mechanically* stable bursting fractures may be neurologically unstable).
3. *Unstable* fractures of the spine may be recognised in the plain films, but if there is any doubt, CAT scanning to show the state of the middle and posterior columns is indicated. Unstable fractures may be accompanied by neurological involvement. If this is incomplete, there is always hope of recovery. There is however the risk that further displacement at the fracture site may jeopardise this, or convert an uncomplicated injury to a complicated one. Treatment is, therefore, vitally important.
4. The commonest spinal injury *by far* is the flexion compression wedge fracture.
5. In practice, the most frequently encountered problems are the recognition of such a fracture and to decide whether it is stable or not.
6. Other types of injury are more often unstable than stable.

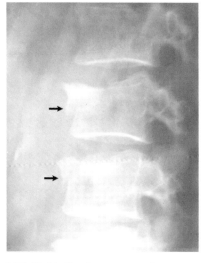

105. Stable flexion compression (wedge) fractures (a): Flexion compression (anterior wedge) fractures are most commonly observed in lateral radiographs and are caused by pure flexion forces. (Illus.: Flexion compression fractures of two vertebrae: note the difference in height between the anterior and posterior margins of each vertebral body.)

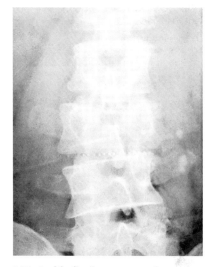

106. Stable flexion compression fractures (b): Less commonly, when there is a rotational element added to forward flexion, vertebral wedging may be apparent in the AP projection (lateral wedging). (Illus.: Lateral wedging of L3 resulting in a traumatic scoliosis.) This form of wedging is often associated with root compression on the narrowed side, and these injuries have a poorer prognosis regarding ultimate functional recovery and freedom from pain.

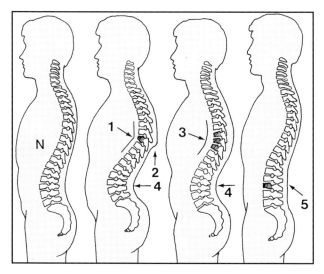

107. Interpreting the radiographs (a): In the thoracic spine, a flexion compression fracture with anterior wedging of a single vertebra will lead to localised kinking (1) with or without a localised overlying kyphotic prominence (2). Multiple fractures in the thoracic spine, especially when wedging is slight in each of the affected vertebrae, will lead to a more regular kyphosis (3). In either of these circumstances, the increased thoracic curvature will tend to produce an increased lumbar lordosis (except where the lumbar spine is arthritic) (4) and/or hyperextension in the hip joints. In the case of the lumbar spine, there may be obliteration or reversal of the normal lumbar lordosis (5). (Compare with the normal profile, N.)

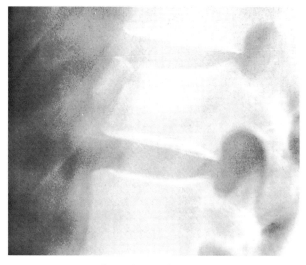

108. Interpreting the radiographs (b): In the commonest flexion compression fractures, the anterior border of the vertebra will measure less than the posterior border. The crushing of the anterior portion may be quite regular, or may result in a marginal shearing fracture (generally the anterior superior corner) (Illus.). If the *posterior* margin appears to show a decrease in height (compared with the heights of the vertebrae above and below) this is evidence of greater violence, and raises the possibility of an element of burst fracture, with the risk of bony fragments encroaching on the vertebral canal. If this is suspected, a CAT scan to clarify the issue is recommended.

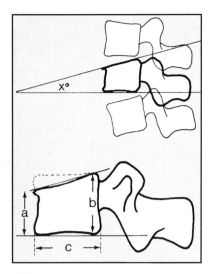

109. Interpreting the radiographs (c):
Assess the amount of wedging; the fracture is likely to be stable if the height of the anterior margin still amounts to two-thirds or more of the posterior margin or, putting this another way, if the degree of wedging is 15° or less, or if the width of the body divided by the difference in the heights is greater than 3.75, i.e.

$$x < 15°, \text{ or } \frac{c}{b-a} > 3.75.$$

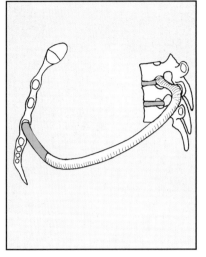

110. Interpreting the radiographs (d):
In the case of the upper eight thoracic vertebrae, note any associated fractures of the sternum or ribs. Each of the upper thoracic vertebrae is linked by ribs to the sternum, and *appreciable* wedging cannot take place without involvement of these structures.

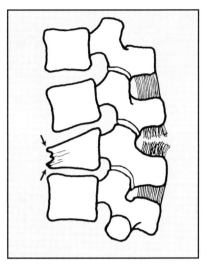

111. Unstable fractures (a): Marked wedging (20° or more, or collapse of the anterior margin to less than half the posterior) points to damage to the posterior ligament complex, and therefore to instability. (Note however that if the *posterior* margin is reduced in height a greater degree of wedging is possible prior to posterior complex rupture – but in the presence of this finding, the possibility of a burst fracture should be investigated, e.g. by CAT scanning.)

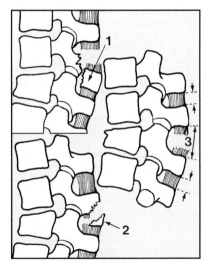

112. Unstable fractures (b): Look for other evidence of damage to the posterior ligament complex and associated structures fundamental to spinal stability. Note especially any avulsion fracture of a spinous process (1), avulsion-fracture of the tip of a spinous process (2), and wide separation of the vertebral spines at the level of injury (3). In the cases illustrated, the possibility of the additional involvement of the facet joints should be considered.

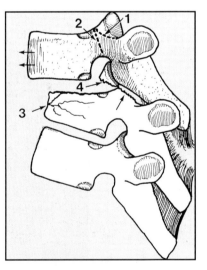

113. Unstable fractures (c): Examine the radiographs carefully for evidence of fractures at the level of the facet joints (1) or pedicles (2). A comminuted fracture of a vertebral body (3) with involvement of these structures (Illus.: Facet joint fracture, 4) is generally unstable; bilateral pedicle fractures are invariably unstable. If there is any doubt regarding the integrity of the articular processes, CAT scans may give valuable additional information.

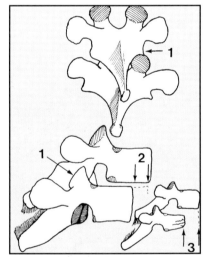

114. Unstable fractures (d): Look for shift of one vertebra relative to another. This is an invariable sign of instability. Vertebral displacement patterns include the following: (a) Ruptured posterior ligament with unilateral facet joint displacement (1), in the lateral projection, the degree of forward shift is about a third or less (2); (b) Bilateral dislocated facet joints, often with a vertebral body fracture and a greater degree of displacement (3).

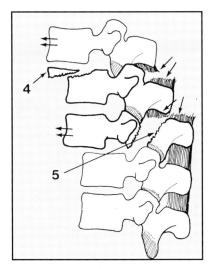

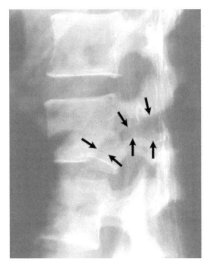

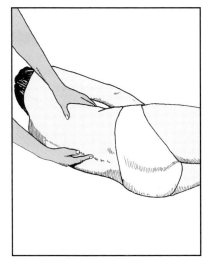

115. Unstable fractures (e): Shearing fracture of a vertebral body (4); Bilateral neural arch fractures and traumatic spondylolisthesis (5). *Note:* In all these injuries there is damage to the posterior ligament complex. If there is any remaining doubt the following additional radiographs should be taken: 1. Oblique projections; 2. A further lateral, *supervised*, in slight flexion; 3. If available, and most usefully, an MRI scan.

116. Unstable fractures (f): *Seat belt injuries (Chance fractures)*: These result from failure of the posterior and middle columns *in tension*. In the plain films the points to note are widening of the interpedicular distance in the AP, and, in the lateral, increased distance between the spinous processes. These are indicative of a significant degree of posterior ligament complex disruption. In the example, failure has occurred through the vertebral body and the spinous process (Type 3 of the patterns shown in Frame 10.)

117. Unstable fractures (g): The radiographs may give unequivocal evidence of instability. In other cases where there is the *slightest* suspicion of the posterior ligament complex being involved, that structure must be carefully examined clinically. Press firmly between successive spines, preferably in slight flexion. If the interspinous ligaments are torn, a boggy softness will be felt instead of the normal resistance to pressure. An increased gap between the spinous processes may also be noted.

120. Treatment of unstable fractures, with or without a neurological lesion (a): The primary aims of treatment are:
1. To reduce any displacement that is present.
2. To prevent any recurrence of displacement (with risks of neurological disasters) until stability is regained.
3. To treat any major neurological problem and its complications (see later).

Stability may be achieved by:
1. Spontaneous anterior fusion.
2. Healing of the torn posterior ligament complex (which can seldom be relied upon, especially in cases uncomplicated by fracture).
3. By internal fixation with or without fusion.

Generally speaking *internal fixation of all unstable fractures* is *preferred*, to facilitate nursing and permit early mobilisation. However, as union of a spinal fracture usually results in stability, if the fracture can be reduced and held till this occurs, conservative treatment is often possible especially where there are no facilities for internal fixation and early mobilisation. Conservative management may also be undertaken in other cases to give the patient time to recover from their injuries (to the spine and elsewhere) and to allow a thorough assessment of the case to be made. Surgical treatment may then be undertaken as an elective procedure.

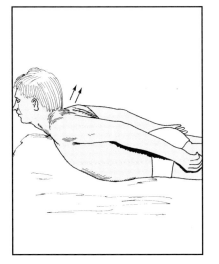

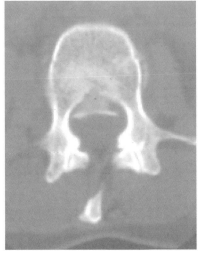

118. Treatment – Stable fractures (a):
1. Admit for bed rest in recumbency.
2. Prescribe analgesics as required, and as soon as pain is under control commence vigorous extension exercises. The patient may then be mobilised, and may often be allowed home after a week, especially if wedging is minimal. Some form of back brace may be helpful initially in reducing pain and encouraging mobility.

119. Treatment – Stable fractures (b): Burst fractures are usually stable and if this is confirmed may be treated as described in the previous frame. If there is instability, internal fixation may be considered. In the face of a neurological problem some advise decompression (e.g. with removal of the affected vertebral body, clearance of the canal, and the insertion of 3 strut grafts and a bridging plate), but unfortunately there is little to suggest that this has any benefit, and it is difficult to justify as the complication rate is 75%.

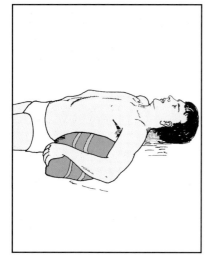

121. Treatment (b): Reduction can generally be achieved by gently extending the spine with a pillow or a sandbag at the level of injury. (If this is unsuccessful, or if there are locked facets, open reduction will be required.) After reduction, further care is dependent on the nature of the injury and the availability of equipment.

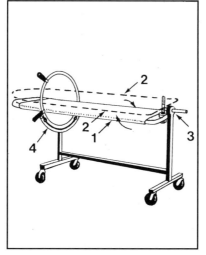

122. Treatment (c): The patient may be nursed in a Stryker frame. This is now seldom used, but is available in some centres. This special bed allows the patient to be rotated from the supine to the prone position with minimal nursing effort. During the manoeuvre, the patient is sandwiched between two mattresses (1, 2) which are locked together, and turned round a pivot at one end (3) and a quadrant (4) at the other. The frame is then locked and the uppermost mattress removed.

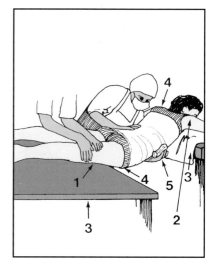

123. Treatment (d): Alternatively, where instability is minimal *or* as a follow up to a period in a Stryker frame, a POP jacket may be applied. The sedated but conscious patient supports himself by the thighs (1) and shoulders (2) between two tables (3) while the plaster is applied over stockinet (4). Felt and wool are used to protect the bony prominences prior to the application of slabs and encircling bandages (5). The patient is lifted on to pillows and the cast trimmed when dry. Instead of a cast, an orthosis may also be used.

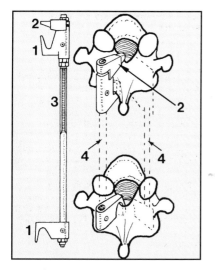

124. Treatment (e) – Internal fixation (i): This is generally the treatment of choice for unstable fractures. It may be combined with open reduction (necessitated, for example, by locked facets) and with bone grafting. The AO Locking Hook Rod system illustrated may be used between T3 and T10. The hooks (1) snug against the laminae, and can be locked to them as required (2). They are fixed to paired partially threaded rods (3, 4) which may be bent to fit the contours of the spine.

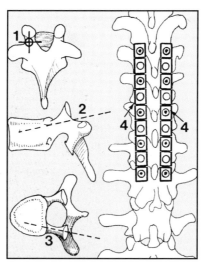

125. Internal fixation (ii): Most other systems use screws passed through the pedicles into the vertebral bodies. The entry point (1) is below the facet close to the upper margin of the transverse process, with the track through the pedicle inclined downwards (2) and medially (3) at an angle which varies with the vertebral level. Great care must be taken (by probing and image intensifier control) to see that the spinal canal is not entered. AO notched plates (4) and 4.5 mm screws may be used from T6 to S1.

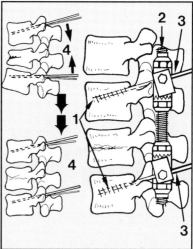

126. Internal fixation (iii): Paired Schanz screws (1) and *internal* fixators (2) may also be employed. After careful introduction, the upper and lower pairs of screws are locked to fixators, one on each side of the spinous processes. One fixator can be linked to the other across the midline. The ends of the pins are cut off (3) so that all can be buried. Angulation can be corrected (4) before the fixator is tightened. Bone chips can be packed into the collapsed vertebra through a small funnel.

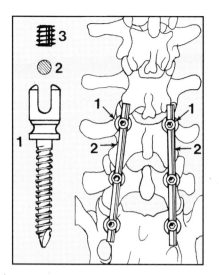

127. Internal fixation (iv): The Oswestry pedicle screw system can be used from T10 to S1, and employs rigid self-tapping pedicle screws (1). These are inserted after the accuracy of their proposed paths has been confirmed with probing and the use of an image intensifier. The pedicle screws are linked with connecting bars (2) which can be bent to suit the local contours, before being locked with square socket grub screws (3) in the threaded ends of the pedicle screws.

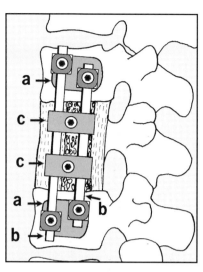

128. Internal fixation (v): The Kaneda Anterior Spinal system may be used from T10–L3 to treat spinal instability caused by fracture, and as an adjunct to spinal fusion where decompression with removal of a vertebral body has been performed. Tetra spiked contoured plates (a) help spread axial loads. Smooth rods (b) are anchored with spinal screws to the vertebral bodies, and to one another by transverse couplers (c).

129. Treatment of unstable fractures with a complete, irrecoverable cord lesion: In theory the need for open reduction and internal fixation of the spine becomes of less importance when an associated cord lesion is found to be complete, and in the past such injuries were treated conservatively.

Nevertheless, particularly if the spine is grossly unstable, internal fixation may be indicated on the following grounds:
1. To facilitate nursing;
2. To prevent or minimise spinal deformity which, if marked, may compromise respiratory function and the ability to sit up, to use a wheelchair, and complete a satisfactory programme of rehabilitation;
3. To permit earlier mobilisation;
4. To reduce the risks of chronic back pain from nerve root involvement.

If the spine is not wildly unstable, and first-class nursing is available, there is less need for internal fixation, and the treatment is then of the accompanying paraplegia.

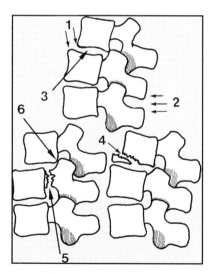

130. Other injuries (a) – Retrospondylolisthesis: This lesion (1) occurs most especially at T12–L1, and may follow a distally sited blow (2). There may be shearing through the disc (3), the vertebral body (4) or the pedicles (5) so that the articular processes impinge on the vertebral body (6). Any neurological involvement is seldom complete, but as the posterior ligament complex is damaged, instability may be present; these injuries should be treated with respect.

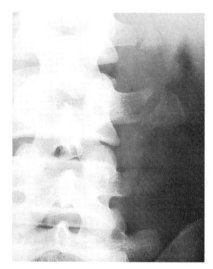

131. Fractured transverse processes: In the lumbar region these may result from direct trauma, avulsion (quadratus lumborum), or, in the case of L5, be associated with a sacro-iliac disruption (which may involve the L5 nerve root). They may accompany fracture–dislocations of the spine. Multiple fractures may be complicated by retroperitoneal haemorrhage, shock, paralytic ileus or renal damage, all of which will require appropriate treatment. No treatment apart from rest is needed for uncomplicated transverse process fractures.

132. The management of spinal paralysis
The aims of treatment are:
1. To prevent the well known sequelae of spinal injuries,
2. To obtain maximal physical recovery and mental readjustment with, ideally,
3. Complete physical independence and
4. Return to full-time employment.
These ideals can be most fully realised through the special resources and environment of a spinal cord injury unit, and no effort should be spared in having the patient transferred to such a unit at the earliest possible opportunity. Pending transfer, and assuming the injury has been dealt with in an appropriate fashion, it is vital that attention is paid to the skin, bladder and other problems as detailed in the following pages.

TREATMENT OF THE SKIN

If pressure is applied to the skin it becomes ischaemic; if pressure is maintained, necrosis from tissue anoxia results. The skin of the elderly is thin, and least able to tolerate pressure. Poorly nourished skin, anaemia, and local skin damage such as abrasions (which increase oxygen demand) are also adverse factors. The most important points, both of which are amenable to treatment, are: 1. The *duration* of ischaemia, 2. The *amount* of pressure applied to the skin.

Duration of skin pressure The duration of pressure applied to any one area is in practice regulated by regular turning of the patient. During the initial weeks of treatment it is essential that the patient does not lie for longer than 2 hours in one position. If the patient is being nursed on a Stryker frame, then they alternate from the prone to the supine; if they are being nursed in bed, then they alternate between lying on each side and in the supine position. It is important to note that regular turning of the patient should start from the time of injury; irreversible damage may be done on the day of admission when other problems allow this vital aspect of treatment to be overlooked for some hours.

Amount of skin pressure The amount of pressure applied to the skin is obviously important: if the body weight is locally concentrated then ischaemia will be complete. If the skin loading is reduced by being spread over a large area, then ischaemia will be less severe and more tolerable. Because of these loading factors, pressure sores tend to commence over bony prominences – the sacrum, the trochanters, the heels, the elbows and the malleoli. Particular attention should be paid to these areas, and local padding over the ankles and elbows may help. To distribute the body weight more evenly, the patient may be nursed on pillows laid across the bed from head to foot. When the patient is lying on their back, additional pillows laid horizontally may be used to support the elbows and arms. Pillows may also be placed under the legs so that the heels are relieved of pressure. When the patient is lying on their side, a pillow may be placed between the legs and the legs positioned in such a way that the malleoli and knees are free from pressure. In some centres, water beds or sand beds are used to help distribute the loads on the skin.

It is important to preserve the tone and general condition of the skin. If it becomes moist it becomes susceptible to bacterial invasion. If it is subjected to friction through contact with rough, unyielding surfaces, local abrasions may occur. Local injury of this nature increases tissue demands and may initiate the production of pressure sores. To prevent this: 1. Unstarched, soft bed linen should be used and non-porous surfaces avoided. Nursing the patient on sheepskin is sometimes advocated. 2. The skin should be protected from incontinence. 3. Skin hygiene should be maintained by frequent, thorough cleansing with soap and water. After washing, the skin must be thoroughly dried.

If pressure sores occur, substantial undermining of the skin may conceal the often considerable extent of each lesion. Preventative measures should be tightened up, and any underlying anaemia corrected. Any local sloughs or sequestra should be removed. If the area involved is small, healing may be achieved with local dressings, going through the stages of granulation and contraction. If a large area is involved, rotational flaps usually afford the best means of closure. If sores persist, they are frequently followed by progressive anaemia, deterioration in general health and well being, and often amyloid disease.

TREATMENT OF THE BLADDER

Note first the neurological control of the bladder, detailed in the following frames, (a)–(c).

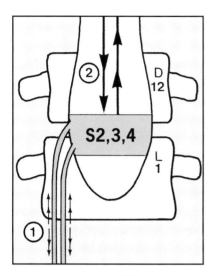

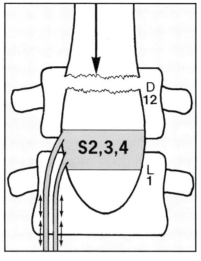

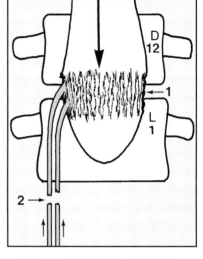

Neurological control of the bladder (a): *Note:*
(i) Autonomic fibres controlling the detrusor muscle of the bladder and the internal sphincter travel from cord segments S2, 3 and 4 to the bladder via the cauda equina (1).
(ii) Under normal circumstances bladder sensation and voluntary emptying are mediated through pathways stretching between the brain and the sacral centres (2).

Neurological control of the bladder (b): If the cord is transected above S2 (e.g. by a thoracic spine fracture), voluntary control is lost, but the potential for coordinated contraction of the bladder wall, relaxation of the sphincter and complete emptying remains. (Normally 200–400 mL of urine is passed every 2–4 hours, the reflex activity being triggered by rising bladder pressure or skin stimulation) – (automatic bladder or cord bladder).

Neurological control of the bladder (c): Injuries which damage the sacral centres (1) or the cauda (2) prevent coordinated reflex control of bladder activity. Bladder emptying is always incomplete and irregular, and occurs only as a result of distension. Its efficiency varies with the patient's state of health, the presence of urinary infection and muscle spasms (autonomous or isolated atonic bladder). In summary, the effects on the bladder are dependent on the level of injury.

Prevention of overdistension The long-term aims of treatment are to minimise the effects of chronic bladder distension such as renal failure, bladder calculi, and chronic infection. The immediate problem is the prevention of overdistension of the bladder while minimising the risks of infection. The methods available include:

1. *Intermittent catheterisation:* If properly performed during the acute phase on a regular 4–6 hour basis, with a full aseptic ritual, the risks of infection are probably lowest with this method. It is however very demanding on staff.
2. *Indwelling catheterisation:* This is probably the commonest method employed, but is almost invariably accompanied by some degree of urinary infection.
3. *Intermittent suprapubic cystostomy using plastic tubing:* This method is demanding on staff and facilities, and carries the risk of pelvic infection.

Mechanical emptying of the bladder by one of these methods is usually required for 3–4 weeks, after which, in the appropriate lesions, automatic function will be starting to take over. A bladder retraining programme may then be initiated. The bladder emptying profile, i.e. when most urine is produced, should be assessed first. A constant fluid intake is adhered to, then the aim should be provide the most efficient way of emptying the bladder. Ultrasound and urodynamic analysis may be used to judge the completeness of bladder emptying. After an initial IVP, this is repeated at yearly intervals, along with a urine culture, estimation of the serum urea and creatine, and the performance of a creatine clearance test.

TREATMENT OF THE BOWEL

At the end of the period of spinal shock there is a slow but incomplete recovery of peristalsis. The bowel is emptied with cathartics, aperients and suppositories, and a bowel retraining programme commenced, the aim being to achieve emptying every second day, and avoid overstretching of the bowel and megacolon. Emptying is enhanced by taking advantage of the gastro-colic reflex, but also using abdominal skin and sphincter stimulation and suppositories. Should megacolon develop a colostomy or an ileostomy may become necessary.

TREATMENT OF SPASTICITY

With the return of the spinal reflexes spasticity of the trunk and limb muscles may develop. The aim should be to prevent contractures and maintain a full range of joint movements by physiotherapy and appropriate medication: diazepam is often of value.

TREATMENT OF PAIN

Neuropathic pain, often accompanied by disturbing hyperaesthesia, may develop at or below the level of injury. This is best managed through the combined efforts of a pain management team.

OTHER TREATMENTS

Physiotherapy and occupational therapy These measures should be commenced without delay, attention being paid to the following aspects of management:
1. **The chest:** The risks and effects of respiratory infection should be minimised by deep-breathing exercises, the development of the accessory muscles of respiration, assisted coughing, percussion and postural drainage.
2. **The joints:** Mobility should be preserved in the paralysed joints by passive movements. This must be done with caution if there is any spasticity; overstretching must be avoided to minimise the risks of myositis ossificans.
3. **The unparalysed muscles:** These should be developed for compensatory use, e.g. shoulder girdle exercises to make unaided bed–wheelchair transfers possible.
4. **Other measures:** Depending on the level of the lesion the patient may require assistance in some or all of the following areas:
   (i) Regaining balance for sitting or standing;
   (ii) Tuition in calliper walking (or gait improvement in partial lesions);
   (iii) Overcoming problems of dressing;
   (iv) Help with alterations and adjustments within the home to permit wheelchair use;
   (v) Industrial retraining or other measures to help return to employment.

SELF-TEST

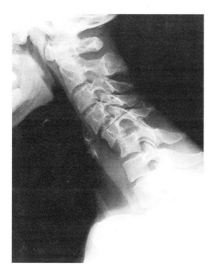

133. Describe the lesion shown. Is the injury stable or unstable?

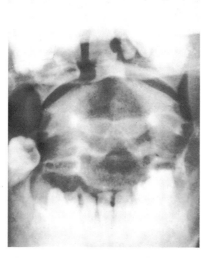

134. Describe this through-the-mouth view of the first two cervical vertebrae.

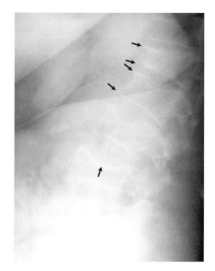

135. This lateral radiograph is of an elderly patient complaining of pain in the back after lifting a heavy weight. What does the radiograph show?

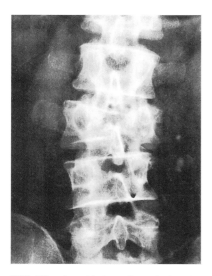

136. What does this AP radiograph show? Which two neurological complications are most likely to be associated with the injury?

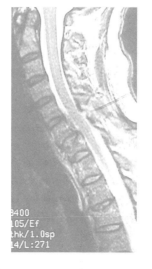

137. What does this MRI scan show? Is the injury stable?

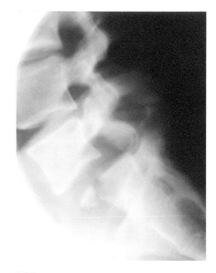

138. Describe this injury. What treatment would be required?

ANSWERS TO SELF-TEST

133. Dislocation of C5 on C6 with bilateral locked facets. 50% forward shift is present and the injury is unstable. There is no accompanying fracture.

134. There is a congenital deformity of the odontoid process (hypoplasia). No fracture is present and there is no evidence of other injury. The shadow lying above the hypoplastic odontoid process is that of one of the incisors. This is a common finding which is sometimes misinterpreted as a fracture.

135. Flexion compression fractures (anterior wedge fractures) of L1 and L2 and probably L3. Central ballooning of the disc into L4. Gross demineralisation of the spine, probably secondary to osteoporosis or osteomalacia (i.e. these are pathological fractures).

136. There is a burst fracture of L3, with marked wedging, a vertical split through the vertebral body, and separation of the pedicles. The structures most at risk are: 1. The L3 nerve passing through the neural foramen on the wedged side of the spine; 2. The cauda equina within the spinal canal.

A CAT scan would help clarify how much bony material has been extruded into the canal; in practice, burst fractures in this region have generally a very good prognosis, even in the face of gross extrusions.

137. There is a flexion (anterior compression) fracture of C7. There are additional, less obvious fractures of T1, T2 and T3. Those affecting T1 and T2 are of hairline pattern. There is disruption of the posterior ligament complex, so that the injury is an unstable one.

138. Anterior dislocation of L5 on the sacrum, with bilateral locked facets, and a fracture of the anterior margin of the first piece of the sacrum. This is a fracture–dislocation of the flexion-distraction type. Open reduction was required.

CHAPTER

11

The pelvis, hip and femoral neck

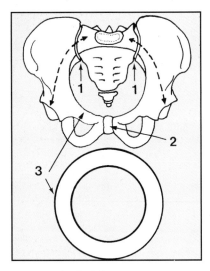

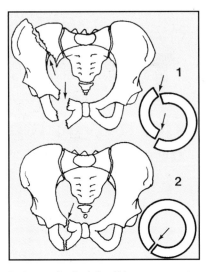

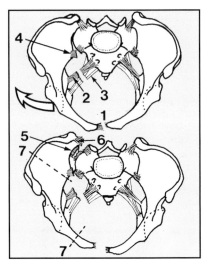

1. General principles (a): The two wings of the pelvis are joined to the sacrum behind (1) by the very strong sacroiliac ligaments. In front they are united by the symphysis pubis (2). This arrangement forms a cylinder of bone, the pelvic ring (3) which protects the pelvic organs and transfers the body weight from the spine to the limbs. (The dotted line indicates the path of weight transfer.)

2. General principles (b): If the pelvic ring is broken at two levels, the pelvis may be free to open out or displace proximally (1), carrying the limb with it. Isolated (single) injuries of the ring (2) do not have this tendency. This simple concept underlines the main consideration in classifying pelvic fractures, namely to decide whether the injury is *stable or unstable*. Conversely, if there is a major pelvic displacement, the pelvic ring must be broken at two levels even if on first inspection only one is obvious.

3. Anatomical considerations (a): If the pelvis is subjected to splaying forces, the weak symphysis tends to give first (1); with greater violence, the sacrospinous (2), the sacrotuberous (3), and the anterior sacroiliac ligaments (4) rupture, so that the halves of the pelvis can externally rotate. If the pelvis is subjected to vertical shear forces, the interosseous (5) and posterior sacroiliac ligaments (6) are torn, leading to dislocation of the sacroiliac joint and proximal migration of the hemipelvis. In many injuries local fractures replace ligament tears (7).

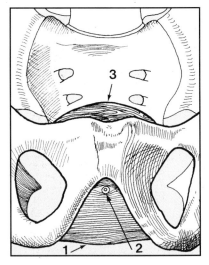

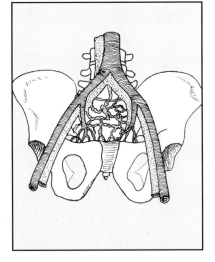

4. Anatomical considerations (b): The urogenital diaphragm (1) is pierced by the membranous urethra (2), and the bladder lies behind the pubic bones. Fractures of the pelvis, especially in the region of the symphysis and pubic rami, are often associated with damage to the urethra or bladder; rarely, there may be involvement of the rectum.

5. Anatomical considerations (c): The pelvis is richly supplied with blood vessels which are frequently damaged by fractures. *Internal haemorrhage is often severe, leading to shock which can be rapidly fatal.* NB: Shock should be *anticipated* in pelvic fractures and merits *first consideration* (see p. 33). In the region of the sacroiliac joint the lumbosacral trunk and the sacral nerves are also susceptible to injury.

6. Classification of pelvic fractures: In both the Tile and the AO classification three clearly defined Types are recognised: *Stable* fractures are classified as Type A; fractures which are *rotationally unstable but vertically stable* fall into Type B; and fractures which are both *rotationally and vertically unstable* form Type C. In Tile's widely used classification the subgroups are as follows:
A1: Fractures of the pelvis not involving the pelvic ring.
A2: Stable, minimally displaced fractures of the pelvic ring.
B1: Anteroposterior compression fractures (open book).
B2: Lateral compression (ipsilateral).
B3: Lateral compression (contralateral).
C1: Unilateral vertically unstable.
C2: Bilateral vertically unstable.
C3: Associated with acetabular fracture.
Diagnosis: Fractures of the pelvis commonly occur in falls from a height and from crushing injuries. *Screening films of the pelvis should be taken* in every case of multiple trauma (especially in the unconscious patient), unexplained shock following trauma, blunt abdominal injury, and femoral shaft fractures. Instability is best assessed by pelvic inlet and outlet films and by CAT scan. If the software for 3-D reconstructions (imaging) is available, this greatly facilitates interpretation of the exact relationship of the bony elements involved.

7. Summary of treatment guidelines:

There are two clear issues involved in the management of any major pelvic fracture:

1. *Initial procedures (IP)* to reduce internal haemorrhage. These include the application of an external fixator and perhaps a pelvic clamp.

2. *Definitive treatment (DT)* of the fracture. Both goals may in some cases be achieved by the same measures. The present tendency is for increasing use of open reduction and internal fixation.

A1 and **A2** (Tile's classification):
IP and *DT*: Conservative treatment may be followed in the majority of cases.

B1
IP: Apply an external fixator.
DT: Use an external fixator; or internally fix the symphysis pubis unless there is a contraindication (such as increased risk of infection from a supra-pubic drain).

B2 and **B3**
IP: Use an external fixator if the patient is haemodynamically unstable.
DT: Conservative, unless there are multiple injuries or difficulty in pain control, making nursing difficult.

C1 and **C2**
IP: External fixator (and if necessary a pelvic clamp) plus skeletal leg traction.
DT: Internal fixation (e.g. by sacral bars, application of reconstruction plates).

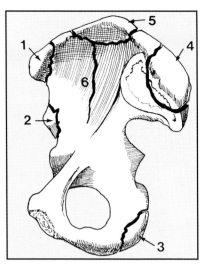

8. A1: Fractures not involving the pelvic ring – Avulsion fractures (a):

Sudden muscle contraction, especially in athletes, may avulse the anterior superior spine (sartorius) (1), the anterior inferior spine (rectus femoris) (2), the ischial tuberosity (hamstrings) (3), the posterior spine (erector spinae) (4), and the crest (abdominal muscles) (5). The crest and blade (6) may also be fractured by direct violence. In all cases there is localised tenderness, and symptomatic treatment is all that is usually required.

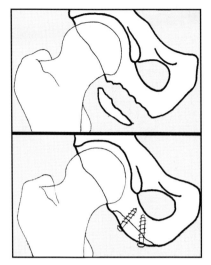

9. A1: Fractures not involving the pelvic ring – Avulsion fractures (b): In

the case of the ischial tuberosity, non-union is an appreciable risk, and if this occurs there may be problems with chronic pain and disability. To prevent this, open reduction and internal fixation have been advocated, and this is especially indicated if there is much separation of the fragments (2 cm or more).

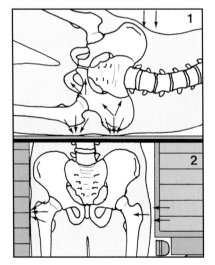

10. A2: Minimally displaced, stable fractures of the pelvic ring (a): These,

like many other pelvic fractures, may result from a fall on the side (1), force being transmitted through the trochanter or iliac crest, or from crushing accidents (e.g. from reversing vehicles (2), rock falls etc.), or through violence transmitted along the femoral shaft (e.g. road accidents, falls from a height, etc.). Other stable injuries may follow anterior compression forces.

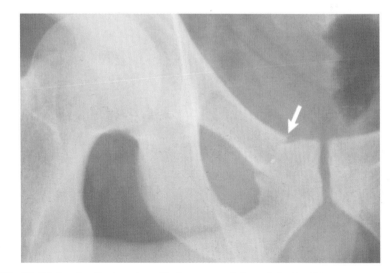

11. A2: Minimally displaced, stable fractures of the pelvic ring (b): By far the

commonest fracture is one involving the superior pubic ramus. This is seen frequently in the elderly patient following a fall on the side. Osteoporosis or osteomalacia are frequently contributory factors. *This injury is often missed* and should always be suspected if there is difficulty in walking after a fall, and a femoral neck fracture has been excluded. Clinically there will be tenderness over the superior ramus, and pain on side-to-side compression of the pelvis; movements of the hips may be relatively pain-free. Radiographs of the hip may fail to visualise the area and full pelvic films are required. Treatment is by bed rest for 2–3 weeks until the pain settles and mobilisation can be commenced.

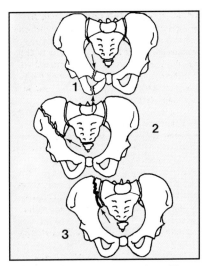

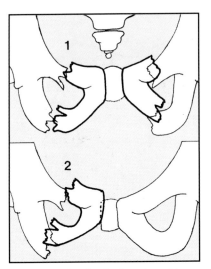

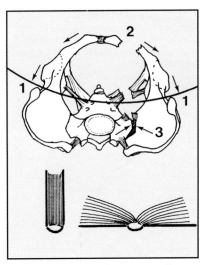

12. A2: Minimally displaced, stable fractures of the pelvic ring (c): Other fractures of this type include: (1) fractures of two rami on one side; (2) fracture of the ilium running into the sciatic notch; (3) fracture of the ilium or sacrum involving the sacroiliac joint. The nature of these injuries often suggests at least momentary involvement elsewhere in the ring: nevertheless, assuming that they are uncomplicated, they may be treated as in the previous frame.

13. A2: Minimally displaced, stable fracture of the pelvic ring (d): Many quadripartite (butterfly) fractures (1) of the pelvis, and double fractures of the rami with symphyseal involvement (2) are stable. They usually result from AP compression of the pelvis which is insufficient to disrupt the anterior sacroiliac ligaments: the posterior part of the pelvic ring remains intact and rigid, while the loose anterior fragment is only slightly displaced. *Anticipate shock and damage to the urethra*, but otherwise treat with 6 weeks' recumbency.

14. B1: Anteroposterior compression, rotationally unstable, vertically stable fractures (a): These injuries frequently result from run-over incidents where the wheel of a motor vehicle forces the anterior superior iliac spines backwards and outwards (1); they may also occur when the pelvis is compressed by falling rock or masonry which pins the patient to the ground. The ring fails *anteriorly* (e.g. at the symphysis or through two rami) (2), *and posteriorly* (3). The pelvis opens out (hence the term 'open-book' fractures).

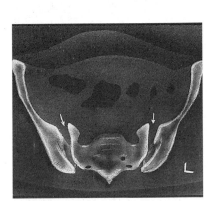

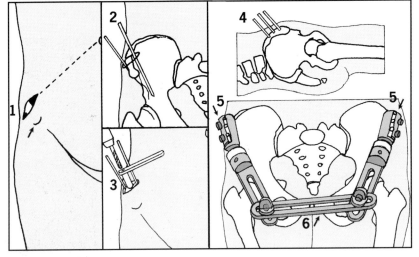

15. B1 (b): As the pelvis opens out the sacrospinous and sacrotuberous ligaments are torn, and CAT scans may show anterior widening of the sacroiliac joints. The posterior sacroiliac ligaments remain intact, so that there is no vertical instability. *Treatment:* 1. Where the posterior damage is minimal and the anterior gap does not exceed 2.5 cm, treat by bed rest and monitor the symphyseal separation by repeated radiographs. 2. If the separation exceeds 2.5 cm, more active treatment is required.

16. Treatment (a) – External fixation (a): An external fixator may be required to deal with the haemodynamically unstable patient, and for definitive treatment. Fixation pins may be inserted (a) in the iliac crest, or (b) in the anterior inferior iliac spine. The iliac crest is exposed 2.5 cm posterior to the ASS through a 1.5 cm incision directed towards the umbilicus (1). Separate the subcutaneous fat down to bone with forceps, and identify the inner and outer tables. As the space between them is small, their orientation must be clearly defined. To do this, carefully introduce a 1.6 mm K-wire on each side to act as a guide, keeping its tip against the bone (2). The crest is then drilled between them, using a guide (3) to protect the soft tissues. The fixation pins may be self-drilling threaded Schanz pins of 5–6 mm in diameter, inclined at 45° to the body axis (4). Preferably two further pins, 2 cm apart are introduced in a similar manner on each side. They are connected to bars parallel to the crest (5). Before tightening the connector (6), close the pelvic gap by manual compression or by turning the patient on their side. This technique is suited to the emergency room, as the use of an image intensifier is not required.

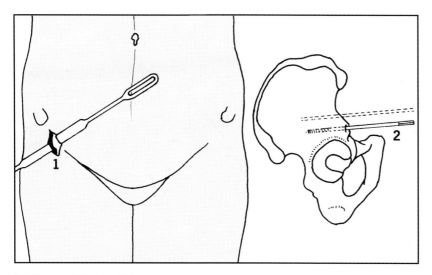

17. External fixation (b): Here a screw is inserted into the anterior inferior iliac spine on each side. The quality of the fixation is better (and, as is aptly remarked, it is easier to close a book from the front than the top). *Method:* A 2 cm incision is made 3 cm distal and slightly medial to the ASS. The tissues are parted down to bone with artery forceps and separated with small retractors, taking care to avoid damage to the lateral femoral cutaneous nerve (1). Use a drill sleeve while starting drilling the cortex. The screw should lie between the bony cortices, and above the acetabular roof (2). Its position should be checked with an image intensifier (although some rely on K-wire guides as previously described). Use a single 6 mm self-drilling or similar screw, inserted to a depth of 40–50 mm (and, if preferred, a second, inserted 2 cm proximal to the first). Reduction may be carried out under intensifier control, e.g. with distancing manipulation forceps applied to the screws, rotation of the hips to correct any rotation of a hemipelvis, and turning the patient on their side and/or applying side pressure to close the pelvis before final tightening of the connectors. A curved radiolucent carbon fibre connector may also be used.

18. Aftercare – The pins: 1. Clean the wounds and the visible parts of the pins with sterile water daily, and dress until the wounds are dry. If there is a colostomy, the pin sites must be protected at all times.
2. If there is any inflammation round the pins, take a bacteriological swab, clean the area, and administer antibiotics.
3. If there is a purulent discharge, enlarge the skin incisions at the pins to establish drainage, and if necessary perform an aggressive debridement and lavage. In severe cases the affected pin may have to be removed; then, if the remaining pins do not afford sufficient fixation and re-siting is not possible, treat the fracture by conservative methods at least until pin-track healing has been obtained.
4. Pin loosening may often be dealt with by re-siting.
Physiotherapy: This should be started without delay to lessen the risks of DVT. The patient can usually be allowed to sit up after a week, and often start partial weight-bearing with a frame at three weeks.
Removal of the frame: Trial removal of the connecting bar may be carried out when there is radiological evidence of early union. Otherwise do not attempt at less than 9 weeks where there has been a symphyseal disruption, or 6 weeks in other cases. If pain occurs, replace the connector; if there is none after a week, remove the bars and the pins.

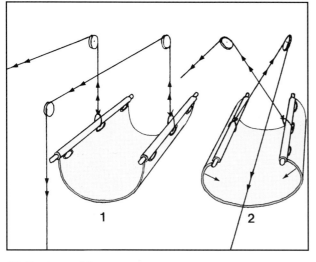

19. Treatment (b): If the patient is not haemodynamically unstable, conservative treatment is also possible using a canvas pelvic sling. The upper edges of the sling are reinforced with steel rods and eyelets, and it may be padded with wool prior to being positioned under the pelvis. Weights in the order of 4–8 kg are applied through pulleys in a Balkan beam (1), resulting in an inward thrust on the sides of the pelvis. If check radiographs show the reduction is incomplete, the weights may be increased or the traction cords crossed (2). The treatment should be continued for 6 weeks, taking the usual precautions over skin care; weight-bearing can generally be allowed after 8 weeks.

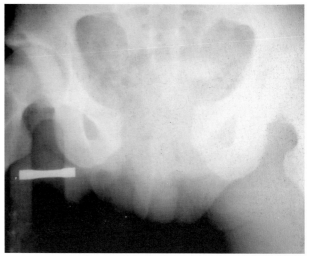

20. Treatment (c): This radiograph shows a Type B1 open book fracture of the pelvis with wide separation at the symphysis pubis. Indications for open reduction and internal fixation of the symphysis include: 1. A symphyseal gap of 3 cm or more; 2. An associated S-I joint disruption; 3. A posterior pelvic disruption which requires stabilisation; 4. A locked symphysis. An in-dwelling catheter should be introduced prior to surgery, but note that the presence of a supra-pubic catheter or a colostomy are absolute contraindications for surgery in this region.

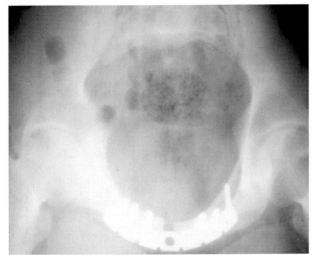

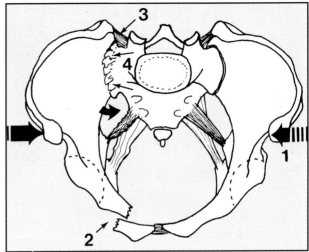

21. Treatment (c) cntd: Check radiographs of the previous case show complete reduction of the symphyseal disruption which has been held with a reconstruction plate. This has been applied to the superior aspects of the pubic bones with three screws on each side. In similar cases, if there is any instability in the vertical plane, a second anterior plate may be required, although anterior plating is generally best avoided as there is some risk of the screws penetrating the retro-pubic space. (Meticulous care must be exercised in performing surgery in this area to lessen the risks of infection and disabling symphyseal osteitis.)

22. Ipsilateral lateral compression injuries (B2): Violence to the side of the pelvis (1) may cause fracture of the rami (2) or overlapping of the pubic bones; the posterior sacroiliac ligaments remain intact (3), and the hemipelvis hinges round them, often with crushing of the anterior margin of the sacroiliac joint on the same side as the rami (4). Tissue elasticity often leads to spontaneous reduction, so that in most cases no fixation is needed. In the remaining cases, an external fixator may be used to control any instability. Nevertheless an external fixator will be required in any case where there is a problem with haemodynamic instability, and should also be considered in cases of multiple injury, or where there is a problem with pain on mobilisation. Open reduction is required in the rare tilt fractures where bone protrudes into the perineum.

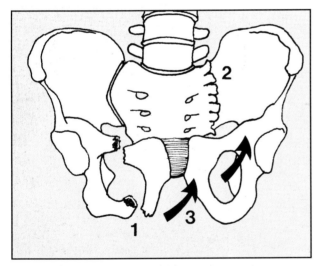

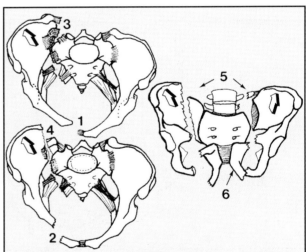

23. Contralateral compression injuries (bucket handle fractures) (B3): Two rami fracture (1) opposite the posterior injury (2) (or there is a butterfly fracture). The hemipelvis rotates (3), causing leg shortening without vertical migration. The majority are stable so that in most no fixation is needed. As in the previously described B2 cases, an external fixator may be used to control any frank instability or considered as suitable for dealing with leg shortening in excess of 1.5 cm. An external fixator will be required in any case where there is a problem with haemodynamic instability, and should also be considered in cases of multiple injury, or where there is a problem with pain on mobilisation.

24. Rotationally and vertically unstable injuries (C1, 2 & 3) (a): The pelvic ring is completely disrupted at two levels or more. *Anteriorly*, in the *unilateral (C1)* injury the symphysis is disrupted (1) or the rami fractured (2). *Posteriorly*, there is total loss of continuity between the sacrum and pelvis. This may result from complete ligamentous rupture and dislocation of the sacroiliac joint (3); or it may involve fractures of the posterior iliac spines (4), the ilium at other levels, or the sacrum. In *bilateral (C2)* injuries (5), there is extensive disruption (often with an anterior butterfly fracture (6)) involving both sides of the pelvis, so that both are free to migrate proximally.

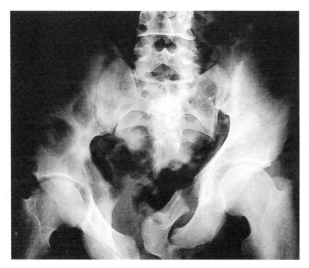

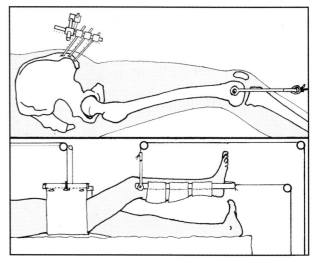

25. Rotationally and vertically unstable injuries (b): On the radiographs the most obvious sign of vertical instability is the proximal migration of a hemipelvis. In addition, there may be avulsion of the transverse process of L5, and avulsion of the tip of the ischial spine. In the CAT scan, posterior displacement of a hemipelvis by more than 1 cm is diagnostic. Note in the above radiograph gross vertical instability on the left, with fracture of both rami and dislocation of the sacroiliac joint. There is in addition disruption of the symphysis pubis and a fracture through the sacrum on the right (most noticeable at the inferior margin of the sacroiliac joint). Although not clearly shown, the transverse processes of L5 are fractured on both sides. This is a C2 (bilateral) fracture.

26. Rotationally and vertically unstable injuries (c) – Initial procedures (IP): These serious injuries are often associated with life-threatening internal haemorrhage and other complications. In the initial stages, prompt application of an external fixator and skeletal traction may be sufficient to control blood loss, but in some cases a C-clamp (see next frame) or other measures will be required. Prior to surgery, or if surgery is considered inadvisable, control rotational instability with an external fixator or a canvas sling, and proximal migration of the hemipelvis with skeletal traction (up to 20 kg) applied through a supracondylar or tibial Steinman pin.

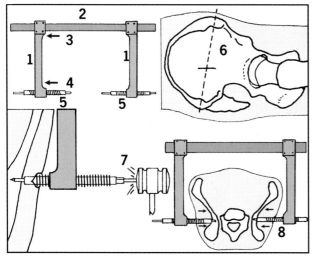

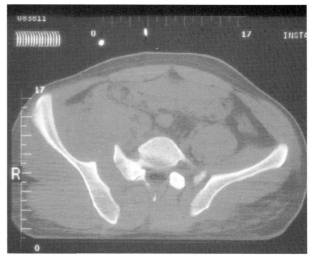

27. The anti-shock pelvic C-clamp: This consists of side-arms (1) which can be moved freely along a cross bar (2) when pressure is applied proximally (3), but lock when subjected to any distal force (4). Hollow bolts (5) which screw into the side arms are designed to carry Steinmann pins. *Method of application:* Make a skin incision on each side approximately 6 cm or so from the posterior superior iliac spine, on a line connecting the posterior superior iliac spine with the anterior superior iliac spine (6), and slide the side-arms until the threaded bolts enter the wounds. Anchor each bolt by hammering a Steinmann pin a depth of 1 cm into bone (7). Bring the bolts into contact with the pelvis by approximating the side-arms with pressure from above. Tightening the bolts with a spanner will now close the S-I joints (8).

28. The anti-shock pelvic C-clamp cntd: This CAT scan shows marked widening of the right sacroiliac joint. This was associated with disruption of the symphysis pubis and haemodynamic instability. In this case, as in others with similar pathology, it was considered important to stabilise the pelvis as soon as possible both from circulatory considerations and from the point of view of facilitating nursing during the initial period following the injury; this is especially important in cases of multiple injury.

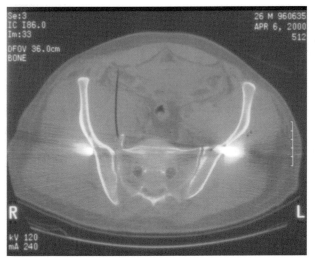

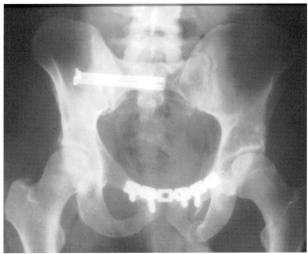

29. The anti-shock pelvic C-clamp cntd: Application of a C-clamp was successful in stabilising both the sacroiliac joint disruption and the haemodynamic instability. (Note that in the CAT scan only the tips of the C-clamp screws are showing in the plane of the cut.)

Definitive treatment (DT) (a): Any secondary definitive treatment procedure is usually advised within the subsequent five days; protracted use of external fixation carries the risk of pin track infections and ultimately makes nursing less easy. The interval can be used with profit to stabilise the patient, to allow appropriate radiographs to be taken, and to obtain and check any specialised equipment required for the intervention.

30. Definitive treatment (DT) (b): *Illustrated:* The definitive treatment of the case shown in Frames 28 and 29, using a reconstruction plate for the symphysis and two screws to secure the sacroiliac joint. Note that surgery should only be undertaken by the experienced, because of the high operative morbidity: problems include uncontrollable haemorrhage, infection, wound breakdown, and neurological damage. *Anterior approaches,* which seldom give problems with wound healing, may be used to internally fix most fractures and dislocations in the region of the sacroiliac joints, to apply reconstruction plates to the ilium, to plate the rami and symphysis, and to reconstruct certain acetabular fractures.

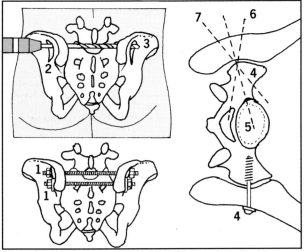

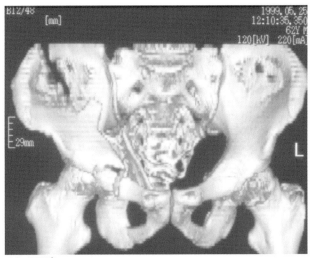

31. Definitive treatment (DT) (c): *Local posterior approaches* may be used to treat dislocations of the sacroiliac joint, and fractures of the sacrum in Type C injuries. In the latter, the safest method of stabilising the sacral fracture is by means of sacral bars (1), inserted through small incisions (2), after cross-drilling (3). **(DT) (d):** The sacroiliac joint may be stabilised by screws running into the lateral masses (ala) of the sacrum (4). The position and direction of these screws must be determined with the greatest care, and it is advisable to visualise the ala directly *and* to use an image intensifier. In some cases, however, it is possible to carry out the procedure percutaneously using guide wires and cannulated screws. **(DT) (e):** Where the sacrum is fractured, fixing screws must engage the body of the sacrum (5) to obtain the necessary purchase. Again the utmost care must be taken to avoid broaching the sacral canal (6) or entering the pelvis anteriorly (7). The use of an image intensifier is mandatory. *Formal posterior approaches* (e.g. Kochers's) may be needed in acetabular reconstructions where there is involvement of the posterior column. *Note: In Type C3 injuries the acetabulum takes priority.*

32. (DT)(f): *Formal posterior approaches* (e.g. Moore's) may be needed in some acetabular reconstructions where there is involvement of the posterior column or sciatic nerve involvement (see p. 274).

Type C3 injuries – Definitive treatment (DT): *In Type C3 injuries the acetabulum takes priority in the assessment and in any proposed reconstruction.* (See also Frame 39 et seq.) The 3-D reconstruct above shows a Type C3 injury which would be difficult to interpret fully with plain X-ray films. On the right there is a vertical fracture of the ilium running into the sciatic notch, and fractures of the pubic rami. There is a comminuted fracture of the acetabular floor involving both columns (see later). The anterior part of the ilium and the roof of the acetabulum are rotated. There is no substantial proximal migration of the right hemipelvis.

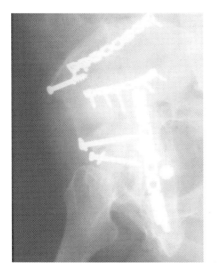

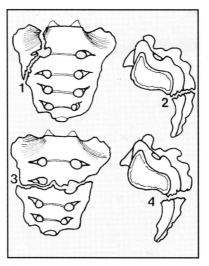

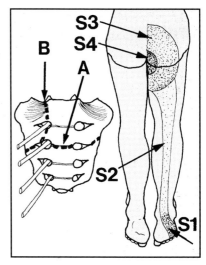

33. Type C3 injuries – Definitive treatment (DT) cntd: This radiograph shows the previous case after surgical intervention. Note the extensive use of reconstruction plates and cancellous bone screws to hold the many elements involved in the fracture.

34. Fractures of the sacrum (a): The ala of the sacrum (1) may be fractured as a result of either side-to-side or anteroposterior compression of the pelvis. *Transverse fractures* of the sacrum usually result from falls from a height on to hard surfaces. These fractures may be undisplaced (2), or they may be associated with some lateral (3) or anterior displacement (4).

35. Fractures of the sacrum (b): In some cases of both horizontal (A) and vertical (B) fractures there may be involvement of sacral nerve roots, leading to sensory disturbance, weakness in the leg(s) or saddle anaesthesia and incontinence. Treatment of the sacral fractures is symptomatic, with 2–3 weeks' bed rest. In the majority of cases the neurological disturbance is transitory (generally being a lesion in continuity), but some advocate early investigation by CAT scan, and dependent on the results, a laminectomy.

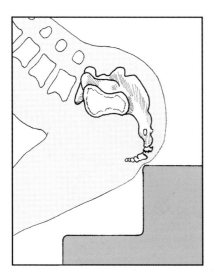

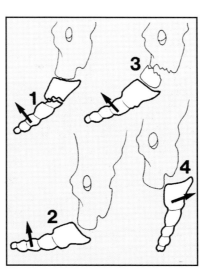

36. Coccygeal injuries (a): The coccyx is usually injured by a fall in a seated position against a hard surface, e.g. the edge of a step. There is local pain and tenderness, and sometimes pain on defaecation. Sitting on hard surfaces is always painful. (Note that coccygeal pain may also be caused by lumbar disc prolapse, pelvic inflammatory disease, chordoma and other tumours of the sacrum.)

37. Coccygeal injuries (b): The main patterns of injury are: (1) Fracture of the coccyx, with a varying degree of anteversion; (2) Anterior subluxation of the coccyx; (3) Anterior displacement of the coccyx secondary to fracture of the end piece of the sacrum; (4) Rarely, posterior subluxation of the coccyx.

38. Diagnosis:
1. Clinically, there is local tenderness.
2. When there is anterior subluxation, the prominent sharp edge of the sacrum may be obvious on palpation.
3. The displacement may be detected on rectal examination.
   The diagnosis is confirmed by localised radiographs of the region, although film quality may be poor in the obese patient.

Treatment:
1. Sitting on hard surfaces should be avoided, and initially the patient should use an inflatable rubber ring cushion. The patient should not be allowed to become constipated.
2. If symptoms become chronic, local short-wave diathermy or ultrasound may be tried; alternatively, the painful area may be injected with a long acting local anaesthetic, e.g. 10 mL of 0.5% bupivacaine hydrochloride (Marcaine®).
3. If all conservative measures fail, excision of the coccyx should be considered.

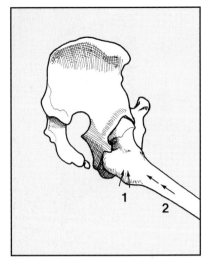

39. Fracture of the acetabulum/central dislocation of the hip: In this group of injuries the pelvis is fractured as a result of force transmitted through the femoral head. This may occur from a blow or fall on the side (1) or when force is transmitted up the limb (2) via the foot, as in a fall from a height or through the knee as in a car dashboard injury.

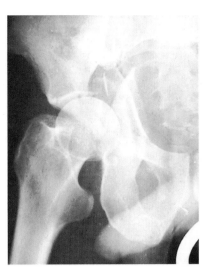

40. Diagnosis (a): The fracture is easily diagnosed by routine radiographs which reveal characteristic disturbance of the acetabulum. There are, however, many patterns of injury due to variations in the amount and direction of the causal force. Pending full assessment, the patient should be treated for any accompanying shock, and skin traction (*c.* 4 kg) applied to the limb.

41. Diagnosis (b): When the hip joint is seriously disorganised, open reduction and internal fixation of the fragments can give good results. Nevertheless, it is clear that a very careful analysis of these fractures is necessary to select those cases suitable for such treatment. The first screening procedures should be: 1. A standard AP projection of the *pelvis* showing both hips on the one film, along with; 2. A lateral projection of the affected hip.

If there is any significant displacement of the fragments or the femoral head, an attempt should then be made to answer the following questions, as discussed in following frames:
1. Is the anterior column intact?
2. Is the posterior column intact?
3. What damage has the acetabular floor sustained?

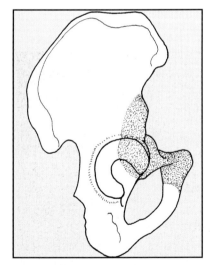

42. Is the anterior column intact? (a): The anterior column is the mass of bone which stretches downwards from the anterior inferior iliac spine, and includes the pubis and the anterior part of the acetabular floor. To help clarify this, CAT scans are invaluable, but if this facility is not immediately available, then a three-quarter internal oblique view of the hip should be obtained.

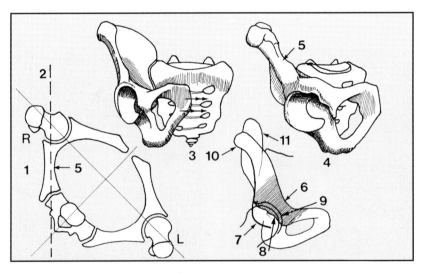

43. Is the anterior column intact? (b): Foam wedges are placed under the buttock on the *affected* side until the pelvis is tilted at 45° (1). The rotation of the pelvis from the AP plane (3) to the oblique position (4) places the blade of the ilium in profile (5) to the central ray (2). The radiographic appearances are complex, especially if the fracture is badly displaced, but note on the films the state of the shaded portion (6) which represents the anterior column. Note also the easily identified posterior margin of the acetabulum (7), its less obvious anterior margin (8) and its floor (9). (10 and 11 are the anterior superior iliac spine and the iliac crest.) *Isolated fractures of the anterior column are uncommon, but are important to recognise as they require an anterior surgical approach for reduction.*

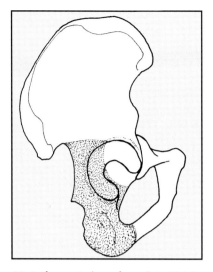

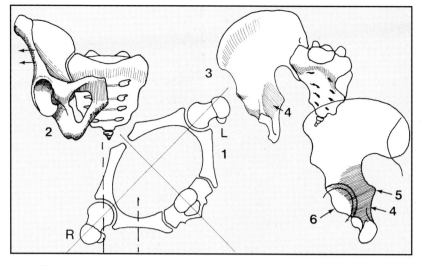

44. Is the posterior column intact? (a):
The posterior column stretches upwards from the ischial tuberosity to the sciatic notch, and includes the posterior part of the acetabular floor. To clarify this a second oblique projection is often helpful (three-quarter external oblique projection).

45. Is the posterior column intact? (b): The pelvis is tilted 45° towards the injured side by sandbags under the good side (1). This rotation of the pelvis from the normal position (2) to the oblique (3) throws the area of the posterior column (4) away from the rest of the pelvis. Note on the radiographs the area of the posterior column (shaded), the ischial spine (5), and the anterior lip of the acetabulum (6). Careful study of the AP, lateral and two 45° obliques may allow you to assess the state of the columns, but if there is still some doubt a CAT scan (especially if there is the facility for 3-D imaging) will usually reveal the main elements involved and any displacement of the femoral head with great clarity; it should be used without hesitation if available. If not, stereoradiography or intensifier screening may be of further help.

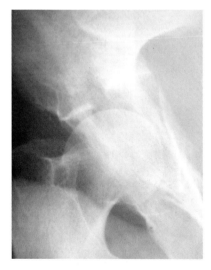

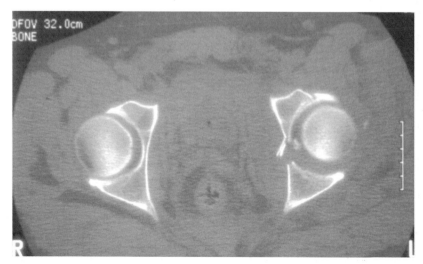

46. What damage has the acetabular floor sustained? (a): The radiograph shows gross comminution of the acetabulum. The degree of acetabular disruption, and the extent of comminution may be further elucidated by CAT scans or 3-D reconstructions.

47. (b): This CAT scan shows an intact hip on the right. On the left there is disruption of the medial part of the floor of the acetabulum, with an appreciable gap between the main fragments. There is comminution of the floor, with a bone fragment – equivalent to a loose body – lying between the femoral head and the main anterior fragment. There is a fracture of the anterior acetabular margin; this is not seen to be significantly displaced at this level of cut.

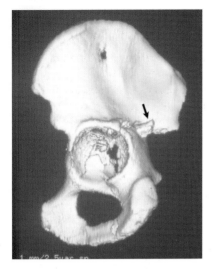

48. (c): A 3-D reconstruction of the previous case confirms the degree of comminution of the acetabular floor. This also shows with great clarity a backward projecting spike of bone in the region of the greater sciatic foramen. (This was held responsible for an accompanying sciatic nerve palsy, and was removed at open operation, during which internal fixation of both disrupted anterior and posterior columns was carried out.) You may now be in a position to relate your findings to the AO classification of acetabular fractures.

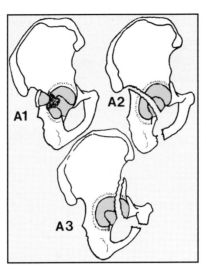

49. AO classification of acetabular fractures – Type A: In Type A fractures one column only is involved, the other remaining intact.
A1: Fractures of the posterior wall and certain variations; these injuries may be associated with posterior dislocation of the hip (see p. 280).
A2: Fractures of the posterior column and variations.
A3: Fractures of the anterior column and variations.

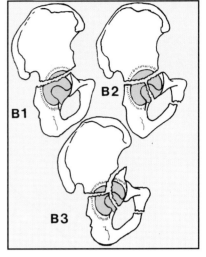

50. AO classification of acetabular fractures – Type B: In Type B fractures the main fracture line lies transversely. Part of the acetabular roof always remains in continuity with the ilium.
B1: Transverse fracture with or without involvement of the posterior acetabular wall.
B2: A vertical fracture added to the transverse fracture forms a T-fracture, of which there are several variations.
B3: A vertical fracture added to the transverse fracture involves the anterior column.

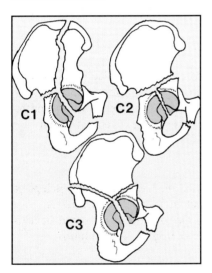

51. AO classification of acetabular fractures – Type C: In Type C fractures both columns are involved, and no part of the acetabulum remains in continuity with the ilium.
C1: The portion of the fracture involving the anterior column extends to the iliac crest.
C2: The portion of the fracture involving the anterior column extends to the anterior border of the ilium.
C3: The fracture involves the sacroiliac joint.

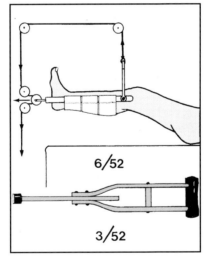

52. Treatment (a): Is the displacement of the fracture minimal (i.e. less than 2 mm) or is the acetabular floor highly fragmented? If so, treat the injury conservatively with traction (e.g. Hamilton–Russell of 3 kg) for 6 weeks, with active hip movements during this period; weight bearing may be permitted after a further 3 weeks. Some loss of hip movements is inevitable, but overall function is often very good. Further treatment will only be required if secondary osteoarthritis supervenes.

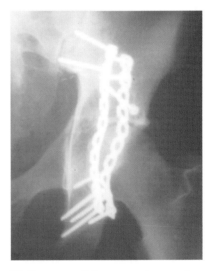

53. Treatment (b): Is there a fracture of one or both columns, with displacement in excess of 2 mm? Is there a fracture of the acetabular floor without gross comminution? Is open reduction and internal fixation technically feasible, and is it likely to lead to reasonable restoration of the acetabulum? If so, then this must be considered. (The illustration is of a case where a badly displaced acetabular fracture involving both columns has been satisfactorily treated by open reduction and internal fixation with reconstruction plates.)

54. TREATMENT (c) – GENERAL CONSIDERATIONS

Open reduction of acetabular fractures is seldom easy. An extensive exposure is always required, and attendant haemorrhage is a common problem. There is often great difficulty in obtaining a substantial improvement in the position of the bone fragments and in subsequently holding them, so that operating time can be very long, increasing the risks of infection and delayed wound healing. There is the danger of exacerbating or producing sciatic nerve problems and of causing heterotopic ossification, avascular necrosis of the femoral head, or chondrolysis of the hip. Such surgery may be contraindicated in the elderly, obese or the unfit. In children and adolescents open reduction is rarely indicated and then not always rewarding. As these fractures are of highly vascular cancellous bone, the vigorous processes of repair may render reduction impossible if surgery is delayed for much longer than a week or so.

The results of open reduction and internal fixation of acetabular fractures are known to be surgeon dependent, and the final decision as to whether surgery should be considered (and this is especially so in borderline cases) should be made by someone with a wide experience of these cases. In some situations this may mean seeking an opinion from elsewhere, or transferring the patient to another unit.

INSTRUMENTATION

Appropriate instrumentation is essential, and the AO Group has developed specialised pelvic reduction clamps and pushers. Schanz pins may be used like a joystick to help lever bone fragments into position. If possible the operation should be performed on a radiolucent table so that full use may be made of an image intensifier.

IMPLANTS

A wide range of implant materials should be available, including cancellous, cortical and cannulated bone screws. Reconstruction plates (3.5 mm and 4.5 mm) permit bending (with appropriate irons) in two planes to accommodate any contour that may be encountered There is a range of reconstruction plates pre-bent in various arcs.

EXPOSURES

The choice of surgical exposure depends on which columns and which parts of the acetabulum have been involved (and, in the case of other pelvic fractures, which parts must be stabilised). One or both columns may have to be tackled. In the latter situation, the anterior may be dealt with first, especially if it is the most displaced.

ANTERIOR APPROACHES

Tile recommends an approach which combines the most desirable features of the Smith Peterson and the ilio-inguinal approaches. This gives wide access, from the lateral two-thirds of the superior pubic ramus anteriorly, to the sacroiliac joint posteriorly.

The incision This is shaped like a question mark, with the *proximal* limb lying 1 cm above and parallel to the outer one third of the inguinal ligament; it extends posteriorly along the iliac crest. The *distal* limb extends down to meet and follow the lateral border of sartorius.

Development:

1. The thick fascia of external oblique is divided 1 cm above and parallel to the outer third of the inguinal ligament and along the iliac crest. Carry the dissection down and divide the internal oblique and transversalis at their attachment to the iliac crest; identify and preserve the lateral cutaneous nerve of thigh.
2. Perform an osteotomy of the anterior superior iliac spine 1 cm proximal to its tip. To aid its later replacement, drill and tap it for a 6.5 mm screw *before* dividing the bone.
3. Mobilise the iliacus from the inner wall of the pelvis. (Do not strip both surfaces of the ilium during the same procedure otherwise there is risk of devitalising the bone and causing avascular necrosis.)
4. Retract the anterior superior iliac spine and by blunt dissection open up the interval between sartorius and tensor fascia lata.
5. Identify the two heads of rectus femoris and insert stay sutures close to their origins. Divide and reflect the straight head from anterior inferior iliac spine, and the reflected head from the anterior part of the acetabulum.
6. Ease the iliacus from the superior pubic ramus.
7. Identify and divide the iliopectineal fascia to facilitate further exposure. Flex and internally rotate the hip to give better access to the superior pubic ramus. In some cases it may be desirable to osteotomise the anterior inferior iliac spine and reflect this and rectus femoris distally.

Posterior approaches There are a number of posterior approaches to the hip which are similar in principle (Kocher, Langenbeck, Stookey, Moore, etc.).

The incision In the Moore approach, in which the patient is prone with a sandbag placed under the hip, the skin incision starts well lateral to the posterior superior iliac spine, bisects the tip of the greater trochanter in the midline, and extends 7.5 cm (3″) down the lateral aspect of the femur.

Development:

1. The incision is deepened over the trochanter to expose the extensive subtrochanteric bursa, and the opening is extended proximally by splitting the fibres of gluteus maximus. Distally, divide the aponeurotic insertion of gluteus maximus by a vertical incision, and extend this distally to divide its attachment to the linea aspera.
2. The sciatic nerve is identified, and if required taped with saline-soaked ribbon gauze and safely positioned without traction. Extension of the hip and flexion of the knee help relieve tension on the nerve.
3. Stay sutures are inserted in the short rotators (internal oblique and the gemelli, and, if necessary for greater access, piriformis proximally and the obturator externus distally) prior to their division close to the femur.
4. Keeping proximal to the quadratus femoris (to avoid the medial femoral circumflex artery supplying the femoral head), the short rotators are reflected medially to expose the acetabulum from the sciatic notch to the ischium.
5. If further exposure of the ischium is required (e.g. to facilitate the placing of a Schanz pin), identify and preserve the pudendal nerve and artery.

6. The ilium can be exposed by reflection of the gluteus maximus and medius. The exposure may be facilitated by abduction of the hip. To access still more of the lateral aspect of the acetabulum, an osteotomy of the greater trochanter may be carried out. To expose more of the acetabular floor, an osteotomy of the ischial spine may be performed. This approach may also be caried out with the patient in the lateral position.

Combined exposures The two above exposures may be combined (an even wider exposure is described by Carnesale). Both are extensile, and may be extended distally to expose the femur.

55. COMPLICATIONS OF PELVIC FRACTURES

1. HAEMORRHAGE

Substantial internal haemorrhage is common, particularly where there is disruption of the pelvic ring and proximal migration of the hemipelvis (Type C injuries). Shock must be *anticipated* in all but the most minor of fractures. (See page 308 for details of the management of major fluid loss.) Internal haemorrhage may be greatly reduced by the prompt stabilisation of the pelvic fracture by application of an anterior external fixator with, if required, a posterior pelvic anti-shock C-clamp. Such emergency procedures are often life-saving, and should be carried out in any significant pelvic fracture where there is haemodynamic instability.

Bruising appearing in the scrotum or buttock, or spreading diffusely along the line of the inguinal ligament, is indicative of a major internal haemorrhage. In the abdomen, a large retroperitoneal haemorrhage may be felt as a discrete mass on palpation (and may be further evaluated with a CAT scan and/or ultrasound examination). If the peritoneum on the posterior abdominal wall has been breached, blood may escape into the abdominal cavity. Intraperitoneal haemorrhage may also result (rarely) from the tearing of mesenteric vessels. This is a serious complication and may be suspected by loss of bowel sounds, abdominal guarding, a progressive increase in abdominal girth, and a blood-stained peritoneal tap; it is an indication for abdominal exploration. Where haemorrhage is extraperitoneal, exploration is generally unprofitable and likely to aggravate blood loss; pelvic stabilisation and fluid replacement remain the mainstay of treatment.

Ischaemia in one leg is a grave sign and may be due to rupture or intimal damage to an iliac artery. If the patient's condition will permit, exploration of this vessel is indicated.

In the uncommon case of a severe retroperitoneal haemorrhage, where in spite of a massive transfusion programme losses continue to gain over replacement, exploration may have to be reconsidered. It is seldom that a single bleeding source can be found, the haemorrhage generally arising from massive disruption of the pelvic venous plexus; then, packing of the wound for 48 hours may give control. Occasionally, successful results have also been claimed from ligation of one or both internal iliac arteries. Where the problem is considered to be due to small-bore arterial bleeding, this may sometimes be brought under control by selective embolisation using image intensifier angiography.

2. DAMAGE TO THE URETHRA AND BLADDER

Incidence Out of every 100 fractures of the pelvis, roughly 5 are likely to have a urinary tract complication; more than two-thirds involve the urethra. Butterfly fractures are the main cause of urethral damage, whilst displaced fractures of the hemipelvis are generally responsible for the sharp edge of a superior pubic ramus rupturing the bladder.

Types of injury *Rupture of the membranous urethra* Many of the cases are partial ruptures, with an intact portion of the urethral wall still connected to the bladder. Less commonly, there is complete rupture with the bladder losing all continuity with the urethra; the bladder often displaces proximally.

Extraperitoneal rupture of the bladder This is usually caused by a sharp spike of bone penetrating the anterior wall.

Intraperitoneal rupture of the bladder This may result from the same mechanism, but only occurs if the bladder is full at the time of injury.

Rupture of the penile urethra Injuries of this type generally follow a fall astride a bar or similar object.

Diagnosis

1. Suspicion should be particularly aroused if the radiographs show either of the fractures described.
2. The presence of perineal bruising is highly suggestive.
3. The presence of blood at the tip of the penis is diagnostic.
4. If there is no penile blood, and damage to the bladder or urethra thought possible but not probable, the patient should be asked to attempt to pass urine. (The dangers of urinary extravasation have been exaggerated in the past and are no longer considered to be of import.) If clear urine is passed, no further investigation or treatment is required. A positive chemical test for blood in the presence of macroscopically clear urine should in these circumstances be ignored. If after several tries the patient fails to pass urine, they should be re-assessed. The palpability of the bladder should be determined and catheterisation considered.
5. Catheterisation carries the risk of converting a partial urethral tear into a complete one, and of introducing infection. A diagnostic catheterisation should be approached with caution: a full aseptic regimen should be followed, and a fine catheter employed. The procedure should be quickly abandoned if the catheter cannot be introduced with ease. If the tap is dry, this suggests intraperitoneal rupture of the bladder; if blood-stained urine is obtained, this suggests an extraperitoneal tear of the bladder or a partial tear of the urethra; if blood only is obtained, this suggests a major tear of the posterior urethra.
6. If there are strong grounds for suggesting significant damage to the bladder or urethra (e.g. penile blood) a urethrogram should be performed in preference to catheterisation. The end of a syringe containing 20 mL of 45% Hypaque® is introduced into the urethra and injected; the penis is closed off with the fingers and radiographs taken. The volume injected may be doubled if required. The following are common findings:
   (a) The bladder shadow is clearly outlined without spillage: *no significant abnormality is likely to be present.*

(b) The bladder is partly filled and there is extravasation of the radio-opaque dye to the side: this suggests *extraperitoneal rupture of the bladder.*

(c) The bladder fails to fill, and there is extravasation of the dye into the pelvic floor: there is *rupture of the membranous urethra.*

(d) The bladder fails to fill, and there is extravasation of dye beneath the pelvic floor: there is *rupture of the penile urethra.*

Treatment *Intraperitoneal rupture of the bladder* The bladder is explored and the tear located and sutured. The bladder is drained subsequently with a Foley catheter.

Extraperitoneal rupture of the bladder The bladder is explored and the diagnosis confirmed. The rupture is repaired and drained by by-pass (suprapubic) catheterisation.

Incomplete tear of the urethra If there is evidence of tearing of the membranous urethra, but the bladder is undisplaced, it is likely that some urethral tissue remains in continuity; a suprapubic drain is inserted and the urethrogram repeated after 10 days. If the circumstances are favourable, a Foley catheter may be introduced at this stage and the suprapubic catheter withdrawn. Later serial bouginage may be required.

Complete rupture of the urethra If the bladder is floating free it must be drawn down to position. This may be achieved by opening the bladder and rail-roading a Foley catheter downwards. After the balloon has been inflated, the catheter may be used for applying gentle traction. The bladder is drained by a suprapubic catheter which is kept in position for several days. The retropubic space may require separate drainage.

Rupture of the penile urethra An incision is made over the tip of a catheter passed to the level of the obstruction. The catheter is then passed into the bladder through the other end of the urethra. If this cannot be located, the bladder will require opening and the distal end of the urethra identified by instrumentation from above. The urethra is then repaired, using the catheter as a stent. Delayed repairs are in the majority of cases associated with severe strictures (requiring complex urethroplasty), and should be avoided.

3. INJURY TO THE BOWEL

The rectum may be torn in open fractures with perineal involvement, and rarely in closed injuries of the central dislocation of the hip type. Injury to the small bowel (mesenteric tears or shearing injuries of the wall leading to infarction or perforation) may be produced by crushing injuries of the pelvis. Bowel involvement may be suspected in the closed injury by abdominal rigidity, loss of bowel sounds, loss of liver dullness and distension. Exploration and a defunctioning colostomy are essential.

4. RUPTURE OF THE DIAPHRAGM

Routine radiography of the chest should be performed in all major fractures of the pelvis, and the standard AP projection should eliminate this often-missed complication. If a rupture is confirmed, a thoraco-abdominal repair through the bed of the eighth rib should be undertaken as soon as the patient's general condition will permit.

5. PARALYTIC ILEUS

This complication may result from disturbance of the autonomic outflow to the bowel due to the accumulation of a retroperitoneal haematoma. Treatment by nasogastric suction and intravenous fluids usually brings rapid resolution within 2–3 days.

6. LIMB SHORTENING

Shortening of one leg may result from persistent proximal displacement of the hemipelvis (Type C injuries) or from rotation of the hemipelvis in contralateral lateral compression fractures (Type B3 injuries). Clinical measurement of the amount of shortening is difficult: leg length as measured from the anterior superior spine to the medial malleolus is unaffected, heel-blocking techniques are rather unsatisfactory and the measurement of the distance from the umbilicus or xiphisternum to the medial malleolus somewhat inaccurate. The amount of shortening may be judged with greatest accuracy from the radiographs by noting any discrepancy between the level of the iliac crests on the AP film (after making a little allowance for film magnification effects). A correction (raise) should be made to the footwear if there is shortening of over 1.25 cm ($\frac{1}{2}''$).

7. NEUROLOGICAL DAMAGE

Neurological damage may involve:
1. The lumbosacral trunk at the triangle of Marcille where there are fractures involving displacement of the hemipelvis;
2. Isolated sacral nerves in fractures of the sacrum;
3. The sciatic nerve itself as it passes behind the hip.
   Investigation by CAT scan and 3-D reconstructions may be helpful.
   Lesions in continuity predominate, and some persistent disability is the rule. Exploration is seldom indicated unless a mechanical cause amenable to treatment can be demonstrated.

8. IMPOTENCE

Impotence occurs in about a sixth of major pelvic fractures, and in about half of those cases in which there is rupture of the urethra. It is frequently permanent. The cause may be due to neurological damage, but some consider this complication to be related to penile vascular insufficiency.

9. OBSTETRICAL DIFFICULTIES

Even in the case of quite marked post-fracture pelvic distortion, natural childbirth is rarely affected to a degree requiring caesarian section. Where there has been a symphyseal disruption, this may recur, persist, and warrant surgery.

10. PERSISTENT SACROILIAC JOINT PAIN

Sacroiliac pain is a common complication of pelvic fractures, especially where there has been clear involvement of a sacroiliac joint (e.g. in open book fractures, Type B1) and may be permanent. Where there has been a sacroiliac joint dislocation, the risks of severe, disabling pain are particularly high and are related to the degree of persisting displacement. In some cases consideration of local fusion is merited.

11. **PERSISTENT SYMPHYSEAL INSTABILITY**

This is a rare complication and an indication for internal fixation; screening may be of help in confirming the diagnosis.

12. **OSTEOARTHRITIS OF THE HIP**

Central dislocation of the hip is not infrequently followed by this complication. It is dealt with along routine lines. Many cases may come to and are suitable for total hip replacement, and prior reduction of a major displacement will render this easier.

13. **MYOSITIS OSSIFICANS**

Myositis ossificans is seen most frequently after operative intervention or where there is an accompanying head injury. The treatment is along the lines previously indicated.

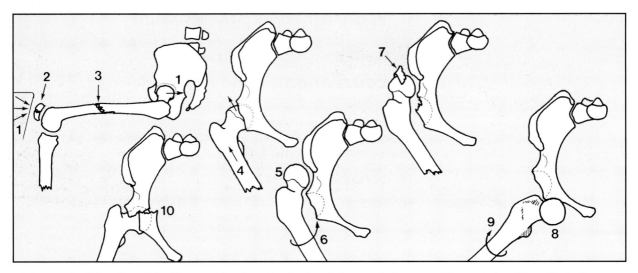

56. Traumatic dislocation of the hip: The hip may dislocate as a result of force being transmitted up the femoral shaft. This most commonly occurs as a result of dashboard impact in road traffic accidents (1). Note that this mechanism may be responsible for simultaneous fracture of the patella (2) or of the femoral shaft (3). Force transmitted up the limbs from falls on the foot, force applied to the lumbar region (e.g. in roof falls on kneeling miners) and rarely force applied directly to the trochanter may also cause the hip to dislocate. If the leg is flexed at the hip and adducted (4) at the time of impact, the femur dislocates posteriorly (5), internally rotating at the same time (6). In some cases, the posterior lip of the acetabulum is fractured (7). If the hip is widely abducted, anterior dislocation may occur, even without any axial transmission of force (8); the femur externally rotates (9). Note that, if the femur is in some other part of the abduction/adduction range, these mechanisms may be responsible for central dislocation type fractures of the pelvis (10). A congenital reduction in the normal degree of anteversion of the hip is a common finding in those who suffer posterior dislocations of the hip.

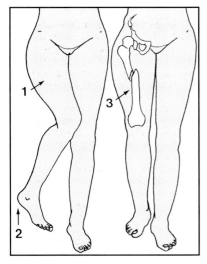

57. Posterior dislocation of the hip – Diagnosis: In a typical posterior dislocation, the hip is held slightly flexed, adducted and internally rotated (1). The leg appears short (2). Few other injuries are associated with the agony accompanying posterior dislocation, and this is almost as diagnostic as the deformity. Pain is less severe if the acetabulum is fractured, and the deformity may be concealed if there is an associated femoral fracture (3).

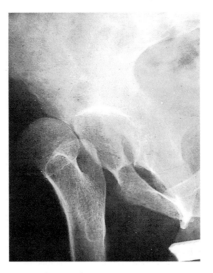

58. Radiographs (a): The diagnosis is confirmed by radiographs of the hip; the deformity is usually obvious on the AP projection, but dislocation cannot be *excluded* with one view (c.f. dislocation of the shoulder); a lateral projection is helpful in confirming the distinction between an anterior and posterior dislocation, and *essential* if no abnormality is obvious on the AP film (Illus.: Obvious posterior dislocation).

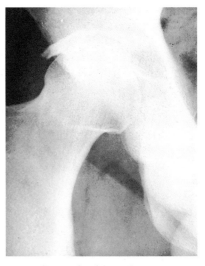

59. Radiographs (b): Acetabular rim fractures may be produced by the shearing force of the backward travelling femoral head (see Frame 56 (7) above). The fragment may be small (Illus.), when it is seldom of consequence. It may be large or comminuted, in which case there is increased risk of sciatic nerve palsy, instability in reduction and later osteoarthritis.

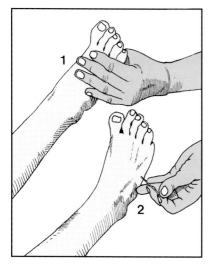

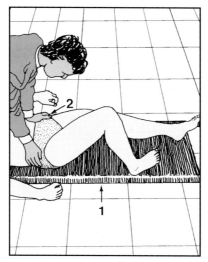

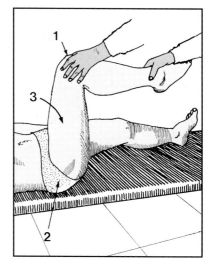

60. Sciatic nerve involvement: The presence or absence of damage to the sciatic nerve should be sought in every case, and particularly where an acetabular rim fracture is present. Enquire about numbness or burning sensations in the limb and, as a minimal screening, test the power of dorsiflexion in the foot (1) and appreciation of pin-prick sensation in the leg below the knee (2).

61. Reduction (a): Reduction should be carried out as soon as a general anaesthetic can be arranged. The complication rate is lowest in those treated within the first 6 hours of the injury. The key to success is *complete* muscle relaxation; the anaesthetist should be reminded of this and of the need to transfer the patient on a stretcher canvas on to the floor to allow the hip to be manipulated (1). An assistant should kneel at the side of the patient and steady the pelvis (2).

62. Reduction (b): When the patient is fully relaxed (and the administration of suxamethonium chloride (Scoline®) just prior to manipulation is often invaluable) the knee (1) and hip (2) are flexed gently to a right angle, at the same time gently correcting the adduction and internal rotation deformities (3). (*Note:* The assistant's hands, vital to the reduction, have been omitted from this and subsequent drawings for clarity.)

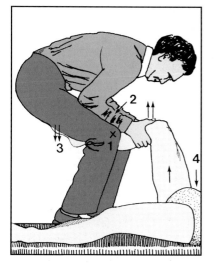

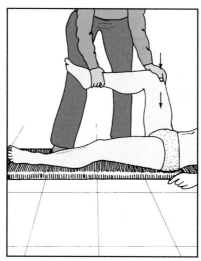

65. Reduction check radiographs (e): Check radiographs should be taken in two planes (and most advocate routine post manipulation CAT scans) to check the reduction and eliminate the presence of loose bodies and any associated bony injury. The following possibilities arise:
1. The dislocation has been fully reduced.
2. The dislocation and a rim fracture have both been reduced, and the hip is stable clinically. (In both 1. and 2. further treatment is conservative.)
3. Although the femoral head is concentric with the acetabulum, the joint space is increased. This should be elucidated further (with a CAT scan, tomography or arthroscopy). Persistent displacement of this type may be due to a trapped bone (rim) fragment or infolding of the labrum. A trapped bone fragment should be removed by surgery, as if left it will lead to rapid onset of osteoarthritis. Excision of a trapped labrum is advocated but the grounds for this are less clear; there would seem some justification for a 'wait-and-see' approach.

63. Reduction (c): The head of the femur should now be lying directly behind the acetabulum and just requires to be lifted forwards. The force required is variable, but great leverage can be obtained by gripping the leg between the knees (1) resting your forearms on your thighs (2) and flexing your knees (3). The assistant keeps the pelvis from lifting by downward pressure (4). Reduction usually occurs with an obvious 'clunk'.

64. Reduction (d): Reduction is often less striking when there is a rim fracture, and when a rim fracture is present (shown by the radiographs) the stability of the reduction should always be checked by downward pressure on the femur. Gross instability is an indication for open reduction and internal fixation of the rim fracture.

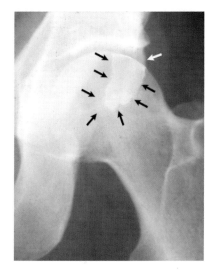

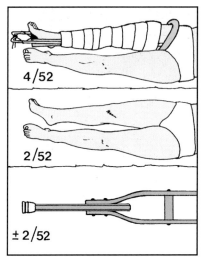

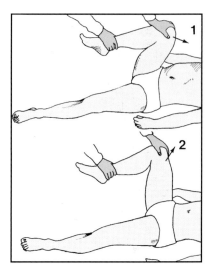

66. Check radiographs cntd:
4. There is persistent displacement of a fracture involving more than 20% of the rim, or the hip is unstable (Illus.: Note rim fragment situated near upper lip of the acetabulum).
5. There is a displaced fracture of the rim with a persisting sciatic palsy.

Operative reduction and internal (screw) fixation of the fragment are indicated in 4. and 5.; in 5. early intervention offers the best chance of recovery. However, the results of rim fixation in children and adolescents are often poor.

67. Aftercare: Some advocate splintage and/or traction to rest the hip in an effort to reduce the risks of complications. A common regimen is fixed (skin) traction in a Thomas splint for 4 weeks and bed mobilisation for a further 2 weeks before weight bearing. (Others however advise much shorter periods of recumbency, e.g. of 1 week, and the value of both traction and splintage have been disputed.) If there is a rim fracture, weight bearing should be deferred until about 8 weeks post-injury.

68. Alternative methods of reduction – Bigelow's method: Failure to reduce a posterior dislocation of the hip by the method described is uncommon and generally due to insufficient muscle relaxation; nevertheless, if failure occurs, Bigelow's method may be tried. In essence, the hip is reduced by a continuous movement of circumduction which may be broken down into five stages: (1) The hip is fully flexed and then (2) abducted.

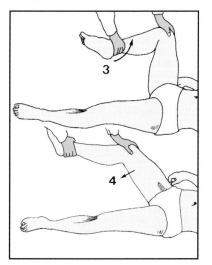

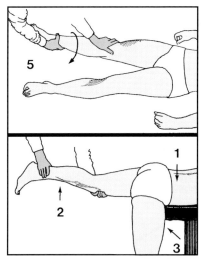

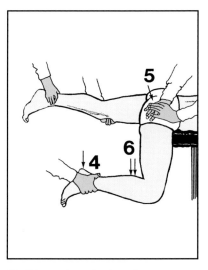

69. Bigelow's method cntd: After flexing and abducting the hip, the joint is smoothly externally rotated (3) and then gradually extended (4).

70. Bigelow's method cntd: As extension of the hip progresses, the external rotated limb is turned into the neutral position (5).
Stimson's method: This is occasionally attempted when a general anaesthetic must be withheld or where there is an associated femoral fracture. The patient is turned into the prone position (1). The end section of the theatre table is removed and the unaffected leg held by an assistant (2). The pelvis is supported by the end of the table (3).

71. Stimson's method cntd: The leg is flexed at the knee and held at the ankle in the neutral position (4). The hip may be reduced by direct pressure over the head of the femur (5) or, if the femur is intact, by downward pressure on the upper calf (6). This may be done manually or by the stockinged foot; the latter procedure allows simultaneous application of pressure over the head of the femur, as at (5).

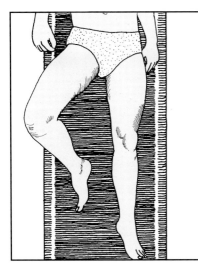

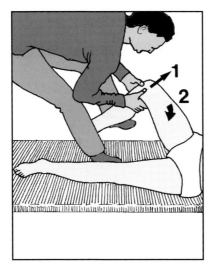

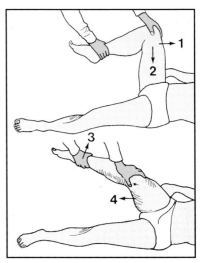

72. Anterior dislocation of the hip:
Anterior dislocation of the hip is less common than posterior dislocation. The leg is usually held abducted and in external rotation. There may be swelling and later bruising in the groin. Anterior dislocation may be complicated by femoral vein compression (with the risks of thrombosis and embolism), by femoral nerve paralysis or femoral artery compression. (Persistent absence of the peripheral pulses after reduction is an indication for exploration.)

73. Reduction: Proceed as for posterior dislocation, with the well-anaesthetised patient on the floor, *and an assistant steadying the pelvis.* Flexing the hip (1) and correcting the abduction and external rotation (2) convert an anterior dislocation into a posterior dislocation. At the end of this procedure the head of the femur is lifted up as before into the acetabulum. (The subsequent management is as Frame 67.)

74. Reduction – Bigelow's method: This method is less reliable for routine use, but may be tried in the difficult case. Circumduction of the hip is again carried out in the following order of movements:
(1) Fully flex; (2) Adduct the hip;
(3) Internally rotate; (4) Extend; (5) Bring into the neutral position.

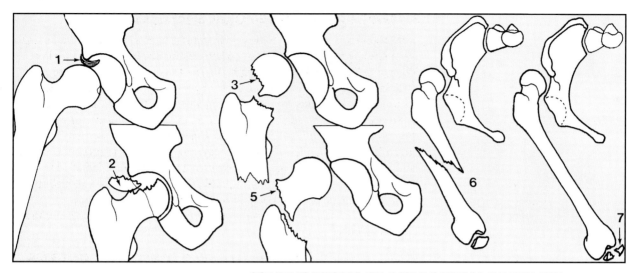

75. COMPLICATIONS OF DISLOCATION OF THE HIP

1. IRREDUCIBLE DISLOCATION

This may result from in-turning of the labrum or by bony fragments trapped in the acetabulum (Illus., 1). Open reduction is necessary, *but be certain* that the patient has been *completely* relaxed during the attempts at closed reduction. (Note that if there is a *delay* in excess of three hours in attempting the reduction of an anterior dislocation, some advocate prior exploration of the femoral vein to remove any thrombus that may have developed, and thereby reduce the risk of embolus.)

2. FRACTURE OF THE FEMORAL HEAD

Osteochondral fractures of the femoral head may remain displaced after reduction of the hip. Small fragments should be excised, but large fragments (Illus., 2) should be replaced and secured with a cancellous screw or other device. Late osteoarthritis is common.

3. INTRACAPSULAR FRACTURE OF THE FEMORAL NECK
(Illus., 3)

The risks of avascular necrosis are extremely high, and the following treatment should be considered: 1. In the frail elderly, excision of the femoral head, and replacement with a Thomson or similar prosthesis. 2. In the middle-aged, total hip replacement. 3. In the young, open reduction and internal fixation through a posterolateral approach.

4. SLIPPED UPPER FEMORAL EPIPHYSIS COMPLICATING HIP DISLOCATION

Treat as 3 (3.).

5. EXTRACAPSULAR FRACTURE OF THE FEMORAL NECK
(Illus., 5)

1. The fracture should be dealt with first by open reduction and the insertion of a pin and plate or similar device. This can be taxing due to difficulty in interpreting control films in unfamiliar planes of rotation. 2. The dislocation may then be reduced, usually with ease, by closed manipulation; alternatively, open reduction may be considered.

6. **FRACTURE OF THE FEMORAL SHAFT** (Illus., 6)

1. It is sometimes possible to treat both injuries conservatively, reducing the hip dislocation by Stimson's method and treating the femoral fracture in a Thomas splint. 2. If Stimson's method fails, it may be possible to apply sufficient traction to the upper fragment by a substantial threaded screw inserted into the greater trochanter percutaneously. 3. It is more satisfactory to expose the femoral shaft and reduce the dislocation by means of a heavy duty bone clamp applied directly to the upper fragment (temporarily insert a large diameter Küntscher nail into the proximal fragment to prevent the bone being crushed with the clamp, and use the linea aspera for orientation). Thereafter the femoral shaft may be internally fixed. (Plating is thought to carry a lesser risk of being complicated by myositis ossificans than intramedullary nailing in this particular situation, although many prefer the latter with cross-screwing.)

7. **FRACTURE OF THE PATELLA AND OTHER KNEE INJURIES** (Illus., 7)

The dislocation should be reduced by any of the methods described and the knee injury treated on its own merits (e.g. a comminuted fracture of the patella should be treated by excision).

8. **SCIATIC NERVE PALSY**

This complicates about 10% of dislocations of the hip. Fortunately three out of four are incomplete, and about half recover completely. If no improvement follows reduction of the hip, exploration is advisable within the first 24 hours of injury if there is a large or comminuted rim fracture which may possibly be causing persistent local pressure on the nerve. In other cases the indications for exploration are less clear, and some treat this complication expectantly by conservative methods. (If the patient is being treated in a Thomas splint, this should be fitted with a foot piece to hold the ankle in the neutral position. When the patient is mobilised, a drop foot splint may be required and precautions must be taken to avoid trophic ulceration in the foot.) Others advocate exploration in all cases where a sciatic palsy is still present after reduction, considering that if no other pathology is found, decompression of any haematoma in the region of the nerve will facilitate recovery.

9. **AVASCULAR NECROSIS**

The inevitable tearing of the hip joint capsule accompanying dislocation of the hip may disturb the blood supply to the femoral head; in about 10% of cases this may lead to avascular necrosis. Dynamic MRI scanning of the hip (using an intravenous paramagnetic contrast agent) gives a good assessment of the blood supply of the femoral head when performed as early as 48 hours after the injury. Radiographic changes however are slow to appear – usually, but not always, within 12 months of injury. Clinically, persistent discomfort in the groin and restriction and pain on internal rotation are suggestive of this complication. Avascular necrosis of the head of the femur leads to secondary osteoarthritis of the hip. It is thought that forage arthroplasty (where the femoral head is drilled), if carried out before there is subchondral bone collapse, may encourage revascularisation.

10. SECONDARY OSTEOARTHRITIS OF THE HIP

This is the inevitable sequel to avascular necrosis, but may also occur when dislocation of the hip is accompanied by a fracture involving the articular surfaces. (Failure to observe such an injury may be prevented by performing an early CAT scan.) It is also seen in cases where scoring of the femoral head is observed in open reductions.

It may occur as a late complication, sometimes as long as 5–10 years after injury; the cause then is less clear, but may possibly arise from articular cartilage damage concurrent with the initial injury. (An MRI scan at an early stage may sometimes confirm potentially harmful articular cartilage damage.) The incidence of secondary osteoarthritis rises to nearly 40% in manual workers who continue with their former occupation. In the young patient hip fusion may be considered, but generally total hip replacement is the treatment of choice.

11. RECURRENT DISLOCATION

This complication is rare; operative fixation of a large acetabular rim fragment in the hip which is demonstrated to be unstable clinically may largely avoid it. Otherwise a bone-block type of repair may have to be considered.

12. MYOSITIS OSSIFICANS

This is seen most frequently following exploration of the hip, or when the dislocation is accompanied by head injury. It may lead to virtual fusion of the hip. The risk of this complication ensuing may be minimised in the following ways:

1. Avoid surgery if possible, but if surgery is essential, then the prophylactic use of indometacin should be considered (see Ch. 5).
2. Splint the hip following reduction.
3. Avoid passive movements of the hip in the head injury case with limb spasticity. Late excision (say after 1 year) of a discrete bone mass, with prophylactic radiotherapy, may restore function, but the recurrence rate in other circumstances is high.

13. LATE DIAGNOSED DISLOCATION

This is a euphemism for missed dislocation. Always suspect dislocation of the hip as a possible accompaniment of fracture of the patella or femur.

1. If discovered within a week of injury manipulation may be attempted.
2. After a week and up to several months good results have been claimed by heavy (up to 18 kg) skeletal traction for up to 3 weeks under sedation. When radiographs show the femoral head level with or a little beyond the acetabulum, the leg is placed in abduction and the traction decreased; this is generally successful in restoring the head to the acetabulum. If this fails, open reduction may be attempted; in either case pessimism regarding the eventual outcome is often unjustified, many cases achieving a good result without avascular necrosis ensuing.
3. After a year, open reduction is unlikely to be feasible and an upper femoral (Schanz) osteotomy may be considered.

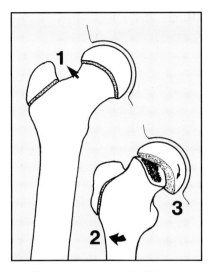

76. Slipped upper (proximal) femoral epiphysis: This condition occurs in adolescence; the term is to some extent a misnomer as in fact it is the femoral shaft which moves proximally (1) and externally rotates (2) on the epiphysis. Only occasionally in advanced cases is there movement of the epiphysis relative to the acetabulum (3). There is never any juxta-epiphyseal fracture (i.e. it is a Salter–Harris Type I lesion).

and in severe cases there may be shortening and an external rotation deformity. Radiographs confirm slipping, and there may be evidence of remodelling and new bone formation.

   Acute-on-chronic: There is a long history of chronic disability on which are superimposed acute symptoms (due to an increase in the slip).

Classification (b): Two more recent classifications (clinical and radiographic) are of prognostic value, and differentiate between so-called stable and unstable slips.

   Clinical Classification: A stable slip is said to be present when walking (albeit with crutches) is possible. In unstable slips walking, even with crutches, is not possible, and this group has the worst prognosis.

   Radiographic Classification: Attention is paid to the presence or absence of a hip joint effusion on an ultrasound examination, and to the presence or absence of metaphyseal remodelling in the plain radiographs. In the stable slip, there is no effusion, but evidence of remodelling; in the unstable slip there is an effusion and no remodelling suggesting an acute event.

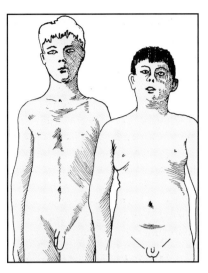

77. Aetiology: Both biochemical and mechanical factors may be involved. *Biochemical/hormonal factors* have long been suspected for the following reasons: 1. The condition is commoner in males, and virtually unknown in females after the menarche; 2. It occurs at adolescence; 3. Those affected are often adipose and sexually immature, showing features of the Fröhlich's syndrome, or are very tall and thin, suggesting increased production of growth hormone, and it is common in children who are receiving growth hormone supplements;

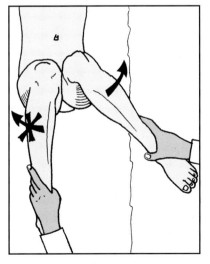

78. Diagnosis (a): The condition should be *suspected* in any adolescent with a history of limp and occasional groin or knee pain, especially if overweight or belonging to one of the body types described. Examination of the hip shows loss of internal rotation, often accompanied by pain, at every stage in the condition. In severe cases there is restriction of flexion and abduction, the limb is held in external rotation, and there may be some shortening.

4. Some cases are associated with juvenile hypothyroidism (with lowered thyroxin and thyroid-stimulating hormones), or hypogonadism; 5. It is often bilateral; 6. In less than 30% is there a history of injury (there is no hereditary tendency).
Mechanical factors may include 1. Increased femoral anteversion; 2. Increased obliquity of the epiphyseal plate (physis); 3. Increased acetabular depth; 4. Increased shear stresses on the epiphyseal plate secondary to obesity.

Classification (a): The traditional classification recognises four categories: 1, Pre-slip; 2, Acute slip; 3, Chronic slip; 4, Acute-on-chronic slip.

   Pre-slip: There is a history of leg weakness, pain in the groin or knee especially on exertion, and some loss of internal rotation in the hip. Some widening of the epiphyseal plate may be detected in the radiographs, but nothing else.

   Acute: The duration of symptoms is less than 3 weeks. There is restriction of movements in the hip, often with an external rotation deformity, and pain may prevent weight bearing. There may be a history of a traumatic incident, but this is often of a trivial nature. The radiographs show evidence of slipping.

   Chronic: There is a history of pain in the groin or knee in excess of 3 weeks. (Symptoms have usually been present for months or even years.) There is restriction of movements in the hip in several planes,

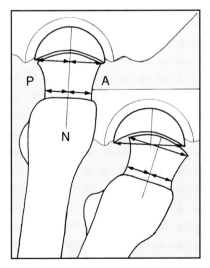

79. Diagnosis (b): The earliest radiographic signs are to be found in the lateral projection. A line drawn up the centre of the neck should normally bisect the epiphyseal base of the head; if it fails to do so, a slip is present, and the percentage and angle of the slip should be noted. (Illus. 15–20%, 17° slip.) **Mild slip:** less than 33%, or 30°. **Moderate slip:** 33–50% or 30–50°. **Severe slip:** more than 50% or 50°.

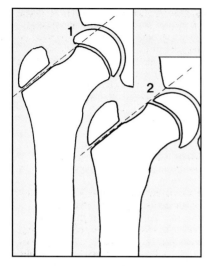

80. Diagnosis (c): In the AP view slip is less obvious, but nevertheless may be detected with experience. Radiographs of both hips should be taken to allow comparison and detect an early silent slip on the other side. In the normal hip (1) a tangent to the neck should cut through a portion of the epiphysis. When slip is present (2) this is no longer the case. (A similar construction (with similar findings) may be used in the lateral, with a line drawn tangent to the posterior part of the neck.)

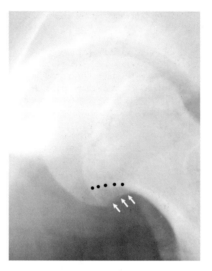

81. Diagnosis (d): Look for radiographic evidence of new bone formation (buttressing). This may be found in the region of the inferior and posterior aspects of the metaphysis. The latter is shown in the illustration, lying between the dotted line (which denotes the original line of the neck), and the arrows. This finding is indicative of chronicity.

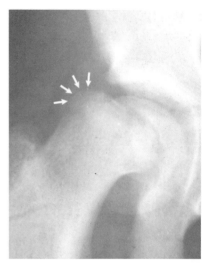

82. Diagnosis (e): Remodelling at the superior (illustrated) and anterior aspects of the metaphysis also indicates chronicity. An ultrasound examination should be carried out; the presence of an effusion indicates an acute episode. These radiographic features along with the patient's ability to weight bear should allow the slip to be classified as stable or unstable. Finally CAT and MRI scans may help diagnose early avascular necrosis and chondrolysis.

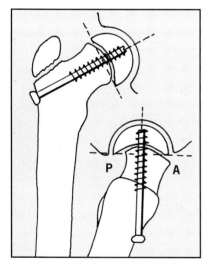

83. Treatment (a): The aim is to stabilise the slip and avoid avascular necrosis and chondrolysis. In stable cases, where slips are generally not severe, in situ fixation is advised using a single percutaneous cannulated screw (6.5 to 7.4 mm) inserted through a small incision carefully placed so that the screw lies in the centre of the head perpendicular to the physis, without penetrating the head postero-superiorly (and thereby endangering the capital blood supply or risking chondrolysis).

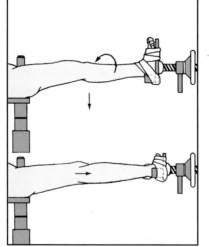

84. Treatment (b): In unstable cases with severe slipping there is controversy over management. Many advocate pinning in situ; others perform an open reduction or a manipulation. Both are said to be associated with an increased incidence of avascular necrosis and the former is probably best avoided. Any attempts at manipulation must be mild, applying *light* traction in mid abduction and turning the leg into internal rotation. Accept any correction to 30% or less, and pin in that position. *Never attempt to correct a chronic slip.*

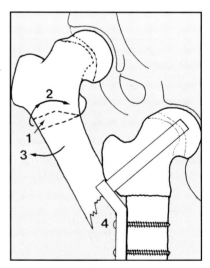

85. Treatment (c): Other methods include: (i) Conservative treatment, with 12 weeks in a hip spica; this runs the risk of further slipping, chondrolysis, and pressure sores; (ii) Immediate corrective osteotomy and internal fixation; the risks of avascular necrosis are high. (iii) *After epiphyseal union,* a subtrochanteric osteotomy with excision of an anterolateral wedge (1) is a valuable procedure, allowing correction of rotation (2), adduction (3) and extension. This may then be held with a nail or blade plate (4).

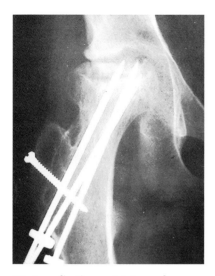

86. Complications – (a) Avascular necrosis: This is a serious complication in the adolescent, and is seen most often in:
1. Acute unstable slips;
2. Where there has been over-reduction of the deformity by forcible manipulation (especially where there has been a misguided attempt to reduce the chronic element of an acute-on-chronic slip);
3. Where pins have penetrated the superolateral quadrant, damaging the blood supply to the head;

4. Where there has been an osteotomy of the femoral neck.

Treatment: If discovered early (e.g. by CAT and MRI scans) a period of non-weight bearing with crutches for several months may help to reduce the deformation of the head which occurs through joint transmitted pressure when the bone is soft and in the early stages of revascularisation. Physiotherapy and anti-inflammatories may help optimise the preservation of joint movements. In the well established case a difficult choice may have to be made between:
1. The uncertain results of osteotomy;
2. The difficulty of hip arthrodesis and the risks of late secondary osteoarthritis in the knee, other hip and spine;
3. The risks and long-term uncertainties of total hip replacement.

(The accompanying illustration is of a case treated by open reduction (with reflection of the greater trochanter) and multiple pin fixation. Neither procedure would be presently advocated by the authors.)

(b) Chondrolysis: This is said to be present if the joint space is reduced on the affected side to half or less of that on the good (or, in bilateral cases, a reduction of the space to less than 3 mm). The cause is not known, but contributory factors include penetration of the head by the fixation materials, severe slips, prolonged pre-slip symptoms and subtrochanteric osteotomy performed prior to epiphyseal closure.

Treatment: This follows the same lines as those employed in cases of established avascular necrosis.

(c) Involvement of other hip: In keeping with the aetiology, the other hip may be affected at any time. This is particularly liable to be missed when the patient is being rested in bed during treatment of the primary complaint. Routine radiography of both hips is advised, particularly in the recumbent patient. If the second hip is involved, treatment is pursued along the lines already described.

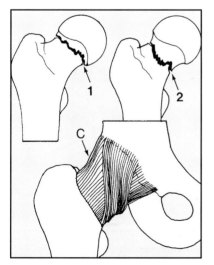

87. Fractures of the femoral neck – Level of fracture (a): Four sites of fracture are well recognised, the most important being: (1) subcapital and (2) transcervical. The distinction between these two is rather blurred, as rotation in the plane of the X-rays may be misleading. It is clear, however, that both lie within the joint capsule (C) and are well described as *intracapsular fractures*.

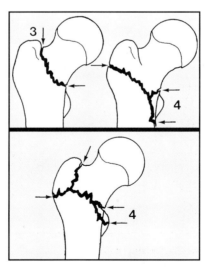

88. Level of fracture (b): The other common sites of fracture are *extracapsular*. In the *intertrochanteric* or *basal* fracture (3) the fracture line runs along the base of the femoral neck between the trochanters. In *pertrochanteric* fractures (4) the fracture line involves the trochanters, one or both of which may be fractured or separated, so that in effect this is often a comminuted fracture.

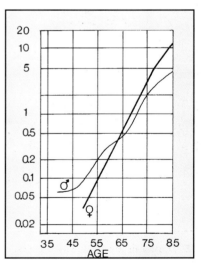

89. Incidence: The *y*-axis of the graph represents the yearly incidence per 1000 population and shows that below the age of 60 the fracture occurs most frequently in men, generally from industrial trauma. The incidence increases with age, and in later life is three times commoner in women, where hormone-dependent osteoporosis and a degree of osteomalacia are contributory factors. The fracture is seen from time to time in children.

90. Aetiology: In middle aged women, a number of factors associated with an increased incidence of hip fracture have been recognised. These include:
1. Having a previous fracture, sustained when above the age of 50, following minor trauma.
2. Having a maternal history of hip fracture.
3. Being a current smoker.
4. Having a low body weight.

Mechanism of injury: A fall on the side is the commonest cause.

Risk factors: There are a number of factors (many of which are correctable), which are associated with a higher incidence of this fracture. These include:
1. Poor eyesight.
2. Slow gait.
3. The taking of hypnotics, sedatives and diuretics.
4. Neurological problems including Parkinson's disease and stroke.
5. Foot deformities and arthritis.
6. Weakness of the lower limbs.
7. Loose carpets or slippery flooring.
8. A decrease in bone mineral density.
9. An elevated rate of bone turnover.

Prevention:
1. The risks of any ageing patient sustaining this fracture should be kept in mind, and any of the risk factors detailed above (e.g. poor eyesight) should be treated as thoroughly as possible. Exercise should be encouraged, and the patient advised against smoking and high alcohol consumption.
2. Calcium and vitamin D supplements in the elderly, especially if housebound, are cost-effective in reducing the incidence of this fracture.
3. In post-menopausal women, HRT (hormone replacement therapy) should be considered if the patient is known to be suffering from osteoporosis or is otherwise in a high risk category.
4. Where the risks are considered to be particularly high, and low bone mineral density has been discovered, bisphosphonates may be considered.
5. Where the patient is very frail, and particularly if there is any unsteadiness of gait, the wearing of padded under garments (eg 'HipSavers') has been demonstrated to dramatically reduce the incidence of these fractures.

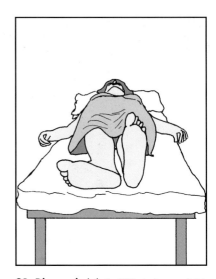

91. Diagnosis (a): Inability to bear weight after a fall, particularly in an elderly patient, with or without pain in the hip, is most likely to be due to this common fracture which must be excluded in every case by radiographic examination; fractures of the pubic rami or distal limb fractures are less common causes of this primary complaint. External rotation of the limb, sometimes with a little shortening, is a valuable (but not invariable) sign.

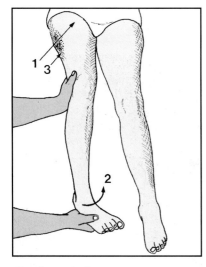

92. Diagnosis (b): *Tenderness* will be found over the femoral neck anteriorly (1) and in extracapsular fractures over the greater trochanter. *Pain* is produced by rotation of the hip (2). *Bruising* (3) is a *late* sign in extracapsular fractures, and is absent in acute injuries and in intracapsular fractures. Rarely, with an undisplaced fracture, the patient may be able to bear weight.

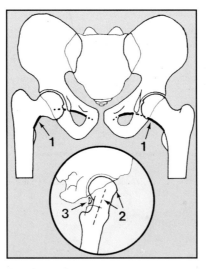

93. Diagnosis (c): An AP radiograph of the pelvis with a lateral of the affected hip are best for screening of this area. Generally the fracture line is obvious but if not, look for asymmetry in Shenton's lines (1) and in the lateral, angulation of the head with respect to the neck (2) or fragmentation (3). If there is any remaining doubt, a localised AP view should be taken; if this appears negative, re-examine by MRI scan after 48 hours, or repeat the plain films after 1–2 weeks.

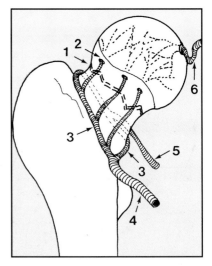

94. Intracapsular fractures: These are prone to complications for two clear reasons: (a) The blood supply to the femoral head may be disturbed by intracapsular fractures (1), leading to *avascular necrosis*. A dynamic MRI bone scan gives the earliest indication of this complication. Note the main supply penetrates the head close to the cartilage margin (2) and arises from an arterial ring (3) fed from the lateral and medial femoral circumflex arteries (4 and 5). A small portion of the head is inconstantly supplied via the ligamentum teres (6).

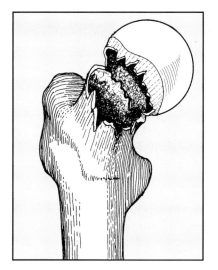

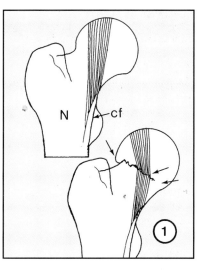

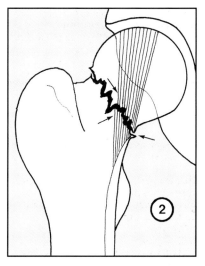

95. Complications cntd: (b) The head fragment is often a shell containing fragile cancellous bone, and affords poor anchorage for any fixation device. Inadequate fixation may lead to *non-union*. Note that any connection between non-union and avascularity is tenuous – the head is often viable in non-union, and avascular necrosis is seen most frequently in united fractures.

96. Complications cntd: It follows that complications are most frequent in proximally situated and displaced fractures. Any displacement should be assessed along the lines laid down by Garden which, amongst other things, take into account disturbance of the weight-carrying trabeculae radiating from the calcar femorale. *In Garden Type 1 fractures*, the inferior cortex is not completely broken, but the trabeculae are angulated (abduction fracture).

97. Garden Type 2 fractures: In Type 2 injuries the fracture line is complete; the inferior cortex is clearly broken. The trabecular lines are interrupted but are not angulated. In both Type 1 and Type 2 fractures there is no obvious displacement of the fragments relative to one another.

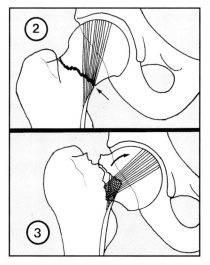

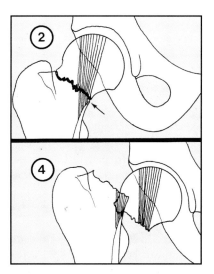

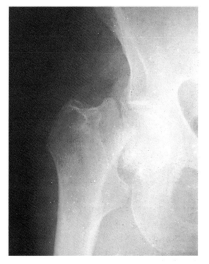

98. Garden Type 3 fractures: Here the fracture line is obviously complete. There is rotation of the femoral head in the acetabulum, i.e. the proximal fragment is abducted and internally rotated. This may be apparent from the disturbance in the trabecular pattern. The fracture is *slightly displaced*. (Garden Type 2 injury is included for comparison.)

99. Garden Type 4 fracture: The fracture here is fully displaced, and the femoral head tends to lie in the neutral position in the acetabulum. (Type 2 injury is included for comparison.) Garden Type 3 and 4 fractures of the femoral neck carry the worst prognosis.

100. Garden classification cntd: The radiograph shows a typical subcapital Garden Type 4 fracture. The femoral head is lying in the acetabulum in the neutral position.

101. **TREATMENT**

IMMEDIATE MANAGEMENT

In the initial assessment the following points should be considered and where appropriate, documented:

1. **Risk of pressure sores:** Where this is high, a large cell, alternating pressure mattress or similar pressure-decreasing bed should be used: otherwise soft surfaces (e.g. fleeces) should be used to protect the sacrum and heels.
2. **Hydration and electrolyte balance:** Set up an intravenous line and initiate an appropriate replacement regime.
3. **Pain:** This should be controlled to allow regular changes of patient position and reduce immobility, and hence the risks of pressure sores and respiratory complications. *Pain relief should be administered prior to the X-ray examination.*
4. **Core body temperature:** Any reduction should be corrected and the patient kept warm.
5. **Continence:** Catheterisation may be needed if the patient is incontinent.
6. The patient's **mental state**, **previous mobility** and **overall function**, and the **social circumstances** should also be noted.
7. **The X-ray investigation** should be carried out expeditiously, and if possible the patient should be transferred to the ward within an hour of admission.

SURGICAL MANAGEMENT

1. **General principles**

Intracapsular fractures may be treated by:
1. Reduction and internal fixation;
2. Primary replacement of the femoral head (hemiarthroplasty);
3. Bipolar arthroplasty;
4. Total hip replacement;
5. Conservative measures.

In the case of young and middle aged adults, most centres advocate closed reduction and internal fixation of all grades of intracapsular fracture. (For the management of fractures of the femoral neck *in children* see Frame 129.)

In the fit, older patient Type 2 fractures are also usually treated by closed reduction and internal fixation. Type 1 fractures are generally treated in the same way in order to avoid the risks of disimpaction, but in a very few centres are managed conservatively, reserving surgery for those cases where subsequent disimpaction occurs.

In the elderly fit patient, internal fixation is usually extended to include fractures of Types 3, and often Type 4, the view being that if the complications of avascular necrosis or non-union supervene, that the patient will be able to tolerate a secondary procedure (usually a total hip replacement). Where the risks of either of these complications are considered in the otherwise fit elderly patient to be particularly high (e.g. in a badly displaced, proximally situated Type 4 fracture) then a primary total hip replacement procedure may be considered, although in fractures of the hip this procedure carries an increased risk (10–20% risk) of dislocation.

Where the patient is less fit, with a life expectancy of perhaps a few but not many years, where there is poor mental alertness, previously reduced mobility from other causes such as arthritis, and/or the risks of complication are also thought to be high, a hemiarthroplasty or bipolar arthroplasty may be considered. In the case of the hemiarthroplasty, uncemented stems are associated with a higher rate of thigh pain, poorer overall function, and a higher rate of revision. On the other hand, the use of cement may cause intraoperative hypotension and elevation of pulmonary artery pressure. The risks of these complications must be anticipated, and may be reduced by lavage of the medullary canal and the use of modern cementing techniques.

In the case of unipolar and bipolar arthroplasties, the latter may give a marginally better result in the more active patients within the particular group where hemiarthroplasty is the treatment of choice, especially after the second year. Many such devices may be converted into a total hip replacement at a later date. In choosing such a device care should be taken to select one which does not permit dissociation of the components should dislocation occur.

2. Investigations

The following investigations may prove invaluable in assessment and are performed routinely in many centres: 1. A chest radiograph and, if there is a productive cough, a sputum film and culture; 2. Electrocardiograph; 3. Full blood count, with at some stage grouping and cross-matching of blood for surgery; 4. Estimation of the serum urea and electrolytes; 5. Routine charting of fluid input and output.

3. General treatment

1. *Preliminary skin traction* (3–4 kg) may help to relieve initial pain but its ability to minimise further displacement of the fracture has not been shown.
2. *Analgesics* appropriate to the patient and the level of pain should be repeated. *Tranquillisers and hypnotics* may also be required but administered with caution.
3. *Intravenous fluids* should be continued, with consideration given to any concurrent respiratory or cardiovascular problems. (A raised serum urea is clearly associated with a poor prognosis in femoral neck fractures.) Whole blood or packed cells may be required if the patient is markedly anaemic. The type and quantity of replacement are determined by the urinary output, the urea, electrolyte and haemoglobin levels, and the respiratory and cardiac state. Oral fluids are encouraged.
4. *The physiotherapist* may give valuable assistance in the management of the moist chest.
5. *Nursing* of the highest standard is required if, in particular, pressure sores are to be avoided, especially in the heavy patient who is afraid to move because of pain.
6. *Antibiotics* may be prescribed where there is a heavy purulent spit or frank urinary tract infection; although treatment may be started immediately, bacteriological confirmation must be sought.

While it has been established that the mortality rate for operative treatment of a hip fracture is higher where the procedure is not carried out within the first 24 hours, delay is justified if it can bring the patient into the optimal medical state prior to surgery.

4. **Surgical factors** For the lowest mortality and morbidity, the following points should be noted:
1. Both the surgeon and anaesthetist should be experienced in this field.
2. Regional (spinal/epidural) is generally better than general anaesthesia.
3. Posterior approaches with the patient in the prone position should generally be avoided.
4. Antibiotic prophylaxis over a minimum period of 24 hours is recommended.
5. Prophylactic measures against thromboembolism should be taken when appropriate.

5. **Postoperative care**
In summary, attention should be given to the following:
1. Monitor and relieve pain.
2. Give oxygen for the first 6 hours following surgery, and as long as hypoxaemia persists (assessed by oximetry).
3. Keep the patient well hydrated and correct any electrolyte imbalance or anaemia.
4. Give postoperative physiotherapy, especially if there is any evidence of constrictive airways disease.
5. Mobilise the patient as early as possible, and preferably within the first 24 hours.
6. Adopt a multidisciplinary approach to the rehabilitation of the patient.

6. **Internal fixation devices** A large number of systems have been developed for the internal fixation of intracapsular fracture. None meets all criteria that are desirable in this exacting situation: some have advantages under particular conditions and circumstances, and some in others. Most of the design problems relate to the softness of the bone and restricted size of the proximal fragment; it is often difficult to grip it in a manner that will not further imperil its dubious blood supply, while at the same time holding the fragments in close, reliable and continuing proximity, without penetration of the femoral head or extrusion of the device.

The AO dynamic hip screw addresses most of the difficulties encountered in this exacting area, and it and its variations are in widespread use for the treatment of most femoral neck fractures (but see later for alternative methods). It is inserted like the majority of devices by a *blind procedure*, i.e. the fracture site is not exposed (although the fracture, its reduction, and the placement of the device are visualised with the use of an image intensifier).

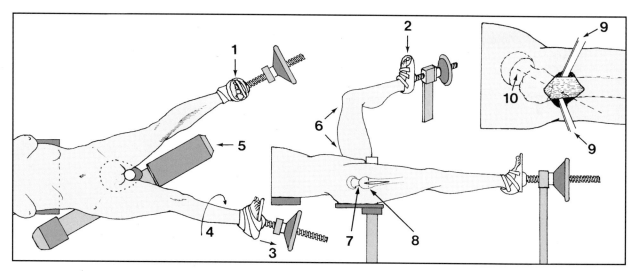

102. The lateral approach for blind (closed) nailing procedures:
The patient is placed on an orthopaedic table and the feet secured, either with 10 cm calico bandages to the foot platforms (1) or by the use of foot cases (2). If the fracture is displaced it is reduced by applying traction (3) and internal rotation (in the case of most intracapsular fractures) (4). The position is checked in two planes by an image intensifier (5). If there is difficulty in abducting the sound leg to give sufficient access for the intensifier head for the lateral, some

improvement may be gained by slightly dropping the injured leg (i.e. by extending the hip) and raising the other. Alternatively the sound leg may be positioned clear of the intensifier head by flexing it at the knee and hip (6); traction in this position is, however, less effective as pelvic tilting is unopposed. Failure to achieve reduction may be regarded as an indication for a replacement procedure.

The incision is made in the line of the femur, commencing between the tip of the greater trochanter (7) and the trochanteric ridge (8); its length is dependent on the build

of the patient and the size of any plate; small can always be extended. The incision is deepened through the vastus lateralis; this is reflected with a rugine, and the bone exposed using spike retractors (9) which help control any bleeding.

The next stage is to insert a carefully positioned guide wire which is used to guide the definitive fixation device. Ideally it should lie either centrally or slightly towards the inferior and posterior parts of the femoral neck, and pass through the centre of the femoral head (10).

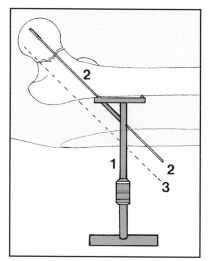

103. Insertion of AO dynamic hip screw (a): An angle guide (1) is used to position the guide wire at an angle to the femoral shaft which corresponds with the geometry of the device. The outer bone cortex is drilled and the guide wire (2) is inserted; its position is checked in two planes with the intensifier. A second guide wire (3) may be inserted well out of the way above the first, in order to steady the head and avoid losing the reduction during the insertion of the device.

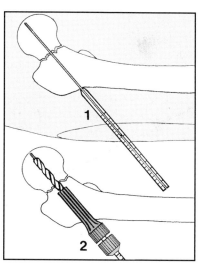

104. DHS insertion (b): A device (1) which measures the protrusion of the guide wire is used to gauge the length of the screw required (usually 10 mm less than the distance between the shaft and the head margin). The DHS triple reamer (2) is adjusted to the size of the screw, and used to cut a tapping hole for the screw, a hole for the plate sleeve, and a bevel for its shoulder. If the bone of the head is dense, it may be tapped for the screw.

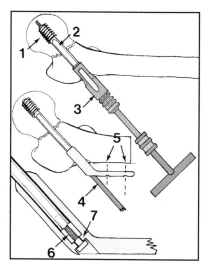

105. DHS insertion (c): The screw (1) is inserted with a guide (3) and its position checked; flats in its stem (2) which permit sliding must be aligned with keyways in the plate sleeve. The guide wire is removed and the plate driven home with an impactor (4). It is screwed to the shaft (5) with AO cortical screws. A compression screw (6) which threads into the stem of the DHS screw and abuts on a shoulder (7) in the sleeve may be used to draw the fragments together. A screw parallel to the main screw may be used to prevent rotation.

106. Aftercare: After surgery fluid and electrolytes should be carefully monitored and appropriate pain relief medication should be prescribed. Give oxygen for the first 6 hours, and thereafter for as long as there is pulse oximetry evidence of hypoxaemia. If there is constrictive airways disease then the patient should have pre- and postoperative physiotherapy.

In most cases the patient can be allowed to sit out of bed the day following surgery. Early (i.e. within the first week) weight bearing does not seem to affect the union of intracapsular fractures in a material way, and should therefore be encouraged as soon as the patient's general condition will permit. Once sound wound healing is underway the patient may be allowed home if mobility and social circumstances will allow. A domiciliary assessment by an occupational therapist is often invaluable in making a decision in this respect.

Out-patient attendances (e.g. at 6 weeks, 3 months and 6 months), with check radiographs, should be arranged until the patient is independent; thereafter, they should be seen at intervals of 6 months to 1 year for a total of 3 years to allow detection of avascular necrosis, which may be late in declaring itself. (Note that if a titanium DHS screw is chosen, MRI scans may be used to detect avascular necrosis at an early stage.)

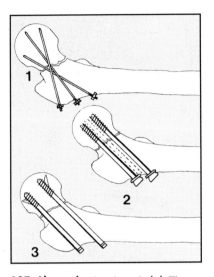

107. Alternative treatments (a): There are many other methods described for fixing these notoriously difficult fractures. These include: (1) Moore or Knowles pins (a minimum of 3) can be of value in children as they have the least effect on the blood supply of the femoral head; (2) Three self-tapping parallel screws, inserted percutaneously, are often favoured, particularly in Garden 1 and 2 fractures; (3) Two hybrid screws, which have extending wings controlling rotation and backing-out, have also been recommended for intracapsular fractures.

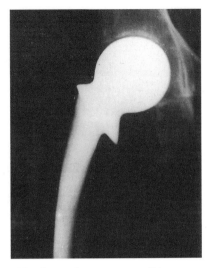

108. Alternative treatments (b): In a frail patient over 65, who is not likely to have a long or very active life, and who has a fracture with a high risk of non-union or avascular necrosis (e.g. a Garden 3 or 4 fracture), a hemiarthroplasty may be performed, e.g. with a Moore or Thompson prosthesis (Illus.); the latter is preferred where the calcar femorale is poor. Cemented stems seem to give the best results. A Hardinge approach is recommended. There is a tendency to late, slow erosion of the acetabulum.

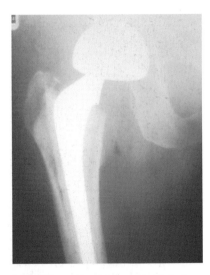

109. Alternative treatments (c): In the frail elderly patient who has a reasonable expectation of remaining mobile for a number of years, then a bipolar hemiarthroplasty may be considered. Where such a procedure is performed the results after two years are generally better than those following a unipolar arthroplasty. The pattern chosen should not allow separation of the components should dislocation occur.

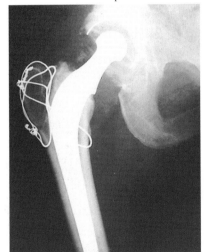

110. Alternative treatments (d): A total hip replacement is appropriate in the fit older patient, particularly with a Garden 3 or 4 fracture, who has medium or high activity levels, or previous joint disease, and has a reasonable life expectancy. It gives better results after 3 years than a hemiarthroplasty, and is the best treatment for a failed nailing. There is a 10–20% risk of dislocation, but if this is isolated a good prognosis can be expected. The most important consideration is the patient's fitness for this more major procedure.

111. Alternative treatments (e): All impacted fractures (Garden 1 and some Garden 2) may be treated conservatively, and this is an important consideration, especially where in an ageing population these fractures are on the increase, and where surgical time is in heavy demand. Overall a lower mortality rate has been claimed in those treated conservatively as opposed to surgically.
Method:
1. The leg is rested in a gutter splint until pain settles (usually after about a week).
2. Partial weight bearing with crutches is then commenced, and continued for 8 weeks, after which full unsupported weight bearing may be allowed.
3. Check radiographs are taken 2 days after the start of mobilisation, and thereafter every 2 weeks until the eighth week.
4. If the fracture disimpacts and becomes unstable (a 14% incidence only is claimed) then active treatment becomes necessary, when a hemi- or total arthroplasty may be performed. Disimpaction is seen most often in those over 70, especially those in poor general health, or in the younger patient with a low life expectancy. The problems of prolonged recumbency in the elderly may nevertheless follow this line of treatment.

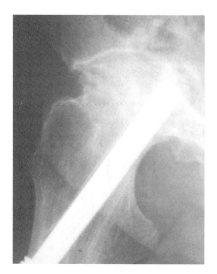

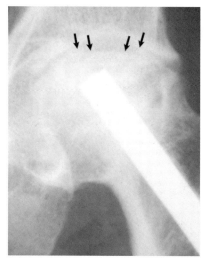

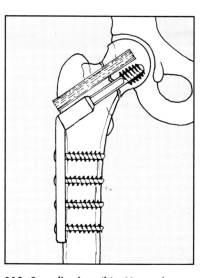

112. Complications (a) – Avascular necrosis: In most cases, the cause is the interruption of the blood supply to the femoral head by the fracture. A bulky internal fixation device may further disrupt the blood supply. It is commonest in Grade 3 and 4 fractures. The onset of pain, limp, deteriorating function and restriction of movements may be delayed for many months. X-ray changes usually appear within the first year, but may be delayed for as long as 3 years. The whole femoral head may be involved with increased density, loss

of sphericity, joint space narrowing and secondary OA lipping. Changes may show only in the weight bearing portion of the head ('superior segmental necrosis') where there is a characteristic double break in the contour of the femoral head. Dynamic MRI scans may permit an early diagnosis. *Treatment:* Control mild symptoms with analgesics. In severe cases in the young patient a MacMurray osteotomy should be considered; in the older patient a total hip replacement is usually advised.

113. Complications (b) – Non-union: This is most often seen in Grade 3 and 4 fractures, especially if missed or where the quality of fixation has been poor. In the younger patient, even where the diagnosis is late (e.g. at 6 months) internal fixation and bone grafting (e.g. with a Dynamic Hip Screw and fibular graft) may be considered, and in some quarters *primary* treatment with pinning and grafting is recommended for high-risk fractures.

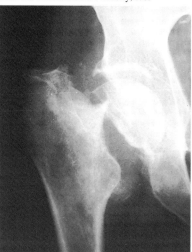

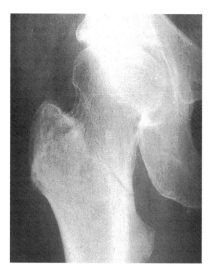

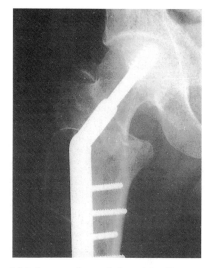

114. Non-union cntd: In the older patient, especially in the untreated fracture where the fracture has come seriously adrift (Illus.), or where there is pronounced rounding of the bone ends, sclerosis, or marked cystic changes in the neck, prosthetic replacement of the femoral head (hemiarthroplasty), or total hip replacement are the treatments of choice. A Pauwel's osteotomy is a useful procedure both in the young and in the old (up to the age of 70) for whom a total hip replacement is a fall-back procedure.

115. Intertrochanteric basal neck fractures (a): Fractures of this type occurring at the base of the neck have the following points in their favour 1. They are extracapsular, and in the adult are not associated with avascular necrosis. 2. Because of the size of the neck and head fragments, good internal fixation can usually be achieved; non-union is extremely rare, and early weight bearing after internal fixation is usually possible.

116. Intertrochanteric basal neck fractures (b): *Operative treatment:* The patient is placed on the orthopaedic table, and if the fracture is displaced, traction in the neutral position will generally achieve reduction. The proximal femur is exposed as previously described, and the fracture secured either with a Dynamic Hip Screw and a long (e.g. 7-holed) plate, or a one-piece blade or nail plate.

117. Intertrochanteric basal neck fractures (c): *Aftercare*: 1. The patient can usually be allowed to sit out of bed by the second day. 2. Stitches are removed about the 10th day. 3. If, as is usual, good fixation of the fracture has been obtained, the patient can be gradually mobilised during the first week. Full weight bearing is often achieved within the first 3 weeks. 4. The patient is discharged home as soon as a satisfactory level of independence has been regained. 5. Thereafter the patient attends as an outpatient at intervals of 4–6 weeks. 6. As soon as check radiographs show sound union of the fracture, the patient may be discharged from further attendance (again assuming a good functional result). The fixation device is not removed unless the patient is young (e.g. under the age of 45) or the device is giving rise to symptoms.

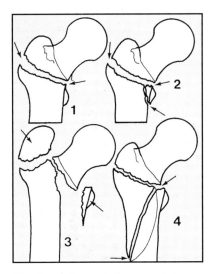

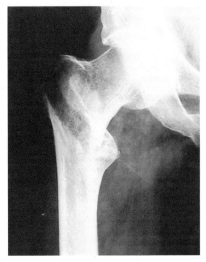

118. Pertrochanteric fractures (a): These lie distal to the intertrochanteric line, and several patterns are common (see the AO classification on p. 301 for fuller details). The fracture line may pass through the mass of the greater trochanter and run to the lesser trochanter with (2) or without (1) its separation. It is often highly fragmented, with separation of the greater and usually the lesser trochanter (3). It may be continuous with a spiral fracture of the proximal femoral shaft (4).

119. Pertrochanteric fractures (b): *Treatment*: Where there is little or no fragmentation (as in 1 & 2 in Frame 118), stability is not a problem, and a Dynamic Hip Screw with a long plate will give adequate fixation. If the fracture requires preliminary reduction on the table, analysis of the radiographs will indicate whether the limb should be internally rotated, externally rotated, or placed in the neutral position.

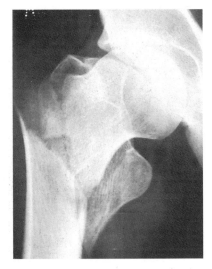

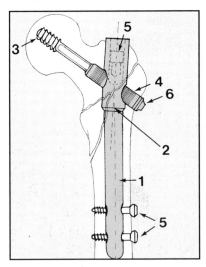

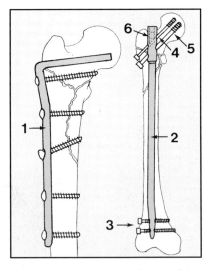

120. Treatment cntd: In the unstable fracture (3 in Frame 118 and Illus.), it is difficult to obtain strong reliable fixation. The stresses on any fixation device are high, and mechanical failure is common. A Dynamic Hip Screw with a long plate is nevertheless often successful, and this may also be used in fractures involving the proximal femur, especially in conjunction with neutralising screws.

121. Treatment cntd – Alternative fixation devices (a): The Gamma nail, Illus., (or Richards hip screw), used for pertrochanteric and proximal subtrochanteric fractures, has an IM nail (1), angled (2) to suit the proximal femoral canal, and a lag screw (3). A sleeve (4) with keyways for the lag screw is held with a set screw (5). Rotation of the IM nail is prevented with distal locking screws (5) located with a jig, and the fragments can be compressed with a compression screw (6). Fracture distal to the nail tip may occur with these devices.

122. Alternative fixation devices (b): Where more of the proximal shaft is involved, a blade plate (1) or 95° Dynamic Condylar Screw may be used. With further involvement of the shaft, a Russell–Taylor reconstruction (locking) nail (2) offers considerable versatility. This has slots distally for 6.4 mm locking screws (3). The proximal end accepts 6.4 mm (4) and 8 mm (5) cancellous screws. A nail locking screw (6) is available. It is of value in pathological subtrochanteric fractures in tumours and in ipsilateral shaft fractures.

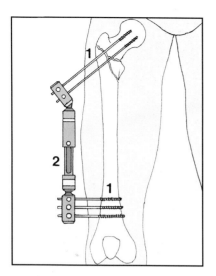

123. Alternative fixation devices (c):
Schanz screws (1) in combination with an external fixator (2) are of particular value in the management of open injuries in this region. This treatment is also advocated in many closed fractures, especially where resources are low. Surgical trauma and blood loss are minimal; the technique is straightforward, quick and inexpensive, and mobilisation on crutches, non-weight bearing, can usually be started after 48 hours. The average time to union is 16 weeks.

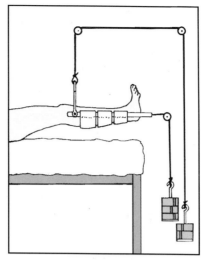

124. Conservative treatment: As union is seldom a problem in intertrochanteric and pertrochanteric fractures, they can be successfully treated by bed rest and traction. A Thomas splint may be used if desired for additional support. This form of treatment may be adopted if, for example, the patient is unfit for anaesthesia, or there are problems with other injuries; the risks must outweigh the advantages of early mobilisation.

125. Aftercare in pertrochanteric fractures: In stable fractures (e.g. 1 & 2 in Frame 118) with high quality internal fixation, the patient may be mobilised early, with weight bearing at any stage. In less stable injuries the decision when to permit weight bearing is even more dependent on the rigidity of the form of fixation employed. In the very unstable fracture premature weight bearing may lead to mechanical failure of the internal fixation device, and it is often wise to advocate non-weight bearing with crutches until callus appears and is seen to be offering appreciable local reinforcing support.
Complications: The commonest complication is failure of fixation, with the hip drifting into coxa vara (usually secondary to cutting out of the fixation device). If this occurs before much callus has appeared, it can usually be corrected by returning the patient to bed and applying skeletal traction of 5–7 kg. This is maintained until union is established. Alternatively, a further attempt at internal fixation may be made. If coxa vara is discovered late, the position has usually to be accepted. In some cases a corrective osteotomy or a hip replacement procedure may have to be considered.

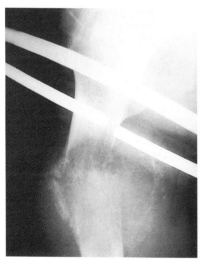

126. Subtrochanteric fractures:
Fractures at this level are often pathological (e.g. from metastases). If the patient's general condition is very poor, pain relief may be obtained by traction in a Thomas splint (Illus.). In all other cases, internal fixation is advocated with, for example, a Russell–Taylor reconstruction nail. Where there is a large osteolytic defect, acrylic cement packed into it will give much additional support to the internal fixation device, and immediate mobilisation may be possible.

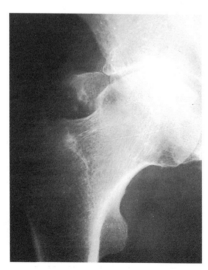

127. Trochanteric fractures: Isolated fractures of the greater (Illus.) or lesser trochanters may result from sudden muscle contraction (avulsion of gluteus medius, or iliopsoas insertions). Fractures of the greater trochanter may also result from direct violence. Symptomatic treatment only is required, and the patient may be mobilised after a few days' bed rest.

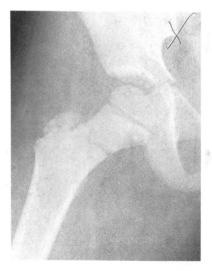

128. Fractures of the femoral neck in children (a): These uncommon injuries result from severe violence, and have been classified by Delbet into 4 types:
Type I: Subcapital (trans-epiphyseal)
Type II: Transcervical (Illus.)
Type III: Cervicotrochanteric (basal)
Type IV: Pertrochanteric.

129. Fractures of the femoral neck in children (b):

Type I: Subcapital: These are fracture-dislocations with the capital epiphysis being extruded from the joint. Avascular necrosis is virtually inevitable.

Treatment: In a child under 10, manipulative reduction should be attempted, followed by the application of a hip spica. In the older child, or where closed reduction fails, open reduction and internal fixation with transepiphyseal pins should be carried out.

Type II: Transcervical: This is the commonest injury. If undisplaced, avascular necrosis is uncommon, but if displaced the incidence is very high (60%).

Treatment: If the fracture is undisplaced and the child is under 10, a hip spica should be applied and maintained until the fracture has united. In the older child internal fixation which does not transgress the growth plate should be considered (e.g. with a small hip screw, multiple cancellous screws or Knowles pins; the latter have the disadvantage of not offering any compression). If the fracture is displaced, manipulative reduction and internal fixation may be required. Capsulotomy is sometimes advocated in an effort to reduce intracapsular pressure and diminish the risks of avascular necrosis.

Type III: Cervicotrochanteric: In these injuries (and also in Group IV fractures) the incidence of avascular necrosis is lower, but coxa vara and non-union may occur.

Treatment: Treat as Group II injuries.

Type IV: Pertrochanteric: The deformity should be controlled by skin traction for 3–4 weeks until callus begins to appear, and then a hip spica should be applied and maintained until union is complete. Over the age of 10 internal fixation may be considered, and some advise that in this age group a primary subtrochanteric osteotomy lessens the risks of non-union and coxa vara.

Complications

Avascular necrosis: The extent is highly variable, and the fracture should be treated expectantly. Sometimes a hip fusion may have to be considered.

Non-union: A subtrochanteric osteotomy, usually using some form of internal fixation, is generally successful in achieving union.

Coxa vara: This may be treated with a corrective osteotomy.

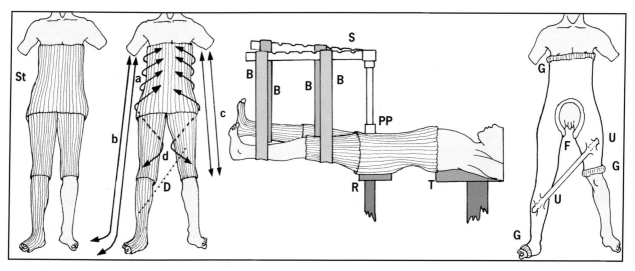

130. Hip spica application:

1. The child should be sedated, and while still in bed, apply stockinet in sections to the affected leg (from the toes to the knee), to both thighs, and to the trunk (St). Now get ready a number of plaster slabs: (a) 3-4 slabs (10–15 cm (4″–6″) wide) sufficient in length to encircle the trunk, and meet in the midline anteriorly; (b) Anterior and posterior slabs (10 cm (4″)), stretching from the toes to the level of the nipple line on the affected side; (c) Anterior and posterior slabs for the good side, stretching from above the knee to the nipple line; (d) A groin reinforcing slab for each side (10–15 cm (4″–6″)): each slab should run in a spiral direction from the lower abdomen near the midline round the lateral, posterior and medial aspects of the thigh. Also cut to length a piece of wooden (or plastic) dowelling, e.g. a broom handle, approximately 2.5 cm (1″) in diameter, to stretch from mid tibia on the affected side to mid thigh on the other (D). This, by triangulation, improves the strength of the cast enormously, and later can serve as a handle to help lift the child.

2. Now transfer the child to an orthopaedic table equipped with a child's pelvic rest (R) and perineal post (PP). The table should be adjusted so that the trunk below the scapulae is clear (T). The legs must be supported in such a way that movement (and the risk of cracking the plaster) is minimised. This may be done with a separate assistant to hold each leg. Alternatively, support each leg with wool bandage (B) slings tied to a scissors fitment (S) attached to a pole inserted in the perineal post. (After the cast has been applied and has set, the slings are cut flush with the plaster and a few turns of plaster bandage used as a local reinforcement.

3. Apply wool roll generously to cover all areas. In the older or very thin child the bony prominences may be first protected with felt pads in the same areas as recommended for a plaster jacket (see p. 57).

4. Now apply plaster bandages, thoroughly covering the entire area to be incorporated in the plaster. For best results, and to avoid problems with premature setting, it is best to have two staff applying the bandages, and two dipping. Then apply the slabs, starting at the trunk; one operator holds one end of the slab, and passes the other under the patient to the other operator; the slab is then stretched and wrapped round the trunk, meeting in the midline. The anterior slabs may be passed between the verticals from the slings. Girdering may be used to reinforce the groin area. After all the slabs have been applied, apply the finishing layers of plaster; cover the dowel with a layer of plaster and anchor its ends with a figure of eight of plaster bandages (U). Throughout the application of the plaster, stop frequently to smooth down and consolidate the layers. Now cut any suspension bandages and make good any local defects; remove the perineal post, and trim the cast in the perineal area in the front (F); turn back the stockinet in all areas, and secure with a few turns of bandage (G).

5. Transfer the patient back to bed, to lie on pillows supporting the plaster during the drying out period. At a later stage trim the cast generously posteriorly, and protect the raw plaster with waterproof adhesive tape to prevent soiling.

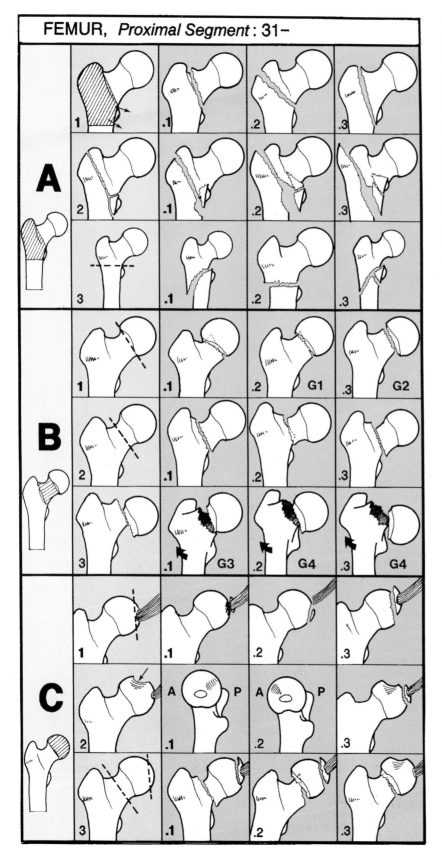

FEMUR, *Proximal Segment* : 31–

131. AO classification of fractures of the femur, proximal segment (31–):

Type A fractures involve the trochanteric area (bounded by the intertrochanteric line and the line separating the diaphysis from the proximal segment, at the level of the distal limit of the lesser trochanter).

A1 = Simple fractures beginning anywhere in the region of the greater trochanter, and ending above or below the lesser trochanter: .1 the fracture runs along the intertrochanteric line; .2 it passes through the greater trochanter; .3 it passes below the lesser trochanter.

A2 = Multifragmentary fractures starting anywhere on the greater trochanter and running into the medial cortex which is broken at two levels: .1 with one intermediate fragment; .2 with several intermediate fragments; .3 with the medial border of the fracture extending more than 1 cm below the lesser trochanter.

A3 = The fracture line extends from below the greater trochanter to above the lesser trochanter: .1 simple oblique; .2 simple transverse; .3 multifragmentary.

[*Note*: Avulsion fractures of the greater and lesser trochanters cannot be classified with other Type A fractures, and have a separate classification, namely 31–D1.]

Type B fractures involve the femoral neck.

B1 = Minimally displaced subcapital fractures: .1 impacted with 15° or more valgus; .2 impacted with less than 15° of valgus; .3 non-impacted fractures.

B2 = Transcervical fractures: .1 basal; .2 adduction pattern; .3 shear pattern.

B3 = Displaced subcapital fractures: .1 moderate varus displacement with external rotation; .2 moderate displacement with shortening and external rotation; .3 marked displacement.

Type C fractures involve the femoral head; they are rare, and are generally seen as a complication of posterior dislocation of the hip.

C1 = Split fractures: .1 avulsion of the ligamentum teres; .2 with detachment of the ligamentum teres; .3 with a large fragment.

C2 = Depressed fracture of the head: .1 posterior superior; .2 anterior superior; .3 depression with a split fracture.

C3 = Fracture of the head and the neck: .1 split fracture with a transcervical fracture; .2 split fracture with a subcapital fracture; .3 depressed fracture with a fracture of the neck.

Note: 1. The distinction between fractures in Type B is somewhat arbitrary as the great majority of fractures within this group are of a common pattern, the apparent radiological differences being due to differences in positioning or projection.

2. The AO group observe the following approximate equivalents with the Garden Classification:

Garden 1 = 31–B1.2
Garden 2 = 31–B1.3
Garden 3 = 31–B3.1
Garden 4 = 31–B3.2 or 31–B3.3

SELF-TEST

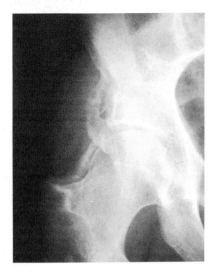

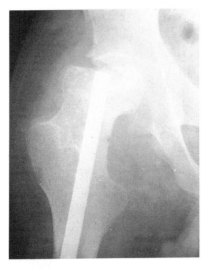

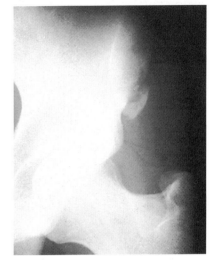

132. Following a head injury and a dislocation of the hip which was reduced by manipulation, this patient complained of persistent pain and stiffness in the hip. What is the cause of this?

133. Nine months after internal fixation of a femoral neck fracture by a trifin nail this patient complained of pain in his hip.
(a) What is the source of his complaint?
(b) What was the level of the fracture?
(c) Has it united?
(d) What deformity of the femoral neck existed before the injury?

134. This radiograph is of a young man who was complaining of severe pain in the hip and difficulty in weight bearing after a sudden sprint while playing football. What abnormality is present?

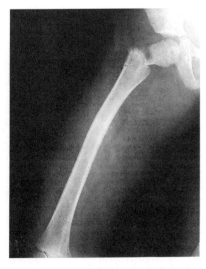

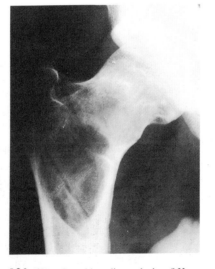

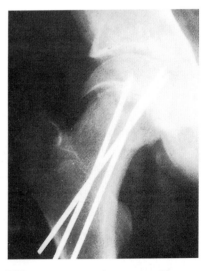

135. This radiograph is of a child who complained of pain in the hip and inability to weight bear after a fall from a tree. What injury is present, and what complications might ensue from this?

136. What does this radiograph show? How would you treat this?

137. What pathology is present, and how has it been dealt with?

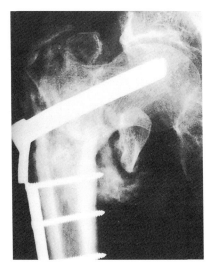

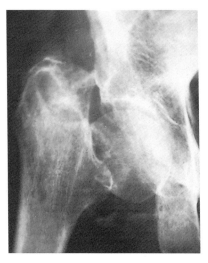

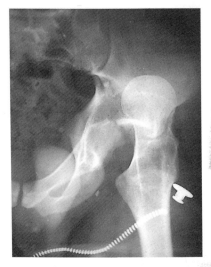

138. What fracture has occurred here? What treatment has been carried out? What is the result?

139. What complication is present in this untreated intracapsular fracture of the femoral neck?

140. What injuries are present? How might this be treated?

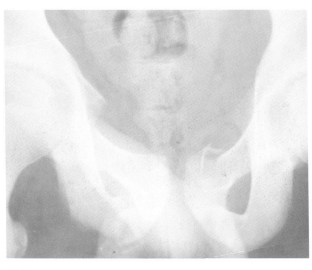

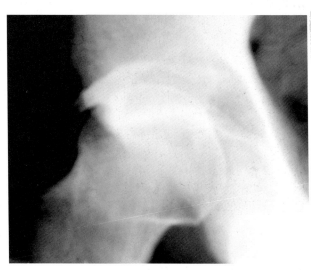

141. What is this fracture? What complication may be present?

142. What injury is present?

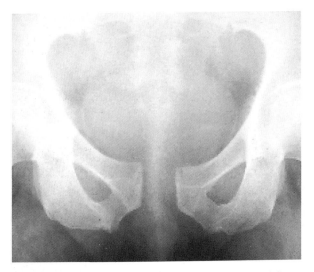

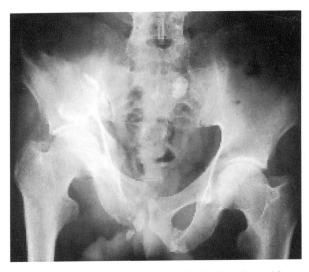

143. What abnormality is present? Assuming this is the only injury, how would you treat it?

144. What class of pelvic fracture is showing in this radiograph?

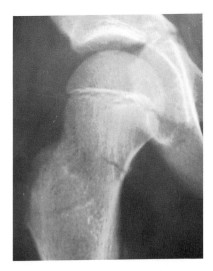

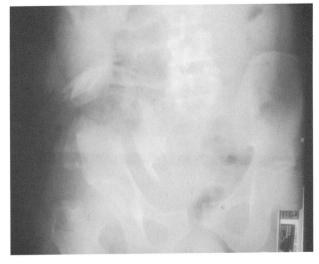

145. Describe this injury in a child of six. How might it be treated?

146. What class of pelvic fracture is showing in this radiograph?

ANSWERS TO SELF-TEST

132. Myositis ossificans.

133. (a) Avascular necrosis with bone collapse.
(b) Subcapital.
(c) Yes.
(d) Coxa valga (secondary to poliomyelitis).

134. Avulsion fracture of the anterior inferior iliac spine (rectus femoris).

135. Delbet Type III (cervicotrochanteric or basal) fracture of the femoral neck with displacement. Possible complications include avascular necrosis, delayed or non-union, and coxa vara.

136. There is a multilocular cyst involving the femoral neck and proximal femoral shaft, with a fracture running across it. This is an undisplaced (as yet) extracapsular fracture of the femur in a case of fibrous dysplasia. The diagnosis would have to be confirmed by biopsy; normally the area would be curetted, packed with bone chips, and the fracture secured with a Dynamic Hip Screw and long plate, or a blade-plate.

137. Slipped proximal femoral epiphysis. There is some persisting deformity. The position has been accepted (a lateral would be required to confirm the extent of the slip) and held with three pins, one of which may be penetrating the head. Screw fixation might be a preferable procedure.

138. This is an unstable pertrochanteric fracture which has been treated with a one-piece nail-plate device. This has broken (due to the severe stresses it has been subjected to), but the fracture has gone on to unite, albeit in coxa vara.

139. Non-union.

140. There is an obvious dislocation of the hip. In addition there is a fracture of the floor of the acetabulum. Further radiographs and a CAT scan would be required to clarify the extent of the latter, but the impression is of a comparatively undisplaced transverse fracture through the acetabular floor. Assuming this impression is confirmed, the dislocation would be reduced by manipulation; the acetabular fracture would then be reassessed by a postoperative CAT scan; if displacement of the fracture is minimal, then conservative management with traction and early hip movements would be advocated.

141. This is a quadripartite (butterfly) fracture of the pubic rami; there is risk of damage to the urethra or bladder.

142. This shows a posterior dislocation of the hip which was unstable due to an associated fracture of the acetabular rim; the fragment in question can be seen lying in proximity to the upper and outer quadrant of the femoral head. The hip was reduced, and to maintain the reduction, the rim fragment had to be exposed through a posterior approach and screwed back into position.

143. There is a symphyseal separation of just under 2.5 cm. This should be treated by bed rest until the pain settles. The separation should be monitored by repeated radiographs, and more active treatment pursued (e.g. with the use of an external fixator or by internal fixation) should deterioration occur.

144. Examination of the symphysis shows a degree of overlap. The sacroiliac joints appear intact, but there is a fracture involving the blade of the pelvis and the floor of the acetabulum on the right; the hemipelvis is displaced proximally. This is a Tile Type C3 injury.

145. There is an undisplaced crack fracture of the femoral neck in a child (Delbet Type II injury). This may be treated by the application of a hip spica.

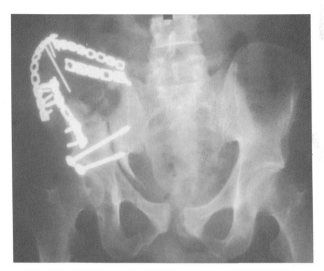

146. The right hemipelvis is vertically and rotationally unstable, but the acetabulum is intact: this is therefore a Tile Type C1 fracture. After successful resuscitation the injury was treated by open reduction and held with long cancellous screws and reconstruction plates.

CHAPTER

12

Fractures of the femur and injuries about the knee

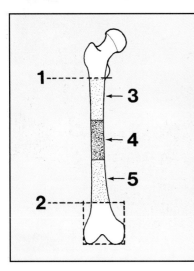

1. Classification: In the AO classification system the femoral shaft is defined as in effect stretching between the inferior margin of the lesser trochanter (proximal segment) (1) and the upper border (2) of a square containing the distal end of the femur (the distal segment). For descriptive purposes the shaft (or diaphyseal segment) may in turn be divided into proximal (3), middle (4), and distal thirds (5). The proximal third is sometimes referred to as the subtrochanteric zone.

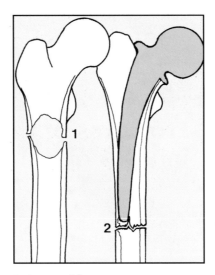

2. Causes of fracture: Considerable violence is usually required to fracture the femur, and the common causes include road traffic accidents, falls from a height, and crushing injuries. Pathological fractures may also occur: the commonest cause is senile osteoporosis but metastatic deposits, especially in the subtrochanteric region, are frequently seen (1). Stress concentrations and bone erosions at the stem ends of prostheses may also be responsible (2).

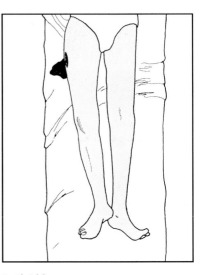

3. Fluid loss: In a closed fracture, loss of half to one litre of blood into the tissues, with accompanying shock, is common. Fractures open from within out occur classically in the proximal third. Blood replacement is often required in closed fractures, and normally essential in open ones; grouping, cross-matching and setting up of an intravenous line should be done routinely (except in children). In the transport of patients to hospital, temporary splintage will help reduce local bleeding and shock.

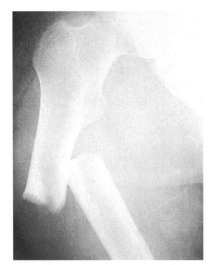

4. Diagnosis: This seldom presents any difficulty; weight bearing is impossible and there is abnormal mobility in the limb at the level of the fracture. The leg is often externally rotated, abducted at the hip, and shortened. Radiographs confirm the diagnosis. It is most important to exclude fracture of the patella, dislocation of the hip, fracture of the neck of the femur, and acetabular fracture; only good quality radiographs should be accepted.

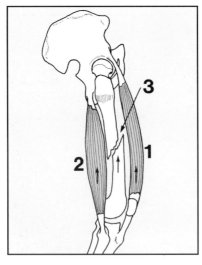

5. Conservative treatment: Femoral shaft fractures are frequently treated conservatively, and the first principle to appreciate is that the large muscle masses of the quadriceps (1) and hamstrings (2) tend to produce displacement and shortening (3). Traction can overcome this, and is the basis of most conservative methods of treatment.

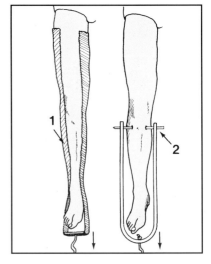

6. Traction methods – (a) Skin traction: Skin traction with adhesive strapping, is used in children and young adults. There are occasional problems with skin sensitivity and pustular infections under the strapping. (Non-adhesive tapes may sometimes be used for short periods of light traction.)
(b) Skeletal traction: Skeletal traction using a Steinmann pin through the tibial tuberosity is preferred in the older patient with inelastic skin and where heavy traction is required. There are occasional problems with pin track infections.

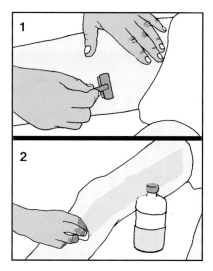

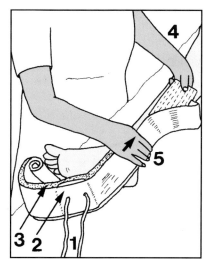

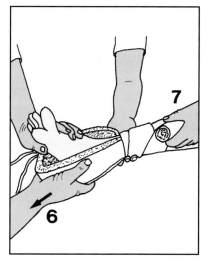

7. Applying skin traction (a): With the exercise of care and gentleness this can usually be done without an anaesthetic. (1) Begin by shaving the skin. (2) It is then traditional to swab or spray the skin with a mildly antiseptic solution of balsam of Peru in alcohol. This may facilitate the adhesion of the strapping.

8. Applying skin traction (b): Commercial traction sets use adhesive tapes which can stretch from side to side but not longitudinally. They come supplied with traction cords (1) and a spreader bar (2) with foam protection for the malleoli (3). Begin by applying the tape to the medial side of leg – do this by peeling off the protective backing with one hand (4) while pressing the tape down and advancing the other (5).

9. Applying skin traction (c): The leg is internally rotated and the tape applied to the outside of the leg, preferably a little more posterior than on the medial side. The tapes should extend up the leg as far as possible, irrespective of the site of the fracture. Now apply traction to the leg (6) and finally secure the tapes throughout their length with encircling crepe bandages (7).

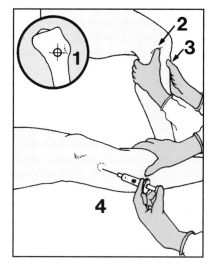

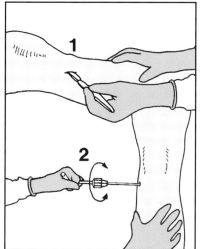

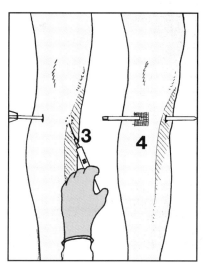

10. Applying skeletal traction (a): The preferred site is the upper tibia a little under 2 cm (1″) posterior to the prominence of the tibial tuberosity (1). It is important to avoid the knee joint, and the growth plate in children: so begin by carefully identifying it by flexing the knee (2), noting its relationship to the tuberosity (3). If a general anaesthetic is not employed, infiltrate the skin and tissue down to periosteum with local anaesthetic (e.g. 2–3 mL of 1% lignocaine) (4).

11. Skeletal traction (b): Now make a small incision in the skin (1) enough to take the traction pin only; insert it until the point strikes bone. Drive the pin through the lateral tibial cortex by applying firm pressure and twisting the chuck handle (2). You should feel it penetrate the outer cortex and pass quickly with little resistance till it meets the medial cortex. Stop at this stage.

12. Skeletal traction (c): Infiltrate the skin down to periosteum on the medial side, using the lie of the pin to guide you to the expected exit area (3). Drive the pin through the medial cortex, and make a small incision over the tenting skin to allow it to come through. Protect the openings with gauze strips soaked in Nobecutane™ or a similar sealant (4). Try to insert the pin at right angles to the leg.

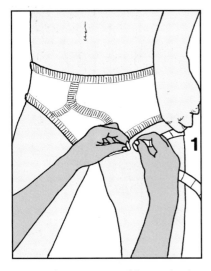

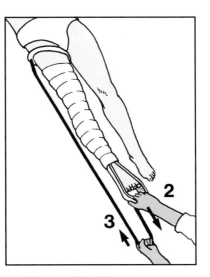

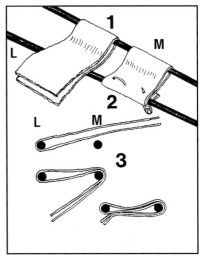

13. Traction systems – Skin traction in a Thomas splint (a): The most important decision in selecting a Thomas splint is the ring size. To save time (e.g. before anaesthesia) the uninjured leg may be measured (1), and an allowance of 5 cm made for swelling, present and anticipated. It is nevertheless wise to have readily available a size above and below the estimate in case of inaccuracies.

14. Thomas splint (b): Anaesthesia will be required in the adult. Applying traction with one hand on the spreader bar (2) the selected splint is pushed up the leg (3). It should reach the ischial tuberosity (or more likely the perineum) and it should be possible to pass one finger beneath the ring round its complete circumference. If the ring is too large or too small, maintain traction while the next size is tried.

15. Thomas splint (c): The choice of soft furnishings and their method of application is often made with a fanaticism that may amaze the uncommitted. Slings to bridge the side irons may be formed from strips of 15 cm (6″) wide calico bandage (1). It is traditional to secure these with large safety pins inserted from below, close to the outer iron (2). Sometimes spring clips are used. A double bandage thickness ensures greater rigidity (3).

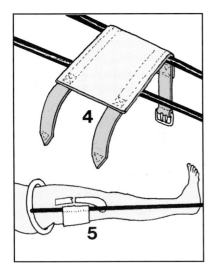

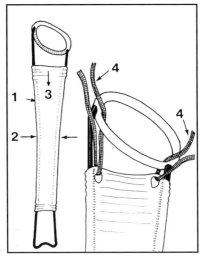

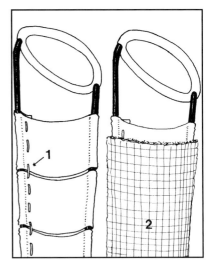

16. Thomas splint (d): The sling placed directly beneath the fracture (5) should preferably be unyielding, and one of canvas with web and buckle fastenings (4) is often favoured in this situation. It is customary to apply the splint with the master sling in position; the other slings are then attached and adjusted to the contours of the limb. Less satisfactorily, perhaps, the splint is applied with all the slings already in position.

17. Thomas splint (e): Calico and canvas slings can drift, separate, or ruck, and many prefer the smoothness of an unbroken circular bandage, stretched in double thickness over the splint (e.g. Tubigrip™) (1). This has the disadvantage of 'waisting' the splint (2), being less than firm under the fracture and tending to drift distally (3). The last may be prevented by anchoring it to the ring with ribbon gauze or bandage (4).

18. Thomas splint (f): If multiple slings are used, any tendency for them to separate may be minimised by pinning each to its neighbour (1); any tendency to distal drift may be prevented by attaching the top sling to the posterior half of the ring. A layer of wool should be placed between the slings and the limb to smooth out any unevenness (2) (not necessary with circular woven bandage). In all cases, a large pad (e.g. of gamgee) should be placed directly beneath the fracture to act as a fulcrum.

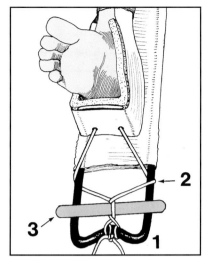

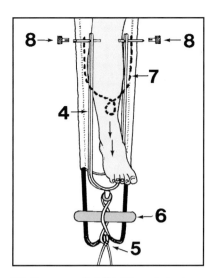

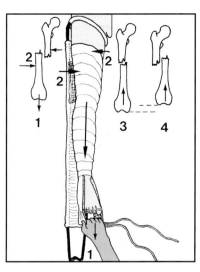

19. Thomas splint (g): In long oblique fractures and those with apposition, no manipulation will be needed and the traction system may be completed by, for example, tying the cords to the end of the splint (1). The convention of passing the medial cord under the corresponding iron helps to control the tendency to lateral rotation (2). A Chinese windlass (of spatulae or a metal rod) may be used to take up slack (3).

20. Thomas splint (h): Where skeletal traction is being used a metal loop (4) (Tulloch–Brown loop) allows a direct pull to be made in the line of the limb. The loop may be tied to the end of the Thomas splint (5) and tensioned with a windlass as previously described (6). A stirrup (7) may be employed to prevent springing of the loop. Protect the sharp ends of the pin with caps (8).

21. Thomas splint (i) – Manipulation: With the exception of the young child, manipulation is advisable if there is loss of bony apposition. With the splint in position, but unattached, an assistant applies strong traction (1) while pressure is applied in the directions deduced from the radiographs (2). When the traction is eased off, the limb remains the same length if a hitch has been obtained (3) but telescopes if not (4).

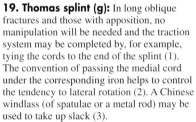

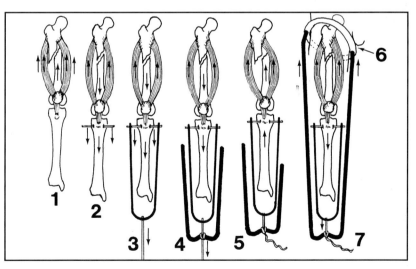

22. Thomas splint (j): After the traction cords have been attached, the end of the splint can be raised temporarily on a pillow (1) while the limb is bandaged to the splint, using, for example, 15 cm (6″) crepe bandages (2). Note gamgee or wool padding behind the fracture to act as a fulcrum (3), behind the knee to keep it in slight flexion (4), and along the shin to avoid sores (5).

23. Thomas splint (k): The system described is normally referred to as fixed traction in a Thomas splint. The basic principles are straightforward, but it is important that they are thoroughly understood. Muscle tension (mainly quads and hams) tends to produce shortening (1); this can be overcome by traction, for example through a Steinmann pin (2) aided by a loop and traction cord (3). If the traction cord is tied to a ringless Thomas splint, the reduction is maintained so long as a pull is kept on the cord (4); redisplacement occurs if the cord is released (5). This proximal migration is normally prevented by the ring (6) so that the reduction is maintained even when the traction cord is released (7). Note that muscle tone = tension in traction cord = ring pressure.

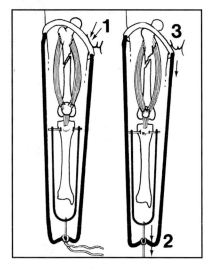

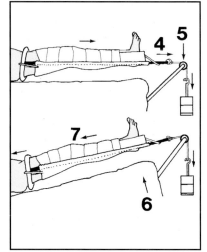

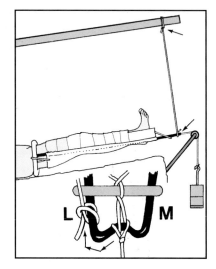

24. Thomas splint (l): The pressure of the ring of the Thomas splint tends to produce sores (1) (especially in the perineal, groin and ischial tuberosity regions) and must be relieved (3). This is done by applying traction (*c.* 3 kg/8 lb) to the anchored cords (2). If ring pressure is unrelieved, *increase the traction weights*.

25. Thomas splint (m): The traction weights have a tendency to pull the patient down towards the foot of the bed (4). This may continue till the splint comes to rest on the traction pulley (5). This may be countered if it becomes a problem by raising the foot of the bed (6), when the traction weight is balanced by the upward component of the patient's body weight (7).

26. Thomas splint (n) – Supporting the limb and the splint (i): To allow the patient to move about the bed and prevent pressure on the heel, it is desirable to support the splint; this may be done most simply by tying a cord from the end of the splint to an overhead bar of the Balkan beam bed. The position of the suspension cord may be adjusted from near the midline to either side. (Illus.: Lateral attachment to control external rotation.)

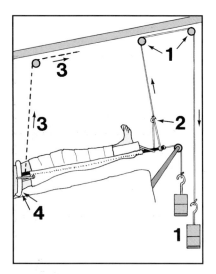

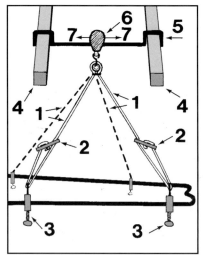

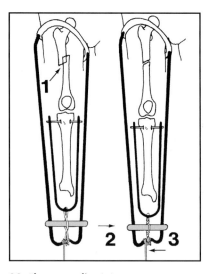

27. Thomas splint (o) – Supporting the splint (ii): Some prefer a lively system which can be achieved in various ways, e.g. by weights and a system of pulleys (1). The suspension cord may be arranged in Y-fashion to straddle both irons of the Thomas splint (2). Support for the proximal end of the splint (3) is less clearly an advantage although often pursued – it may cause extra pressure beneath the ring (4).

28. Thomas splint (p) – Supporting the splint (iii): Another form of lively splint support ('the octopus ') consists of elastic Bunjee cord (1), which can be adjusted with tensioners (2). The cords are attached to the splint with G-cramps (3) and to cross members of the Balkan beam (4) by means of a bar (5) along which a pulley (6) is free to move, allowing easy movement up and down the bed (7).

29. Thomas splint (q): Check radiographs should be taken after the application of a Thomas splint, after any major adjustment, and thereafter at fortnightly intervals till union.

Corrections: (i) If there is persistent shortening (1) tighten the windlass in a fixed traction system (2). This will inevitably increase ring pressure, and must be compensated by increasing the traction weight (3). (Soft tissue between the bone ends may nevertheless thwart reduction.)

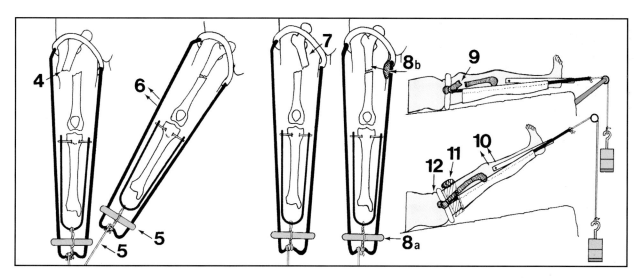

30. Thomas splint (r) – Corrections: (ii) Where the proximal fragment is abducted (4) the position may be improved by increasing the traction (5) and abducting the leg (6). The position of the ring traction pulley and the splint supports will require corresponding adjustment. **(iii)** If the proximal fragment is adducted (7) increase of traction alone (8a) may lead to an improvement in the position. It may be helpful to apply side thrust with a pad (8b) between the leg and the medial side iron. **(iv)** Flexion and/or abduction of the proximal fragment (9) due to unresisted psoas and gluteal action is frequently a very painful complication. In the young patient, raising the splint (10) and/or abducting the leg and bandaging a local pad in position (11) may bring the fragments into alignment, but this manoeuvre is less certain in the older patient where internal fixation is frequently advisable for femoral fractures at this level and of this type. In any patient in whom this conservative technique is practised, care must be taken to avoid pressure in the region of the anterior superior iliac spine (12).

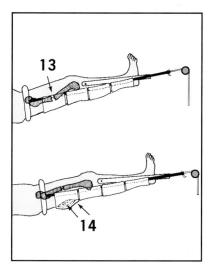

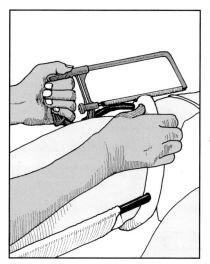

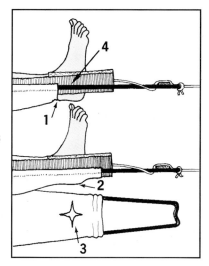

31. Thomas splint (s) – Corrections: (v)
Perhaps the commonest residual deformity requiring and amenable to correction is backward sag at the fracture site (13). If a continuous posterior support is used, the padding behind the fracture should be increased in thickness. If separate slings are used, the sling behind the fracture should be tightened and/or the padding behind the fracture increased (14).

32. Thomas splint (t) – Aftercare (i):
During the first 72 hours following fracture, swelling of the thigh from haematoma and oedema may render the ring tight round its circumference. (Normally it should be easy to put a finger under the ring at any point.) To avoid changing the splint, split the ring with a hacksaw, ease the ends apart, and protect them with adhesive strapping.

33. Thomas splint (u) – Aftercare (ii):
The following items should be checked daily. Look for impending pressure sores (and take appropriate action). In the *Achilles tendon* region if the slings stop at this level (1); under the *heel*, if the heel is included (2) (if a circular woven support is used, a cruciate incision in it at heel level is prophylactic (3)); over the *malleoli* (4).

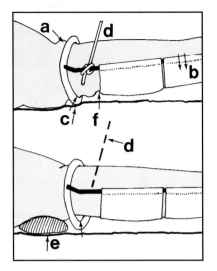

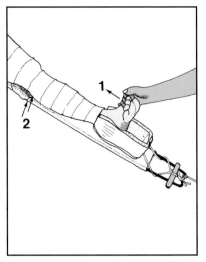

36. Thomas splint (x) – Aftercare (v): In those cases where skeletal traction is employed, look for:

1. Loosening of the Steinmann pin; this may require recentring; other treatment is seldom required, so that traction may be continued. 2. Pin-track infection; a wound swab should be sent for bacteriological examination and the appropriate antibiotic administered. If infection is marked, the traction site may have to be abandoned. 3. Shifting and digging-in of the loop; adjust with padding.

During the period a patient spends in bed they should practise quadriceps and general maintenance exercises. Splintage in children should be continued until union (6–12 weeks). In adults, mobilisation of the knee joint and/or the patient may be possible before union is complete.

34. Thomas splint (v) – Aftercare (iii):
The ring area: Good nursing care is vital to avoid skin breakdown. In addition, for circumferential tightness, split the ring; for perineal pressure, increase the ring traction weight; for anterior spine pressure (a), lower the splint (b); for pressure below the ring (c), decrease or remove any support weight (d) and place a pillow above the ring (e); pad the edge of the sling if needed (f).

35. Thomas splint (w) – Aftercare (iv):
Check daily for weakness of ankle dorsiflexion (1), indicative of common peroneal nerve palsy and necessitating careful inspection of the neck of the fibula where the cause is generally felting of the wool padding which then transmits pressure from the side iron (2). Repad, and fit a Sinclair foot support or similar if the palsy is complete: expect recovery in 6 weeks.

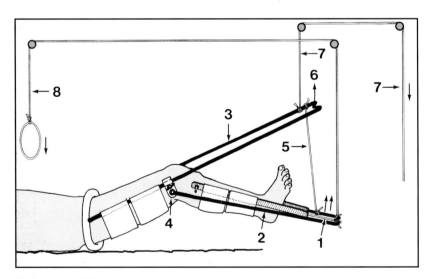

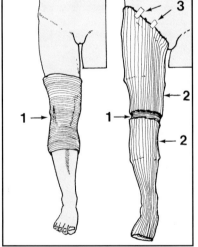

37. Early mobilisation techniques (a): Where there is abundant callus and the fracture cannot be sprung, splintage may be discarded and the knee mobilised until there is sufficient mature callus to allow weight bearing.
(b): *The Pearson knee-flexion piece:* this may be used as soon as some stabilising callus appears at the fracture site.
Method: The traction cord (1) is transferred to the Pearson attachment (2) which is fixed to the Thomas splint (3) and hinges at the level of the knee axis (4). An adjustable cord (5) may be used to gradually advance the range of permissible knee flexion. The end of the Thomas splint is raised (6) and supported (7) while a cord (8) may allow the patient to assist knee extension manually.

38. Early mobilisation techniques: (c) – Cast bracing (i): After 4–8 weeks in a Thomas splint, cast bracing may be considered, especially in fractures of the distal half. Many techniques are practised. In a typical procedure the patient is sedated with diazepam, a sandbag placed under the buttocks, and a cast sock drawn over the knee (1). Circular woven bandages (stockinet) encase the limb in two sections (2) and are taped in position (3).

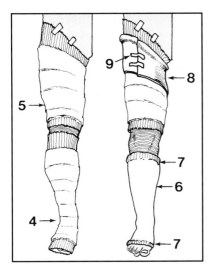

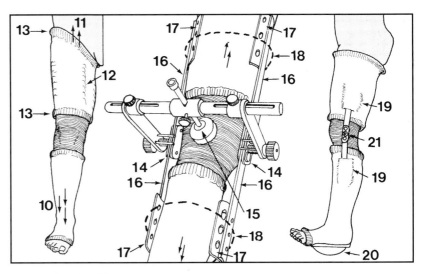

39. Cast bracing (ii): A layer of wool roll is used to protect the bony prominences below the knee (4) and as a single layer of padding in the thigh (5). A below-knee plaster is then applied (6) and completed by turning back and incorporating the circular woven bandage (7). An appropriately sized bucket top of polythene is selected (8), trimmed as required and taped in position (9).

40. Cast bracing (iii): Traction is applied to the leg (10), the bucket is pulled well into the groin (11), a plaster thigh piece applied, moulded in a quadrilateral fashion (to prevent rotation) (12) and completed (13). Maintaining traction in 10° flexion, polycentric hinges (14) are carefully positioned with a jig which is centred on the patella (15). The side-stays (16) are adjusted until the fixation plates (17) lie snugly against the upper and lower plaster components. Large encircling jubilee clips (18) may be used to hold the hinges in position while the jig is removed and flexion function checked. The hinges are plastered in position (19) and a rocker or boot applied (20). The hinges can be unlocked by removal of 2 set screws (21).

41. Cast bracing (iv): The cast brace affords moderate support of the fracture, and mobilisation of the patient may be commenced – at first using crutches and with the hinges locked. After 1–2 weeks or as progress determines, flexion can be permitted and the crutches gradually discarded. The brace is worn until union is complete.

A number of commercially produced cast-bracing kits are available using materials other than plaster of Paris (e.g. the bucket may be formed from pre-cut plastic sheet which can be temporarily softened by heating and moulded to shape; resin plaster bandages and polyethylene hinges can be employed). In many cases these render the technique comparatively simple, with the result that the so-called weight-relieving calliper, tubed into the patient's shoe, is now much less frequently employed for early mobilisation than in the past.

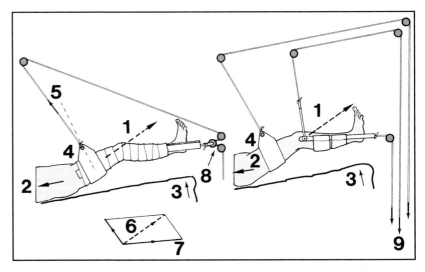

42. Other methods of treating fractures of the femur – Hamilton–Russell traction: This is particularly applicable in the conservative treatment of bilateral fractures; it is a form of balanced traction where the pull on the limb (1) is countered by the body weight (2) through the bed being raised (3). The fracture and distal fragment are supported by a padded canvas sling (4), angled slightly towards the head (5) to counter a tendency to distal drift. The theory behind the classical arrangement is that the line of pull on the femur is the resultant (6) of a parallelogram of forces, where the horizontal component (7) is doubled because of the pulley arrangement (8). Friction losses spoil the theory, and many prefer direct control of all forces (9). This method of treatment, although often useful, gives restricted support to the fracture. Note that balanced traction can be carried out using a Thomas splint bandaged to the limb, but unattached to any of the traction cords.

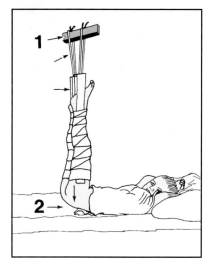

43. Gallows traction: Children up to the age of 3 years (or 4 if very small and light) are ideally treated by this method, which may sometimes be used at home if the circumstances are suitable. Traction tapes are applied to both legs and fixed to an overhead beam (1) so that the child's buttocks are just clear of the bed (2), making nursing easy. The body weight is responsible for the traction. *Gallows traction should not be used in the older child as there is the risk of vascular spasm and peripheral gangrene.*

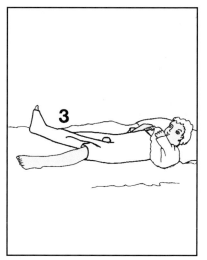

44. Hip spica: Stable femoral shaft fractures may be supported by a plaster hip spica (3); this must include the injured leg to the toes, the other leg to above the knee, and extend to above the nipple line ('one and a half hip spica'). A hip spica may be used for the fretful child where good nursing care is available at home (with fortnightly out-patient reviews) or for the badly infected open injury in the adult. (See p. 300 for application details.)

45. Intramedullary (IM) nailing (a): In many centres internal fixation by intramedullary nailing is considered the preferred treatment for femoral shaft fractures in the adult. The prime advantage is that it generally permits early mobilisation of the patient, thereby lessening the risks of pulmonary, circulatory, renal, joint and other complications, while promoting muscle activity, joint movements and functional recovery. It may also alleviate problems of bed occupancy (which is the historic reason for its introduction). Intramedullary nailing is of particular value in cases of multiple injuries, where its use is advocated if the patient's general condition will allow.

The main patterns of nail in common use include:
1. Plain intramedullary nails (Küntscher, clover-leaf and other patterns) which are inserted without preliminary reaming, or with reaming limited to removal of any medullary tight spots which might interfere with their passage.
2. AO (or other intramedullary nails of similar pattern) which are inserted after a thorough reaming, which is carried out to ensure that the nail has a tight fit throughout the length of the medullary canal. (Note, however, that reaming is generally not advised in most Grade III open femoral fractures.)

3. Interlocking nails (e.g. Grosse–Kempf, Russell–Taylor and others) where rotation of the upper, lower, or both bone fragments is prevented by horizontal screws; these are passed through openings in the intramedullary nail and engage cortical bone on either side. The use of interlocking nails is advocated in the presence of instability (eg from comminution); this may be deduced from study of the radiographs, being by definition a feature of AO Type C fractures. Instability may also accompany certain Type B fractures, and may not become apparent until sometime during the course of surgery.
4. In children, flexible Nancy nails which do not breach the epiphyseal plates may be employed.

Nailing is usually carried out by a closed ('blind') technique, with the fracture not being exposed unless reduction cannot otherwise be obtained. Plain nails may also be inserted from below (i.e. with the entry point being accessed through the knee joint). Most patterns of titanium nails are stronger than those of stainless steel and are less prone to fracture, especially if unprotected weight bearing is permitted before bony union is advanced.

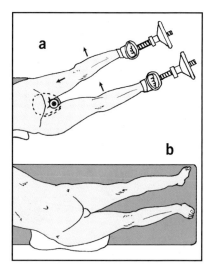

46. IM nailing (b) – Positioning: Careful positioning is required to give proximal access and to allow two-plane visualisation of the fracture with an image intensifier. (a) Traction may be applied through foot pieces or a traction pin, on an orthopaedic table with a perineal post. The affected leg is adducted, while the good leg is flexed and abducted at the hip. (b) Alternatively the operation is performed on a radiolucent table, with a pillow under the buttock (and with or without a perineal post). The leg is positioned by an assistant.

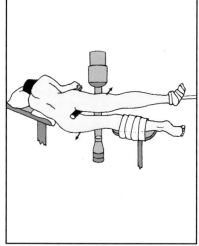

47. IM nailing (c) – Positioning cntd: Again, an orthopaedic table may be used with the patient in the lateral position. A horizontal perineal post is employed and used to permit effective skeletal or foot support traction. The good leg is extended at the hip while the affected leg is flexed at the hip to allow access for the C-arm and the heads of the image intensifier.

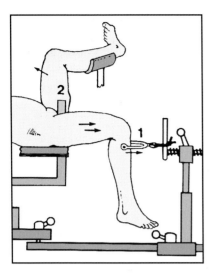

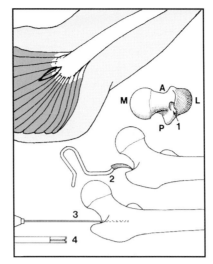

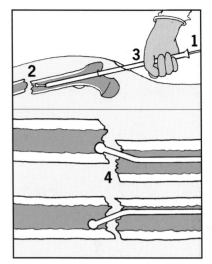

48. IM nailing (c) – Positioning cntd:
Alternatively, using an orthopaedic table, the good leg may be flexed at the hip and externally rotated, to give access for the image intensifier. Traction may be applied on the affected side in the line of the limb through a Steinmann pin (1), with the perineal post offering counter-traction (2). The affected side is adducted at the hip.

49. IM nailing (d): The greater trochanter is exposed through a 6–8 cm lateral incision; the piriform fossa (1) is identified with a finger, and the medullary canal entered through it, using an awl (2). The position is confirmed with the intensifier before enlarging the opening. Alternatively a guide wire (3) held in the chuck of an introducer may be used and the opening may be enlarged with a cannulated cutter (4). It may be necessary to slightly trim a medially overhanging trochanter using bone nibblers.

50. IM nailing (e): Initially the aim is to reduce the fracture and pass a guide wire (1) across the fracture (2) into the distal segment. To gain purchase on the proximal fragment, a small diameter nail (3) may be slipped over the guide wire. If one angled at its tip is used, this may if rotated facilitate the reduction (4). The length and diameter of the intended nail may be determined prior to surgery by X-ray using a suitable calibrated rule.

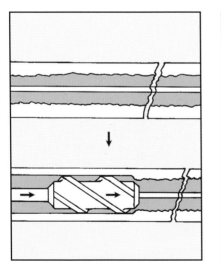

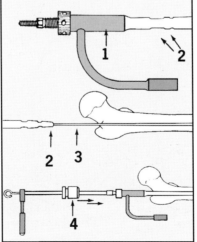

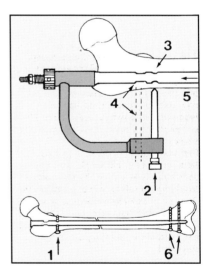

51. IM nailing (f): Reaming is frequently, but not always, undertaken before insertion of the nail. This may be merely to remove any tight spots, or it may aim to remove sufficient bone to ensure that ultimately there will be good contact between the nail and bone over a reasonable length of the shaft. Techniques vary, but often a reaming rod is substituted for the guide wire; cannulated flexible reamers of increasing diameter are then fed over the reaming rod until the desired bore has been achieved.

52. IM nailing (g): The nail is then inserted. (The choice of nail length and diameter is preferably made with X-ray studies prior to surgery.) Instrumentation varies with the devices employed, but generally an insertion handle (1) is attached to the chosen nail (2) and the nail threaded down the guide wire (3). A so-called slap hammer (4) is then usually employed to drive the nail home.

53. IM nailing (h): Interlocking screws may then be inserted (1, 6), but first confirm the absence of any rotational deformity (the second toe, patella and anterior superior iliac spine should be in alignment). The insertion handle usually doubles up as a jig (2) to allow easy placement of the cross-screws. The corresponding holes in the nail may be circular (3) or slotted (4) giving static or dynamic locking (where some telescoping is possible (5)). Distal locking screws may be inserted using the intensifier for location purposes.

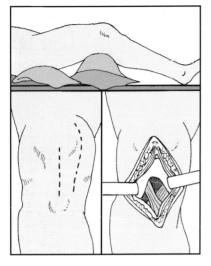

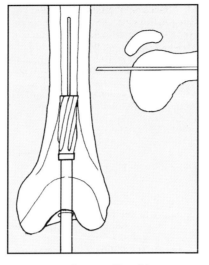

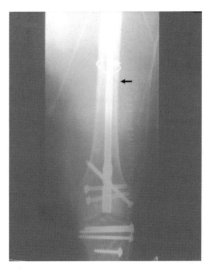

54. Retrograde IM nailing (a): This can be of value in obese patients, in cases of multiple injury, and where there are additional fractures round the femoral or tibial condyles which have to be dealt with at the same time. The knee is flexed over a pillow to about 45°. The intercondylar notch is exposed either through a patellar tendon splitting incision or through a medial parapatellar incision, with lateral displacement of the patella.

55. Retrograde IM nailing (b): A guide wire is then inserted and its position checked in two planes with the image intensifier. A reamer is threaded over the guide wire, and this is used to prepare the bone to accept the intramedullary nail which is expanded over a short length at its hilt.

56. Retrograde IM nailing (c): After the nail has been introduced, static or dynamic locking screws may be inserted at the distal end; proximal static locking may also be carried out. Short nails are available for supracondylar fractures (including after some knee replacements) and for some distal femoral fractures after hip replacements. (Illus.: Femoral mid-shaft fracture with cerclage wiring and a locked IM nail, plus fractures of the proximal tibia treated by open reduction and cross-screwing.)

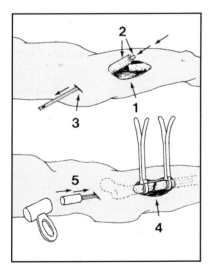

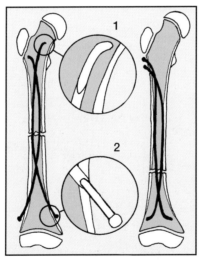

57. Retrograde IM nailing from the fracture site: Plain, clover-leaf and some other pattern intramedullary nails may be inserted by a retrograde technique after exposure of the fracture. This can be of value where image intensification is not available. The fracture is exposed (1) and the selected nail driven up the proximal fragment (2) until it presents at the buttock where it is delivered through a small incision (3). The fracture is reduced (4), and the nail driven back down (5) across the fracture site into the distal fragment.

58. IM nailing in children: While conservative treatment is generally advocated for shaft fractures in children, stable fractures of the femur may be treated with Nancy nails using the principle of 3-point fixation. They range from 2–4 mm in diameter and are flexible. They are bent to fit, and have flattened ends (1) to engage in cancellous bone and control rotation; the other, protruding ends are atraumatic (2). They are inserted through small 2 cm incisions (medial and lateral supracondylar for mid-shaft fractures, lateral for distal shaft fractures).

59. Other methods of fixation – External fixators: Fractures of the femur are less easy to control with external fixators than those of the tibia, owing to the magnitude of the stresses at the fracture site from the weight of the limb. Nevertheless the technique is often useful in the management of highly contaminated open fractures, and can be replaced under suitable circumstances by an IM nail at up to 10 days post-trauma. (See also Frame 82.) Some cases of open fracture are suitable for treatment by thin wire methods (e.g. Ilizarov, p. 78).

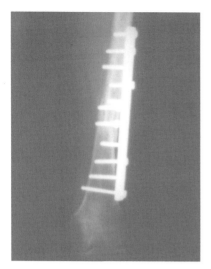

**60. Other methods of fixation –
Plating:** This is particularly useful for rapid, rigid fixation in an ischaemic limb requiring vascular repair. Plating incurs a slightly increased risk of infection and non-union. Compression plating is recommended, with screws engaging 8 cortices above and 8 below the fracture. There should be no gaps at the fracture site, and if possible an interfragmentary screw should be inserted. Compression plating with bone grafting is sometimes used in the treatment of non-union after intramedullary nailing.

61. Aftercare following IM nailing:
Postoperatively, and preferably when the patient is still on the table, the knee should be checked for instability. On return to the ward the limb should be supported on a Braun frame, gutter splint, or Thomas splint. Postoperative radiographs should include good quality views of the proximal and distal femur to exclude any condylar or missed subcapital fractures.

After the first few days care is dependent on the quality of fixation. If a tight fitting, large diameter nail is used, and if rotation is well controlled by interdigitating fragments or cross-screws, no external splintage is necessary. The knee may be mobilised and the patient allowed up on crutches. To avoid the risks of the nail bending or undergoing fatigue fracture many prefer to defer weight bearing for 8–10 weeks or until some callus appears. (Shorter periods may be considered when stronger titanium nails are used.) Where the fixation is less sound, a period of a few weeks with the leg cradled in a Thomas splint may be thought desirable.

After union of the fracture, but not before 12–18 months, the nail is removed routinely in all but the very frail to reduce the risk of a comparatively minor injury causing a fracture of the femoral neck (from local stress concentrations at the end of the nail).

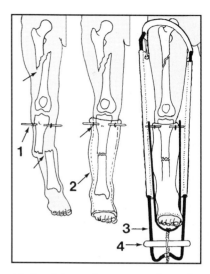

62. Special situations – (a) Ipsilateral fracture of the femur and tibia: The complication rate for these combined injuries is high, irrespective of treatment. To allow early mobilisation, internal fixation (e.g. by intramedullary nailing) of both fractures is often preferred. Where conservative treatment is indicated (e.g. in children) a Steinmann pin is inserted proximally (1), the tibia manipulated, and a below-knee cast applied incorporating the pin (2). A Thomas splint (3) with traction through the pin (4) controls the femoral fracture.

63. Special situations cntd:

(b) Fracture in the confused patient:
Where there is a head injury or a senile confusional state, a patient being treated conservatively may try to remove their own splint; it is possible to prevent this by encircling it with plaster bandages laid on top of the normal crepe bandages (Tobruk splint). This procedure may also be used to give extra security when a patient is in transit.

(c) Metastatic fracture: If death is not imminent, intramedullary nailing is advised to relieve pain. Acrylic cement packed round any defect may give sufficient support to allow the patient to bear weight.

(d) Femoral shaft fracture with (acute) ischaemia of the foot: Nearly all will respond to reduction of the fracture, which should be carried out under circumstances which will permit exploration should reduction fail. If the femoral artery is in fact divided, compression plating through the exploratory incision will usually give the rigid fixation that is required prior to vessel reconstruction.

(e) Femoral shaft fracture with nerve palsy: The majority are lesions in

continuity, the common peroneal element being most often affected. If there is reason to believe that there may be nerve *division*, exploration and internal fixation may have to be undertaken.

(f) Fracture of the femoral neck and shaft: This combination of injuries must be excluded in every case; note too that the ring of a Thomas splint may obscure the affected area. If the shaft fracture is proximal, both fractures may be treated by a dynamic hip screw and long plate. In many cases a Russell–Taylor reconstruction nail may be suitable, although it gives less satisfactory compression of the femoral neck fracture.

(g) Femoral neck fracture with dislocation of the hip: See p. 284.

(h) Fractures of the femoral shaft and patella: Note the following important points: 1. Early mobilisation of the knee is essential for retention of function. 2. Avoid patellar excision when mobilisation of the knee is going to be delayed. 3. Avoid if possible exposure of the femoral fracture and the creation of tethering adhesions between the femur and quadriceps.

The ideal management of this difficult combination of injuries is IM nailing of the

femoral fracture and immediate treatment of the patella appropriate to the type of fracture sustained. If the femoral fracture must be treated conservatively, it is best to leave even badly displaced or comminuted patellar fractures to unite by fibrous union; mobilise the knee as early as possible; excision of the patella can then be carried out as a late secondary procedure when no further flexion can be gained.

(i) Open fractures: Inspection of the fracture site to exclude intramedullary contamination should be part of the initial debridement. If internal fixation is indicated (especially with multiple injuries) the infection rate in Grade I and Grade II injuries is said to be no greater after a meticulous debridement and closed nailing than in closed fractures. Grade IIIA fractures with good skin cover and no medullary contamination can be nailed in reasonable safety if reaming is avoided. Grade III B & C open fractures are generally best treated initially with an external fixator.

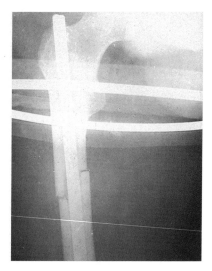

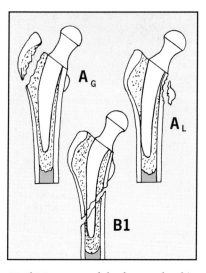

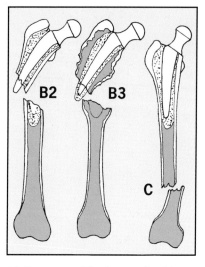

64. Other fractures of the femur – (a) Fractures of the upper third: It is often hard to control fractures at this level by conservative measures (but see Frame 30). Severe, prolonged pain is often a further problem, and is due to the psoas and glutei causing involuntary movement of the proximal fragment. In the adult internal fixation should certainly be considered (Illus.: Nailed femur in Thomas splint). Some cases are suitable for fixation with a pin and long plate, aiming to get three screws at least distal to the fracture.

65. (b) Fractures of the femur after hip replacement (i): The Vancouver classification of these fractures (Duncan & Masri) is well established. Three Groups, some with subdivisions, are recognised: **Type A:** These are the trochanteric fractures (incidence 4%), and are subdivided into A_G and A_L depending on which trochanter is involved. **Type B:** These occur round or just distal to the stem of the prosthesis. In **B1** the prosthesis is stable (incidence 16%).

66. Fractures of the femur after hip replacement (ii) – Vancouver classification cntd: **Type B2:** Here the prosthesis is unstable (38%). **B3:** The bone stock is inadequate. This is the most serious and hardest to treat (32%). **Type C:** The fracture occurs well below the stem (9%). *Treatment:* **Type A:** If the fracture is stable, conservative management will generally suffice. If the fracture is unstable, then open reduction and internal fixation is generally advised (e.g. with a Dall–Miles cleat and cable grip system).

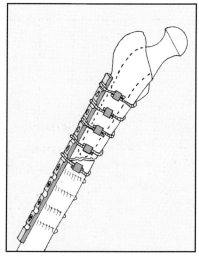

67. Fractures of the femur after hip replacement (iii) – *Treatment cntd:* Operative treatment has been advised for all other fractures, generally with bone grafting to encourage union. **B1:** The Dall–Miles system is often recommended. Proximally, cerclage cables are attached to cable sleeves which sit in slots in the plate which is attached to the shaft distally with screws. While additional screws may be inserted obliquely on either side of the prosthetic stem, broaching the original cement mantle is not particularly recommended.

68. Fractures of the femur after hip replacement (iv) – B2: In this group where there is instability, removal of the original prosthesis and replacement with a long-stemmed device is usually advised. This may require supplementing with cerclage wires or cables, along with routine bone grafting. **B3:** In this most challenging group the treatment of each case must be decided on its merits. Several strategies have been described: 1. The proximal femur may be replaced with an allograft along with a long stemmed prosthesis. This requires supplementation with bone grafting and often cerclage wiring. The patient's own proximal femur may be retained and used as vascularised autograft (by bivalving it and wrapping it round the allograft). 2. In some cases a less major procedure may be possible; the canal may be cleared of debris, fresh cement inserted, taking care to avoid cement extrusion between the fresh fracture surfaces. A plate is then used, with cerclage wiring and screws through the shaft and the new cement mantle. 3. In the older patient, the proximal femur may be resected and replaced with a custom prosthesis (of tumour-replacement type). **C:** Here open reduction and internal fixation are recommended. The selection of the most appropriate fixation device is dependent on the exact site and the particular features of the fracture. These include plates (such as the Liss plate); screw, nail and blade plates; and short cross-pinned intramedullary nails inserted in the retrograde fashion.

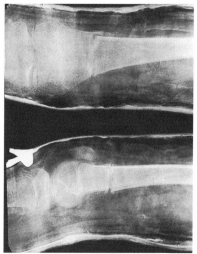

69. (c) Supracondylar fractures (Type A fractures of the distal segment) (i): (*See Frame 84 for full AO classification*) In children, fractures in the distal third of the femur are frequently only minimally displaced, and may be successfully treated by the application of a cylinder plaster. Weight bearing should not be permitted until evidence of early union appears on the radiographs, but during this period the patient may be mobilised with crutches.

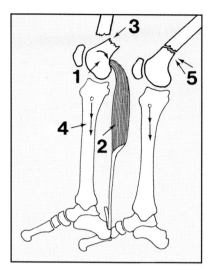

70. Supracondylar fractures (ii): In the adult, especially, supracondylar fractures have a strong tendency for the distal fragment to rotate (1) under the continuous pull of the gastrocnemius (2) into a position of posterior angulation (anterior tilting) (3). If these injuries are being treated conservatively, this cannot be controlled by traction in the line of the limb (4). It is necessary to flex the knee and maintain the traction over a fulcrum (5).

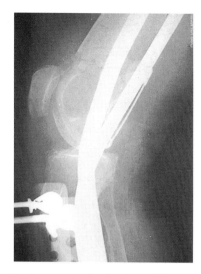

71. Supracondylar fractures (iii): The necessary degree of knee flexion may be obtained using a Pearson knee flexion piece, or better still by bending the Thomas splint at the level of the fracture (Illus.). Mobilisation of the knee should be started as early as possible, as the risks of knee stiffness from the development of tethering adhesions (between the quadriceps muscle and the fracture) is high.

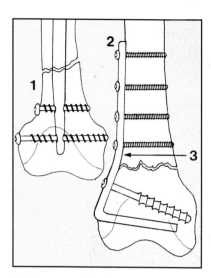

72. Supracondylar fractures (iv): To allow early mobilisation of the knee and lessen the risks of stiffness many prefer internal fixation of these potentially difficult fractures. If the fracture is proximally situated, an interlocking intramedullary nail may be used (1). Many other devices are suitable: these include (a) a Liss plate; (b) a condylar blade-plate (2) (these are available in a number of sizes, and are elbowed (3) to fit the curve of the lateral femoral condyle).

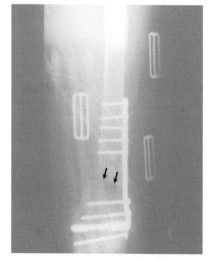

73. Supracondylar fractures (v) – Internal fixation devices cntd: A combination dynamic screw and plate is another method of fixation. The radiograph shows such a device being used to internally fix a supracondylar fracture which has occurred distal to the stem of a hip replacement (Type C fracture).

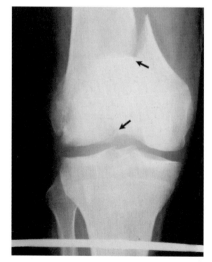

74. (d) Unicondylar fractures (AO Type B fractures) (i): Where the displacement is slight (Illus.) these injuries may be treated successfully by conservative measures. Traction in a straight Thomas splint may be used for the first 1–2 weeks, but thereafter mobilisation should be started early, either with a Pearson knee-flexion piece or with Hamilton–Russell traction. *Many however prefer to treat all fractures of this type by internal fixation.*

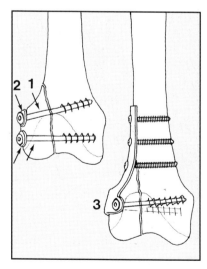

75. Unicondylar fractures (ii): If there is a significant displacement with disturbance of the contours of the articular surfaces of the knee, then internal fixation is certainly indicated. Where the bone is of good texture, use two cancellous screws (1), with washers (2) to prevent the heads sinking. A well-contoured buttress plate (3) and cancellous screws can be used if the bone is very soft, or where the fracture has occurred in the presence of a knee joint replacement.

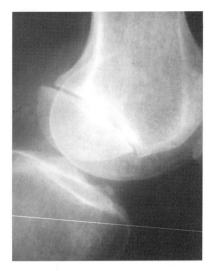

76. Unicondylar fractures (iii): Shearing fractures which are entirely intra-articular frequently fail to unite if treated conservatively, possibly due to dispersal of the fracture haematoma by the synovial fluid. Non-union may cause knee instability. These fractures may be held with two cancellous screws with their heads sunk below the level of the articular surface. Thereafter a 6 week period of non-weight bearing in a plaster cylinder is advised before vigorous mobilisation.

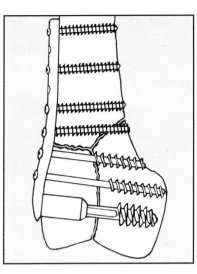

77. (e) T- and Y-condylar fractures (AO Type C fractures) (i): Undisplaced fractures may be treated conservatively or surgically, with the latter generally allowing earlier mobilisation of the knee. If there is no gross fragmentation, a dynamic condylar screw may be used. The procedure requires an extensive exposure and is seldom easy: in many cases this is due to extensive comminution which in practice is often found to be greater than suggested by the radiographs.

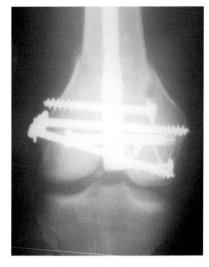

78. T- and Y-condylar fractures (ii): Some cases are amenable to treatment with a retrograde IM nail in combination with interlocking and additional cross-screws to secure the other components of the fracture (Illus.). Using a short stemmed nail, such a procedure may be used in some fractures of the femur (e.g. Type C fractures) associated with hip replacements. Ilizarov methods, including hybrid fixation systems (see p. 78) may also be employed, and are of especial value in elderly patients with osteoporotic bone.

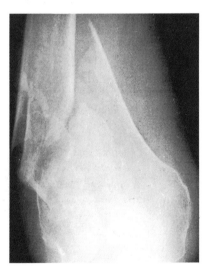

79. T- and Y-condylar fractures (iii): Where there is a great deal of comminution, the aim should be to restore the alignment of the knee and mobilise it as early as possible. Hamilton–Russell traction or other conservative methods may be employed. Attempts at open reduction of the fracture itself are not likely to be rewarding, but fine-wire fixation using Ilizarov techniques or a hybrid system may be used. Irrespective of treatment the results in this pattern of fracture are often poor.

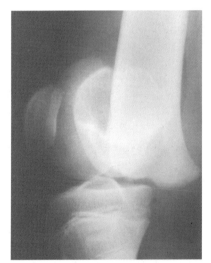

80. (f) Displaced femoral epiphysis: This injury usually results from hyperextension, and there is risk of vascular complications; reduction should be carried out expeditiously by applying traction, flexing the knee to a right angle and pressing the epiphysis backwards into position. The knee should be kept in flexion for 3 weeks in a plaster slab, and for a further 3–5 weeks in a plaster cylinder in a more neutral position. Alternatively, after reduction the epiphysis may be stabilised with two K-wires across the growth plate.

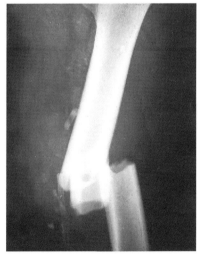

81. (g) Segmental fractures: These are uncommon in the femur, but are associated with a high incidence of non-union at one level. Fracture exposure may lose the tenuous blood supply to the intermediate segment. Although they may be treated conservatively (dealing with each complication as it arises), closed nailing, if reduction can be accomplished, is a more attractive alternative. A nail, locked at both ends, should be used. Static nailing may be converted at a later stage to dynamic nailing if union is delayed.

82. COMPLICATIONS OF FRACTURES OF THE FEMUR

Among the many complications which may accompany this fracture the following should be noted:

1. **Oligaemic shock** See page 33.

2. **Fat embolism** See page 103.

3. **Compartment syndromes** Involvement of the fascial compartments of the thigh is extremely uncommon because of their large volume and because they blend with those related to the muscles round the hip, allowing extravasation beyond their limits. This complication is seen most often after intramedullary nailing, and the possibility of its occurrence kept in mind. (For details of pressure monitoring and treatment, see p. 99.)

4. **Slow or delayed union** These are common complications, and if the fracture is being treated conservatively, may necessitate prolonged immobilisation of the knee, with risk of permanent stiffness. Where the fracture is being treated by intramedullary nailing, if the nail is not a close fit, undue movement may be occurring at the fracture site; this is particularly likely to be the case in distal fractures. Revision nailing, with reaming (which is said to have an osteogenic effect) and the insertion of a wider nail usually result in union. Where a locked intramedullary nail is used, conversion from static to dynamic locking (by removal of the appropriate interlocking screws) may encourage union.

5. **Non-union** In fractures being treated conservatively, this is generally dealt with as soon as it is confidently diagnosed, by intramedullary nailing and bone grafting. If non-union occurs in a fracture which has been treated by intramedullary nailing, bone grafting will also usually be required. In addition, the quality of the fixation must be reviewed, and if this is found wanting, it must be dealt with. In some cases this will involve replacing the nail (after reaming the canal) with one of a larger diameter. Rotational instability must be controlled, and the use of interlocking screws is desirable. In some cases, in order to obtain compression of the fragments, the use of a dynamic compression plate may be considered.

6. **Malunion** In conservatively treated fractures persistent lateral angulation is the commonest deformity, and if 25° or more, then correction by osteotomy and intramedullary nailing should be considered. Angulation in the lateral plane seldom gives rise to much difficulty. Nearer the knee, angulation showing on the AP radiographs may give rise to instability, difficulty in walking and secondary osteoarthritis of the knee. Each case must be assessed on its own merits, but again corrective osteotomy/osteoclasis should be considered.

Where intramedullary nailing has been carried out, angulation showing on the AP or lateral projections is seldom a problem in midshaft fractures unless there has been failure of the fixation device. Moderate and usually acceptable angulation in these planes may occur in distal third fractures.

Rotational deformity in cases treated by intramedullary nailing may require correction. If recognised when the fracture is still mobile, this may be dealt with by revision of the placement of the interlocking screws. If union has occurred, a rotational osteotomy may be performed and maintained with a reamed interlocking intramedullary nail.

7. **Limb shortening** Moderate shortening in the adult should be corrected by shoe alteration to within 1–2 cm (1/2″) of the limb discrepancy. In the carefully selected, more severe case, lengthening may be considered using a modified Ilizarov technique over an intramedullary nail.

In children, any difference in leg length usually corrects (or indeed overcorrects) spontaneously within 6–18 months of the injury, and alteration to the shoes is seldom required. Only rarely in epiphyseal injuries is there progressive shortening.

8. **Knee stiffness** This is a common complication of femoral and tibial fractures, and of injuries to the extensor mechanism of the knee. Among the factors which are involved are the following:

(a) *Quadriceps tethering:* If the quadriceps becomes adherent to a femoral shaft fracture, it becomes unable to glide over the smooth distal shaft in the normal fashion. This results in fixation of the patella and restriction of movement in the knee. The closer the fracture is to the knee, the more important is this effect. Surgical intervention tends to aggravate this tendency (unless it can be followed by rapid mobilisation). Some advocate the use of a continuous passive motion machine in the immediate postoperative period.

(b) *Fractures involving the knee joint:* Fractures which involve the articular surfaces may give rise to intra-articular and periarticular adhesions, or may form a mechanical block to movement. Early mobilisation is especially desirable where a fracture involves the joint, and the use of continuous passive motion equipment is often advocated.

(c) *Prolonged immobilisation:* Fixation of the knee for an undesirably long period, for example by delay in union, may lead to stiffness, and this effect is particularly marked in the elderly.

9. **Infection** Infection may sometimes supervene in femoral shaft fractures treated by intramedullary nailing. Sometimes the source is obvious (e.g. from a contaminated open wound where the initial debridement has been unsuccessful or insufficiently scrupulous), but often it may unaccountably follow a meticulously performed closed procedure. The course of treatment must be individually determined, but the following guidelines usually apply:

1. The causal organism should be isolated, and the appropriate antibiotic administered in effective doses for an adequate length of time.
2. If the infection has become established, it is unlikely to respond unless the fracture is firmly supported, and a most thorough debridement carried out under antibiotic cover.
3. If the fixation afforded by the nail remains good, the nail may be retained, but here, as in those cases where the fixation is poor, removal of the nail is often advocated. At the time of the debridement and after removal of the nail, the canal may be reamed (to permit the later insertion of a larger (by 2–2.5 mm in diameter) nail), and irrigated thoroughly with 10 L of saline; a drainage hole placed in the distal femoral cortex facilitates the fluid flow. The limb is placed in traction or an external fixator applied. Intravenous antibiotics are administered. A repeat debridement may be required in 48 hours. If negative post-debridement cultures are obtained then repeat nailing may be performed; if not, then it will be necessary to continue with an external fixator, although it may be difficult to maintain

a good hold on the fracture as Schanz pins in the metaphysis have a tendency to loosen.

AFTERCARE

1. **Immediate postoperative** See Frame 61.

2. **Quadriceps exercises** Stability in the knee and extension power are dependent on a good quadriceps. It is important that the muscle is not allowed to waste, and quadriceps exercises should be started as soon after the injury as possible, and intensified on removal of any fixation. (Amongst the few exceptions are injuries to the extensor mechanism, where quadriceps exercises are usually delayed for 2 weeks in case early contraction endangers a repair.)

3. **Flexion exercises** These should also be commenced as soon as possible, provided the means can be devised to support the fracture fully. Flexion should not be permitted unless stress on the fracture can be reduced to a safe level or where healing can be more or less guaranteed (e.g. tibial table fractures).

4. **Discarding walking aids** Walking without the support of sticks or crutches is frequently followed by an improvement in flexion, and such supportive measures should be discontinued as soon as the state of union and the patient's balance will allow.

5. **Physiotherapy** Ideally, quadriceps and flexion exercises should be supervised by a physiotherapist with access to aids and facilities such as weights, slings, local heat and hydrotherapy, but basically the patient should be instructed in quadriceps and flexion exercises, and the importance of performing these frequently should be stressed. Passive mobilisation of the patella in appropriate cases may also be helpful. Physiotherapy should be continued until an acceptable functional range has been achieved (see below) or until a static position has been reached. For this it is necessary to record the range of movements in the knee with accuracy; this should be done initially at weekly and then at monthly intervals. A measurable gain in range, no matter how small, is an encouragement to the patient to further effort; and on the other hand the absence of any improvement should make it clear to them that to continue treatment is not justifiable.

In routine cases treated by intramedullary nailing, recovery of a full range of flexion is achieved in the majority of cases in 12 months, with most of the gain occurring in the first three months.

NOTES

Acceptable functional range What is acceptable obviously varies considerably from case to case, being dependent on the gravity of the injury, the age of the patient, occupation, athletic or outdoor pursuits, hobbies, etc., but the basic aim is a stable knee which places little restraint on normal everyday activities. The following factors are important.

Lack of extension Loss of extension, both active and passive, may be found, e.g. in an angulated supracondylar fracture of the femur, or where there has been previous osteoarthritis in the knee. Such losses are seldom severe enough to cause appreciable disability, usually being compensated at hip and ankle. If the knee can be passively but not actively extended, this is known as an *extension lag*. Extension lag frequently gives rise to 'giving way' of the knee. It is common to some degree after most cases where a patellectomy has been performed, but usually recovers if quadriceps exercises are intensified.

Where extension lag is due to quadriceps tethering, quadriceps exercises should also be encouraged. The patient in most cases of persistent lag learns to compensate for the disability by using the hip extensors to keep the knee straight while standing.

Lack of flexion Appreciable disability follows if flexion to 100° (i.e. 10° more than right-angle flexion) cannot be obtained, and 100° should be the aim. Flexion to 80–90° will permit sitting in inside seats (i.e. non-aisle seats) in public transport, cinemas, etc., but will not allow the patient to kneel. Less than 100° will cause difficulty with steps, deep tread and narrow stairs, and if both knees are affected, rising from armless chairs.

Where flexion has just become static at less than 100°, manipulation of the knee under general anaesthesia should be considered. This is best avoided, however, after patellectomy and quadriceps tendon and patellar ligament repairs because of the risks of secondary rupture. Gains in flexion by manipulation are seldom high, and late manipulations are usually very unrewarding. Arthroscopy should be considered, with division of any intra-articular adhesions.

Where 80° or less flexion is possible and the position static, the patient's functional disability and functional requirements should be carefully assessed. If there is a marked deficit, quadricepsplasty should be considered. In this procedure the vasti are divided close to the knee so that their tethering effect is eliminated; rectus femoris then becomes the sole extensor of the knee. This often gives a useful gain (often in the region of 40°) although sometimes this is at the expense of an extension lag, and always with some loss of power.

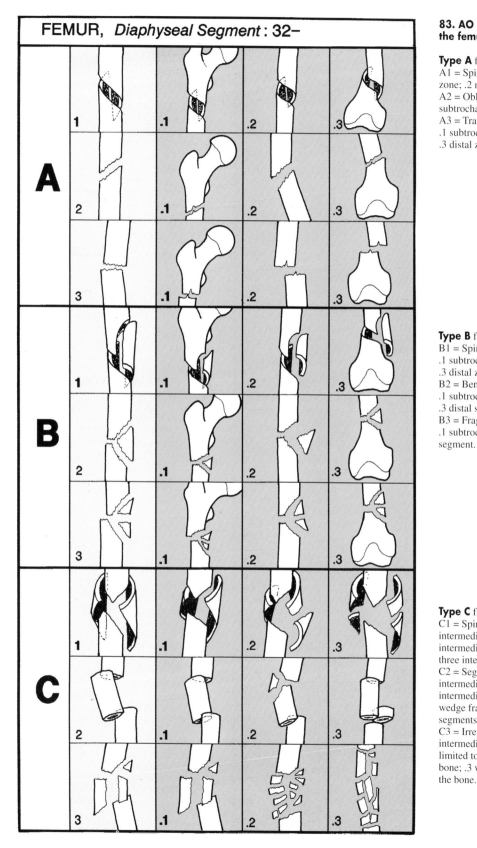

FEMUR, *Diaphyseal Segment : 32–*

83. AO classification of fractures of the femur, diaphyseal segment (32–):

Type A fractures are simple.
A1 = Spiral fractures: .1 subtrochanteric zone; .2 midshaft; .3 distal zone.
A2 = Oblique fracture (30° or more): .1 subtrochanteric; .2 midshaft; .3 distal zone.
A3 = Transverse fractures:
.1 subtrochanteric; .2 midshaft;
.3 distal zone.

Type B fractures are wedge fractures.
B1 = Spiral wedge fractures:
.1 subtrochanteric; .2 midshaft;
.3 distal zone.
B2 = Bending wedge fractures:
.1 subtrochanteric; .2 midshaft;
.3 distal segment.
B3 = Fragmented wedge fractures:
.1 subtrochanteric; .2 midshaft; .3 distal
segment.

Type C fractures are complex.
C1 = Spiral fractures: .1 with two
intermediate fragments; .2 with three
intermediate fragments; .3 with more than
three intermediate fragments.
C2 = Segmental fractures: .1 with one
intermediate segment; .2 with one
intermediate segment and an additional
wedge fracture; .3 with two intermediate
segments.
C3 = Irregular fractures: .1 with two or three
intermediate fragments; .2 with shattering
limited to less than a 5 cm length of the
bone; .3 with shattering over 5 cm or more of
the bone.

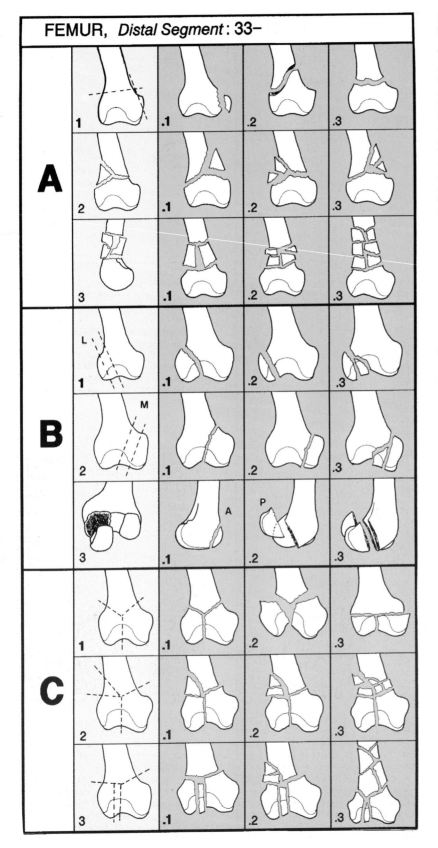

FEMUR, *Distal Segment* : 33–

84. AO classification of fractures of the femur, distal segment (33–):

Type A fractures are extra-articular.
A1 = Simple fractures: .1 avulsion fractures of the medial or lateral epicondyle; .2 fracture of the metaphysis, oblique or spiral; .3 fracture of the metaphysis, transverse.
A2 = Metaphyseal wedge fractures: .1 wedge intact; .2 lateral multifragmented wedge; .3 multifragmented medial wedge.
A3 = Complex metaphyseal fracture: .1 with a split intermediate segment; .2 irregular, but limited to the metaphysis; .3 irregular, and extending up into the diaphysis.

Type B fractures are partial articular.
B1 = Lateral condylar fractures in the sagittal plane: .1 simple through the intercondylar notch; .2 simple through the weight bearing surface; .3 multifragmentary.
B2 = Medial condylar fractures in the sagittal plane: .1 simple through the intercondylar notch; .2 simple through the weight bearing surface; .3 multifragmentary.
B3 = Frontal plane fractures: .1 flake fracture, anterior and lateral; .2 posterior unicondylar; .3 posterior bicondylar.

Type C fractures are complete articular.
C1 = Simple fractures of both the articular surface and the metaphysis: .1 slightly displaced T- or Y-fracture; .2 markedly displaced T- or Y-fracture; .3 distally situated T-fracture with the horizontal element involving the epiphysis.
C2 = Simple fracture of the articular surface, multifragmentary of the metaphysis: .1 with intact wedge; .2 multifragmented wedge; .3 complex.
C3 = Multifragmentary of the articular surface: .1 metaphyseal simple; .2 multifragmentary of the metaphysis; .3 multifragmentary of the metaphysis, extending into the shaft.

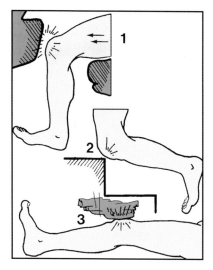

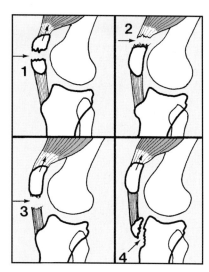

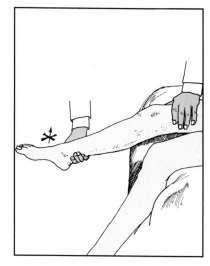

85. Injuries of the patella and extensor mechanism of the knee – Mechanisms (a): The *patella* may be fractured by direct violence, e.g. in road traffic accidents in which the knee strikes the fascia (1) (note the association between fracture of the patella, fracture of the femoral shaft and dislocation of the hip); by falls against a hard surface, e.g. the edge of a step (2); by heavy objects falling across the knee (e.g. falling rock) (3).

86. Mechanisms (b): The patella may also be fractured by indirect violence, i.e. as a result of a sudden muscular contraction (1). This same mechanism may also cause: rupture of the quadriceps tendon (2), rupture of the patellar ligament (3), or avulsion of the tibial tubercle (4).

87. Diagnosis (a): Fracture of the patella should be suspected when there is a history of direct violence to the knee; fracture of the patella and other injuries to the extensor mechanism should be suspected when there is difficulty in standing after a sudden muscular effort (especially when there is a snapping sensation within the knee). In many cases *there is inability to straight leg raise*, and in most cases *there is inability to extend the knee.*

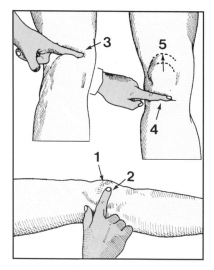

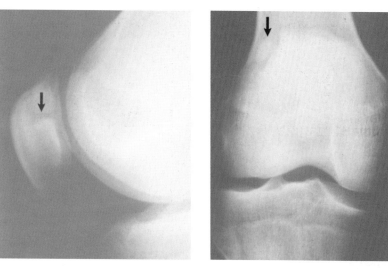

88. Diagnosis (b): Note clinically any of the following: bruising and abrasions (1); the presence and site of tenderness (2); any palpable gap above the patella (3) or beneath it (4); any obvious proximal displacement of the patella (5).

89. Diagnosis (c): In all cases, radiographs are essential to clarify the diagnosis. An AP projection and a lateral (preferably in extension) will generally suffice. In the acute case tangential projections cannot usually be obtained because of pain, but these views are often of value in cases which present late. If there is remaining doubt over the integrity of the patella, oblique projections may be helpful. Do not mistake a congenital bipartite patella (Illus.) for a fracture. This anomaly most frequently affects the *upper* and *outer* quadrant; it may be obvious in one view only. The edges are usually rounded, and this may help to differentiate it from a fracture. Other anomalies, such as tripartite patella, may also be distinguished by similar rounding and absence of local tenderness. Do not mistake non-traumatic patella alta for a ruptured patellar ligament. Ultrasound and MRI scans may be helpful in confirming the diagnosis in cases of rupture of the quadriceps tendon or the patellar ligament.

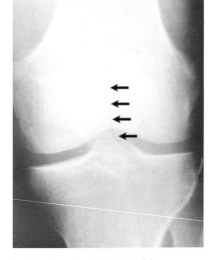

90. Treatment (a) – Vertical fractures:
Fractures of this type are usually undisplaced and stable. They do not show in the lateral radiographs. In the AP view, the overlapping femoral shadow may make them difficult to detect, and in fact these fractures are frequently missed. Conservative treatment only is required.

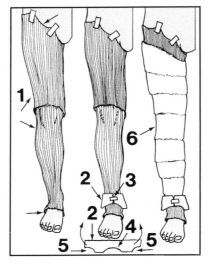

91. Treatment (b): A 6 week period in a cylinder plaster (plaster cylinder, pipestem plaster) is usually advised. *Method:* Apply a layer of stockinet (two pieces) from the hind foot to the groin (1). Protect the malleoli with a piece of felt (2), holding the butt-joined ends with adhesive tape (3). Note concavities for the Achilles tendon (4) and dorsum of the foot (5). Pad the leg with wool (6).

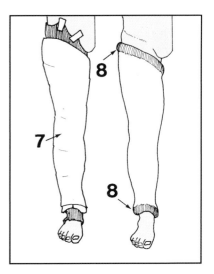

92. Treatment (c): The knee is normally kept in full extension (but not in recurvatum or hyperextension) while 20 cm (8″) plaster bandages are applied (7). A slab is not necessary. The edges of the stockinet are turned back before completion (8). Crutches are usually advised for the first 2 weeks, with a total of 6 weeks in plaster. As an alternative to a plaster cast, many prefer to use a plastic knee splint (e.g. by Zimmer) for about 3 weeks, followed by a further 3 weeks in a hinged knee brace.

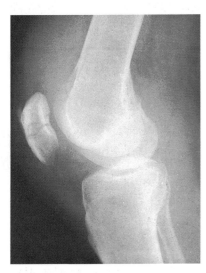

93. Undisplaced horizontal fractures:
Undisplaced horizontal fractures (even with some comminution) may be treated along similar lines with, however, radiographs at weekly intervals for the first 2–3 weeks to exclude late separation. After removal of the plaster or brace at 6 weeks, physiotherapy will be required, and crutches may be needed again for the first few weeks until confidence is regained.

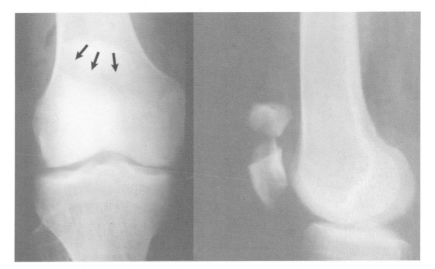

94. Displaced horizontal fractures: Fractures of this type should be explored so that:
1. The exact nature of the pathology may be determined; 2. The appropriate treatment carried out. Knee function after patellectomy is often excellent, but may fall a little short of perfect; although a full range of movements may be regained, there is often a feeling of instability while descending steep slopes, and there may be some weakness in rising from the squatting position. The patella should therefore be preserved, but only if the articular surface can be perfectly restored and maintained in that position until union occurs. In practice, this is only usually possible when there is no fragmentation, and although the radiographs (Illus.) may suggest that only two fragments are present, this can only be confirmed at exploration.

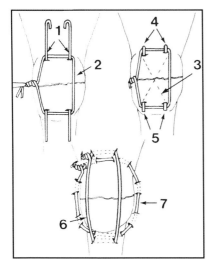

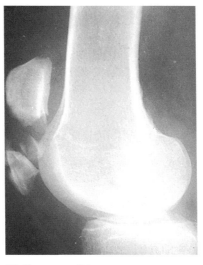

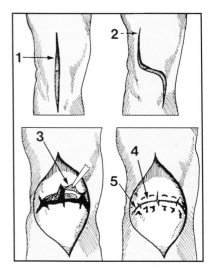

95. Treatment (a): If the joint surface can be restored, the fragments may be held by AO tension band wiring: two hooked K-wires (1) are inserted, round which is looped a wire (2) tightened by twisting. A second wire in a figure of eight (3) may be used (as may a figure of eight with the inferior limb in a hole drilled through the patella). The K-wires are sunk home (4) and trimmed (5). *Pyrford wiring* which uses a wire loop (6) and purse string (7) is strong, but is not advised because of the risks of avascular necrosis of the patella.

96. Treatment (b): If the joint surfaces cannot be restored and held, or if, as illustrated, there is much fragmentation, a complete patellar excision should be carried out, with repair of the quadriceps insertion and lateral expansions (which are invariably damaged). Note, however, that if the damage is confined to one pole of the patella, and the major part of the patella is spared, then good results can be obtained by *partial patellectomy.*

97. Treatment (c): For exploration or excision, the patella may be exposed through a midline vertical incision (best where further surgery is required) (1) or a lazy S (2) with the raising of two flaps. The patellar fragments are carefully dissected free, taking care that every piece is removed (3). The insertion (4) along with the lateral expansions (5) are repaired with mattress sutures and a plaster cylinder applied. Crutches should be used for 4 weeks and mobilisation commenced at 6 weeks.

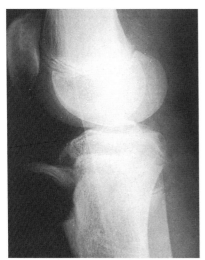

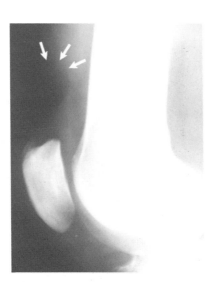

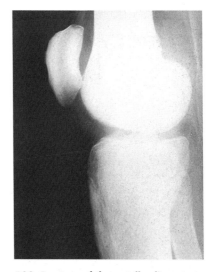

98. Avulsion fractures of the tibial tubercle: In the adult or adolescent near skeletal maturity (Illus.) the displacement, if marked, should be reduced and the tubercle fixed with a screw. If displacement is slight, a 6 week period in a plaster cylinder should suffice. In children, surgery should be avoided if possible because of the risks of premature epiphyseal fusion but, if manipulative reduction fails, open reduction and fixing with a suture may become necessary.

99. Rupture of the quadriceps tendon: The diagnosis is essentially clinical; it may sometimes be suggested by examination of the soft tissue shadows on the radiographs (Illus.), or by ultrasound. The tendon must be re-attached surgically; and it is often necessary to drill the patella to provide anchorage for the sutures. Thereafter a plaster cylinder is applied. Quadriceps exercises are commenced at 2 weeks, weight bearing at 4 weeks and knee flexion at 6 weeks.

100. Rupture of the patellar ligament: The clinical diagnosis may be confirmed by proximal displacement of the patella in the plane films (Illus.), or by ultrasound. The tendon should be repaired, and a quadrilateral wire (through the patella and tibial tubercle, retained for six weeks) will reduce tension in the sutures. With avulsions of the distal tip of the patella, remove the bony fragments and re-attach the ligament (with holes drilled through the patella) and use a tension relieving wire.

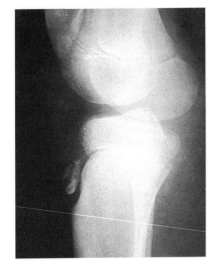

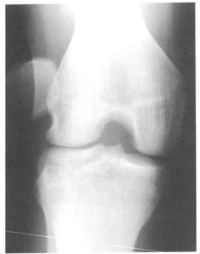

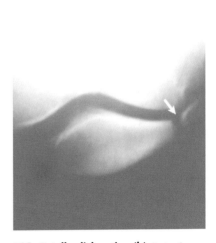

101. Osgood Schlatter's disease: In children, sudden or repeated quadriceps contraction may be responsible for this condition, which is characterised by recurrent pain, tenderness, and swelling over the tibial tubercle. It may be mistaken for an acute injury. While slow spontaneous resolution is the rule, an acute episode may be treated by 2 weeks in a plaster cylinder. Severe persistent symptoms occasionally merit excision of the detached fragment.

102. Acute lateral dislocation of the patella (a): The patella dislocates laterally, often as a result of sudden muscular contraction or a blow on its medial border. It may be reduced (unless of long standing) by applying firm lateral pressure (anaesthesia is seldom required). If a first incident, a 6 week period of plaster fixation is advised; if not, apply a pressure bandage for 1–2 weeks. Some prefer early arthroscopy, washing out blood and any loose bodies, re-attaching any large osteochondral fragment, and early mobilisation.

103. Patella dislocation (b): Lateral dislocation commonly occurs as a first or subsequent incident in the course of recurrent dislocation of the patella, a condition seen most frequently in teenage girls. The presence on the tangential projection of the knee of a marginal osteochondral fracture is diagnostic, but may not be obvious until some weeks after a first incident (which may also be overlooked if spontaneous reduction occurs).

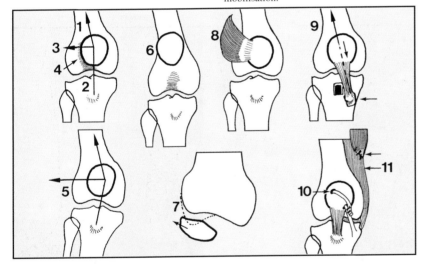

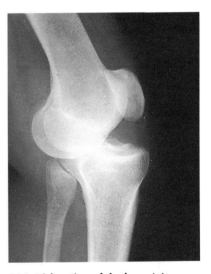

104. Patella dislocation (c): As the femur meets the tibia at an angle, the quadriceps (1) and patellar ligament (2) have a *lateral component* (3) during muscle contraction; this is greater where there is genu valgum (5); it is resisted by the femoral gutter (4). An error in tracking may cause the patella to dislocate. When this *starts in extension*, patella alta (6) or an abnormal quadriceps insertion (8) may be factors. In these particular cases a re-alignment procedure may be required (e.g. Elmslie–Trillat, Hauser (9)) or Galeazzi; in the latter, more suitable in the adolescent, the divided semitendinosus tendon is threaded through a hole in the patella (10), and the stump sewn to semimembranosus (11). Where the dislocation occurs *in flexion* there may be hypoplasia of the patella or lateral femoral condyle (7), with a shallow sulcus and tilting of the patella. Such cases may respond to a lateral tissue (vastus lateralis) release, with or without medial reefing, but they may also require a re-alignment procedure. If there is no tracking problem, ligament laxity is sometimes blamed. Many respond to physiotherapy (concentrating on the oblique fibres of vastus medialis) and the use of a knee brace during athletic activities.

105. Dislocation of the knee (a): Surprisingly, this injury may follow comparatively minor trauma. Most commonly the tibia is displaced anteriorly, but medial, lateral, posterior and rotational displacements are also found. There is inevitably major damage to the ligaments of the knee; all or most may be torn along with the joint capsule. Note that clinical examination has been shown to give a more accurate assessment of ligamentous damage than MRI scanning.

106. Dislocation of the knee (b):
Sometimes there is displacement of the menisci, fractures of the tibial spines, common peroneal nerve palsy and, most seriously, popliteal artery damage.

Treatment: Closed reduction should be carried out as expeditiously as possible. Reduction is generally easy, and may be achieved with traction and the application of pressure over the displaced tibia. Thereafter, these injuries may be treated conservatively or surgically.

In the *conservative management* of these cases, where surprisingly good results preponderate, the leg should be supported after reduction by light traction (2–3 kg/6 lb) in a Thomas splint for 3–4 weeks; this may be followed by a further 4 weeks in a plaster cylinder before mobilisation is commenced.

Surgery is indicated in the following circumstances: 1. If closed reduction fails (generally due to button-holing of the capsule by a femoral condyle); 2. If there is persistent circulatory impairment in the limb after reduction, when popliteal artery exploration is indicated; 3. If there is a common peroneal nerve palsy, also persisting after reduction, and where it is thought that exploration and possible nerve decompression might be of benefit.

In addition, some advocate exploration and ligament repair after closed reduction in all cases of dislocation of the knee. The formal repair may be delayed for some days after the closed reduction.

107. Soft tissue injuries of the knee:
When there has been trauma to the knee and the radiographs show little in the way of bony injury, the possibility of a significant soft tissue injury should be considered. It would be unrealistic to say that injuries of this type are easy to diagnose; they sometimes are, but often cause much difficulty. There is the common clinical picture of pain in the knee, swelling, and difficulty in weight bearing shared by many lesions. Investigation of each case should aim first to localise the injury to a specific structure, although it must be accepted that localising tenderness may be difficult to ascertain where there has been an associated fracture in the region. An attempt should be made to exclude the following:
1. Damage to the extensor apparatus;
2. Lateral dislocation of the patella with spontaneous reduction;
3. Tears of the ligaments of the knee;
4. Meniscus tears.

In some centres, when the injury is suspected of being more than trivial, further investigation is pursued in an aggressive fashion: any haemarthrosis is aspirated, and the soft tissue elements examined directly by arthroscopy, or indirectly by MRI scan. Note that the presence of a substantial haemarthrosis is generally associated with damage to a major structural element. Aspiration is generally required to permit a more meaningful examination, and general anaesthesia is advisable. Any suggestion of locking or other evidence of meniscal damage merits further investigation by arthroscopy or MRI scan (because if a meniscus is torn and suitable for surgical repair, this is best undertaken within 4 weeks of the injury).

If there is no hard evidence to implicate any of the major soft tissue structures (and this is so in the *majority* of cases) a provisional (and rather unsatisfactory) diagnosis of 'knee sprain' or 'sprained ligaments with traumatic effusion' may be made, and the case treated appropriately (e.g. by the application of a crepe bandage support, Jones pressure bandage, or circular woven bandage (Tubigrip®)). The case should be re-assessed at weekly intervals thereafter until either the symptoms have settled completely, or a more accurate diagnosis can be established.

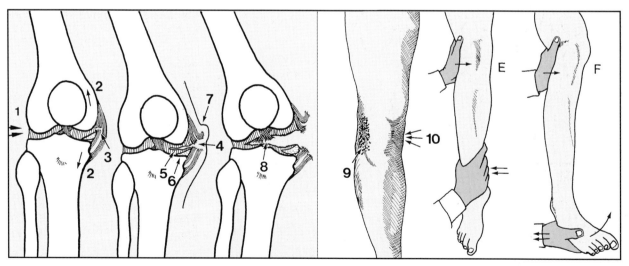

108. Medial ligament injuries:
The commonest cause is a blow on the lateral side of the knee (1) which forces the joint into valgus (2). With slight force, there is partial tearing of the medial ligament (knee sprain) and the knee remains stable on clinical testing. With greater violence, the deep portion of the ligament ruptures (partial tear) (3); stressing the knee in 30° flexion with the foot internally rotated (F) causes more opening up of the joint than normal, but stressing the joint in extension (E) has no effect. There may be clinical evidence of rotatory instability. With greater violence, superficial *and* deep parts of the ligament rupture (4) and the tear rapidly spreads across the posterior ligament (5). The medial meniscus (6) may also tear. When the knee is stressed in extension (E) slight to moderate opening up will be noted, and if the edge of the ligament rolls over it may be felt subcutaneously (7). With severe violence, the cruciates (especially the anterior cruciate) rupture (8) and the joint opens widely on stressing as at (E). Bruising on the lateral side (9) and medial tenderness (10) are suggestive of medial ligament damage. If there is remaining doubt regarding its integrity, repeat clinical tests after aspiration, or take stress radiographs, comparing one side with the other.

109. Medial ligament injuries (b) – Treatment

(a) Sprain: Crepe bandages or a Jones pressure bandage should be applied and the patient given crutches to use until the acute symptoms have settled: review at least twice.

(b) Isolated tear, with no evidence of 'rolling over' of the medial ligament: POP fixation *with the knee at 45° flexion* for 8 weeks, or the use of a limited motion (30°–60°) knee brace. Review at one week to exclude associated meniscal injury.

(c) Major tear: If isolated and uncomplicated, conservative management may be pursued (e.g. with a limited motion brace) and a good result expected. If under anaesthesia gross instability is found, this is suggestive of posterior capsular tearing and/or involvement of other major structures. Exploration and repair of the medial ligament and posteromedial capsule are then advised. An associated meniscus injury should be carefully assessed and treated on its merits: the meniscus should be preserved if feasible, and in some cases it may be possible to re-attach or repair it. If the anterior cruciate ligament has been detached or torn, it may be re-attached or repaired, or this deferred until later when knee movements have been regained.

Complications of medial ligament injury – (a) Late valgus instability: It

may be possible to improve stability by a reconstructive procedure; semitendinosus may be rerouted and used to reinforce a

defective medial ligament, or a prosthetic ligament replacement may be carried out.

(b) Persistent rotatory instability:

Improvement may follow a medial capsular repair and pes anserinus transposition, although the late results are often disappointing.

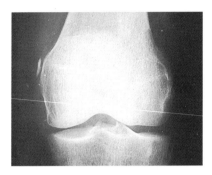

110. Pelligrini–Stieda disease: A valgus strain of the knee may produce partial avulsion of the medial ligament, with subsequent calcification in the subperiosteal haematoma. There is prolonged pain and local tenderness, with limitation of flexion, but no instability. In the acute phase, plaster, immobilisation for 2–3 weeks is advised, followed by mobilisation. Local hydrocortisone infiltrations are sometimes advocated for the chronic case.

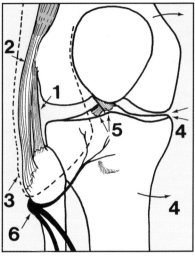

111. Injuries to the lateral ligament

(a): The lateral ligament (1) is part of a complex which includes the biceps femoris tendon (2) and the fascia lata (3) attached to tibia, fibula and patella. All these structures may be damaged if the knee is subjected to a varus stress (4), and with severe violence the cruciates (5) will also be torn. The common peroneal nerve (6) may be stretched or torn.

114. Lateral ligament (c) cntd:

Treatment cntd: 2. If there is instability, operative repair of the ligament and repair of the posterolateral capsule (if involved) is indicated, unless there is a definite, undisplaced fracture which seems likely to go on to union; in such circumstances a plaster cylinder should be applied and retained for 6–8 weeks before mobilisation. 3. Common peroneal nerve palsy, if present, is likely to be due either to a lesion in continuity, or a complete disruption of the nerve over an extensive area. If the ligament is being repaired, the opportunity should be taken to inspect the nerve. (Some advocate exploration of the nerve in all cases, irrespective of the need for repair of the lateral ligament, holding the view that this gives the opportunity of carrying out a local decompression should this be required, and thereby perhaps aiding recovery.) In all cases treatment for drop foot should be started. With a lesion in continuity, recovery usually starts within 6 weeks, but a disruptive lesion carries a poor prognosis.

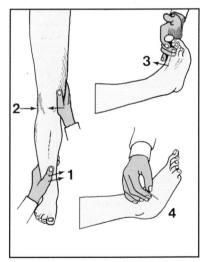

112. Lateral ligament (b): Test the stability of the knee by applying a varus stress with the knee in extension (1), looking for opening-up of the joint on the lateral side (2). Test for common peroneal involvement by looking for weakness of dorsiflexion of the foot and toes (3), and/or sensory loss on the dorsum of the foot and side of the leg (4).

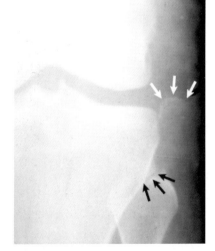

113. Lateral ligament (c): In some cases the radiographs may show tell-tale avulsion fractures of the fibular head or tibia. (Illus.: Note a small undisplaced fracture of the head of the fibula produced by the lateral ligament (the fracture highlighted with black arrows), and a large displaced fragment (indicated with white arrows) avulsed by the biceps.) *Treatment:* 1. If the knee is clinically stable, symptomatic treatment only is required (e.g. a crepe bandage and crutches).

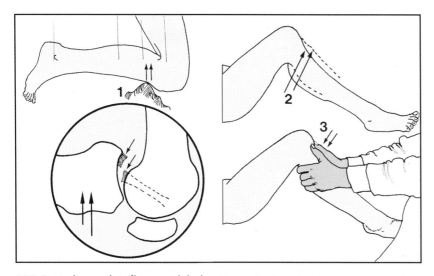

116. Posterior cruciate ligament injuries cntd: (c) Radiographs may show avulsion fractures of the posterior cruciate ligament attachments.

Treatment: If untreated, and instability persists, disability is considerable, and osteoarthritis often advances with great rapidity.
1. If there is an undisplaced fracture of the posterior tibial spine representing an avulsion of the posterior attachment of the ligament, the leg should be kept in a plaster cylinder for 6–8 weeks before mobilisation. (Some however advocate internal fixation irrespective of the pattern of injury.)
2. A displaced tibial spine fracture should be reduced and held with a screw.
3. A detached ligament should be re-attached to bone.

   As the majority of detachments are posterior, procedures 2. and 3. involve a posterior (popliteal) approach to the knee.

115. Posterior cruciate ligament injuries: The mechanism whereby the posterior cruciate ligament is damaged is usually either a fall, in which the tibia strikes a rock or some other object and is forced backwards (1) or from dashboard impact in road traffic accidents. There is often associated damage to the medial or lateral ligaments.

Diagnosis: (a) In most cases there is a striking alteration in the profile of the knee when placed in flexion: the tibia sags backwards (2) and this explains why the anterior drawer test (for the *anterior* cruciate ligament) often gives a false positive; the displaced tibia can be pulled forward to the normal position. (b) The posterior drawer sign may be positive (3). If there is remaining doubt, the knee should be aspirated and examined under anaesthetic.

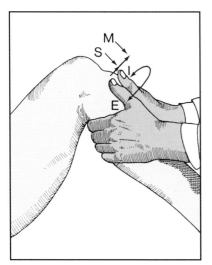

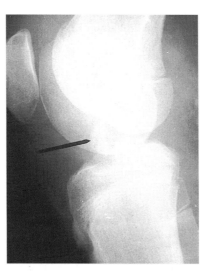

117. Anterior cruciate ligament tears (a): Isolated tears are uncommon (forced flexion or hyperextension injuries); tears of the medial ligament and/or medial meniscus may be associated.

Diagnosis: 1. Note variations in the anterior drawer sign: slight slip + internal rotation of the tibia (S + I) = isolated anterior cruciate tear; slight slip + external rotation (S + E) = medial ligament tear; marked slip without rotation (M) = tear anterior cruciate + medial ligament.

118. Anterior cruciate ligament tears (b): *Diagnosis:* 2. Carefully examine AP and lateral radiographs of the knee, looking for tell-tale avulsion fractures (Illus.: Avulsion of the anterior attachment indicated with pointer). Independently test the medial ligament, and look for evidence of meniscus injury. Consider performing an arthroscopy or MRI to obtain unequivocal evidence of concurrent meniscal and cruciate ligament tears. Radiographs may also be used to assess anterior cruciate function.

119. Anterior cruciate ligament tears (c): *Treatment:* 1. If the anterior tibial spine is undisplaced, treat with a 6–8 week period of fixation in a plaster cylinder. 2. If there is a substantial tibial spine fracture which is displaced, it should be carefully repositioned at open operation and fixed with a screw. 3. If the anterior attachment of the ligament is avulsed, it may be re-attached to bone; it may also be left and the need for a formal reconstruction assessed at a later date on the basis of instability. 4. The results of immediate surgical treatment of tears of the central portion of the anterior cruciate ligament are somewhat uncertain. In some cases, it may be possible to effect a direct repair, but generally the shredding and attenuation of the torn ends render this ineffective. An augmented repair (which seems to give the best results) or a secondary reconstruction may be possible, using for example: (a) A portion of the patellar ligament and part of the patella (used to anchor the end of the 'new' ligament); (b) Part of the iliotibial tract formed into a tube pedicle anchored with a block of bone; (c) the use of semitendinosus, gracilis or both. 5. Associated tears of the medial meniscus and medial ligament take precedence in treatment. Any minor instability may be dealt with by intensive quadriceps building and the judicious use of a dynamic knee brace; if there is any significant instability, surgical reconstruction should be considered.

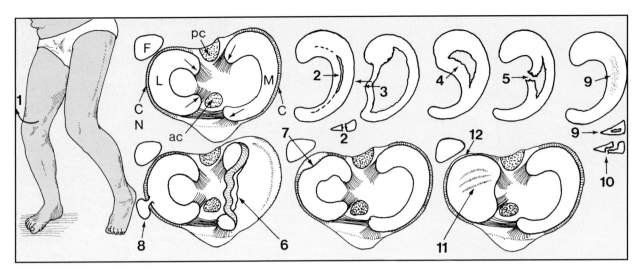

120. Meniscus injuries: In the young adult, the menisci are generally injured as a result of a rotational stress applied to the flexed, weight bearing knee (1). Injury can also result from rapid knee extension (anterior horn tears) and direct violence (cysts). The medial (M) and lateral (L) menisci are attached at their anterior and posterior horns to the tibia, and by coronary ligaments (C) to the femur and tibia. The majority of tears commence as vertical splits in the substance of the meniscus

('longitudinal tear') (2); the free edge may displace centrally, forming a bucket handle tear (3) or a racquet tear of the posterior (4) or anterior horns. The central edge may rupture forming a parrot-beak tear (5). In peripheral detachments the whole meniscus may displace centrally (6) or, more commonly, the posterior horn only of the lateral meniscus is affected (7). Congenital discoid menisci may also become detached (12) with ridging of their upper surfaces (11) – a common condition in children.

Detachments of the anterior horn also occur, but are less common. A meniscus cyst (8) may result from a direct blow (such as a kick) and the lateral meniscus is most commonly affected. Cysts of the medial meniscus must be distinguished from pes anserinus ganglions. In middle age, horizontal tears may occur within the substance of the meniscus (9), sometimes without trauma, and may convert to tears with potential for displacement (10).

121. Diagnosis of meniscus injuries – Note the following points:
1. Acute tears in the young adult generally result from a clear-cut incident of weight bearing stress, often while engaging in an athletic pursuit such as football. There is immediate pain in the knee and difficulty in weight bearing. Initial disability is usually marked, and if the patient has been playing football, they will be unable to continue – this important aspect of the history should be clarified. Locking, if present and shown to be true, is a very important finding.
2. Meniscus tears are very uncommon in women. Dislocation of the patella or chondromalacia patellae should always be eliminated before the diagnosis of a torn meniscus is contemplated in women.
3. Absence of knee swelling may be deceptive. After peripheral tears there is certainly usually a rapidly forming haemarthrosis but there may be no immediate swelling after longitudinal tears (the menisci are avascular). Any reactionary synovitis may appear quite late (e.g. several days) after the initial incident.
4. There is almost invariably joint line tenderness, but as many minor lesions give this finding this is of little diagnostic value apart from localisation to either side of the joint.

5. A springy block to full extension is almost diagnostic of a displaced, bucket handle tear.
6. Some days after the first incident other signs may appear, such as quadriceps wasting and slight oedema in the joint line. When pain subsides, other confirmatory tests such as MacMurray's manoeuvre may give positive results.
7. Radiographs should always be taken to exclude other pathology.
8. In chronic lesions, positive physical signs are often lacking, and further investigation may be required (e.g. by arthroscopy, MRI scan, arthrography, provocative exercises).

Treatment

1. *Locked knee:* Admit at an early date for surgical treatment. Pending admission, a pressure bandage support, crutches, and analgesics may be prescribed. Attempts to unlock the knee are of questionable value.
2. *In other cases where the history and findings suggest a fresh meniscus tear:* Treat conservatively. Remember that peripheral detachments can unite, and that many joint injuries may mimic a torn meniscus yet recover completely. A pressure bandage should be applied, the patient given crutches and advised to practise quadriceps exercises. Analgesics may be required. If the knee fails

to settle within 2 weeks, the usual practice is to perform a diagnostic arthroscopy followed by the procedure appropriate to the findings and available facilities. In general terms, the aim should be to preserve any part of the meniscus that can be made to make a contribution to the proper functioning of the knee (e.g. excision of the central portion only of a bucket handle tear, leaving an intact peripheral rim). Where the meniscus is detached at the periphery, or where there is a tear through the vascular peripheral margin of the meniscus, re-attachment or repair may be carried out. In many cases it is possible to do this using the arthroscope, and without opening the joint: this may make it possible to mobilise the patient at a very early stage, and may shorten the initial period of convalescence. Repair is best undertaken within four weeks of injury. It is not suitable for chronic or horizontal cleavage tears.
3. *Meniscus cysts:* Excise the cyst. In addition, many advocate removal of the associated meniscus which is not infrequently torn.
4. *Horizontal cleavage tears:* Symptoms may resolve with physiotherapy alone, and meniscectomy may frequently be avoided.

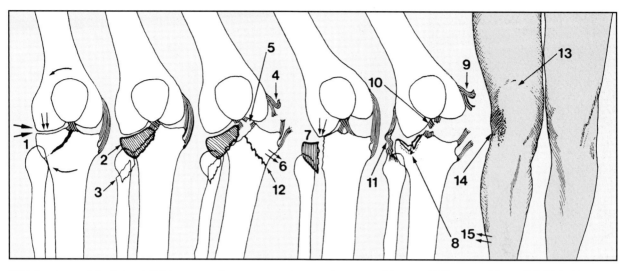

122. Fractures of the lateral tibial table: These generally result from a severe valgus stress, and several patterns of injury are found.

(a) Impact of the mass of the lateral femoral condyle may be responsible for the 'sliding fracture' which passes downwards and laterally from the tibial spine region, the main articular surface remaining intact (1). With increasing violence the tibial fragment is depressed (2) and there may be an associated fracture of the fibular neck (3). In the severe cases there may be rupture of the medial ligament (4), rupture of the cruciates (5), and medial subluxation of the tibia (6).

(b) The 'corner' of the lateral femoral condyle may cause a split fracture (7); or

(c) A crush fracture (8) of the tibial table. In either of these cases there may be tearing of the medial ligament (9), or the cruciates (10), relative lengthening of the lateral ligament (11), or crushing of the lateral meniscus.

(d) A second fracture line (12) may convert any of these injuries into a bicondylar fracture.

(e) Fractures of the medial tibial table are uncommon, but do occur. They may be associated with lateral ligament ruptures and common peroneal nerve palsy. (Their treatment is along similar lines to lateral tibial table injuries.)

Diagnosis (a): The clinical findings of lateral tibial table fracture include: haemarthrosis (13), lateral bruising and abrasions (14), valgus deformity of the knee (15).

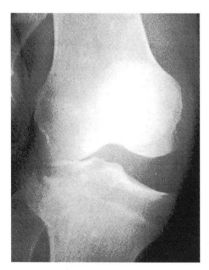

123. Diagnosis (b): This is confirmed by radiographs, an AP view with a 15° tube tilt giving the most information. Measure the maximal depression of any fragment relative to neighbouring intact bone or a line projected from the (intact) medial table. If the medial ligament is suspect (e.g. local tenderness, etc.) stress films (preferably after aspiration and under GA) may be helpful. (Illus.: Small split fracture with stress films showing medial ligament tear.)

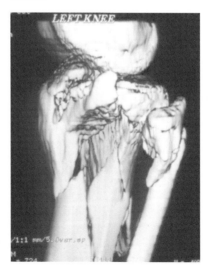

124. Diagnosis (c): The state of the tibial table and the articular surface in particular may be assessed with CAT scans. With 3D reconstructions (Illus.) which can be rotated on the screen it becomes possible to assess the extent of major fragment displacements and the state of the articular surfaces with great clarity.

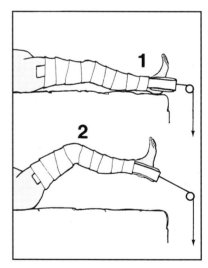

125. Treatment (a): *No ligament damage, no tibial subluxation, and a table depression of less than 10 mm.* Apply skin traction of 3 kg (6–7 lb) (1); quadriceps exercises should be commenced immediately and flexion as soon as pain will permit (2). Traction may often be discontinued after 4 weeks; weight bearing may be permitted after 8 weeks. The late results are generally excellent. Alternatively, fix the lateral table with cannulated cancellous screws inserted percutaneously.

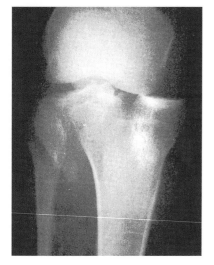

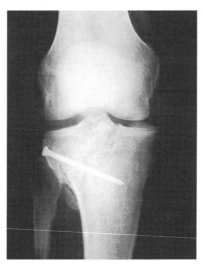

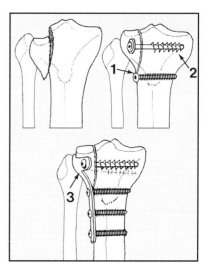

126. Treatment (b): *Fractures displaced by more than 10 mm (i).* If the displacement is more than 10 mm and is not reduced, there will be persistent valgus deformity of the knee, and often some residual instability leading to appreciable disability. Note in the illustration the large lateral fragment and the medial subluxation of the tibia of a degree suggesting some associated damage to the medial ligament.

127. Treatment (c): *Fractures displaced by more than 10 mm (ii).* These injuries should be treated by open reduction and internal fixation. When the fracture has been fixed, the medial ligament should be re-tested, and if found to be ruptured it should be repaired. It may also be possible to re-attach any displaced meniscus using absorbable sutures. (The radiograph shows the previous fracture after open reduction and internal fixation with a single cortical screw: it has gone on to union.)

128. Treatment (d): *Fractures displaced by more than 10 mm (iii).* In some cases more stable fixation can be obtained using a cortical screw to lock the inferior margin of a lateral fragment (1), with one or more cancellous screws to obtain compression (2). If it is thought that the deforming forces are unlikely to be sufficiently countered by these measures, then a T- (3) or L-plate with the appropriate cortical and cancellous bone screws may be used. The AP and lateral alignment of the knee must be carefully assessed.

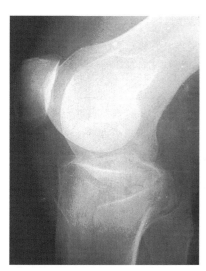

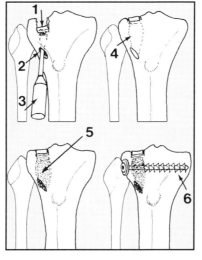

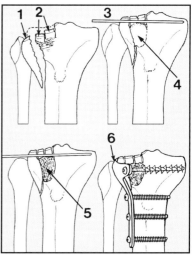

129. Treatment (e): If the articular surface of the tibial plateau is depressed more than 10 mm, even in the absence of depression of the upper lateral tibial margin, the chances of obtaining a good result by conservative treatment becomes less likely. In assessing the indications for surgery, the extent and degree of depression of the lateral tibial plateau may be apparent on AP or lateral (Illus.) radiographic projections; further information on the bony disturbance may be obtained by CAT scans and 3D reconstructions.

130. Treatment (f): It may be possible to elevate the bony depression (1) with its cartilaginous covering by making an opening (2) on the lateral tibial flare through which a narrow punch (3) may be inserted. Elevation inevitably leaves a defect (4) which should be tightly packed with bone grafts (5). It may be necessary to stabilise the fragments with a cross-screw (6). Visualisation may be enhanced by temporary elevation of the anterior horn of the meniscus. Then the ligaments should be tested and dealt with as required.

131. Treatment (g): Where there is depression of both the tibial margin (1) and the upper articular surface (2), reconstruction is technically more difficult. The steps in reconstruction that have been recommended are (i) Reduction of the fracture and temporary fixation with K-wires (3); (ii) Packing the remaining defect (4) with bone grafts (5); (iii) Supporting the fracture with a T- (6) or L-plate and the appropriate cancellous and cortical screws.

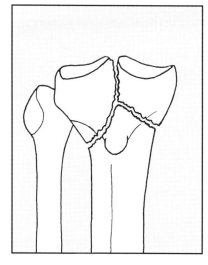

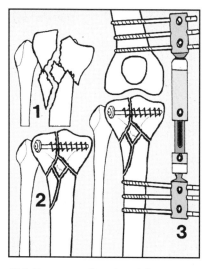

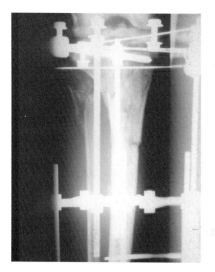

132. Treatment (h) – Bicondylar (Type C) fractures (a): If the displacement is minimal it is often possible to treat injuries of this pattern conservatively. This may be carried out with 6–8 weeks' traction, initially in a Thomas splint, and later, when pain has settled, by Hamilton–Russell or other traction methods which will permit early mobilisation of the knee.

133. Treatment (i) – Bicondylar (Type C) fractures (b): Where there are two main fragments (1) it may be possible to hold these in alignment with one or more cancellous screws (2). Additional support is required: a single buttress plate is usually inadequate, and bilateral plates are best avoided, carrying as they do a great risk of contributing to avascularity of the proximal tibia. An external fixator (3) may be used to maintain length. Later, a hinged link inserted between the pin holders may be employed to allow early knee movements.

134. Treatment (j) – Bicondylar (Type C) fractures (c): Alternatively, and especially where there are more than two main proximal tibial fragments, fixation may be achieved using fine wire methods. In many situations a hybrid system can give good results. (Note in the illustration a combination of a tibial shaft and a tibial plateau fracture, treated by a combination of fine wires and tibial pins.)

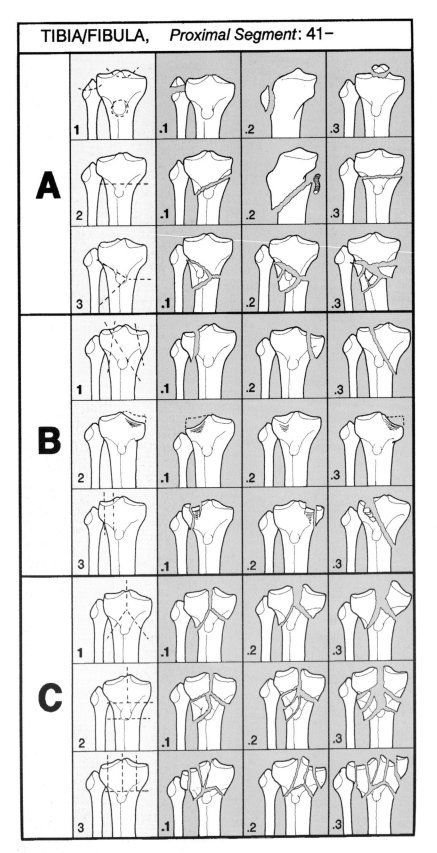

TIBIA/FIBULA, *Proximal Segment*: 41–

135. AO classification of fractures of the tibia/fibula, proximal segment (41–):

Type A fractures are all extra-articular.
A1 = Avulsion fractures: .1 of the head of the fibula (lateral ligament); .2 of the tibial tuberosity (patellar ligament); .3 of the tibial spines (cruciate ligaments).
A2 = Simple metaphyseal fractures:
.1 oblique from side to side; .2 oblique from posterior to anterior, often with vascular damage; .3 transverse.
A3 = Multifragmentary metaphyseal:
.1 wedge intact; .2 fragmented wedge;
.3 complex.

Type B fractures are partial articular.
B1 = Split fractures only: .1 lateral;
.2 medial; .3 including the area of the tibial spines and one tibial table.
B2 = Depressed fractures only: .1 all of the lateral tibial table; .2 part only of the lateral tibial table; .3 part or all of the medial tibial table.
B3 = Combined split and depression:
.1 lateral; .2 medial; .3 oblique, involving the tibial spines and one tibial table.

Type C fractures are complete articular.
C1 = Articular simple, metaphyseal simple:
.1 minimal displacement; .2 one condyle displaced; .3 both condyles displaced.
C2 = Articular simple, metaphyseal multifragmentary: .1 intact wedge;
.2 fragmented wedge; .3 complex.
C3 = Multifragmentary articular: .1 lateral;
.2 medial; .3 both lateral and medial.

SELF-TEST

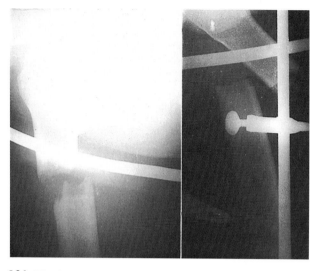

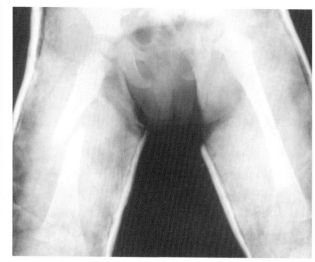

136. What is the level of fracture shown on these radiographs? How is it being treated? Is the position acceptable?

137. Describe the fracture and the method of treatment. Is the position acceptable?

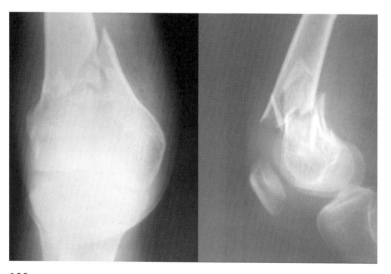

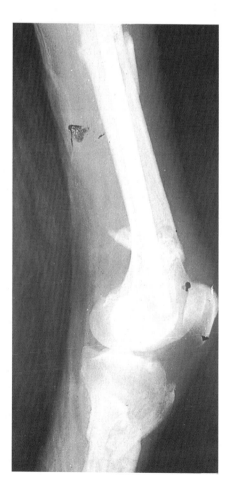

138. (Above) Describe this fracture. What is the unusual feature about the deformity? How might it be treated conservatively?

139. (Right) What fractures are present? What treatment is obvious?

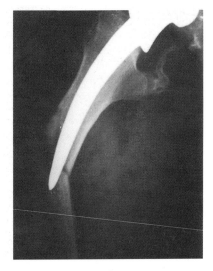

140. What does this radiograph show? How might this be dealt with?

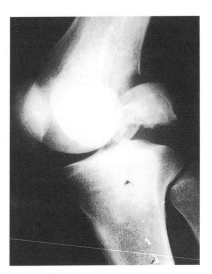

141. What fracture is present? What treatment should be carried out?

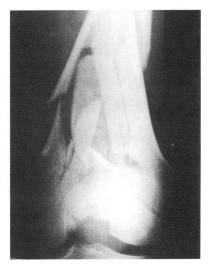

142. What fracture is present? What treatment might be advised?

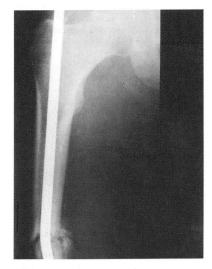

143. What fracture is shown on the radiograph? What complication has occurred, and what is its most likely cause? What would you advise?

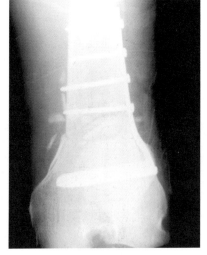

144. What fracture is present? How has it been fixed?

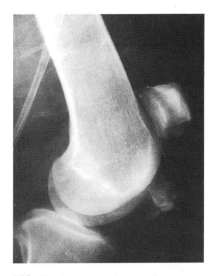

145. What fracture is shown on the radiograph? How might this be treated?

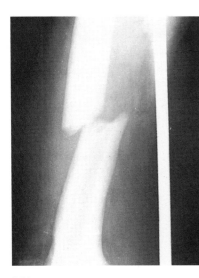

146. Describe this fracture: how is it being treated? Assuming conservative treatment was being continued, would you make any correction?

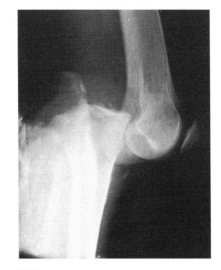

147. What does the radiograph show? What structure is at serious risk?

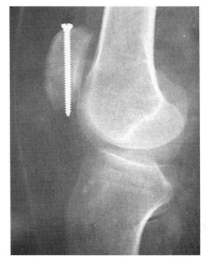

148. What is this fracture? How has it been treated? What alternative treatment might have been carried out?

ANSWERS TO SELF-TEST

136. Proximal third fracture of the femur being treated in a Thomas splint. The proximal fragment is flexed so that there is no bony apposition, and probably soft tissue between the bone ends. The position is unacceptable (risk of non-union or malunion) and internal fixation would be advocated. (AO = 32–A3.1)

137. Oblique fracture of the midshaft of the femur (with shortening and angulation) in a child. It is being treated in a plaster hip spica. The position is acceptable: union is likely to be rapid; the shortening will almost certainly resolve spontaneously; any residual angulation is also likely to disappear with remodelling. (AO = 32–A2.2)

138. Supracondylar fracture of the femur. Angulation is slight, and is in the reverse direction from normal. Traction in a straight Thomas splint might be used and mobilisation commenced at an early date. Alternatively, this fracture might be dealt with by Hamilton–Russell traction and cast bracing or internal fixation with a blade plate, a dynamic condylar screw or an intramedullary nail with interlocking screws. (AO = 33–A1.2)

139. There is a fracture of the midshaft of the femur and a supracondylar fracture, both held in alignment with an intramedullary nail. In addition, there is a fracture of the proximal third of the tibia. Such injuries are typical of high velocity road traffic accidents. (AO = 32–B1.2 + (33–A2.3 or 32–B2.3) + 41–A3)

140. Fracture of the femoral shaft at the level of the tip of a replacement arthroplasty prosthesis (Type B1 fracture). Treat by open reduction and internal fixation, e.g. using a plate and cerclage wiring (such as the Dall–Miles system).

141. Displaced, intra-articular fracture of the medial femoral condyle. Treat by open reduction and internal fixation with countersunk cancellous bone screws; otherwise non-union is likely even if reduction is achieved. Avascular necrosis of the fragment is probable. Were the fragment larger, a buttress plate would be considered. (AO = 33–B2.2)

142. Highly comminuted fracture of the distal third of the femur, with a fracture extending between the femoral condyles. Surgical reconstruction is likely to prove difficult due to the degree of comminution, but might be attempted using for example a screw-plate and cancellous screws. Alternatively conservation management with traction and early mobilisation should be considered. (AO = 33–C3.3)

143. Fracture of the midshaft of the femur, treated by intramedullary nailing. Union is incomplete and the nail has bent, with angulation of the femur because of premature weight bearing. The nail should be removed without delay, and a new nail substituted after reaming. Removal of the nail will obviously be difficult. It may be possible to straighten the bend by forcible manipulation, but if this fails it may be necessary to expose the fracture, saw through the nail and extract the two fragments separately. (AO = 32–A3.2)

144. Supracondylar fracture of the femur supported with a one-piece blade plate and screws. (AO = 32–A3.3)

145. Highly comminuted fracture of the distal portion of the patella, with retraction of the main fragment. The proportion of the patellar surface involved and the degree of comminution militates against preservation, and excision, with repair of the ruptured lateral expansions, would probably be the best procedure here.

146. Fracture of the femoral shaft at the junction between the middle and distal thirds, with posterior angulation (anterior tilting of the distal fragment). It is being treated in a Thomas splint (note the side iron). Traction should be increased, and further padding placed under the fracture to correct the angulation. (AO = 32–A2.2)

147. Dislocation of the knee (posterior dislocation with 90° rotational deformity superimposed). The popliteal artery is in grave danger.

148. A transverse fracture has been anatomically reduced and held with a single cortical screw. This method of fixation is prone to failure due to the magnitude of the distracting forces. A tension band wiring system is to be preferred.

CHAPTER
13
Fractures of the tibia

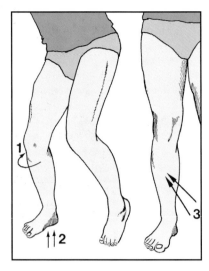

1. General principles (a) – Mechanisms of injury: The tibia is vulnerable to torsional stresses (1) (e.g. sporting injuries), to violence transmitted through the feet (2) (e.g. falls from a height, road traffic accidents), and from direct blows (3) (e.g. road traffic accidents, blows from falling rock, masonry, etc.).

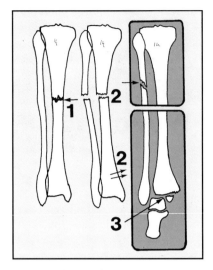

2. General principles (b): Isolated fractures of either the tibia or fibula may occur from direct violence (1), although this is comparatively uncommon. As in the case of the forearm bones, indirect violence leads to fracture of both tibia and fibula (2). Always obtain radiographs of the whole length of the limb to exclude a distal injury accompanying a proximal fracture (3).

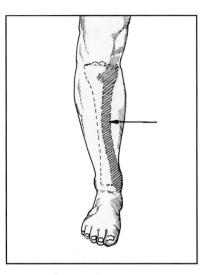

3. General principles (c): Note that a third of the tibia is subcutaneous. There is little to resist the spiky end of a fractured tibia from penetrating the skin; again, any direct violence to the shin is uncushioned, and the skin is readily split; these factors account for the fact that tibial fractures are often open (either from within out or from without in).

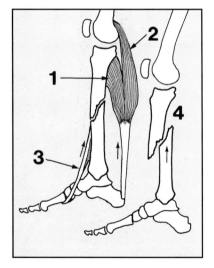

4. General principles (d): Partly because of its triangular shape, and partly because of the frequency of injury caused by torsional forces, oblique and spiral fractures of the tibia are common. Muscle tone in the soleus (1), gastrocnemius (2) and tibialis anterior (3) tends to produce shortening and displacement in fractures of this type (4).

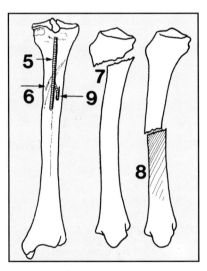

5. General principles (e): The popliteal artery (5) is anchored as it passes under the origin of the soleus at the soleal line (6). It is susceptible to damage in upper tibial fractures (7) and may cause Volkmann's ischaemia of the calf with permanent flexion contracture of the ankle. Fractures of the tibia may be followed by ischaemia of the distal fragment (8) caused by interruption of the blood supply through the nutrient artery (9).

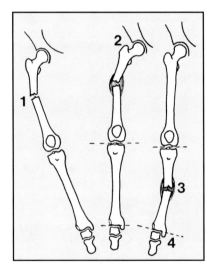

6. General principles (f): It is particularly important to correct angulation in fractures of this weight bearing bone. Unlike angulation in femoral shaft fractures (1), which can be compensated at the hip (2), residual angulation in tibial fractures (3) will throw inevitable stress at the ankle (4) and/or the knee, perhaps leading to pain and secondary osteoarthritis.

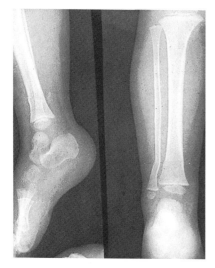

7. Undisplaced fractures (a): In children, owing to the thickness of the subcutaneous fat and periosteum, and the elasticity of the bones, fractures are often of greenstick pattern and closed. In many cases, too, the fractures are minimally displaced. (Illus.: Greenstick fracture distal tibia and fibula, betrayed by fibular kinking and tibial cortical buckling.)

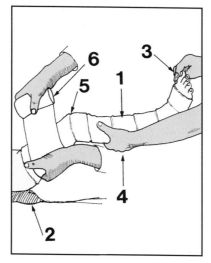

8. Undisplaced fractures (b): When deformity is minimal, apply a long leg plaster immediately over a generous layer of wool (1) (mild sedation only may be required). A sandbag under the buttocks (2) may be helpful, while an assistant holds the toes (3) and supports the calf (4). The knee is slightly flexed (5) and the plaster may be applied in one stage with or without a slab (6).

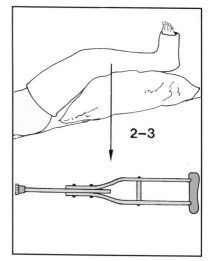

9. Undisplaced fractures (c): Elevation of the leg and a regular, careful check of the circulation is essential, and admission for this is desirable. In a child, non-weight bearing with crutches can usually be allowed as soon as there is no circulatory risk (say 2–3 days post injury). Thereafter the child should be seen every 2–3 weeks (the casualty rate in children's plasters is high).

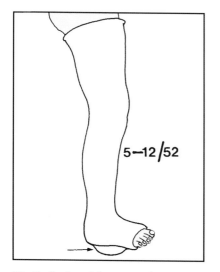

10. Undisplaced fractures (d): A walking heel can certainly be applied when there is evidence of early callus on the radiographs (e.g. after 3–4 weeks in a child of 9 years). Before that a heel may be applied if in your assessment there is no risk of displacement or problems from swelling. Any hesitation may sometimes be dispelled by the appearance of the sole of the plaster which often indicates premature successful weight bearing!

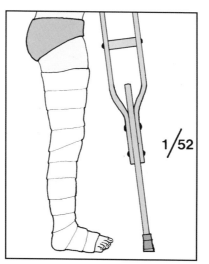

11. Undisplaced fractures (e): The fracture may be assessed for union after say 4–5 weeks in a child of 4 years, 8 weeks in a child of 8, and 8–12 weeks in a child of 12. On removal of the plaster no support for the limb is usually required, but confidence may be raised by a crepe bandage. Crutches for the first few days are advocated as the child often shows timidity in commencing weight bearing and the parents may require reassurance.

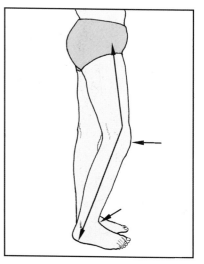

12. Undisplaced fractures (f): The child should be reviewed 2 weeks after removal of the plaster. In most cases he will be walking unsupported, the movements in the knee and ankle will have returned, and the limb lengths will be equal. The child may then be discharged. The parents should be reassured that any residual limp will resolve, and that athletic activities may be resumed say in a further 2 months.

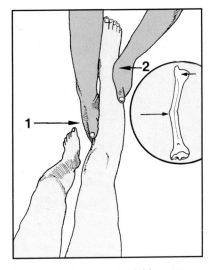

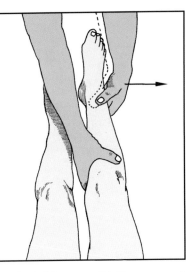

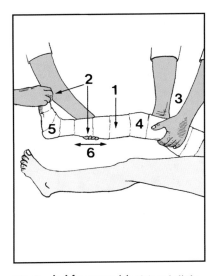

13. Angled fractures in children (a):
These are reduced under general anaesthesia.
One hand is placed over the fracture site (1)
while the other, at the ankle (2), is used to
correct the angulation. Although the AP
plane only is illustrated, obviously any
deformity in the lateral plane should be
similarly corrected.

14. Angled fractures (b): The pressure of
the hand at the ankle should be released, and
any tendency for the deformity to recur noted
(indicating springy intact periosteum). If this
is found, particular care must be taken during
the application of the plaster to maintain full
correction; alternatively, complete tearing of
the periosteum may be obtained by over
correction of the deformity.

15. Angled fractures (c): If there is little
tendency to recurrence of angulation, the
plaster may be applied as follows: wool roll
is wound round the limb from toes to groin
(1); one assistant supports the fracture and
the toes (2) while the second takes the weight
of the thigh (3). The knee is flexed to 15° (4)
and the ankle maintained at right angles (5).
The supporting hands are moved during the
application of the plaster (6). Use a sandbag
under the buttocks.

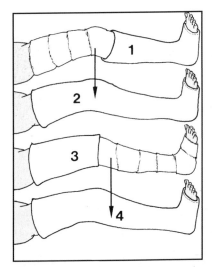

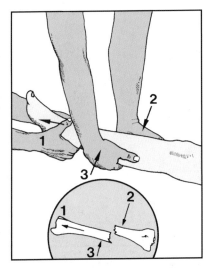

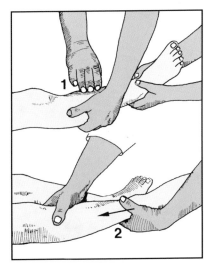

16. Angled fractures (d): If there is a
tendency to re-angulation, the plaster must
be moulded while it sets. Except in the
smallest of children it is difficult to apply a
full length plaster and mould the fracture
within the setting time. A two-stage
technique may be used: *either* apply a below
knee plaster (1), mould and complete the
thigh (2); *or* apply the thigh cuff first (3),
complete the plaster (4) and then mould.

17. Displaced fractures of the tibia (a):
An assistant applies strong traction in the line
of the limb (1) while strong pressure is
applied with the heels of the hands above (2)
and below (3) the fracture to correct the
displacement. The traction is then slackened
off to allow the bone ends to engage.

18. Displaced fractures of the tibia (b):
Checking the reduction clinically can be
difficult. Try palpating the fracture line along
the subcutaneous border (1) or in the case of
a transverse fracture confirm that a hitch is
present by noting resistance to attempted
telescoping (2).

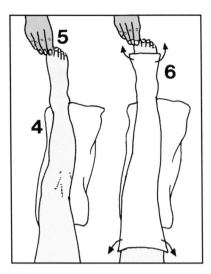

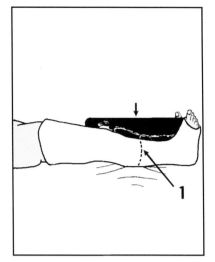

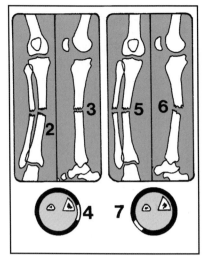

19. Displaced fractures of the tibia (c):
If the reduction obtained by manipulation is somewhat precarious and it is feared that the fracture might slip during the application of plaster, place the limb on a firm pillow (4), steady the leg by holding the toes (5) and apply a thick, anterior, plaster slab (6) tucking the edges well round the limb. When it has set, the leg can then be carefully bandaged into the slab.

20. Wedging (a): Ultimately, if necessitated by circumstance, displacement and even off-ending may be accepted in children. If, however, the radiographs indicate residual angulation, this should be corrected, and this may usually be done by wedging. Begin by marking the plaster circumferentially at the level of the fracture (1) using the radiographs as a guide.

21. Wedging (b): Now carefully work out where the plaster must hinge to correct the deformity. For example, where there is medial angulation (2) and the lateral projection is normal (3), the hinge should lie medially (4). Where there is lateral angulation (5) along with posterior angulation (6) the hinge should be positioned posterolaterally (7).

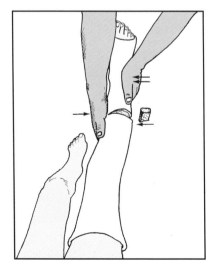

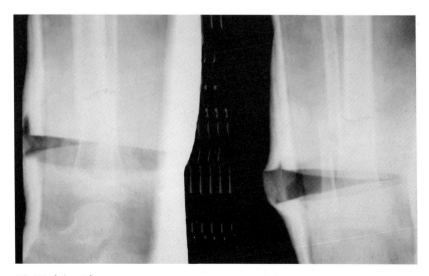

22. Wedging (c): Cut through 7/8 of the circumference of the plaster at the marked level, sparing the hinge; use a plaster saw or a hacksaw with a fine blade. Now spring the plaster 1–2 cm open; maintain the position temporarily by placing a suitably sized piece of previously prepared cork into the mouth of the wedge.

23. Wedging (d): Check radiographs should be taken, and any adjustment made on the result. If a satisfactory correction has been obtained, wool should be packed lightly into the gap on either side of the cork, and the plaster reconstituted locally with a 15 cm (6″) plaster bandage.

(Illus.: A badly angled fracture in the distal third of the tibia has been corrected by wedging. Although the level of the wedge is more distal than it should be, an almost anatomical position has been achieved.) General anaesthesia is not required for wedging, but mild sedation is desirable. Aftercare should follow the lines described for undisplaced fractures.

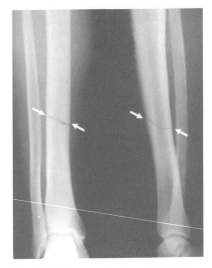

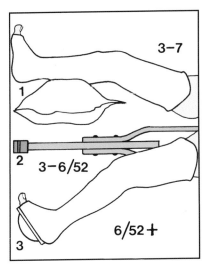

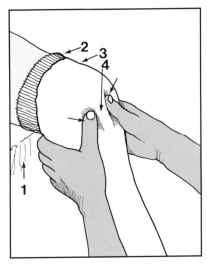

24. Tibial fractures in the adult (a): In the adult many tibial fractures may be treated conservatively, and where good results with few complications are the rule it is unwise to advocate surgery with its additional risks. Conservative treatment may with good reason always be advised for stress, isolated (Illus.) and undisplaced fractures, and for slightly displaced stable fractures.

25. Minimally displaced fractures in the adult (b): A long leg plaster is applied, check radiographs are taken, and the limb elevated (1) for 3–7 days until swelling subsides. The plaster is checked for slackness and changed if required. As soon as the patient has mastered crutches they may be allowed home (2). A walking heel is applied (3) usually after 3–6 weeks (depending on your assessment of stability) and the plaster retained till union.

26. Sarmiento plaster (a): Alternatively, at 4–6 weeks post injury, the long leg plaster is removed and a Sarmiento cast applied. The patient sits on the edge of the plaster table (1), the foot being steadied by the lap of the operator. Stockinet (2) and wool roll are applied, and the plaster extended over the knee (3). It is firmly moulded (before setting) round the patellar ligament (4).

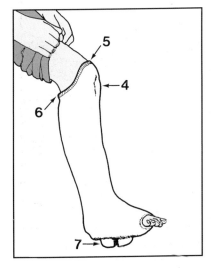

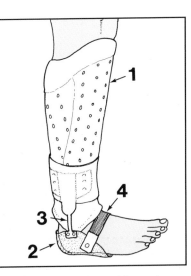

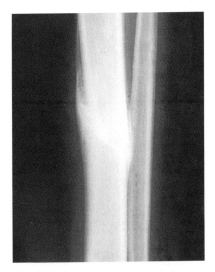

27. Sarmiento plaster (b): The plaster is then trimmed from the upper pole of the patella (5) round to the upper part of the calf (6); check that knee movement is free before turning down the stockinet and finishing in the usual way. A rocker sole may then be applied (7) and weight bearing and knee flexion commenced. The plaster is retained until union is sound.

28. Functional bracing with a gaiter: In the later stages of fixation, or even as early as 4 weeks when instability is not a problem, a supporting gaiter may be used instead of plaster. The type illustrated may be fashioned from perforated Orthoplast™ (Johnson & Johnson) thermoplastic sheet (1). For additional support a plastic heel seat (2) may be secured to the brace with polyethylene hinges (3) and a garter strap (4).

29. Aftercare: 1. Intervals between hospital attendances should not exceed 4 weeks, and the fixation – plaster or brace – changed if it becomes unduly slack.
2. Tibial fractures take an average 16 weeks to unite, but union may be sought in 8–12 weeks in the case of a hairline crack, and after 12 weeks in a transverse fracture. Radiographs should be taken (Illus.: advanced union in tibial fracture) preferably out of plaster.

30. Aftercare cntd:
3. Apparent radiological union should be confirmed by clinical examination.
4. If union is judged sound a crepe bandage support is prescribed for the leg and knee, and full unsupported weight bearing commenced. Sticks or crutches may be required to give confidence over the first few weeks, but the patient should be encouraged to discard these as soon as possible (although the elderly patient may have difficulty in this respect).
5. The patient should be reviewed 2 weeks after plaster has been discarded.

The following problems may be encountered:

1. *The knee.* Pain or discomfort in the knee at the beginning of mobilisation is normal. A small to moderate *effusion* is common. If the period of immobilisation is under 16 weeks, return of flexion is usually rapid. Physiotherapy is nevertheless advisable in the majority of cases to encourage knee flexion, to develop the quadriceps and to help restore the gait to normal.

2. *The ankle.* Slight swelling and oedema of the foot and ankle are usual for several months after tibial fractures. A crepe bandage or circular woven support is advised until this swelling subsides. Gross swelling with marked stiffness and pain in the foot and ankle should suggest Sudeck's atrophy. Swelling which is maximal over the fracture calls for re-assessment of union. Slight *restriction of ankle movements* is common after tibial fractures, but is seldom incapacitating.

3. *Athletic activities. Swimming* may be permitted almost as soon as the plaster has been discarded, and should be encouraged. *Cycling* can be allowed as soon as knee flexion will allow (c. 110°). Golf may be allowed as soon as limb swelling is no longer a problem. *Rugby, football and gymnastics* should not be permitted until endosteal callus is sound, till knee flexion is nearly normal (say 130°) and muscle power is restored.

4. *Return to work.* The patient should be encouraged to return to work as soon as possible, and in sedentary work the patient may do so while in plaster. Factors which may delay return are: (a) Severe persistent oedema in jobs involving prolonged standing; (b) Lack of knee flexion in work involving kneeling; (c) Muscle and functional weakness in jobs involving work at heights.

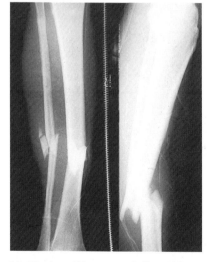

31. Displaced, but potentially stable fracture in the adult: Transverse fractures of the tibia, in particular, are potentially stable if good bony apposition can be obtained. While it is usual to treat injuries of this pattern by closed intramedullary nailing, conservative treatment is also possible. While in the latter mobilisation of the patient generally takes longer and loss of some of the range of knee movements is not uncommon, there is no risk of infection or other problems related to surgery or the implant.

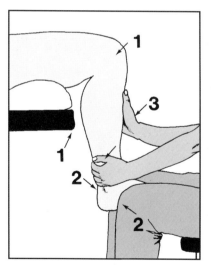

32. Reduction techniques: The fracture may be manipulated as already described for the child. It is often helpful, especially if assistance is limited, to let gravity work to your advantage. The patient's knee is flexed over the end of the table (1), with the thigh supported with a sandbag. Use your own knees to steady or to apply traction to the foot (2). Both hands are then free to manipulate the fracture (3).

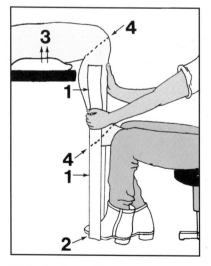

33. Reduction techniques cntd:
Alternatively, it is sometimes possible to apply temporary traction using skin traction tapes (1). The traction may be controlled by the operator's foot on the spreader bar (2) and by elevating the table (3). After manipulation a padded plaster is applied over the tapes from the heel to the knee (4). The tapes are cut, and the foot of the plaster completed.

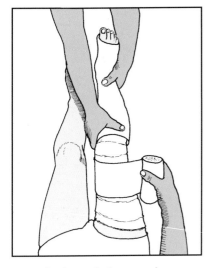

34. Reduction techniques cntd: Once the leg and foot have been encased in plaster, the knee is gently extended to 15°, wool applied to the thigh, and the thigh cuff completed with 20 cm (8″) plaster bandages. Check radiographs are desirable on completion of the below-knee portion of the plaster, and after the thigh cuff has been added.

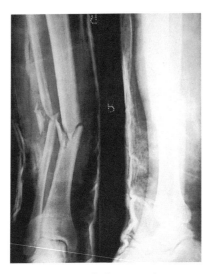

35. Reduction techniques cntd: If manipulation succeeds in bringing the bone ends into apposition, any residual angulation may be corrected within the first few weeks by wedging. (Illus.: Postmanipulation radiograph of the previous fracture (Frame 31). Angulation is marked, and exceeds what is taken as the upper limit of acceptability – this is 15° for fractures in the middle third, and 10° for those in the proximal third. This deformity was easily corrected by wedging and union proceeded uneventfully.)

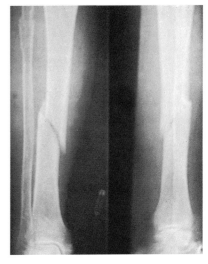

36. Unstable fractures with minimal displacement: Oblique and spiral fractures are potentially unstable. Although they may be managed conservatively along the lines indicated, meticulous supervision is necessary during the first 6 weeks. Slackness in the plaster must be promptly dealt with. Slight slipping of the fracture may be accepted, but if evidence of substantial displacement is found, internal fixation should be considered.

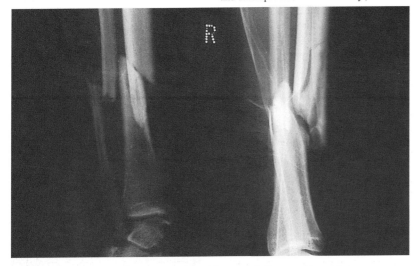

37. Displaced unstable fractures – Closed intramedullary nailing (a): Fractures which are unstable because of their pattern may be manipulated to the best position that can be obtained, and any residual angulation treated by wedging. Nevertheless this method of treatment requires much experienced supervision: shortening is inevitable, union may be delayed, and stiffness in the knee and ankle may become a problem. *For the majority of fractures under normal circumstances closed intramedullary nailing (with interlocking nails) is the treatment of choice.*

Method: The operation is performed as soon as the patient's condition will allow, and prophylactic antibiotic cover is frequently advocated. The fracture must be amenable to reduction by traction, but in practice this is seldom a problem. (If reduction cannot be achieved, the fracture must be exposed and openly reduced.) Traction may be effected manually or by a Steinmann pin through the heel. (A boot may also be used, but its size will interfere with the insertion of any distal locking screws.)

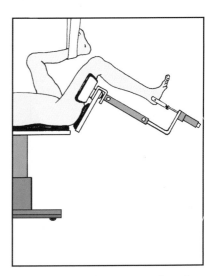

38. Closed intramedullary nailing (b): The leg must be positioned so that traction can be applied while at the same time there is good surgical and image intensifier access. The knee should be flexed, and care must be taken to avoid undue pressure on the popliteal structures. This may be achieved in a number of ways on an orthopaedic table. Illustrated is the use of a Watson–Jones frame after removal of the table end-piece; the good leg is supported clear of the field (e.g. by lithotomy straps).

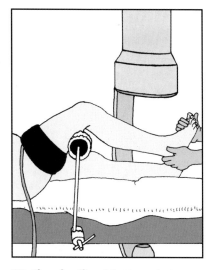

39. Closed nailing (c): Alternatively, a radiolucent table may be used, with a well padded bar to support the thigh; after scrubbing up and skin preparation the limb is draped free. Manual traction is applied when required by an assistant. This gives good access for the surgeon, the assistant and the image intensifier. A pneumatic tourniquet should be available, but it need not be used routinely.

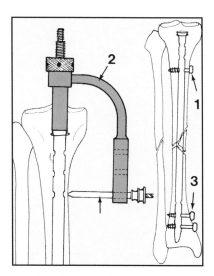

42. Closed nailing (f): The nail should be driven well home to lessen the risks of knee pain. The position for the insertion of proximal locking screws (1) may be determined by use of the insertion handle (2) which doubles as a jig. Due to the cumulative errors caused by nail flexibility and lost motion distal locating jigs are not very successful, and the holes in the nail for distal locking screws (3) are generally best located free-hand using the image intensifier.

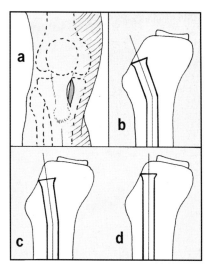

40. Closed nailing (d): The patellar ligament is retracted after making a medial (a) or lateral incision; or alternatively, and often preferred, a patellar tendon splitting incision may be used. The knee joint is not entered. The safe area for insertion of the nail lies anterior to the menisci and proximal to the tibial tuberosity, and lies on a line 2 mm lateral to the most prominent part of the tubercle. The shallower the (Herzog) angle of the nail – (b) 20°, (c) 10°, or (d) 0° – and the longer the tibia – the more proximal must be the entry point.

43. Closed nailing (g): *Aftercare:* Mobilisation of the knee and ankle may be commenced immediately, and as a result complete recovery of movements in these joints is the rule. As regards weight bearing, advice on when this should be permitted is dependent on the nature of the fracture and the quality of fixation. Absence of pain at the fracture site on weight bearing has been said to be a valuable guide as to when full unsupported weight may be taken through the limb. The fracture should be followed up until soundly united, when a decision, based on the usual criteria, should be made regarding removal of the fixation device. Return to work and athletic activities follows along the lines already discussed.

Complications: Knee pain occurs in about 40% of cases, and generally settles on removal of the nail. *Delayed union* may be treated by converting from static to dynamic fixation by removal of the appropriate locking screws, sometimes with an osteotomy of the fibula if it has united. *Hypertrophic non-union* may be dealt with by exchange nailing (removal of the existing nail, re-reaming to a greater diameter, and using a larger nail). *Infection* is uncommon, and should be dealt with along the usual lines, preferably retaining the nail until union has occurred. *Compartment syndromes* may occur, usually within the first 5 days; they must not be overlooked, and should be dealt with promptly (see Frame 52).

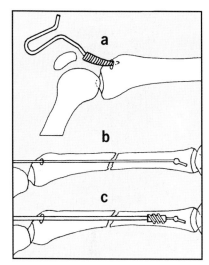

41. Closed nailing (e): The cortex is opened with an awl held parallel to the anterior cortex (a). Check its position; neither it nor the nail should broach the posterior cortex. If the canal is being reamed, then a reaming rod is passed across the fracture (b), and sequential reaming carried out (c). (Exposure may sometimes be needed in proximal tibial fractures to avoid their displacement.) If reaming is not being undertaken, then after measuring and selecting the appropriate length of nail, this is gripped on a holder and inserted.

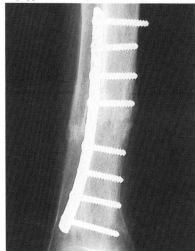

44. Alternative methods of treatment (a): Many fractures may be plated: this can provide rapid, rigid fixation which can be of value in cases requiring arterial repair or bone grafting. (Infection and mechanical failure are possible complications.) A well-contoured dynamic compression plate, with screws engaging 8 cortices above and 8 below the fracture may be used; butterfly and other separate fragments may be secured with interfragmentary screws. Image intensification and an orthopaedic table are not required.

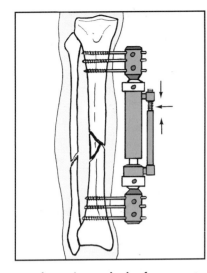

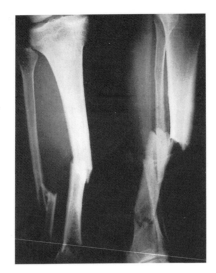

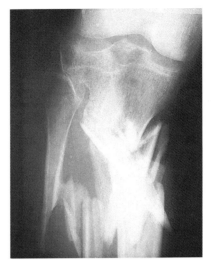

45. Alternative methods of treatment (b): External fixators are of particular value in open fractures. Good support is provided with preferably three threaded cantilever pins on each side of the fracture, with a connector which can give axial compression. The most rigid systems use a total of 12 pins, inserted in pairs at right angles to one another, with two linking bars. At the other end of the scale, tibial length may be preserved in conservatively treated fractures with two Steinmann pins incorporated in the plaster.

46. Special situations (a) – Double (segmental) fractures: Casts give poor support, and non-union at one level is high. (If this occurs it may be dealt with by internal fixation and grafting.) The most useful primary treatment is *closed* intramedullary nailing (taking care to avoid rotation of intermediate fragments with any reaming), with the insertion of proximal and distal locking screws. *Open reduction* and plating carries the risk of further devitalisation of the intermediate segment.

47. Special situations (b) – Gross fragmentation: Where the bone is highly fragmented (as may occur in high energy dissipation situations) the multiplicity of small, detached avascular bone fragments may prevent any meaningful reduction. Alignment may be restored by manipulation, and length and position held by Steinmann pins incorporated in a plaster cast. Alternatively a fine-wire hybrid fixation system (see p. 78) may be employed.

50. Special situations (e) – Displaced fractures in children: These can generally be managed conservatively along the lines already described, but other methods are available. These include the use of an external fixator (with 2 pins on each side of the fracture), plating (with early removal of the plates), and the use of Nancy intramedullary nails which do not cross the growth plates.

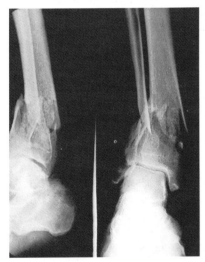

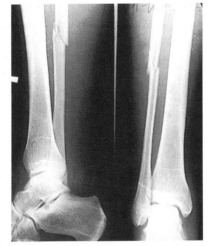

48. Special situations (c) – Fractures of the distal shaft: Many of these fractures can be treated conservatively by reduction and plaster fixation, with or without a Steinman pin through the heel to help maintain alignment. Some permanent restriction of ankle joint movements is common. Alternatively, some can be internally fixed allowing early movements (e.g. by using a buttress plate with proximal cortical and distal cancellous screws) or by a fine-wire/Schanz pin hybrid fixator system. (See also pilon fractures p. 380).

49. Special situations (d) – Isolated fractures of the fibula: The fibula may be fractured by direct violence; symptomatic treatment only is required (e.g. a below-knee walking plaster for 6 weeks). Always ensure, however, that the tibia is not fractured at another level, or that the fibular fracture represents part of a more complex injury to the ankle joint.

SPECIAL SITUATIONS (F) – OPEN FRACTURES

The frequency with which fractures of the tibia are found to be open, and the reasons for this, have been given at the beginning of this section. The AO and Gustilo classifications of open fractures are dealt with separately in Chapter 1; some general guidelines in the management of open fractures (including skin replacement methods) are commented upon in Chapter 3. In this common fracture situation some additional details may require consideration.

INITIAL TREATMENT

1. The limb should be re-aligned if there is gross deformity.
2. The state of the peripheral pulses should be documented. If absent and not restored by re-alignment, there may be need for arteriography.
3. Note if there is absence of sensation in the foot; such a finding may be important if amputation needs to be considered.
4. Document the location and dimensions of the wounds. Remove any gross contaminants (such as grass or leaves). Take a Polaroid photograph of the wounds to avoid any further disturbance before the case is taken to theatre.
5. Take a bacteriological swab and commence antibiotics (for Gram +ve organisms in *all* cases; in addition, commence antibiotics for Gram −ve organisms where there is gross contamination and for anaerobes if there is contamination with soil, river or lake water. If the patient has received tetanus protection within the previous 5 years, no further preventative measures need be taken. If the protection was given over 5 years previously, then booster prophylaxis should be administered. If there has never been any tetanus protection or this is doubtful, then give toxoid along with tetanus immune globulin.
6. Seal the wounds with a sterile dressing.
7. If there is likely to be any problem with skin cover, then consultation with an experienced plastic surgeon is advised at this stage.

TREATMENT IN THEATRE

1. The wound(s) should be extended to allow a thorough inspection of all possible soiled tissue, including the fractured bone ends. Any wound extension should follow the so-called 'safe' incisions (see Frame 52).
2. Non-viable skin should be excised until good dermal bleeding is found. If in doubt, especially over the anterior border of the tibia, leave any doubtful skin until the second inspection.
3. Excise any dead muscle. If there is doubt (and this is often the case), this should also be left until the second inspection.
4. In the case of bone, ideally all devitalised separate fragments should be removed, but any major articular segments (e.g. of the tibial table) should be retained; otherwise retention of completely free segments should be only rarely considered because of the much higher rate of infection.
5. Perform a prophylactic fasciotomy on any muscle compartment directly involved, and consider fasciotomies of the remaining compartments if the injury has been a high energy one.
6. Carry out a thorough lavage, preferably using a pulsatile system, with up to 10 litres of saline followed by 2 litres of bacitracin/polymyxin solution.

7. If contamination has been great, the use of antibiotic beads should be considered.

8. The original wounds should always be left open (although good results following primary closure have been claimed in children where contamination has been minimal). Closure of any wound extension is often permissible at this stage.

FIXATION OF THE FRACTURE

There has been much controversy over the use of internal fixation in the treatment of open fractures, but in many cases the fears expressed of increasing the risks of infection have been shown to be unjustified. In open fractures of Types 1 & 2 (Gustilo) the infection rate following intramedullary nailing using the closed technique has been shown to be low, and no greater than in closed injuries of a similar pattern.

In Grade 3 open fracture it has been suggested that reaming of the medullary cavity is undesirable, and for this reason a solid intramedullary nail has been advocated. The pattern of nail chosen must be of sufficiently small diameter to allow it to negotiate the tibial canal without sticking, and if made of titanium this should prove of adequate strength. Others have shown that in the majority of Grade 3 open fractures the results of nailing (with the use of locking screws) after reaming are comparable in terms of infection with those obtained when external fixators have been employed; and that nailing is better in terms of joint stiffness, malunion, access for plastic reconstructions, and patient preference. Nevertheless, where there has been gross tissue contamination, many would still prefer to use an external fixator or, where applicable, a simple plaster cast support until the situation regarding wound infection has been resolved.

SECOND INSPECTION

This should be performed about 48 hours after the primary procedure. Any necrotic tissue should be excised and irrigation repeated. Further inspections are dictated by the findings at this stage. Once the soft tissue bed is stable, secondary wound closure may be carried out. If any plastic surgical procedure (such as a fasciocutaneous flap, see p. 71 et seq) is going to be needed, the aim should be to get the tissue bed in a state suitable for this by the fifth day, as this greatly increases the chances of success. Split skin grafting is not suitable for bone which has no periosteal cover, or tendon without paratenon. The following techniques have been recommended for consideration in open fractures with substantial skin defects.

Proximal third

1. Proximally based medial or lateral fasciocutaneous flap.
2. Gastrocnemius muscle flap.
3. Free flap.

Middle third

1. Proximally or distally based, medial or lateral fasciocutaneous flap.
2. Anterior compartment muscle flap.
3. Soleus muscle flap.
4. Free flap.

Distal third

1) Distally based fasciocutaneous flap.
2) Free flap.

Ankle

Free flap.

Note also the following:
1. If at inspection there is no indication of infection, an external fixator may be replaced with an intramedullary nail; provided this is done within the first week, the risks of infection are slight. If however there is at any time a pin track infection following the use of an external fixator, reaming of the medullary canal is contraindicated as it carries the almost certain risk of disseminating infection throughout the bone.
2. If there is a bone defect involving more than 50% of the circumference of the bone, and more than 2 cm long, then bone grafting will ultimately be required in all cases; where the bone defect is smaller, healing may occur without grafting.

51. DIAGNOSIS AND TREATMENT OF COMPARTMENT SYNDROMES

This complication is seen most frequently associated with severe soft tissue damage, especially where there has been a high velocity, high energy injury. It is said to occur more frequently after intramedullary nailing, especially where reaming has been carried out, or after prolonged excessive traction over a thigh bar. It is not confined to closed fractures. Close observation is required in all these circumstances, and if treatment is delayed for more than 6 hours there will usually be some permanent damage.

DIAGNOSIS

The first symptoms are of severe or increasing pain or tightness in the leg. The pain is greater than might be expected, even when the limb is immobilised. It is relentless in character, and often not greatly relieved by opiates. The limb is tense and swollen, and there may be induration (a late sign) over the affected compartment. Tenderness is diffuse, and can be elicited some distance from the fracture itself. There is pain on passive stretching of the muscles arising in the affected compartment (e.g. by passive movement of the foot or toes), and there may be muscle paralysis. There may be complaint of sensory disturbance in the leg or foot and this may be confirmed clinically; loss of vibration sense is an early finding. The distal pulses may be reduced or absent.

   The intercompartmental pressures may be monitored; this should be done as close to the fracture as possible. A differential tissue pressure below 30 mmHg is an indication for surgery.

TREATMENT

Prophylaxis Where there is an open fracture with extensive muscle damage, the compartment involved should be widely decompressed at the time of the initial exploration.

Established cases Prompt decompression of *all four compartments* is advised. This is generally best performed through two 'safe' incisions (see following frames for details). (A single lateral incision can give access, but the dissection can be difficult; it is best reserved for cases where there is concurrent damage to the anterior tibial artery, when the viability of the intervening skin bridge might be in doubt.)

Aftercare Often, one of the two wounds may be closed directly, and the other by controlled tension or split skin grafting. If the swelling is marked, both should be left open; then, in most cases, both may be closed after 3–5 days when the swelling has decreased; skin grafting is rarely required.

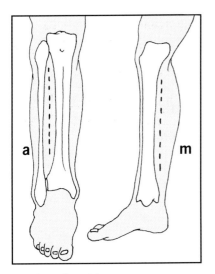

52. The safe incisions: These are designed to avoid the perforating arteries, and should be used for compartment decompressions or to extend existing wounds, especially if fasciocutaneous flaps are going to be required. The anterolateral (a) should be placed 2 cm lateral to the anterior border of the tibia. The medial (m) is made 1–2 cm posterior to the medial border of the tibia. In both cases the incisions are made straight through skin and fascia.

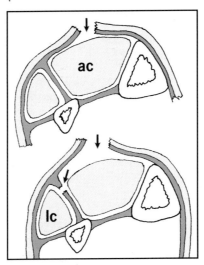

53. Anterior and peroneal compartment decompression: Use a 15 cm 'safe' anterolateral incision. Grasp the investing fascia forming the roof of the anterolateral compartment with Köcher forceps to keep it under tension, and split it longitudinally with blunt scissors – aiming proximally for the patella and distally for the mid-point of the ankle. Then retract the lateral skin flap and divide the anterior peroneal septum to decompress the lateral (peroneal) compartment (ac = anterior compartment; lc = lateral compartment; fascia shown in dark grey).

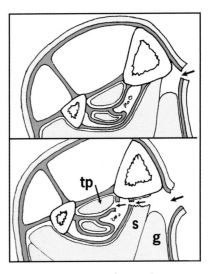

54. Decompression of posterior compartments: Use a 15 cm 'safe' medial incision in the distal part of the leg to open the superficial posterior compartment. Then, to open the deep compartment, separate the soleus from its tibial attachments: begin distally where its tendinous part blends with gastrocnemius, and working proximally detach the soleal bridge from the tibia. Finally the fascial coverings of the three deep bi-pennate muscles may be divided (s = soleus; g = gastrocnemius; tp = tibialis posterior).

TIBIA/FIBULA, *Diaphyseal Segment : 42–*

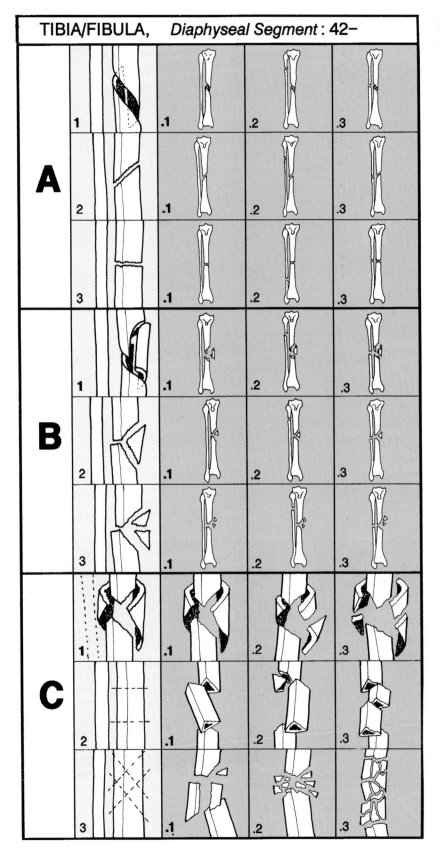

55. AO classification of fractures of the tibia/fibula, diaphyseal segment (42–):

Type A fractures are simple fractures.
A1 = Spiral: .1 fibula intact; .2 fibula fractured at another level; .3 fibula fractured at the same level.
A2 = Oblique fracture (30° or more): .1 fibula intact; .2 fibula fractured at another level; .3 fibula fractured at the same level.
A3 = Transverse fracture (less than 30° of obliquity): .1 fibula intact; .2 fibula fractured at another level; .3 fibula fractured at the same level.

Type B fractures are wedge fractures.
B1 = Spiral: .1 fibula intact; .2 fibula fractured at another level; .3 fibula fractured at the same level.
B2 = Bending wedge fracture: .1 fibula intact; .2 fibula fractured at another level; .3 fibula fractured at the same level.
B3 = Fragmented wedge: .1 fibula intact; .2 fibula fractured at another level; .3 fibula fractured at the same level.

Type C fractures are complex fractures.
C1 = Spiral: .1 with two intermediate fragments; .2 with three intermediate fragments; .3 with more than three intermediate fragments.
C2 = Segmental: .1 with one intermediate segment; .2 with an intermediate segment and additional wedge; .3 with two intermediate segments.
C3 = Irregular: .1 with two or three intermediate fragments; .2 with shattering over a length of less than 4 cm; .3 with shattering over a length of 4 cm or more.

SELF-TEST

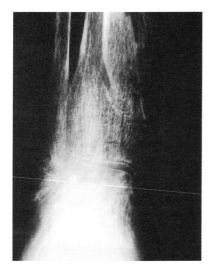

56. What complication has occurred in this uniting fracture of the tibia in the distal third?

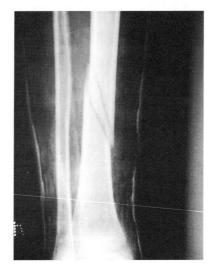

57. What pattern of fracture is present? How is it being treated?

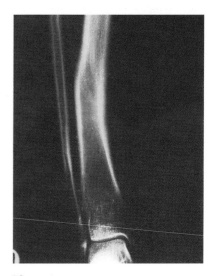

58. What complication is present in this united tibial fracture? What effect will this have?

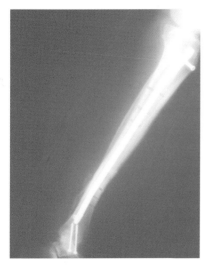

59. What is being treated here at present, and what earlier treatment was employed?

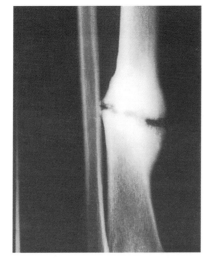

60. What complication is shown in this radiograph of a tibial fracture?

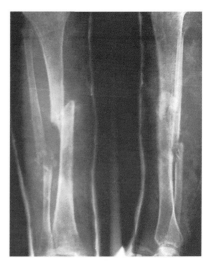

61. These radiographs were taken through plaster 10 weeks after injury. Describe the fracture. What further treatment would you advocate? What is the prognosis?

ANSWERS TO SELF-TEST

56. The radiograph shows the disturbance of bone trabeculation typical of Sudeck's atrophy.

57. This shows a spiral fracture of the tibia at the junction of the mid and distal thirds being treated in plaster. The position in this *single* view appears excellent. (AO = 42–A1.1.)

58. Malunion of the fracture is present with lateral angulation. The plane of the ankle joint is affected, and secondary, degenerative arthritis in it is possible.

59. There is a fracture of the mid-shaft of the tibia, with an associated malleolar injury. The former is being treated with a locked medullary nail, and the latter with cross-screws. The fracture was an open one, and treated originally with an external fixator, the bone scars of the threaded screws being still visible.

60. Hypertrophic non-union is present. (AO = 42–A3.1.)

61. The radiographs are of an oblique fracture of the tibia in the middle third, with an associated fibular fracture at the junction of the middle and lower thirds. Both fractures are uniting, and bridging callus is well formed. The general alignment is good. No correction at this late stage is required: the patient will require to continue with fixation for about another 4 weeks before plaster can be discarded (or a cast brace may be substituted). There will be approximately 1 cm of shortening, but the functional prognosis is excellent. (AO = 42–A2.2.)

CHAPTER

14

Injuries about the ankle

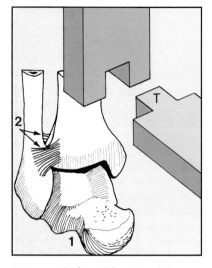

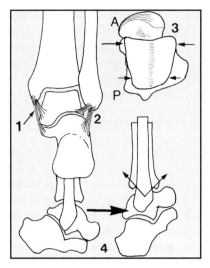

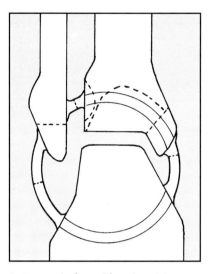

1. Anatomical considerations (a): The ankle joint is often fairly compared with the mortise and tenon joint of the woodworker. The talus (1) resembles the tenon (T), and is supported by the two malleoli and the articular surface of the tibia (the ankle mortise). The lateral malleolus is firmly attached to the tibia by the strong anterior and posterior tibiofibular ligaments (2). The ankle is not quite a true hinge joint; it can permit as much as 18° of rotation through a vertical axis.

2. Anatomical considerations (b): The talus is held in the mortise on the medial side by the very strong deltoid ligament (1), and on the lateral side by the lateral (external) ligament (2). The anterior part of the upper articular surface of the talus is wider than the posterior part (3). When the foot is dorsiflexed, the talus pushes the fibula laterally (4) and is more firmly gripped in the ankle mortise.

3. Anatomical considerations (c): As in the case of the pelvis, the main anatomical structures may be likened to a ring. If this is broken in one place the injury is usually a stable one, and conservative treatment generally indicated. (The dotted lines indicate common sites of failure – the lateral, medial and posterior malleoli; the medial, lateral and anterior tibiofibular ligaments.) Additional breaks in the ring lead to instability, with often the need for surgical stabilisation.

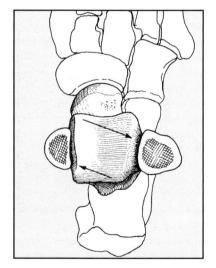

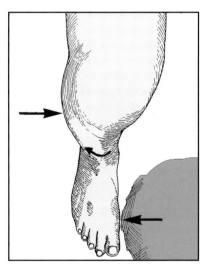

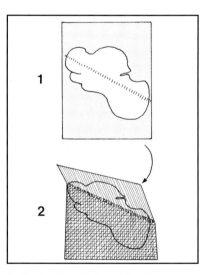

4. Mechanics of injury (a): The *function* of the ankle mortise is threatened if the malleoli are fractured or the tibiofibular ligaments are torn. The *stability* of the talus may also be reduced by rupture of the medial or lateral ligaments. The commonest injury is when the talus is rotated in the mortise, fracturing one or both malleoli.

5. Mechanics of injury (b): External rotation of the talus may be produced in two different ways: 1. The foot may act as a long lever; any rotational force applied to the inside of the foot is transferred to the talus with a mechanical advantage as in any system of levers. Even greater leverage may occur if, for example, the foot is attached to a ski.

6. Mechanics of injury (c): 2. The axis of movement of the subtalar joint is known to run obliquely in the direction of the crease on this paper model (1). Inversion of the heel, represented by folding the paper, results in external rotation of the talus (2) (Rose's torque-converter principle). A common history is of the ankle 'coggling over' on uneven ground.

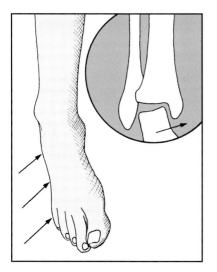

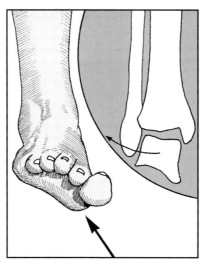

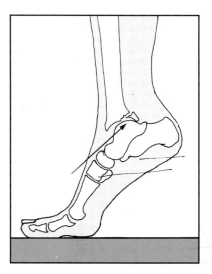

7. Mechanics of injury (d): The talus may be forced into relatively pure adduction as, for example, when the side of the inverted foot strikes the ground heavily. (The external rotation of the talus, produced by inversion of the calcaneus, being countered by the internal rotation of the strike, resulting in net adduction.)

8. Mechanics of injury (e): Similarly, if force is applied to the medial side of the heel and foot, the talus will tend to abduct in the ankle mortise.

9. Mechanics of injury (f): Many injuries occur during the course of walking or running. Under these circumstances there are additional forces transmitted to the posterior part of the inferior articular surface of the tibia (posterior malleolus).

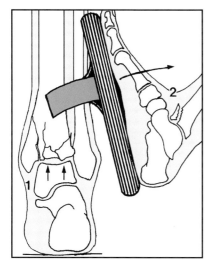

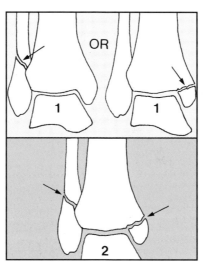

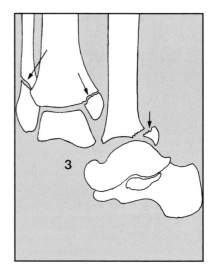

10. Mechanics of injury (g):
Compression injuries may be caused by: (1) falls from a height, forces being transmitted vertically from heel impact, or (2) following rapid deceleration in car accidents – sometimes aggravated by the pedals being driven into the front compartment and the ankle being forcibly dorsiflexed. Comminution is a feature of this type of injury.

11. Classification of ankle fractures: There are several classifications of ankle fractures; for completeness (which none achieves) many are complex to a degree that makes committal to memory nigh impossible. Fractures involving the ankle joint are often loosely referred to as Pott's fractures; although the term is now somewhat archaic, there is some merit in its simplicity: in *first degree* Pott's fractures, one malleolus is fractured (1): in *second degree* Pott's fractures, two malleoli are fractured (bimalleolar fracture) (2).

12. Pott's classification of ankle fractures cntd: In *third degree* Pott's fracture (3) there is a bimalleolar fracture, with in addition a fracture of the posterior part of the inferior articular surface of the tibia – often referred to as the third malleolus. These fractures may also be referred to as trimalleolar fractures.

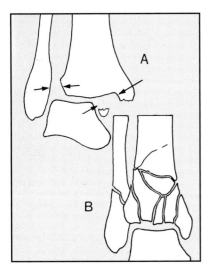

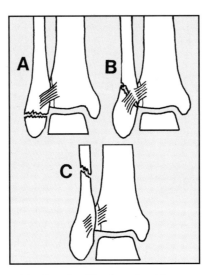

Type C fractures start proximal to the syndesmosis which may be subject to a variable amount of damage. While this classification is simple, it does not take into account injuries to related structures (e.g. an isolated fracture of the fibula is not distinguished from one accompanied by a fracture of the medial malleolus).

15. The AO classification of ankle fractures: This follows the lines of the Weber classification. (It was developed in association with the Weber classification and is sometimes referred to as the AO–Weber classification.) It takes into account damage to other structures. (Interestingly the Groups within each Type tend to follow the Pott's classification.) For full details of this classification, see p. 386.

13. Pott's classification of ankle fractures cntd: These fractures may be qualified by noting the presence of diastasis of the ankle or vertical compression. (A) First degree Pott's fracture with diastasis. (B) Second degree Pott's fracture with vertical compression.

14. Weber classification of ankle fractures: This is based on the level of the fibular fracture, once thought to be the key to all ankle fractures. Type A fractures occur distal to the syndesmosis. Type B fractures start at the level of the tibial plafond; they often spiral in a proximal direction, and usually involve the syndesmosis.

16. The Lauge–Hansen classification of ankle fractures: A fuller and widely accepted classification of ankle fractures is that of Lauge–Hansen, which groups these fractures under double-barrelled headings. The first word in each group title refers to the position of the foot at the time of injury; the second refers to the direction in which the talus moves within the ankle mortise in response to the causal forces. There are five main groups; they have been arranged here in order of frequency and a common terminology of usage has been included.

Order of frequency	Lauge-Hansen classification (and contraction)	Position of foot	Direction of talar movement	Common terminology
1	Supination/lateral rotation (SL)	Inversion	Lateral (external) rotation	External rotation injury without diastasis
2	Pronation/abduction (PA)	Eversion	Abduction	Abduction injury
3	Pronation/lateral rotation (PL)	Eversion	Lateral (external) rotation	External rotation injury with diastasis
4	Supination/adduction (SA)	Inversion	Adduction	Adduction injury
5	Pronation/dorsiflexion (PD)	Eversion	Dorsiflexion	Vertical compression injury

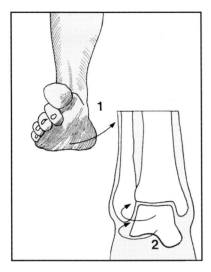

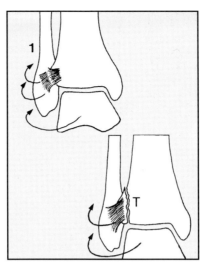

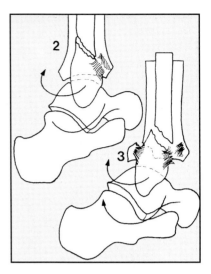

17. Supination/lateral rotation injuries (external rotation injury without diastasis) (a): The foot inverts (1). Due to the torque-converter principle, the talus rotates laterally in the ankle mortise (2). The ankle joint structures are thrown under stress and fail in a regular sequence. As each structure fails, the next is stressed. The number of structures involved is dependent on the magnitude of the forces applied to the joint.

18. Supination/lateral rotation injuries (b): The rotating talus carries the fibula with it, leading first to rupture of the anterior (inferior) tibiofibular ligament (1). Alternatively, the ligament under stress may avulse its tibial attachment (T) (Tillaux fracture).

19. Supination/lateral rotation injuries (c): As external rotation continues, the fibula fractures in an oblique or spiral fashion (2). Note the direction of the spiral. If displacement continues, the fibular fragment drags off the posterior malleolar fragment (3) to which it is attached by the posterior tibiofibular ligament (or the ligament tears).

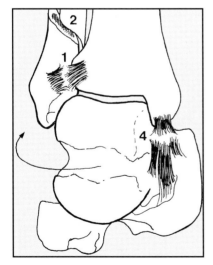

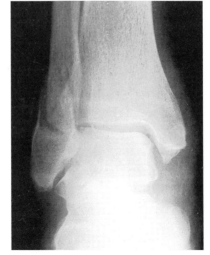

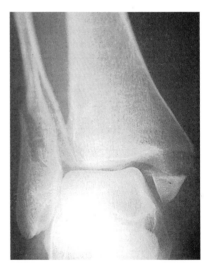

20. Supination/lateral rotation injuries (d): If rotation continues, the fourth structure to fail is the medial ligament or its attachment (the medial malleolus) (4). Such injuries are potentially very unstable and should be carefully distinguished from Stage 1 and 2 lesions.

21. Radiographs (a): A spiral fracture of the fibula at the level shown is typical of an S/L injury: in the lateral radiograph the fracture runs downwards and forwards, and there was no evidence of a posterior malleolar fracture. Although there is very slight incongruity between the upper surfaces of the talus and the ankle mortise, absence of tenderness on the medial side of the ankle suggested this was a Stage 2 or 3 injury.

22. Radiographs (b): The avulsion fracture of the medial malleolus indicates that this is a stage 4 S/L injury. There is lateral shift of the talus in the ankle mortise but the main mass of the fibula maintains its relationship with the tibia, so there is no true diastasis. Nevertheless, this is a very unstable injury.

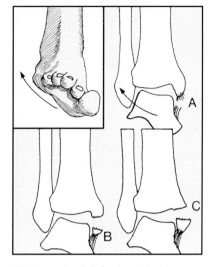

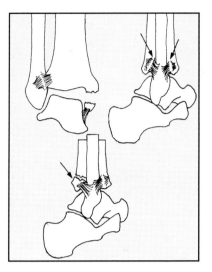

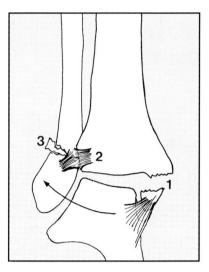

23. Pronation/abduction injuries (abduction injuries) (a): The foot everts and the talus swings into abduction. The first structures to be affected are on the medial side. Either (A) the deltoid ligament ruptures (rare) or there is an avulsion fracture of the medial malleolus. The fragment may be small (B) or large (C). In either case the fracture line runs horizontally.

24. Pronation/abduction injuries (b): In second stage injuries of this type, both the anterior and posterior tibiofibular ligaments rupture. In the case of the posterior tibiofibular ligament, its tibial attachment may be avulsed instead.

25. Pronation/abduction injuries (c): In the third stage the fibula fractures, often close to the level of the joint. Comminution may occur, sometimes with the formation of a triangular fragment of bone with its base directed laterally. The distal fibular fragment is tilted laterally (medial angulation). The fracture line is often horizontal.

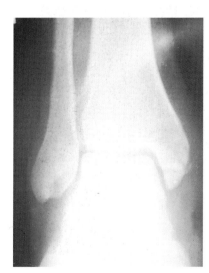

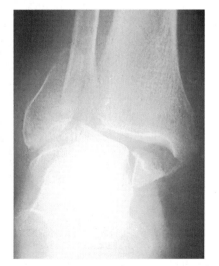

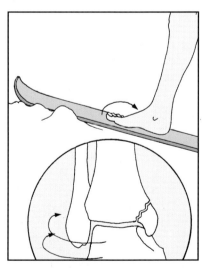

26. Radiographs (a): In this example of a Stage 1 abduction fracture, note the small medial malleolar fragment, the intact fibula, and the undisplaced talus.

27. Radiographs (b): In this Stage 3 abduction fracture, note the direction of talar tilting, the avulsion fracture of the medial malleolus with a large fragment and the distally situated fibular fracture. The latter is not strictly horizontal, and its slightly spiral appearance suggests that there has been a rotational element

28. Pronation/lateral rotation (external rotation with diastasis) (a): The talus is laterally rotated with the foot in the everted or neutral position (i.e. the foot does not invert). The rotating talus in the first stage produces an oblique fracture of the medial malleolus, or ruptures the deltoid ligament.

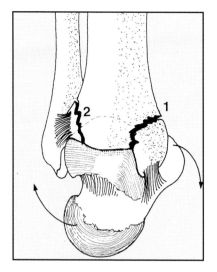

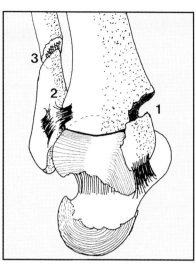

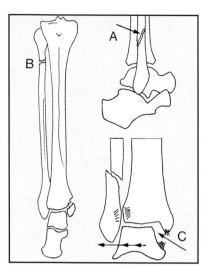

29. Pronation/lateral rotation (b): As the talus continues to twist, it impinges on the fibula. The anterior tibiofibular ligament is put under tension: in the second stage of P/L injuries, its tibial attachment is avulsed (Tillaux fracture) (2) or it ruptures.

30. Pronation/lateral rotation (c): In the third stage, the talus continues to rotate, producing a fracture of the fibula (3) that is spiral or oblique in pattern.

31. Pronation/lateral rotation (d): Note that in the lateral projection (A) the obliquity of the fibular fracture is in the opposite direction to that found in S/L injuries. The fibula may fracture proximally at the neck (B) – the Maisonneuve fracture. By Stage 3, the injury is unstable although stress films may be required to demonstrate diastasis (C).

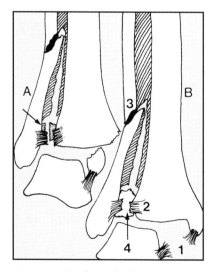

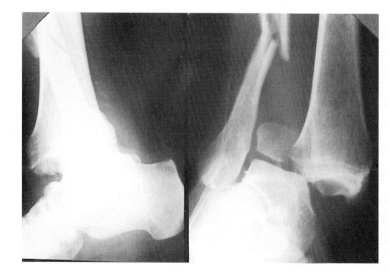

32. Pronation/lateral rotation (e): If the talus continues to thrust laterally against the lateral malleolus, the posterior tibiofibular ligament now ruptures (A) or pulls off its bony attachment (B). The interosseous membrane rips and gross diastasis results (Dupuytren fracture – dislocation of the ankle: Stage 4).

33. Radiograph: Note in the lateral projection:
1. The line of the fibular fracture runs in the opposite direction to the fractures of the fibula found in supination/lateral rotation injuries.
2. The posterior subluxation of the talus.

Note in the anteroposterior projection:

1. The gross lateral displacement of the talus.
2. The obvious disruption which must have occurred in the interosseous membrane.
3. The avulsion of the attachment of the posterior tibiofibular ligament.

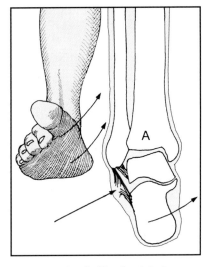

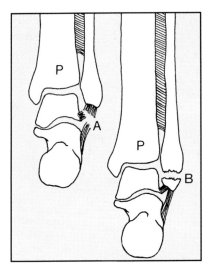

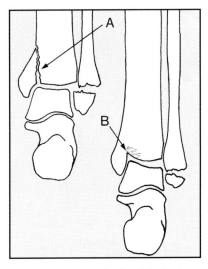

34. Supination/adduction injuries (adduction injuries) (a): The foot inverts, but the tendency to external rotation of the talus as a result of the torque-converter effect is countered by the direction of forces applied to the forefoot by the impact. The overall effect is adduction of the talus in the mortise. If the forces are slight, a partial tear of the lateral ligament results (sprain of ankle).

35. Supination/adduction injuries (b): With more severe violence there will be a complete tear of all three bundles going to form the lateral ligament (A) or there will be an avulsion fracture of the lateral malleolus (with a horizontally running fracture) (B).

36. Supination/adduction injuries (c): In the second stage, the adducting talus strikes the medial malleolus causing a *vertical or high oblique fracture* (A). *Note:* 1. Instead of the medial malleolus being pushed off, there may be a compression fracture of the angle (B). 2. Occasionally the medial malleolus may be broken off without damage first occurring to the lateral ligament.

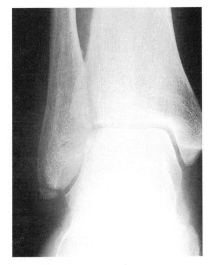

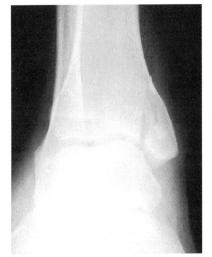

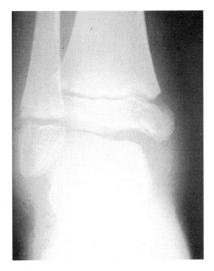

37. Radiographs (a): This radiograph shows quite clearly an avulsion fracture of the tip of the lateral malleolus, typical of a Stage 1 supination/adduction injury.

38. Radiographs (b): Note in a typical Stage 2 injury the fracture line tends to run almost vertically from the medial corner of the ankle mortise. There is some rotation in the radiographic projection so that the fibular shadow overlaps the tibia. The linear opacity near the medial malleolus dates from a previous Achilles tendon repair.

39. Radiographs (c): In this child's ankle there is a greenstick-type fracture of the medial malleolus with some compression of the angle between the medial malleolus and the inferior articular surface of the tibia.

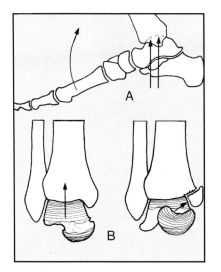

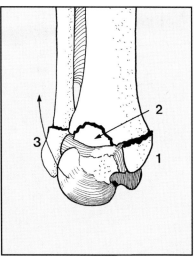

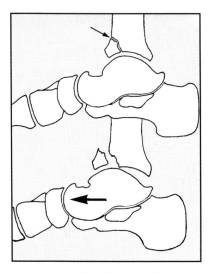

40. Pronation/dorsiflexion (compression injuries) (a): Commonly the foot is dorsiflexed at the ankle in association with an upward compression force – usually from a fall from a height or from a road traffic accident (A). As the talus dorsiflexes, its wide anterior part is forced between the malleoli, shearing off the medial malleolus (B).

41. Pronation/dorsiflexion injuries (b): As violence continues, the anterior tibial margin (2) is fractured, to be followed by the lateral malleolus (3).

42. Pronation/dorsiflexion injuries (c): Fractures of the anterior tibial margin show quite clearly in lateral projections of the joint and help to identify quite clearly this class of fracture. The talus may subluxate anteriorly, carrying the marginal fracture with it.

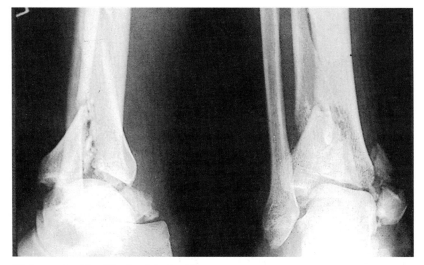

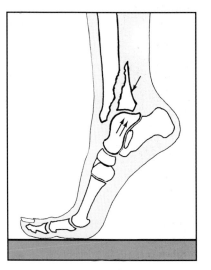

43. Pronation/dorsiflexion injuries (d): With still greater violence the tibia fractures in an irregular fashion, often with great comminution. There may be great irregularity of the inferior articular surface of the tibia. Note in the lateral radiograph the large anterior marginal fracture. In the anteroposterior view note the typical medial malleolar fracture, the gross comminution, and the disruption of the inferior articular surface of the tibia. In this case the fibula has remained intact.

44. Other compression injuries: If a fall occurs on to the plantar-flexed foot, the posterior articular surface of the tibia may be fractured. In addition, fractures of both malleoli (as in typical pronation/dorsiflexion injuries) may occur when the broad anterior portion of the talus is driven between them.

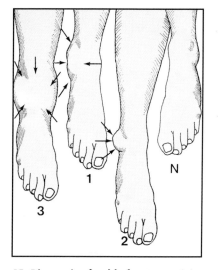

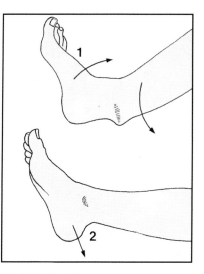

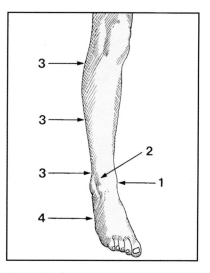

45. Diagnosis of ankle fractures – (a) Swelling: Note the site and distribution of swelling and bruising, e.g. (1) Diffuse swelling in front of the lateral malleolus in many ankle injuries. (2) Egg-shaped swelling over the lateral malleolus shortly after complete lateral ligament tears or lateral malleolar fractures (McKenzie's sign). (3) Gross swelling and bruising in many trimalleolar and compression fractures. *Swelling and bruising which involves both sides of the ankle is highly suggestive of an unstable injury.*

46. (b) Deformity: Note the presence of any deformity. Look for: (1) External rotation of the foot relative to the leg. If the medial malleolus is fractured and laterally displaced, the distal end of the tibia may become quite prominent under the skin. (2) Posterior displacement of the foot, a common feature of posterior malleolar fractures. Deformity is associated with unstable injuries of the ankle.

47. (c) Tenderness: Try to localise tenderness if at all possible. In particular, check: (1) Medial malleolar area; (2) Anterior tibiofibular ligament area; (3) The whole length of the fibula; (4) The base of the fifth metatarsal. (Avulsion fractures following inversion injuries are often confused with ankle fractures.) *Localised (as opposed to diffuse) tenderness on both sides of the joint is also suggestive of an unstable injury.*

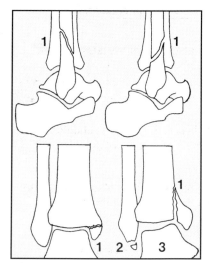

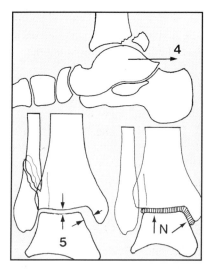

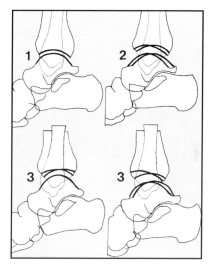

48. Radiographs (a): In grouping , staging and making a decision regarding the treatment of these injuries, note: (1) The site and slope of any fracture. (If in doubt, note the soft tissue shadows, or examine an oblique (Cobb) projection.) (2) Small fragments suggesting avulsion injuries. (If there is some uncertainty about ligament integrity, stress films may be helpful.) (3) Talar tilting.

49. Radiographs (b): Note also any shift of the talus relative to the tibia, e.g.: (4) Posterior subluxation, associated with a posterior malleolar fracture. (5) Lateral subluxation; note that the 'gap' above the talus should be the same as between the medial surface and the medial malleolus.

50. Radiographs (c): Note the following possible appearances in the lateral: (1) Tibia and talus congruent: true lateral projection. (2) Tibia and talus congruent: slight rotation in lateral projection – two pairs of parallel articular shadows. (3) Tibia and talus not congruent.

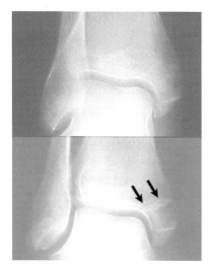

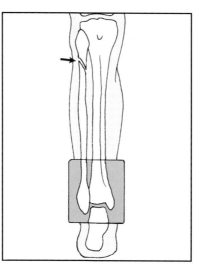

51. Radiographs (d): An oblique projection of the ankle, taken with the foot in 20° of internal rotation (Cobb projection, mortise view) is often helpful in diagnosing hairline fractures of the medial malleolus and Tillaux fractures. It is often advocated that its use should be routine. In the example shown above, contrast the standard AP projection (upper radiograph) with the mortise view of the same case.

52. Radiographs (e): Do not forget that injuries involving the ankle joint may be associated with fractures of the fibula proximal to the area covered by the normal radiographic projections. Transverse and spiral fractures of the fibular shaft are not uncommon, and in the Maisonneuve fracture the fibular neck is involved. If there is any suspicion of a fracture proximal to the ankle joint (e.g. by proximal tenderness, which should always be sought), then the entire fibular shaft should be visualised.

53. PRINCIPLES OF TREATMENT OF ANKLE INJURIES

The first considerations in treatment are:
1. If the fracture is displaced, the normal alignment of the talus with the tibia must be restored.
2. Measures must be taken to see that the fracture does not re-displace, and that the optimum conditions for union of the fracture and damaged soft tissues are established.
3. If the articulating surfaces have been damaged, then these should be treated appropriately to lessen the chances of secondary osteoarthritis developing in the joint.

In assessing each case the main factors to consider are whether the fracture is stable or unstable, and the patient's age.

STABLE INJURIES

Stable injuries have been defined as those which cannot be displaced by physiological forces. Fractures which broach the ring structure of the ankle at one site fall into this category. In the AO classification, A1, B1 and some C1 fractures are stable injuries. Clinically, absence of deformity, minor rather than gross swelling, and bruising, swelling and tenderness confined to one side of the joint are highly suggestive of the injury being stable. On X-ray the pattern of the fracture may confirm the likelihood of it being stable. However, if there is remaining doubt, the joint should be examined under anaesthesia.

Stable injuries have an excellent prognosis almost irrespective of treatment, and should be managed conservatively.

UNSTABLE INJURIES

The more structures which have been damaged, the greater the chances of the fracture being unstable. Clinically, marked swelling, bruising and tenderness on both sides of the joint are suggestive of instability, and the presence of deformity is virtually diagnostic. The pattern of fracture revealed by the radiographs may give a clear indication of the likelihood of instability. In doubtful cases, the joint should be examined under anaesthesia.

While the majority of unstable injuries may be reduced by closed methods, there is often difficulty in holding the position. Any slackening of the plaster must be dealt with promptly; weekly radiographs are essential to monitor the position of the fracture, and any slipping that is detected may require remanipulation. The high level of surveillance that this entails may not be readily available. Again, delayed or non-union of medial malleolar fractures may occur, and the prolonged plaster fixation required may cause problems with the subsequent mobilisation of the ankle. For these reasons the internal fixation of unstable fractures is usually the preferred treatment.

In some situations it is not necessary to fix all of the structures which have been damaged in order to restore stability to the joint. However, as the rigidity achieved with the fixation of what are often quite small bone fragments may sometimes be far from ideal, there is a tendency to fix most, if not all of the elements involved to improve the quality of the overall support.

UNSTABLE FRACTURES IN THE ELDERLY

One of the main problems is that the bone fragments may be small and osteoporotic, so that many of the usual fixation techniques may fail: small malleolar fragments may crumble, and screws cut out, leading to re-displacement. A number of publications have indicated that in this group the results from internal fixation are inferior or at best not better than conservatively managed fractures. Before internal fixation is considered, attention must be paid to the vascular state of the limb and the risks of skin flap necrosis assessed. Careful consideration must also be taken over the methods to be employed; screws should not be used, but tension band wiring may be considered in some cases. In others, K-wires or Rush pins inserted into the fibula percutaneously may be preferable, so long as the tenuous fixation they give is reinforced by a cast.

A guide to some of the methods which may be employed in dealing with the commoner problems in this highly divergent group of ankle fractures is given in the following frames.

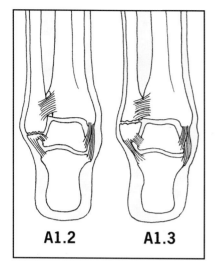

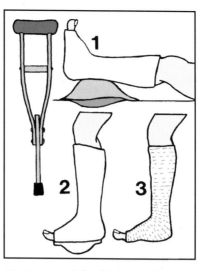

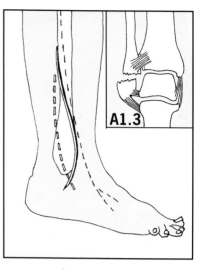

54. Fractures of the fibula distal to the syndesmosis (a): These fractures are classified as Type A in the AO–Weber classification. Type A1 fractures (Illus.) are horizontal and of avulsion pattern. They are caused by adduction or inversion forces. The distal fragment may be small or large. No other major structure is involved, and the injury is an inherently stable one.

55. Fracture of the fibula distal to the syndesmosis (b): If there is no tenderness elsewhere, if the fracture is undisplaced, and if the talar alignment is normal, then the injury may be considered to be stable. Treat conservatively with a below knee cast, elevation of the limb, and crutches (1) for 2–3 days until the swelling subsides, when a walking heel may be applied (2). Retain the cast for about six weeks, with a circular woven bandage (3) until any swelling has resolved.

56. Fracture of the fibula distal to the syndesmosis (c): If there is appreciable separation of the fragments the injury is potentially unstable, and there may be confirmatory evidence of talar tilting. Closed reduction is unlikely to be maintained and there is risk of non-union so internal fixation is advised. An anterolateral incision is to be preferred (but see Frame 58) as the posterior flap has a better blood supply. Avoid damage to the superficial peroneal nerve in the proximal part of the incision.

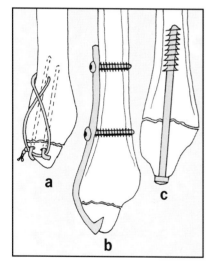

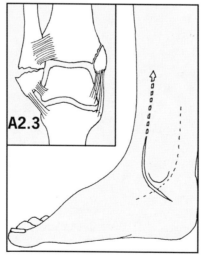

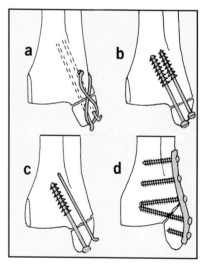

57. Fractures of the fibula distal to the syndesmosis (d): Where the fibular fragment is small, and particularly when the bone is osteoporotic, two K-wires with tension band wiring usually give the best results (a). Alternatively, a Zuelzer (b) or other pattern hook plate can give excellent fixation. Where the fragment is larger, a lag screw may be used (c).

58. Fractures of the fibula distal to the syndesmosis (e): With further adduction the medial malleolus may fracture (Types A2 and A3). Loss of its support leads to marked ankle instability, and internal fixation is the easiest form of management. An extensile anteromedial incision is preferred rather than a posteromedial one, unless a narrow skin bridge will be created if the fibula has also to be exposed or if access to a posterior fracture extension is needed.

59. Fractures of the fibula distal to the syndesmosis (f): If the medial malleolar fragment is small and/or osteoporotic it may be held with K-wires and a tension band (a) or by a hook plate; if the bone quality is good and the fragment substantial, then 2 malleolar screws (b), 2 cancellous screws, or a single screw and K-wire (c) may be used. If the proximal part is comminuted, then some form of plate is desirable (eg DC, T- or clover leaf) (d).

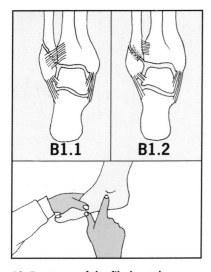

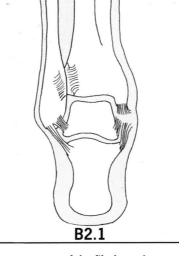

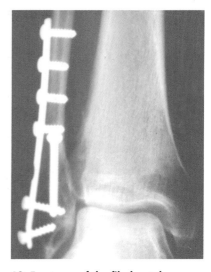

60. Fractures of the fibula at the syndesmosis (a): In Type B1 injuries there may or may not be associated tearing or avulsion of the inferior tibiofibular ligament. These are the commonest ankle fractures and are generally stable. However, it is important to exclude damage to the medial complex. Look for medial tenderness, and if in doubt examine the joint under anaesthesia. If stability is confirmed, then conservative treatment (see Frame 55) gives excellent results.

61. Fractures of the fibula at the syndesmosis (b): If there is associated tearing of the medial ligament (B2.1) the injury is potentially unstable. (The anterior tibiofibular ligament is always torn or its bony attachments avulsed.) An intact medial malleolus however tends to minimise any instability, so that these injuries may be treated conservatively by manipulative reduction (if required), and cast fixation (see Frame 55). Take check radiographs weekly to detect any late slip.

62. Fractures of the fibula at the syndesmosis (c): Some, however, prefer to treat fractures of the fibula which occur at the level of the syndesmosis and which have an associated medial ligament tear, by internal fixation. (So long as the ends of the torn medial ligament are in apposition, suture repair is unnecessary if the ankle is stabilised by either a cast or internal fixation of the fibula.) Here a contoured dynamic compression plate and interfragmental screw have been used.

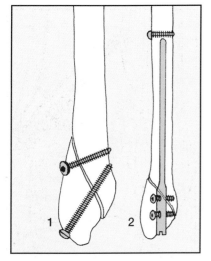

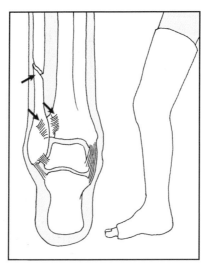

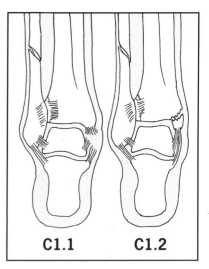

63. Fractures of the fibula at the syndesmosis (d): If the medial malleolus is fractured, internal fixation of both the medial and lateral malleoli is advised. In the case of the medial malleolus the methods described in Frame 59 may be used. In the case of the fibula, methods appropriate to the quality of the bone may be used: these include the methods described in Frames 57 and 62. In addition, interfragmental screws (1); or an SST Small Bone Locking Nail® (2) (with a proximal screw to preserve length) may be used.

64. Fractures of the fibula above the syndesmosis (a): All involve disruption of the anterior tibiofibular ligament. In addition, when the posterior tibiofibular ligament (or its attachments) or the medial complex is involved, the injury is unstable. This is true in the majority of cases. *Stable injuries however do not require surgery.* They may be treated by a cast which can be extended above the knee for extra support. It is important not to miss this small group, and if there is doubt, the joint should be examined under anaesthesia.

65. Fractures of the fibula above the syndesmosis (b): In those cases where there is instability, the pattern and site of the fibular injury vary. Rarely, there is dislocation of the proximal tibiofibular joint rather than fracture. There is associated damage to the medial complex, either in the form of rupture of the deltoid ligament or fracture of the medial malleolus. In unstable injuries the usual treatment is to internally fix any fibular and medial malleolar fracture.

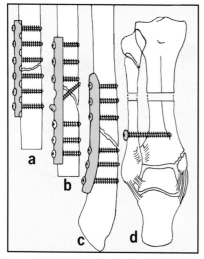

66. Fractures of the fibula above the syndesmosis (c): Most may be held with a Low Contact Dynamic Compression Plate (a); some spiral and comminuted fractures with interfragmentary screws and a neutralising plate (b); and distal fractures by a one-third tubular plate (c). It is vital to ensure that fibular length and rotation are corrected. To avoid the common peroneal nerve, proximal fractures should be treated with a transverse syndesmotic screw above the ankle (with all the holes tapped to avoid compression) (d).

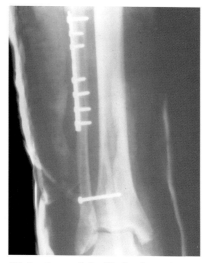

67. Fractures of the fibula above the syndesmosis (d): If the fibula has been perfectly reduced the syndesmosis should close and any displaced avulsion fragment should fall into place. Confirm with check films. Persisting deformity may sometimes be due to problems on the *medial* side of the joint (e.g. soft tissue, or the tendon of tibialis posterior between the bone ends) which may have to be dealt with first. (See also Frames 68 and 69.) Otherwise reduce and hold with a syndesmotic screw (Illus): this should be removed before mobilisation.

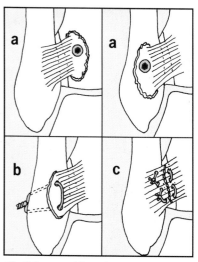

68. Other considerations (a) – Anterior tibiofibular ligament: If possible, any accessible large bone fragment (from the tibial or fibular attachment) should be replaced and held with a small lag screw (a). If the fragment is small a wire loop may be employed (b). If the central portion of the ligament is involved it should be sutured (c). The repair may be splinted with a syndesmosis screw which should be removed at 8 weeks, prior to weight bearing.

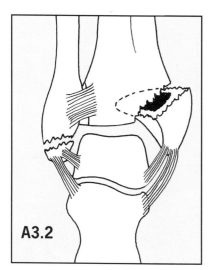

69. Other considerations (b) – Posterior lip (posterior malleolar) fractures (a): These are certain indicators of instability. The presence and position of any posterior malleolar fracture should be determined (e.g. by CAT scan) before any operative procedure is undertaken, as this may govern the best surgical approach. The posterior lip may be formed by a posterior extension of the medial malleolus (Type A3 fractures). If so it may be dealt with by the common medial malleolar fixation techniques.

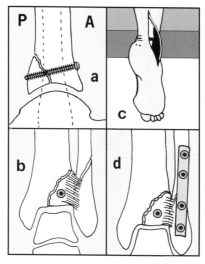

70. Posterior lip (posterior malleolar) fractures (b): If the lip is laterally placed it is likely to have been pulled off by the posterior tibiofibular ligament. If small it need not be fixed; if large, it may be held by a retrograde screw (a). If it is more shell-like it should be secured from behind (b). A posterior approach with the patient in the prone position is recommended (c). The fibular fracture may be fixed through the same incision with a posteriorly placed plate (d).

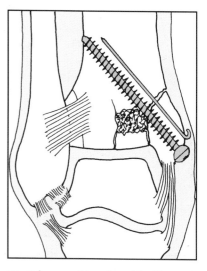

71. Other considerations (c) – 'Corner' fractures: In certain adduction and abduction injuries the inferomedial or inferolateral surface of the tibia or the corresponding part of the talus may be damaged. As a general rule, small loose fragments of bone and cartilage should be removed, but larger fragments with articular cartilage should be retained; it may be necessary to pack any defect with a bone graft.

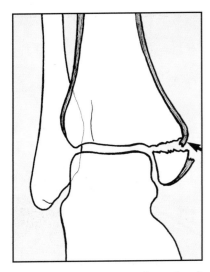

72. Other considerations (d) – Isolated medial malleolar fracture: In an appreciable number of cases a periosteal flap comes to lie between the bone ends. This causes minor but persistent displacement of the malleolar fragment which is not amenable to closed reduction methods; it may lead to non-union, and chronic ankle instability. Open reduction and internal fixation is recommended for all fractures of this pattern (see Frame 59).

73. Other considerations (e):
Timing of surgery: At the earliest opportunity any gross deformity should be corrected by realigning the foot with the leg to lessen the risks of circulatory impairment and of skin necrosis (which is especially great over the medial tibial margin). The complication rate for surgery rises eight fold for the first few days after a delay of over 24 hours. Sometimes, however, especially where the case is seen late, it is may be profitable to delay surgery for 10–12 days (but after a manipulative realignment) to allow swelling and any pressure blistering to subside, thereby improving the chances of uncomplicated wound healing.

Care after surgery: The limb should be well padded and elevated. It is important that the foot is not allowed to become plantarflexed and a removable plastic splint or stout plaster backshell is advised. After a few days this may be removed for short periods to permit mobilisation, provided that this does not jeopardise the fixation. Non-weight bearing, with crutches and a splint or cast, may be permitted when the postoperative swelling has subsided. In most cases it is inadvisable to allow unprotected weight bearing until union is moderately far advanced (usually at about six weeks).

Failure of fixation: If the reduction is lost this is generally the result of the fixation devices cutting out before union has occurred. The deformity must be corrected. While it is sometimes possible to do this by closed methods it may be necessary to remove any fixation device to achieve this. In most cases the bone in the area of the fracture will have become soft and unable to retain screws. The deformity should be reduced manually, and, if necessary, K-wires used to stabilise the fracture. Thereafter close monitoring will be required, with the patient remaining in a cast until union has occurred.

Fractures in the elderly: The results of internal fixation in the elderly are often disappointing, and a number of series in the past have shown these to be usually inferior or certainly no better than conservatively treated fractures. The results are poorer in women than men. The reasons include the quality of the bone fragments, which are often fragile and osteoporotic; poor peripheral circulation leading to problems with wound and fracture healing; excessive stresses through fixation devices due to overweight; and poor anaesthetic risks. Better results are now expected with newer methods which include the use of cannulated screws inserted percutaneously through small stab wounds, and multiple K-wires to help maintain the position of the fracture while the patient remains in plaster until union occurs. Nevertheless it is important to have a sound knowledge of closed methods of treatment for these fractures.

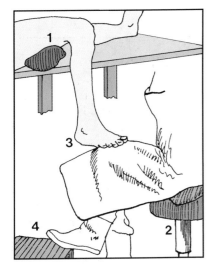

74. Closed treatment of displaced ankle fractures – manipulation (a): Conservative treatment may be proposed if the patient is frail, a poor anaesthetic risk, or the skin and circulation poor. The patient is anaesthetised and the leg abducted over the edge of the table with a sandbag behind the thigh (1). The surgeon's stool (2) or the table should be adjusted until the toes can be steadied with the knee (3). A footstool may be helpful (4).

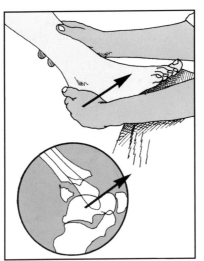

75. Manipulation (b): Carry out a reduction rehearsal. The malleoli generally preserve their relationship with the talus and the foot, so that *in essence it is a case of re-aligning the foot with the tibia.* In most cases, three elements require correction: 1. Begin by correcting any posterior subluxation by grasping the heel and lifting it anteriorly.

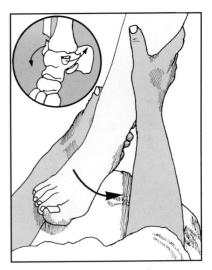

76. Manipulation (c): 2. Still grasping the hind foot, correct any external rotation. It should be noted that little force is required for these corrections, and in many cases re-alignment is completed by sensations similar to those experienced when reducing a dislocation.

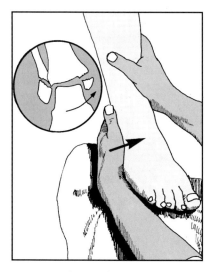

77. Manipulation (d): 3. Finally correct any abduction deformity. *Note:* (i) The appearance of the ankle should be restored to normal. (ii) Overcorrection is difficult or impossible. Repeat the procedure until you can remember the direction of movements and force required for reduction.

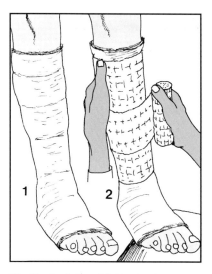

78. Manipulation (e): Now apply wool roll to the limb making sure that the malleolar prominences are well covered (1). Without hurry follow this with two to three 15 cm (6″) plaster bandages from the level of the tibial tubercle to just above the ankle (2).

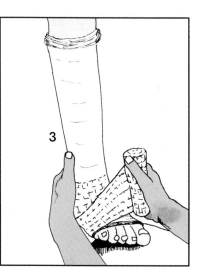

79. Manipulation (f): Smooth the plaster well down and then quickly apply two 15 cm (6″) plaster bandages to the foot and ankle. The toes may be steadied with your knee (3). On completion, you should be left with a plaster which is setting at the calf, but is quite soft and mouldable at the foot and ankle.

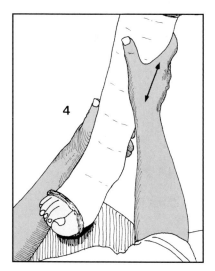

80. Manipulation (g): Now repeat the reduction manoeuvre and hold the limb in the reduced position until the plaster has set (4). Steady the forefoot with the knee (to keep the ankle at right angles) and ease the hands slightly upwards and downwards to prevent local indentation of the plaster. *Extend the plaster above the knee if the fracture is very unstable.*

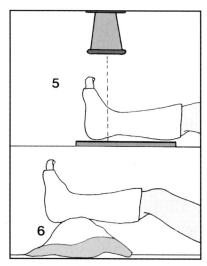

81. Manipulation (h): Check the position of the fracture with radiographs before the anaesthetic is discontinued, and if necessary, repeat the procedure (5). Precautions should be taken over swelling, e.g. elevation, splitting of the plaster (6).

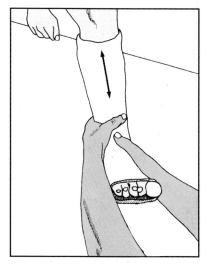

82. Aftercare (a): The plaster should be examined for slackness as swelling subsides. If it becomes slack, it must be changed with care to prevent slipping of the fracture, and general anaesthesia may be necessary. Radiographs should be taken weekly; remanipulation under anaesthesia or internal fixation may have to be considered if there is any slip.

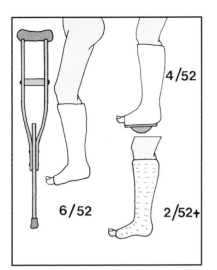

83. Aftercare (b): A walking heel should not be applied before 6 weeks: prior to that the patient may be mobilised, non-weight bearing, with crutches. Plaster fixation should be maintained until union (usually 9–10 weeks in the older patient). Confirm this both clinically and radiologically. Thereafter bandage supports should be worn until swelling subsides. Physiotherapy is often required.

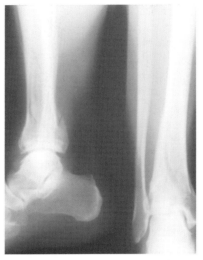

84. Multifragmented compression (or pilon) fractures (a): These potentially most difficult injuries are classified under the AO system as Type B and C fractures of the Distal Tibial Segment. In Type B fractures part of the inferior tibial articular surface is involved; Type C fractures are complete articular fractures (see p. 385). The complexity of the lesion is seldom apparent in plain films, as is the case in this example of a Type C fracture.

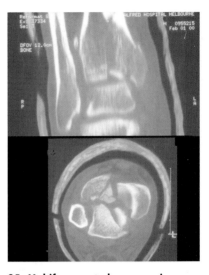

85. Multifragmented compression fractures (b): Analysis by CAT scan is highly desirable where operative intervention is going to be considered. The two views above in the coronal and transverse planes of the previous case give additional information regarding the comminution of the inferior articular surface of the tibia.

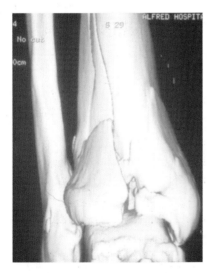

86. Multifragmented compression fractures (c): Still more information may be gained with a 3D reconstruction; the example is again of the previous case. This clarifies the extent of involvement of the distal tibial shaft and the bone immediately proximal to the tibial articular surface.

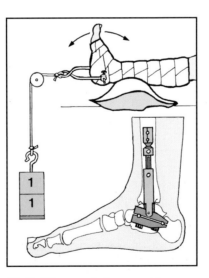

87. Multifragmented compression fractures (d): Where there is gross comminution surgery is unlikely to be profitable, and the aims should be to maintain length and start ankle movements early. This may be achieved with a heel pin and weights (about 2 kg (1)) or a hinged external fixator (2). Weight bearing is deferred until union.

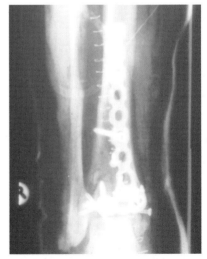

88. Multifragmented compression fractures (e): Surgery may be attempted if there is at least one large articular fragment which can be fixed to the tibial shaft. In the case shown in Frame 86, the medial malleolus and tibial fractures were held with a long medial plate, and the smaller articular fragments secured with additional screws.

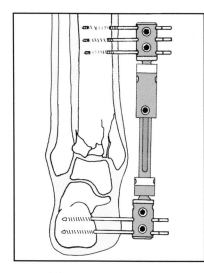

89. Multifragmented compression fractures (f): In some cases it may be thought desirable to delay surgery for 10–12 days until swelling and any pressure blistering have subsided. To maintain length in the interim, an external fixator may be used. Some cases may then be suitable for a limited reconstruction, with screw fixation of the major fragments and, if necessary, fine wire fixation of smaller ones: a hybrid or plain Ilizarov fixator (as in p. 78 and p. 339) may then be employed to hold these and provide overall support.

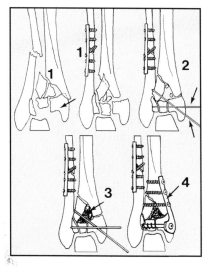

90. Multifragmented compression fractures (g): Other techniques can include the following: (1) Reduction and fixation of any fibular fracture to obtain length and alignment; (2) Reconstruction of the articular surface by placing the fragments over the talar dome and temporarily holding them with K-wires; (3) Packing defects with bone grafts; (4) Fixing the main fragments with a buttress plate (and, if required, cannulated screws).

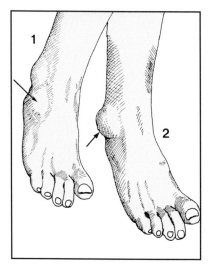

91. Lateral ligament injuries – Diagnosis (a): A soft tissue injury is diagnosed where there is a history of trauma and the radiographs are normal. A history of an inversion injury is obtainable in most lateral ligament injuries. In sprains, swelling and tenderness follow the fasciculi of the lateral ligament (1). In complete tears of the lateral ligament, swelling at first lies over the lateral malleolus (2).

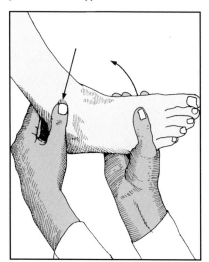

92. Diagnosis (b): If the findings suggest a more substantial injury, grasp the foot and gently abduct the talus in the ankle mortise, feeling for any gap opening up at the outer corner of the joint. Compare with the other side. Excess movement of the talus on the injured side suggests a complete lateral ligament tear. (Note that the test is also positive in tears of the anterior tibiofibular ligament if the foot is not inverted in the *dorsiflexed* position.)

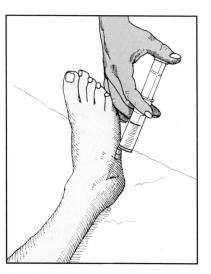

93. Diagnosis (c): If the manoeuvre cannot be performed adequately because of pain, infiltrate the fasciculi of the lateral ligament with local anaesthetic (e.g. 20 mL of 0.5% lignocaine) or administer a general anaesthetic. Repeat the manoeuvre, and for further confirmation, take AP radiographs under stress. The anterior drawer test, with or without stress films, may also be performed.

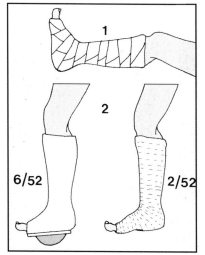

94. Treatment (a): Simple sprains resolve in a few days with local supportive measures (adhesive strapping, crepe bandaging, etc.) rest and elevation (1). Complete lateral ligament tears should be treated either by surgical repair (of both anterior tibiofibular *and* calcaneofibular ligaments) or by plaster fixation for 6 weeks (2), followed by a lighter support till free from discomfort. Alternatively, a hinged ankle brace may be used for the same length of time and will permit early movements.

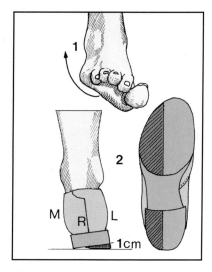

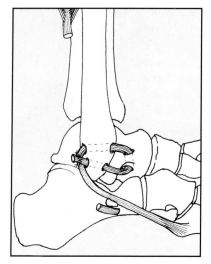

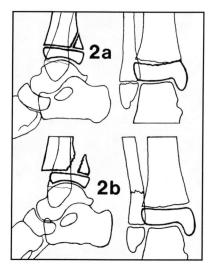

95. Treatment (b): If there is no obvious abnormality, investigate with plain and stress films, MRI scans and arthroscopy. Sometimes tissue thickening in the anterolateral aspect of the ankle may be found and removed with profit. Treat the so-called functional instabilities (thought due to disorders of muscle coordination or proprioception) with physiotherapy to develop the evertors (1) (eg by exercises or a wobble board) and the use of lateral heel and sole wedges (2).

96. Treatment (c): Surgical reconstruction may be required if simple measures fail, and instability has been demonstrated. In the Watson–Jones reconstruction, the peroneus brevis tendon is threaded through holes drilled in the fibula and talus and sewn to itself. The upper stump is sewn to peroneus longus. The tendon replaces the torn ligament, and the success rate of the operation is high. Failure may indicate subtalar laxity.

97. Epiphyseal injuries (a): Salter–Harris Type 1 injuries are rare. In the case of the fibula, a sprain may be mistakenly diagnosed, with traumatic epiphyseal growth arrest sometimes following. The commonest injury is one of Type 2. In either Type 1 or 2, where displacement is minimal (a) a below-knee plaster may be used for 4–6 weeks. Where displacement is appreciable (b) the deformity should be reduced by manipulation prior to the application of a cast.

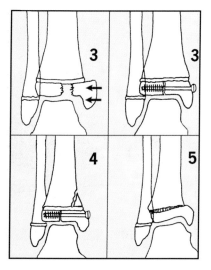

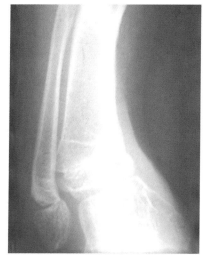

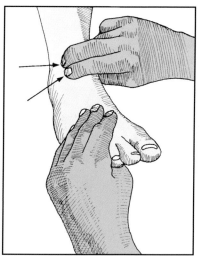

98. Epiphyseal injuries (b): Salter–Harris Type 3 and Type 4 injuries may sometimes be reduced by applying firm local pressure under GA but as re-displacement is common, cross-screwing is generally advised. This may be carried out with a cannulated screw inserted percutaneously with care to avoid transgressing the growth plate. Type 5 injuries should be treated expectantly by manipulative reduction.

99. Epiphyseal injuries (c): Epiphyseal injures (especially those of Type 3 and 4) may be followed by disturbance of bone growth, leading to shortening and deformity. A bony bar may form and bridge the epiphysis and the metaphysis. Its location and extent may be investigated by CAT scan, when consideration should be given to its excision and the filling of the resulting defect. Where a deformity has become well established (Illus.) a corrective osteotomy will be required. (See also p. 90.)

100. Sprain of inferior tibiofibular ligament: Inversion injuries of the ankle may lead to a first stage sup./lateral rotational tearing of the inferior tibiofibular ligament. Pain may be quite severe, and tenderness well localised over the ligament. A 6 week period of plaster fixation is advised. In cases of chronic disability hydrocortisone injections may be tried, or operative reconstruction considered.

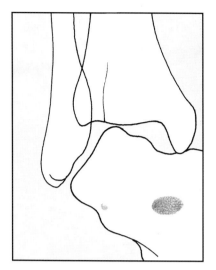

101. Ankle dislocation without fracture: Rarely, the ankle may dislocate without fracture. Although rupture of both medial and lateral ligaments must take place, conservative management by closed manipulative reduction and plaster fixation may achieve a good result. Avascular necrosis of the talus is a minor risk in this situation.

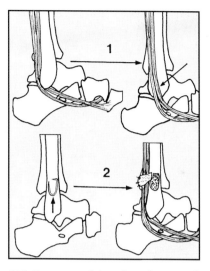

102. Recurrent dislocation of peroneal tendons: This is a rare condition in which eversion causes painful clicking sensations as the peroneal tendons repeatedly snap over the lateral malleolus (1). The condition is associated with a defect in the superior peroneal retinaculum. A flap of bone and periosteum can be used to reconstruct the defective ligament (2).

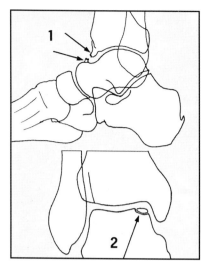

103. Footballer's ankle and osteochondritis tali: Tibial and/or talar osteophytes (1) may arise in footballers from repeated anterior capsular tears, and limit dorsiflexion. Excision for this is seldom indicated, but if symptoms are commanding arthroscopic debridement may be tried. Pain may follow a fresh tear (treat symptomatically by POP fixation) or from early ankle joint osteoarthritis. (Osteochondritis tali (2) – see p. 393.)

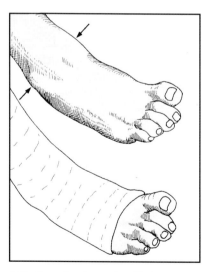

104. Complications of ankle injuries – Swelling: Swelling persisting for weeks or even months after fixation has been discarded is so common as to be an almost normal occurrence. Assuming that the fracture has united in a good position, local supportive measures should be continued until resolution. The patient should be reassured and advised regarding elevation and activity.

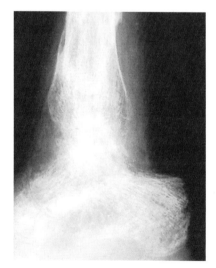

105. Complex regional pain syndrome/Sudeck's atrophy: Where swelling is gross, and especially if the toes are involved, suspect Sudeck's atrophy. There may be glazing of the skin and pain. Radiographs may show typical porotic changes, and confirm union of the fracture. Intensive physiotherapy, continued use of supports and other measures may be required (see Chapters 5, 8). Convalescence may be expected to be slow with occasionally some permanent functional impairment.

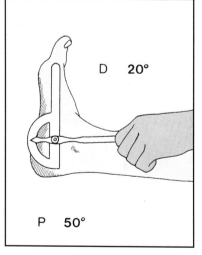

106. Stiffness, 'weakness' and disturbance of gait: Again, assuming sound union, these symptoms generally respond rapidly to appropriate physiotherapy and occupational therapy. Progress may be assessed by charting the range of ankle joint movements. (The normal range is indicated, but compare the sides.) Note also the range in the subtalar joint.

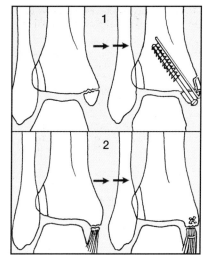
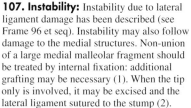

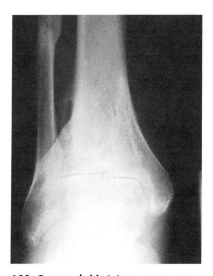

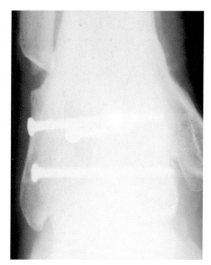

107. Instability: Instability due to lateral ligament damage has been described (see Frame 96 et seq). Instability may also follow damage to the medial structures. Non-union of a large medial malleolar fragment should be treated by internal fixation: additional grafting may be necessary (1). When the tip only is involved, it may be excised and the lateral ligament sutured to the stump (2).

108. Osteoarthritis (a): Considering the incidence of ankle fractures, osteoarthritis is an uncommon complication. It is most likely to follow compression fractures, and fractures with residual diastasis or talotibial incongruity. Note in this example of an old compression fracture the central split in the tibial surface, the broadening of the mortise and the narrowed joint space.

109. Osteoarthritis (b): If symptoms of pain, swelling, stiffness and disturbance of gait are troublesome, then fusion may be advised. In the Crawford–Adams fusion, the articular surfaces are cleared, the fibula is inlaid in the talus and tibia and held in position with cross-screws. Late function is generally good due to persistent midtarsal movement.

TIBIA/FIBULA, *Distal Segment : 43–*

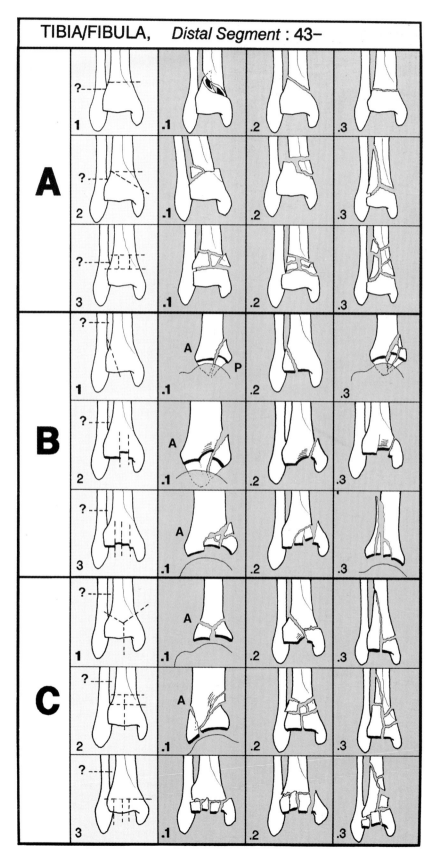

110. AO classification of fractures of the tibia/fibula, distal segment (43–):

Type A fractures are extra-articular.
A1 = Metaphyseal simple, with or without an associated fibular fracture: .1 spiral; .2 oblique; .3 transverse.
A2 = Metaphyseal wedge fracture, with or without a fracture of the fibula: .1 with posterolateral impaction; .2 with an anteromedial wedge; .3 with the fracture extending proximally into the diaphysis.
A3 = Metaphyseal complex, with or without a fracture of the fibula: .1 with three intermediate fragments; .2 with more than three intermediate fragments; .3 with extension into the diaphysis.

Type B fractures are partial articular.
B1 = Pure split fracture with or without a fracture of the fibula: .1 frontal; .2 sagittal; .3 metaphyseal multifragmentary.
B2 = Split fracture with depression, with or without a fracture of the fibula: .1 frontal; .2 sagittal; .3 central.
B3 = Multifragmentary depressed fracture, with or without a fracture of the fibula: .1 frontal; .2 sagittal; .3 metaphyseal.

Type C fractures are complete articular.
C1 = Articular simple, metaphyseal simple, with or without a fracture of the fibula: .1 unimpacted; .2 with some depression of the articular surface; .3 with the fracture extending into the diaphysis.
C2 = Articular simple, metaphyseal multifragmentary, with or without a fracture of the fibula: .1 with uneven impaction; .2 without uneven impaction; .3 with the fracture extending into the diaphysis.
C3 = Multifragmentary, with or without a fracture of the fibula: .1 confined to the epiphysis; .2 confined to the epiphysis and metaphysis; .3 extending into the diaphysis.

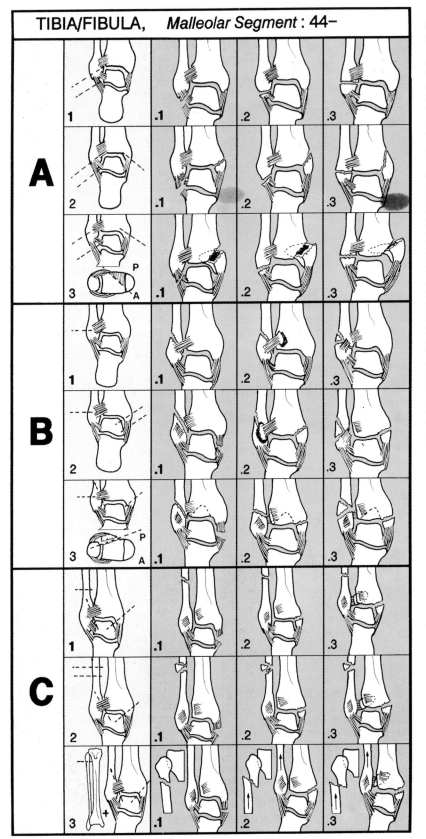

TIBIA/FIBULA, *Malleolar Segment : 44–*

111. AO classification of fractures of the tibia/fibula, malleolar segment (44–): Note the following:

1. At this location the three Types (A, B, C) are selected by where the lateral lesion is placed in relation to the inferior tibiofibular ligaments ('the syndesmotic ligaments').

2. In this exceptional situation, ligament lesions *without any accompanying fracture* have been included.

Type A lesions are infrasyndesmotic.

A1 = Isolated lesions of ligament or bone: .1 complete tear of the lateral ligament of the ankle; .2 avulsion fracture of the tip of the lateral malleolus; .3 transverse fracture of the lateral malleolus.

A2 = Bifocal lesions, with a fracture of the medial malleolus (which may be transverse, oblique or vertical) with: .1 a complete tear of the lateral ligament; .2 avulsion of the tip of the lateral malleolus; .3 transverse fracture of the lateral malleolus.

A3 = Bifocal lesions, with a medial malleolar fracture which extends posteriorly ('round the back') with: .1 a complete tear of the lateral ligament; .2 avulsion of the tip of the lateral malleolus; .3 transverse fracture of the lateral malleolus.

Type B fractures of the fibula are transyndesmotic.

B1 = Where the lateral side of the joint only is involved: .1 simple; .2 with disruption of the anterior syndesmosis (anterior inferior tibiofibular ligament tear or avulsion from the tibia (Tillaux fracture, Illus.) or from the fibula (le Fort fracture); .3 multifragmentary.

B2 = Fracture of the fibula with a medial lesion: .1 simple, with rupture of the medial (deltoid) ligament and disruption of the anterior syndesmosis; .2 simple, with fracture of the medial malleolus and disruption of the anterior syndesmosis (Illus.: le Fort); .3 multifragmentary lateral malleolar fracture with rupture of the medial ligament or a fracture of the medial malleolus.

B3 = Fracture of the fibula with both a medial lesion and a fracture of the posterolateral rim (posterolateral lip; fracture of the posterior malleolus): .1 simple fibula, ruptured medial ligament; .2 fibula simple, fracture of the medial malleolus; .3 multifragmentary fibula with fracture of the medial malleolus.

Type C are bifocal lesions with rupture of the anterior or both anterior and posterior inferior tibiofibular ligaments. The fracture of the fibula is suprasyndesmotic (i.e. above the inferior tibiofibular ligaments), and the medial lesion involves either the medial ligament or the medial malleolus.

C1 = Simple diaphyseal fracture of the fibula; .1 rupture of the medial ligament; .2 fracture of the medial malleolus; .3 with fracture of the medial malleolus and the posterior rim.

C2 = Multifragmentary diaphyseal fracture of the fibula: .1 with rupture of the medial ligament; .2 fracture of the medial malleolus; .3 fracture of the medial malleolus and the posterior rim.

C3 = Proximal fibular fracture (Maisonneuve fracture): .1 without shortening; .2 with shortening; .3 with a posterior rim fracture.

SELF-TEST

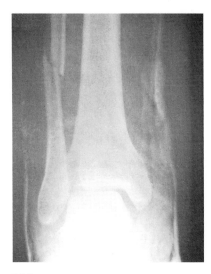

112. This AP radiograph shows the position achieved by closed reduction of a Dupuytren fracture–dislocation of the ankle (P/L (external rotation with diastasis) Stage 4 injury (AO = 44–C1.1)). Is reduction complete?

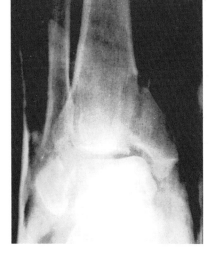

113. Classify this injury. Is the reduction satisfactory?

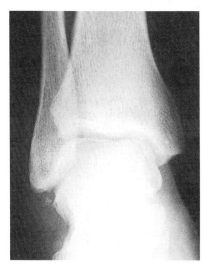

114. This radiograph was taken of a patient complaining of pain in the ankle after an inversion injury. Do you detect any abnormality?

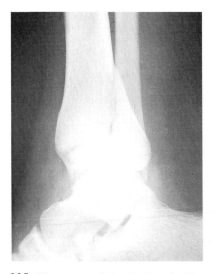

115. What pattern of injury is shown in this lateral radiograph?

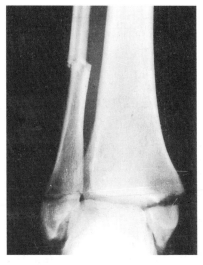

116. What is this injury? What atypical element is present?

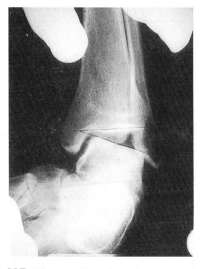

117. What does this radiograph demonstrate?

ANSWERS TO SELF-TEST

112. No: there is persistent lateral talar shift (note the gap between the talus and the medial malleolus) due to slight persistent diastasis. This position would be accepted by a number of surgeons, while others would prefer to reduce and internally fix the fibular fracture and repair the anterior tibiofibular ligament. Any persisting deformity might be dealt with by a cross-screw (syndesmosis screw), removed before full mobilisation is embarked upon. (AO = 44–C1.1.)

113. The vertical fracture of the medial malleolus is typical of a supination/adduction Stage 2 injury (adduction fracture), AO = 44–A3.1. Reduction is incomplete, and there is disturbance of the inferior articular surface of the tibia. Open reduction is indicated.

114. A small opacity is present distal to the tip of the lateral malleolus, and probably represents avulsion of the fibular attachment of the lateral ligament. The fragment is small, and clinical confirmation would be desirable. (AO = 44–A1.2.)

115. This is an epiphyseal injury, in which there is slight backward displacement of the distal tibial epiphysis, along with a small fragment of metaphysis (juxta-epiphyseal fragment), i.e. a Salter–Harris Type 2 injury. There is some evidence on this lateral view of talotibial incongruity, and manipulation would be indicated.

116. This is a pronation/abduction injury with horizontal fractures of the medial and lateral malleoli and lateral displacement of the talus. There are atypically two fractures of the fibula, one through the syndesmosis and one above it. Atypical fracture of the fibula at a higher level, with some of the features of AO = 44–B.2 and 44–C.1 fractures.

117. Although comparison films of the other ankle should be taken, it is almost certain that a complete tear of the external ligament has been demonstrated in this inversion film. (Note the shadows of the lead gloves and the angle of talar tilting which has been marked on the radiograph.)

CHAPTER

15

Foot injuries

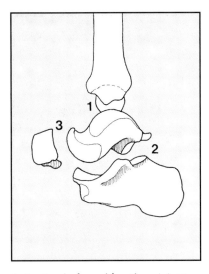

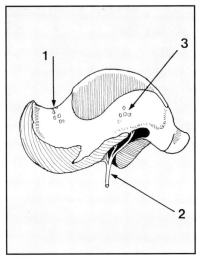

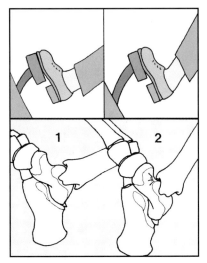

1. Anatomical considerations (a): The talus plays a key role in no less than 3 joints: (1) The ankle joint – articulating with the tibia and fibula; (2) The subtalar joint – articulating with the calcaneus; (3) The talonavicular joint: along with the calcaneocuboid joint, this forms the *midtarsal joint*. Secondary osteoarthritic changes may occur following fractures which cause articular irregularity.

2. Anatomical considerations (b): Secondary osteoarthritis may also follow avascular necrosis which occurs in half of all talar neck fractures. The blood supply of the talus enters at three sites: (1) The neck; (2) The sinus tarsi area; (3) The medial side of the body. The more sources are disturbed, the greater is the risk to the blood supply.

3. Mechanisms of injury: The commonest fracture is of the neck. This may occur in car accidents, when pedal impact (1) forces the talar neck against the tibial margin (2). (There is a long association between this injury and light aircraft crashes where the feet are violently dorsiflexed against the rudder pedals – 'aviator's astragalus'.) The injury may also follow falls from a height in a crouching position.

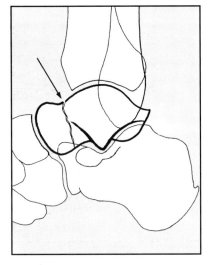

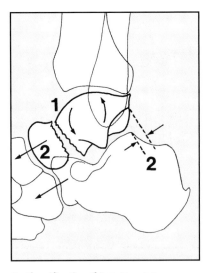

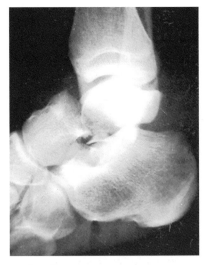

4. Classification of talar neck fractures (a): Talar neck fractures have been classified into four types of increasing severity. In *Type 1* the talar neck is fractured without displacement. Incomplete hairline cracks are not uncommon. Only the blood supply through the neck is affected, and the incidence of avascular necrosis is under 10%.

5. Classification (b): In *Type 2* fractures there is an accompanying subtalar subluxation. The proximal portion of the talus adopts a position of plantar flexion (1). The *head* of the talus maintains its relationship with the navicular and calcaneus (and the rest of the foot) which subluxate forwards (2).

6. Classification (c): Note in the radiographic example a more severe degree of plantar flexion of the proximal fragment, and greater subluxation. The blood supplies through the neck and sinus tarsi are both interrupted, and the incidence of avascular necrosis rises to 50% in fractures of this type.

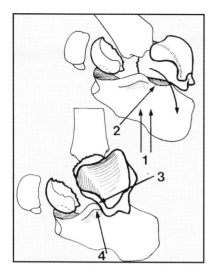

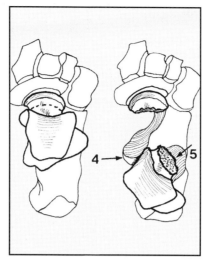

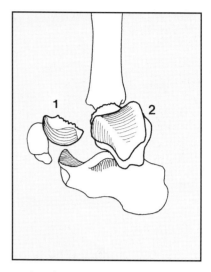

7. Classification (d): *Type 3* injuries. With further dorsiflexion and upward force (1) the tibia is driven between the two talar fragments. The posterior fragment is extruded backwards, while at the same time the convex posterior articular surface of the calcaneus (2) guides it medially. It comes to rest with its medial surface (3) caught on the sustentaculum tali (4).

8. Classification (e): In its final position the main portion of the talus lies on the medial side of the ankle, with its fractured surface (5) pointing laterally. All three sources of blood supply are disturbed. The risks of avascular necrosis are high, rising to 85%.

9. Classification (f): In the rare *Type 4* injury, the head of the talus dislocates from the navicular (1) in association with a Type 3 (2) or a Type 2 injury. The incidence of avascular necrosis here is also high.

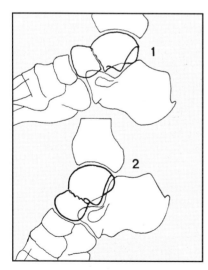

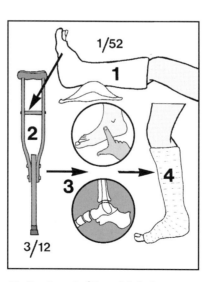

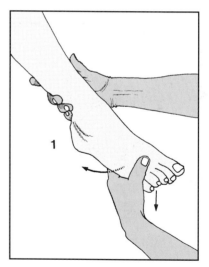

10. Diagnosis: The diagnosis may be suspected from the history, but is made radiologically. Care must be taken to differentiate between Type 1 and Type 2 injuries. If doubt exists, two laterals, one in dorsiflexion (1) and one in plantar flexion (2) should be taken and compared. These will reveal any subluxation (Type 2 illustrated).

11. Treatment of Type 1 injuries: (1) Padded plaster with toe platform and elevation for about a week. (2) Non-weight bearing with crutches for 3 months. (3) The fracture is then assessed out of plaster for union and absence of avascular necrosis. (4) If there are no complications, weight bearing may commence with a light support. Physiotherapy will be required for ankle, subtalar joint and calf.

12. Treatment of Type 2 injuries (a): While some prefer open reduction for all these fractures, closed methods may be attempted: (1) The foot is plantar flexed and everted. (2) A padded plaster is then applied in this position and check radiographs taken. If a satisfactory reduction has been obtained, then conservative treatment may be continued.

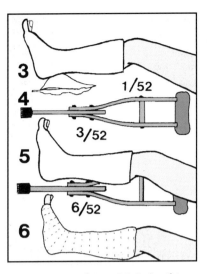

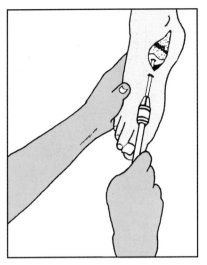

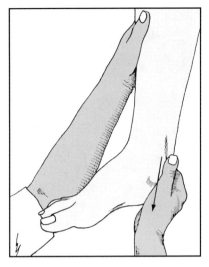

13. Treatment of Type 2 injuries (b): (3) The limb is elevated for a week before (4) non-weight bearing is permitted. After 3–4 weeks the plaster is changed under intensifier control and the foot brought up to a right angle (5). Non-weight bearing is continued for a further 6 weeks. Thereafter, if the fracture is united and there is no evidence of avascular necrosis, weight bearing may be allowed with support (6). Physiotherapy will almost certainly be required.

14. Treatment of Type 2 injuries (c): If closed methods fail in obtaining a reduction, open reduction will be required. The fracture may be secured with a K-wire passed backwards from the head of the talus into the body, with the aftercare being similar to that described in the previous frame. The K-wire may be removed at the change of plaster. For more rigid fixation, a cannulated screw may be preferred.

15. Treatment of Type 3 injuries (a): The displaced portion of the talus is situated subcutaneously, and there should be no delay in reducing it as the overlying skin is tightly stretched over the bone and likely to slough. Facilities for open reduction should be available, but closed methods may be attempted first. Begin by gripping the heel and applying traction to it.

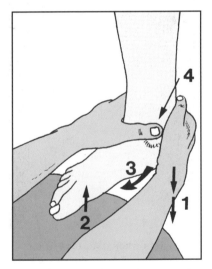

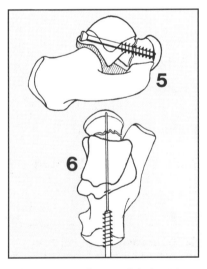

16. Treatment of Type 3 injuries (b): Maintaining traction (1), use the knee (2) to dorsiflex the foot. Pull the heel slightly forward and evert it (3) to open up the space for the talus. Apply strong pressure over the displaced body of the talus (4), pressing laterally, but also slightly anteriorly and downwards. Now plantar flex the foot. If purchase on the heel is poor, a Steinmann pin through the heel and a calliper may be used.

17. Treatment of Type 3 injuries (c): After reduction, proceed with elevation and gradual mobilisation as described in Frame 13 above. If closed reduction fails (as it often does), open reduction will be necessary. The condition of the skin and any planned internal fixation will dictate the incision(s). These fractures may be fixed (best through a posterolateral incision) with one or two cancellous screws passed from behind

through the body of the talus and into the head (5). Cannulated screws may also be used; these can be threaded over K-wires which have been inserted temporarily to hold the reduction (6). The AO group, with an eye to rapid mobilisation, in fact recommend internal fixation along these lines for all talar neck fractures.

Treatment of Type 4 injuries: These uncommon injuries are likely to require open reduction. All fragments should be retained, even if completely detached and obviously avascular. On no account should the talus be excised.

Complications of talar neck fractures (a): – Skin necrosis: The skin may become tightly stretched over a displaced talus and undergo necrosis with late sloughing. *Early reduction is imperative to avoid this complication.*

(b): Open injuries: Thorough debridement of the wound is essential, but again every effort must be made to retain the main fragments. Treatment should follow the usual lines established for the management of open fractures. If sepsis occurs *in conjunction with avascular necrosis,* healing may be obtained only after excision of the avascular fragments.

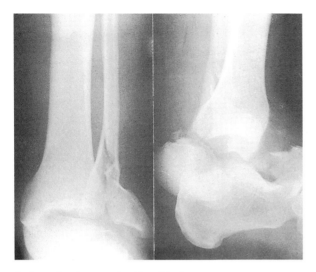

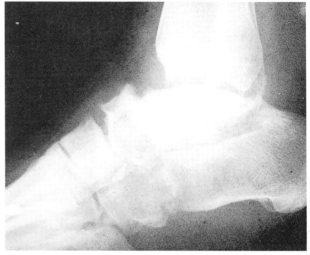

18. Complications cntd – (c) Ankle fracture: Rarely, malleolar fracture may be found complicating talar neck fractures. Closed reduction is here unreliable, and open reduction with internal fixation of the malleolar fracture is desirable. (Illus.: Type 3 fracture with fracture of the lateral malleolus.)

19. Complications cntd – (d) Avascular necrosis: The diagnosis is made from the radiographs. *Increased density* is often apparent by 6 and usually by 12 weeks, but do not be confused by the dense shadows cast by the overlying malleoli in the lateral. Revascularisation always occurs in closed injuries and is usually advanced by 8 months. (Check progress by monthly radiographs.) *Weight bearing before revascularisation is complete is likely to cause marked flattening of the talus (Illus.).* Local supports and physiotherapy will be required. Secondary osteoarthritis is common and should be kept in mind. Because of its key position, avascular necrosis of the talus may lead to osteoarthritis of the ankle, subtalar or midtarsal joints (or any combination of these).

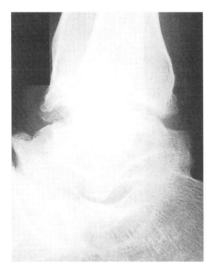

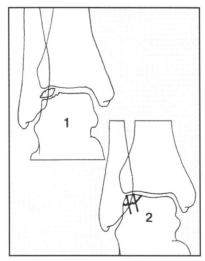

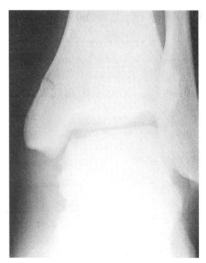

20. Complications cntd – (e) Osteoarthritis: This may occur secondary to avascular necrosis or malunion. Determination of the joints involved is important, and this may be facilitated by the site of the pain and the clinical and radiological appearances. Local anaesthetic infiltration of suspected joints is occasionally helpful. Thereafter the appropriate fusion may be advised. (Where all three joints are involved, as here, all will require fusion.)

21. Other talar lesions – (a) Dome fractures: A fracture may involve a portion of the upper articular surface of the talus (1) as a result of a shearing injury. If undisplaced, this may be treated by a period of 6 weeks in a cast before reassessment by arthroscopy and an MRI scan. If the fragment is substantial and inverted or badly displaced, it should be secured with Smillie pins (2), a Herbert screw, or biodegradable pegs. If the fragment is small, it may be excised and the bone drilled. Thereafter, plaster fixation for 6 weeks is advisable.

22. (b) Osteochondritis tali: This may occur as a sequel to a non-displaced shearing fracture, although frequently there is no history of injury. (Note the lesion on the medial side of the upper articular surface.) Where the fragment is substantial, with appreciable associated pain and swelling, it may be secured with a Herbert screw or a biodegradable dowel. Its base may be drilled in an attempt to encourage revascularisation.

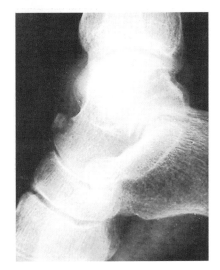

23. (c) Avulsion fractures: Minor avulsion fractures of the talus may result from inversion, eversion, plantar flexion and rarely dorsiflexion strains of the ankle – when flakes of bone are pulled off by ligamentous or capsular attachments. These injuries require symptomatic treatment only (e.g. 2–4 weeks in a below-knee walking plaster).

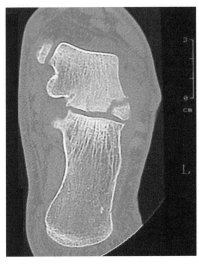

24. (d) Fracture of the lateral process of the talus: These injuries are uncommon (demonstrated here on a CAT scan), but are seen with increasing frequency as a result of snowboarding accidents. The subtalar joint is involved, and they are probably best dealt with by open reduction and internal fixation using a cancellous screw.

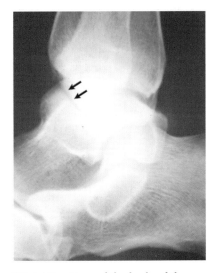

25. (e) Fractures of the body of the talus: The upper articular surface of the talus may be fractured by the same mechanisms which produce compression fractures of the ankle. Vertical splits without significant disturbance of the ankle or subtalar joints (Illus.) may be treated as Type 1 talar neck fractures. If displacement has occurred, accurate reduction and cross-screwing should be carried out. CAT scans are useful in assessing dome fractures.

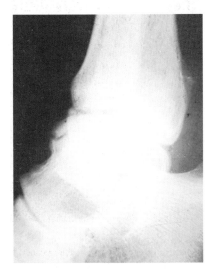

26. Body fractures cntd: Often there is a high degree of comminution. The convexity of the body may be flattened and the talus compressed as it is squeezed between the tibia and calcaneus. Such fractures may also involve the subtalar joint, and there is invariably extensive damage to the cartilaginous surfaces of the ankle joint. Surgical reconstruction is seldom possible.

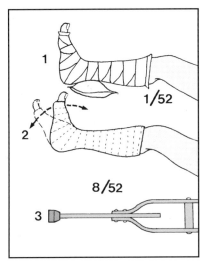

27. Treatment: A typical conservative line of treatment might be: (1) Initial pressure bandaging and elevation. (2) Intensive active exercises as soon as pain and swelling will permit. (3) Avoidance of weight bearing until union is well advanced (about 8–10 weeks). Persistent pain and functional restriction would be indications for ankle fusion.

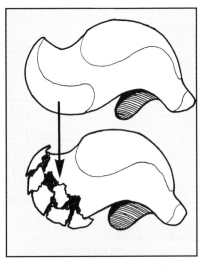

28. (f) Compression fractures of the head of the talus: These fractures are uncommon, but usually highly comminuted and unsuitable for attempts at reconstruction. Early mobilisation of the foot should be the aim, and a regime similar to that described in the previous frame may be followed.

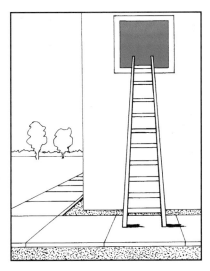

29. Calcaneal fractures – Mechanisms of injury (a): The commonest cause of calcaneal fracture is a fall from a height on to the heels. Important factors include the height fallen, the nature of the ground, and the weight of the patient. The injury is common in slaters, window cleaners and construction workers. Rarely the injury may be produced by impact from below (e.g. a below-deck explosion on a ship).

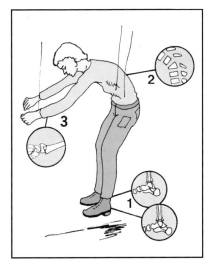

30. Mechanisms of injury (b): Taking into account the commonest cause of injury, it is essential when examining a case of suspected calcaneal fracture that you do not overlook: (1) A similar fracture on the other side; (2) A wedge fracture of the spine (dorsolumbar junction fractures are present in 5% of calcaneal fractures); (3) Upper limb injuries.

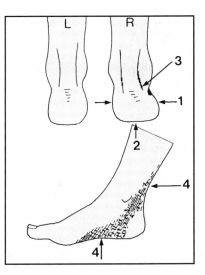

31. Clinical appearance: In major fractures, the heel when viewed from behind appears: (1) wider, (2) shorter and flatter, and (3) tilted laterally into valgus. There is often tense swelling of the heel, marked local tenderness, and later bruising (4), which may spread into the medial side of the sole and proximally to the calf. Weight bearing is usually, but not always, impossible.

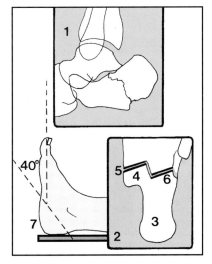

32. Radiographs (a): The most important view is a well-centred and well-exposed lateral projection (1). An axial projection (2) is helpful in visualising the pillar of the heel (3), the sustentaculum tali (4), the anterior talocalcaneal joint (5) and the posterior talocalcaneal joint (6). This film is taken with the tube tilted at 40° from the vertical (7), preferably with the foot dorsiflexed, but pain may force this projection to be abandoned. An AP foot allows visualisation of the calcaneocuboid joint.

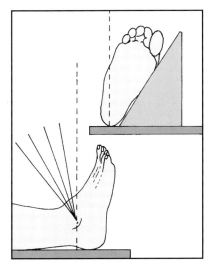

33. Radiographs (b): Oblique projections may be helpful if there is remaining doubt, or to obtain better visualisation of the posterior calcaneal facet. The four projections described by Brodén are particularly valuable for the latter. (The foot is internally rotated 30–40°, with the ankle in the neutral position. Four films, with tube tilts of 10°, 20°, 30° and 40° are taken, with the beam centred on the lateral malleolus.)

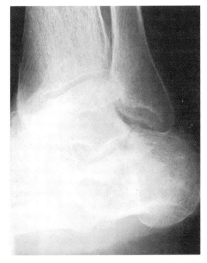

34. Radiographs (c): This oblique projection shows the posterior talocalcaneal joint quite clearly, with a split in the posterior articular surface of the calcaneus.

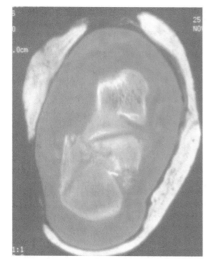

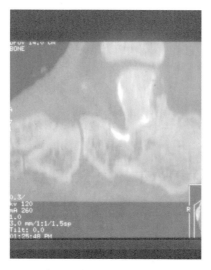

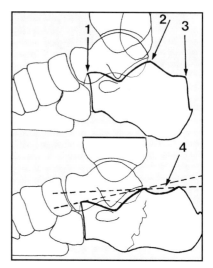

35. Radiographs (d): CAT scans can be of value in assessing the nature and degree of comminution of a calcaneal fracture, and any subtalar and calcaneocuboid joint involvement. Coronal, transverse and sagittal projections have all been used. The coronal projection chosen as a standard to allow useful comparison of cases is made through the widest part of the talus. In the scan above the comminution of the calcaneus and involvement of the subtalar joint is obvious.

36. Radiographs (e): In this sagittal cut of the previous case the downward projecting axe-like lateral process of the talus can be clearly seen, with the extensive calcaneal comminution it has caused. It also gives evidence of alteration to the angles of Bohler and Gissane.

37. Radiographs (f): In the interpretation of calcaneal fractures two common constructions are used: (i) *Bohler's salient angle:* This is formed by the intersection of two lines, both starting from the posterior articular surface of calcaneus (2), with one touching the anterior articular process of the calcaneus (1) and the other the superior angle of the tuberosity (3). The angle normally lies in the 20–40° range, and is decreased (4) in any fracture which flattens the heel, *whether this is extra- or intra-articular.*

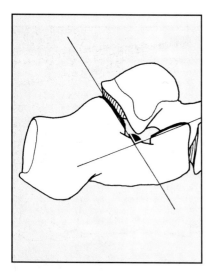

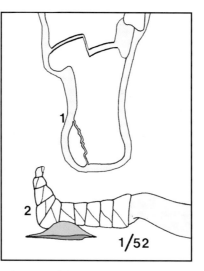

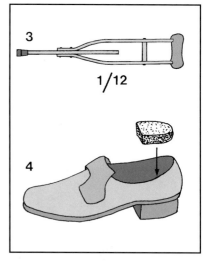

38. Radiographs (g): (ii) *The crucial angle of Gissane:* This is the angle between two bone struts, both of which are obvious in the lateral projection; one lies along the lateral border of posterior articular process of the calcaneus, while the second extends anteriorly to the beak of the calcaneus at the upper margin of the calcaneocuboid joint. A decrease in this angle is indicative of significant disruption of subtalar joint, and this is often also associated with proximal displacement of the prominence of the heel.

39. Types of calcaneal fracture: The key factor in assessing calcaneal fractures is whether or not there is involvement of the subtalar joint. Here the common fracture patterns have been arranged roughly in order of complexity, with the most difficult, the intra-articular fractures, at the end.
A: Vertical fracture of the tuberosity: The subtalar joint is not involved and the prognosis is excellent (1). Nevertheless, swelling may be severe, and should be controlled by firm bandaging over wool and elevation of the limb (2).

40. Vertical fracture cntd: Weight bearing, whilst not harmful, will be painful or impossible, and crutches will be required for some weeks; they may be discarded when pain settles (3). A crepe bandage or similar support may be worn until swelling subsides. Any long-term term heel pain may be controlled with a sorbo rubber heel cushion (4).

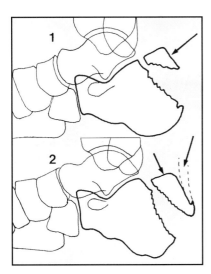

41. *B:* **Horizontal fractures:** These are of two types which must be distinguished. (1) The commoner injury involves the posterior superior angle of the calcaneus without disturbance of the Achilles tendon insertion; it is usually caused by local trauma (e.g. a kick). (2) The second is an avulsion fracture, produced by sudden muscle contraction.

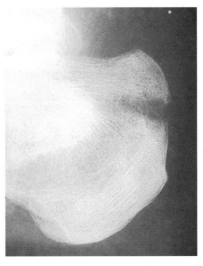

42. Horizontal fractures cntd – Diagnosis: Differentiate between the two main types of horizontal fracture by: 1. Noting the level of the fracture on the radiographs (Type 1 Illus.); 2. Studying the soft-tissue shadows on the radiograph, looking for upward (proximal) retraction of the Achilles tendon; 3. Feeling for a gap between the tendon insertion and the point of the heel.

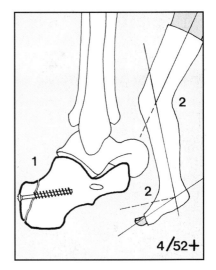

43. Treatment (a): (1) If the fracture is of the avulsion type (or if there is continued doubt) it should be openly reduced and fixed with a screw. (2) To remove stress from the screw, a long leg plaster should be applied with the knee and ankle in flexion. (3) After 4 weeks a below-knee walking plaster may be substituted till the fracture has united (usually about 8 weeks).

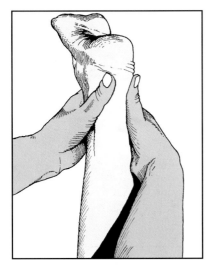

44. Treatment (b): When the fracture is not of the avulsion type, it should be manipulated if severely displaced. Moderate residual displacement can usually be quite safely accepted. Thereafter, a below-knee padded plaster may be applied, and crutches used for the first week or so. A further 5 weeks in a below-knee walking plaster is then all that will be required.

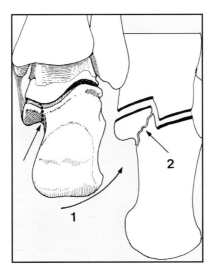

45. *C:* **Avulsion fractures of the sustentaculum tali:** These are generally secondary to forcible eversion of the foot which results in the strong deltoid ligament avulsing the sustentaculum tali to which it is attached (1). They are seen most clearly in axial projections, and indeed may be missed unless this view is taken and examined with care (2). They must be distinguished from major subtalar joint disruptions involving the sustentaculum. Displacement is generally slight, and persisting disability is rare.

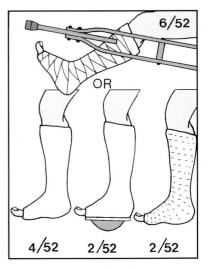

46. Sustentaculum tali cntd: *Treatment:* Healing of the fracture is generally well advanced by 6 weeks. Prior to this the following treatments may be used: 1. A crepe bandage over wool pressure bandage and non-weight bearing with crutches for 6 weeks; or 2. A below-knee padded plaster with crutches initially and then a walking heel; after 6 weeks a circular woven support for a further 2 weeks or so.

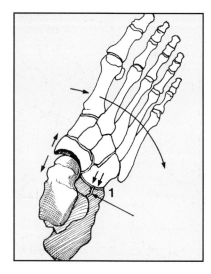

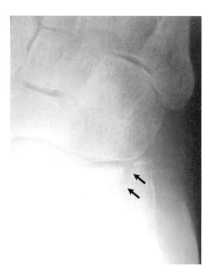

49. Anterior calcaneal fractures cntd:
If there is calcaneal shortening, the mechanisms of the midtarsal joint may be seriously disturbed, leading possibly to pain, restriction of movements in the foot and osteoarthritis. If the patient is elderly or has sustained multiple injuries, it may be wisest to accept these risks, and also treat this injury conservatively. In some other cases it may be possible by open operation and bone grafting to pack up the depressed articular fragments, with the aim of improving function in the midtarsal joint and reducing the risks of secondary osteoarthritis. To control the tendency to recurrence of the collapse it may be advisable to use a small external fixator stretching between the body of the calcaneus and the cuboid.

47. *D:* **Anterior calcaneal fractures:**
This fracture affects the anterior part of the calcaneus which articulates with the cuboid. It may result from (1) Forced abduction of the forefoot in which the cuboid strikes the calcaneus. (2) Forced inversion injuries which have the same effect. (3) As part of a midtarsal dislocation. (4) As part of a major subtalar joint disruption.

48. Anterior calcaneal fractures cntd:
Treatment: If there is no significant compression or shortening of the calcaneus (as in the vertical split illustrated) the injury may be treated conservatively along the lines already indicated for fractures of the sustentaculum tali. If there is evidence of midtarsal instability, treat as for a midtarsal dislocation.

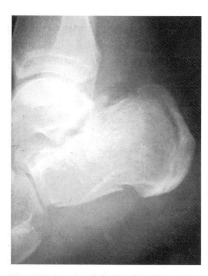

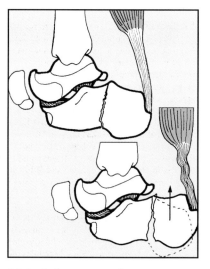

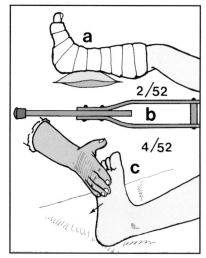

50. *E:* **Fracture of the body of the calcaneus without involvement of the subtalar joint:** The fracture line passes just posterior to the posterior talocalcaneal joint. The crucial angle of Gissane is unaffected, but frequently there is a decrease in Bohler's salient angle. If this is the case (Illus.) then flattening of the heel profile may lead to troublesome localised and persistent heel pain.

51. Body fractures cntd: Due to proximal displacement of the portion of the calcaneus carrying the Achilles tendon insertion, there is slackening of the calf muscles, so that there is weakness of plantar flexion at the ankle, and loss of spring in the step. This slackness is eventually taken up, but recovery is facilitated by *prolonged, intensive physiotherapy* in the form of calf resisting exercises.

52. Body fractures cntd – Treatment (a): If displacement is slight, good results may be obtained by conservative treatment along the following lines: (a) Pressure bandaging, bed rest, elevation and analgesics for 2 weeks. (b) Crutches until graduated weight bearing can be commenced at about 6 weeks. (c) Calf resisting exercises as soon as pain will permit, and continued physiotherapy until maximal recovery. A boot locked in neutral flexion may be used to prevent the development of an equinus deformity.

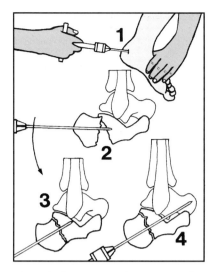

53. Body fractures cntd: Treatment (b):
Severely displaced fractures may be reduced with a Steinmann pin (1) inserted into the heel and used as a lever (2). If required the pin may be driven across the subtalar joint (3) into the head of the talus, following the axis of the joint (4). The pin may then be incorporated in a plaster sabot, thereby permitting early ankle and (some) subtalar joint movements.

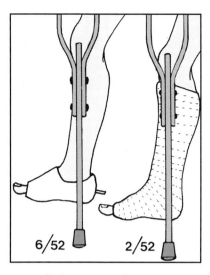

54. Body fractures cntd – Treatment (c): The sabot and spike may be removed after 6 weeks and non-weight bearing exercises continued for a further 2 weeks before full weight bearing. Pin-track infection is not uncommon, and at the first sign the pin should be removed and antibiotic treatment commenced. *Because of this risk, many prefer to treat these injuries with cannulated screws inserted percutaneously,* and certainly pin and sabot treatment is contraindicated if there is any doubt about the peripheral circulation.

57. Classification: The position of the common fracture lines, their associated bony fragments, and the degree of comminution result in enormous variations in these injuries. In spite of this there have been many attempts at classification; more have appeared since the introduction of CAT scanning which use coronal and transverse images: the preferred cut of the former is at the level of the widest part of the talus, and provides information on shape of the heel, the posterior facet, and the sustentaculum tali; the latter show the calcaneocuboid joint, the sustentaculum tali and the posterior facet. *The Zwipp Classification* starts (in the fashion of Neer in the shoulder) by describing 2, 3, 4 and 5 part fractures; these are subsequently modified by the number of joints involved. In the *Sanders Classification* four Types are described. Type I includes all non-displaced articular fractures. Type II comprises two part fractures affecting the posterior facet; there are subdivisions dependent on the site of the fracture. Type III, again with subdivisions, includes three part fractures. Type IV fractures are highly comminuted with four or more parts. In the *Crosby and Fitzgibbons Classification,* which is useful but no doubt unattractive to some because of its simplicity, three Types are recognised: Type I: non-displaced; Type II: displaced; Type III: comminuted.

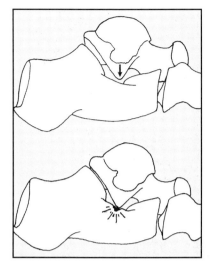

55. *F:* Fractures of the body of the calcaneus with involvement of the subtalar joint: This is the most serious and potentially disabling group of calcaneal fractures. *Pathomechanics:* The majority of these injuries result from the transmission of forces up through the heel, bringing the calcaneus into violent contact with the downward projecting lateral process of the talus: this axe-like area of bone initiates a fracture on the lateral aspect of the sinus tarsi; the process is aggravated if the foot is everted at the time of impact.

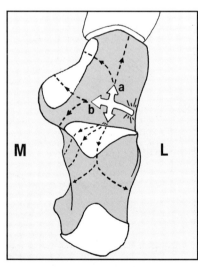

56. Fractures involving the subtalar joint cntd: Propagation of the fracture usually results in the formation of two primary fracture lines. Line (a) splits the calcaneus into medial and lateral fragments: anteriorly this may involve the calcaneocuboid joint or the anterior facet; posteriorly it usually divides the posterior facet: the position and number of splits vary. Line (b) tends to divide the calcaneus into anterior and posterior portions, often extending anteriorly to split the medial facet.

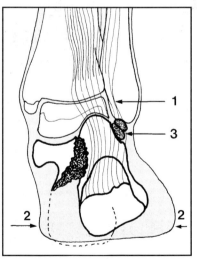

58. Associated extra-articular problems: If uncorrected, proximal displacement of the mass of the heel may result in slackening of the calf muscles (1) with weakness of plantar flexion. Lateral displacement may cause broadening of the heel (2) and heel pad pain. The deformity may be unsightly, and call for special footwear. There may be impingement symptoms from the lateral malleolus or the peroneal tendons (3). On the medial side, entrapment of the tibial nerve may occur. Swelling may also give rise to compartment syndromes.

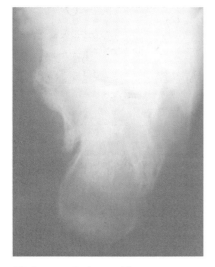

59. Intra-articular problems:
Uncorrected severely displaced fractures lead inevitably to loss of movements in the subtalar joint (and often the midtarsal joint), with pain, impaired foot function and gait disturbances. Secondary osteoarthritic changes often lead to further pain and stiffness. These problems may cause an acquired fear of heights, difficulty in returning to any former employment which involved working at heights or walking on uneven surfaces, and alcoholism.

In cases where there is gross comminution (Sanders type IV), primary arthrodesis may be considered. If crushing has been severe then the possibility of a compartment syndrome must be kept in mind. Careful clinical supervision and pressure monitoring are important in these cases, and decompression may be required (see later).

Treatment after union: 1. Physiotherapy and occupational therapy should be continued until nothing more can be gained. 2. Treat pain under the heel with a sorbo pad. 3. Broadening of the heel may require surgical footwear. 4. Impingement symptoms with sharply localised pain and tenderness beneath the lateral malleolus may respond to local surgery (excision of any exostosis and freeing the peroneal tendons). 5. Persistent pain and limp, due possibly to secondary subtalar osteoarthritis, require careful assessment. Symptoms should be unremitting, persistent for 6–9 months *at least*, and unresponsive to physiotherapy, before surgery is contemplated. Fresh radiographs should be compared with the original films to confirm subtalar joint involvement, and assess the calcaneocuboid joint. If the subtalar joint only is involved, a subtalar fusion is advised. If there is any involvement of the calcaneocuboid joint, a full triple fusion will be necessary (fusion of the subtalar, calcaneocuboid and talonavicular joints).

60. Treatment of intra-articular fractures:
Undisplaced fractures: Where there is minimal displacement these should be treated conservatively (e.g. see Frame 46).

Displaced fractures : Conservative treatment is also usually advised in displaced fractures in the elderly; in the presence of marked osteoporosis and gross comminution; in severe open fractures and cases where there is major soft tissue involvement such as blistering; where the circulation is impaired; and in the poorly controlled diabetic.

In other cases reduction and internal fixation should be considered. It should be noted that the technical difficulties may be formidable and the results surgeon-dependent. The procedure is carried out under X-ray control. The calcaneus may be approached through a lateral L-shaped incision, protecting the peroneal tendons and sural nerve within the anterior flap. Sanders recommends that the depressed superolateral part of the posterior facet is elevated first; if it is in several pieces it may be possible to reconstruct it with biodegradable pins. The main mass of the calcaneus is then levered downwards and medially to correct its lateral displacement; then correct the angle of Gissane. Once a satisfactory reduction has been confirmed by X-ray this is held by

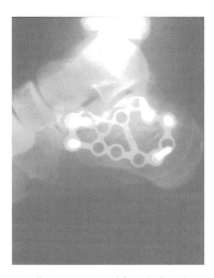

cancellous screws passed from the lateral cortex towards the sustentaculum. The posterior tuberosity is reduced, and then a low profile lateral plate used to stabilise the tuberosity, the posterior facet and the anterior process. (The radiograph shows the calcaneal fracture illustrated in Frames 35 and 36 held with a Timax™ Pe.R.I™ plate and screws.) A cast is worn for three weeks, and a plastic boot locked at 90° (to prevent an equinus deformity) for a further six weeks. Exercises out of the boot are commenced immediately.

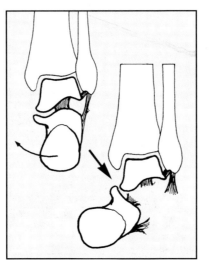

61. Peritalar dislocation – Pathology (a): Forcible inversion of the plantar flexed foot throws stress on the lateral ligament of the ankle and the talocalcaneal ligament. If the strong talocalcaneal ligament ruptures, the talus remains in the ankle mortise and a subtalar dislocation results.

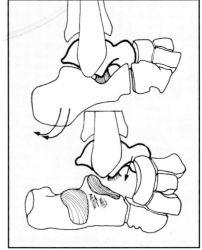

62. Pathology (b): The forefoot remains with the calcaneus and the talonavicular joint dislocates: as the talus remains in position this injury is often described as a peritalar dislocation. It may be accompanied by fractures of the malleoli. The talus, freed from its attachments, goes into plantar flexion (and this is the position in which the foot must be placed during the initial stage of reduction).

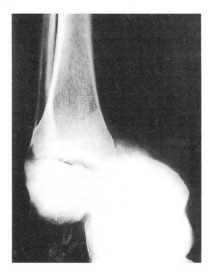

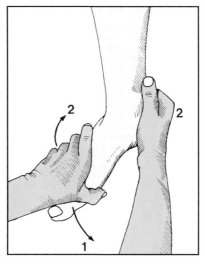

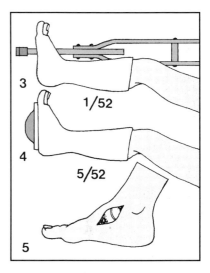

63. Diagnosis: The diagnosis may be suspected clinically, but is always confirmed by radiographs. Note in the example how the talus has maintained its normal relationship with the tibia and fibula (somewhat concealed by the slight obliquity of the radiographic projection). Note that avascular necrosis of the talus does not occur in this condition, but late subtalar osteoarthritis is common.

64. Treatment (a): Reduction is generally easy: Under general anaesthesia (1) Plantar flex the foot. (2) Grasp the heel and the forefoot, apply a little traction, and swing the foot into eversion. In difficult cases use a Schanz pin (held in a T-bar) temporarily inserted in the calcaneus to obtain better leverage.

65. Treatment (b): Thereafter (3) apply a padded below-knee plaster with the ankle at right angles and the foot in slight eversion. (4) A walking plaster may be applied after a week and retained for a further 5 weeks. Open reduction is necessary if manipulation fails, and the talonavicular joint should be exposed first (5) as difficulty is usually due to button-holing of that joint. Instability may be controlled with K-wire.

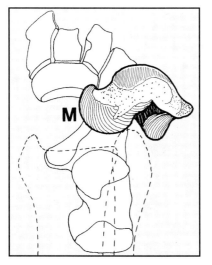

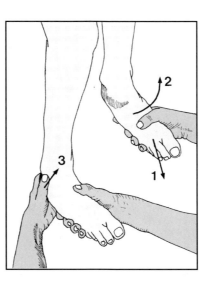

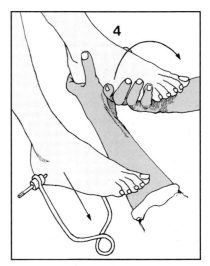

66. Total dislocation of talus – Pathology: With greater violence than shown in Frame 61 there is complete rupture of all the other ligamentous attachments of the talus. The talus dislocates out of the ankle mortise and comes to lie subcutaneously in front of the ankle and on the lateral side of the foot. The head of the talus points medially and its calcaneal surface is directed posteriorly. (Rarely, eversion injuries lead to medial dislocation of the talus.)

67. Treatment (a): Manipulative reduction should be attempted under general anaesthesia. It is imperative that delay is avoided, as there is always risk of skin sloughing where it is tightly stretched over the talus. The following technique may be employed: (1) Plantar flex the foot. (2) Invert the foot strongly. (3) The posterior part of the talus, lying laterally, should be pushed in a posteromedial direction.

68. Treatment (b): (4) When the talus starts to move into place, evert the foot. If these measures fail, use a Steinmann pin through the calcaneus to apply preliminary traction and control inversion. Occasionally open reduction may be required. (5) Thereafter apply a padded plaster. Avascular necrosis is almost inevitable. (Further care is as detailed in Frame 19.)

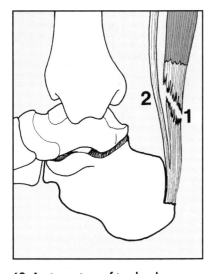

69. Acute rupture of tendocalcaneus:
Rupture may follow sudden muscle activity
(e.g. jumping or sprinting). It is especially
common in the middle aged when
degenerative changes are appearing in the
tendon. It may be precipitated by local
steroid injections. Usually the site is 4–8 cm
above the insertion; rupture is complete (1)
and the plantaris is spared (2). There is
sudden pain with difficulty in walking and
standing on the toes.

SURGICAL TREATMENT

This gives the most satisfactory results where
there is a delay of a week or more in making
the diagnosis or initiating treatment. It is
often also advocated for the young athletic
patient. The tendon is approached through a
vertical incision, 2 cm medial to the midline,
taking great care in the handling of the soft
tissues. A general anaesthetic, a tourniquet,
and the prone position are preferred. The
ends of the ruptured tendon will be found to
come together when the foot is plantar
flexed. It is held in that position during
suturing. Absorbable, non-absorbable or
Bunnell pull-out sutures may be inserted: all
have their advocates and all are effective, but
the frequency of wound breakdown is an
added incentive for the use of absorbable
sutures. Fascia lata may be used if there is
much fraying of the tendon. After wound
closure a long leg plaster cast is applied with
the knee and ankle in flexion. At 3 weeks the
skin sutures may be removed and a below-
knee plaster applied for a further 3 weeks
with the ankle in a more neutral position.
Discharging wounds are managed with
patience along established lines, and only
rarely require grafting.

Good results have also been claimed for
less invasive percutaneous techniques: it is
sutured through several small stab wounds,
using a hollow needle to guide the suture
material. Apart from not being able to view
the repair, there is the disadvantage with this
technique of not being able to 'freshen up' or
carefully align the ruptured tendon ends.

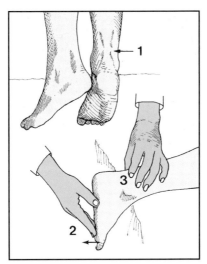

70. Diagnosis: The history and age of the
patient may be suggestive. Clinically there
may be: (1) a visible gap in the tendon; (2)
weakness of plantar flexion against
resistance; (3) lack of 'firmness' on side-to-
side pressure at the site of the rupture, again
when the foot is being plantar flexed against
resistance. Soft tissue radiographs,
ultrasound examination or an MRI scan may
show a defect in the continuity of the tendon.

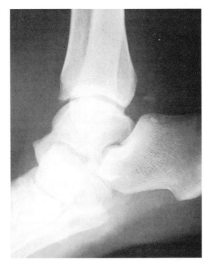

72. Midtarsal dislocations (a):
Dislocation of the talonavicular portion of
the midtarsal joint may accompany subtalar
dislocations. The inversion mechanism has
been described (see Frame 61). The subtalar
joint may reduce (incompletely)
spontaneously, so that the talonavicular
dislocation is the main feature (Illus.).

71. TREATMENT OF RUPTURE OF TENDOCALCANEUS

Both conservative and surgical measures
have their advocates, but neither guarantees
freedom from complications such as re-
rupture, weak plantar flexion, ankle stiffness,
poor wound healing (often taking months)
and deep vein thrombosis.

CONSERVATIVE TREATMENT

This is often advised for all cases seen within
48 hours, but is also particularly suitable for
the elderly, frail or poor anaesthetic risk
patient. The aim is to hold the foot in plantar
flexion in order to approximate the tendon
ends and keep them there until healing is
advanced. A long leg plaster is applied with
the knee in about 45° of flexion and the ankle
in a little plantar flexion. After 4 weeks a
below-knee plaster is substituted, with the
ankle still in a little plantar flexion. After a
further 4 weeks the plaster can be discarded,
weight bearing permitted, and physiotherapy
to improve the gait and calf strength
commenced. An inside shoe lift may be used
to reduce dorsiflexion stresses on the healing
tendon. The incidence of re-rupture is
commonest in conservatively treated cases.
Alternative conservative measures include
the use of a functional brace with the foot in
45° plantar flexion, with a prolonged,
complex regime of physiotherapy.

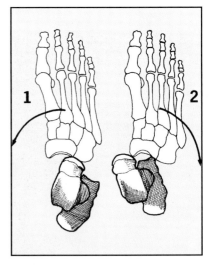

73. Midtarsal dislocations (b): The
midtarsal joint lies between the talus and
calcaneus posteriorly, and the navicular and
cuboid anteriorly. *Both* elements of the joint
may be disrupted as a result of (1) adduction
or (2) abduction forces applied to the
forefoot.

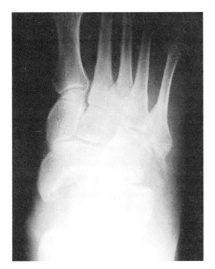

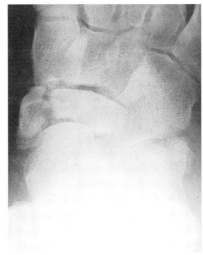

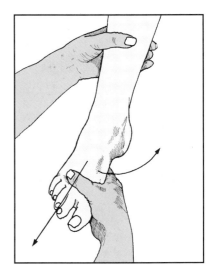

74. Midtarsal dislocations (c): As in any other dislocation, abduction or adduction midtarsal dislocations are associated with ligament rupture or small avulsion fractures, but the talus, calcaneus, navicular and cuboid may escape significant fracture. (Illus.: Adduction midtarsal dislocation with small avulsion fracture of cuboid.) Midtarsal dislocations are not infrequently missed in the context of other injuries, and a CAT scan or screening may be helpful in further defining the pathology.

75. Midtarsal dislocations (d): On the other hand, a midtarsal dislocation may be associated with fracture of any of the components of the joint. The navicular is most frequently involved. (Illus.: An abduction type midtarsal dislocation with fractures of the navicular and cuboid.) When this is the case, reduction is more likely to be unstable, and secondary arthritic changes commoner.

76. Treatment: 1. Under general anaesthesia, traction is applied to the forefoot. 2. Maintaining traction, the forefoot is aligned with the hindfoot (abduction injury illus.). 3. If there is instability, stabilise the forefoot with percutaneous K-wires. 4. Apply and split a padded plaster, and elevate the limb. 5. Start non-weight bearing with crutches after 1–2 weeks, and remove any wires at 3–4 weeks. *Take weekly radiographs* to detect late subluxation. 6. Discard plaster and mobilise after 6–8 weeks.

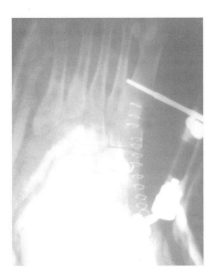

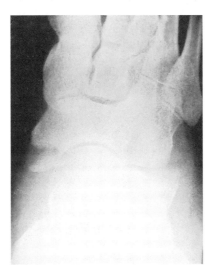

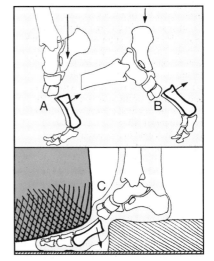

77. Treatment cntd: If manipulation fails, open reduction may be required. (Illus: A navicular fracture has been screwed, and a small external fixator applied medially to help stabilise the reduction and the bone repair.) *Complications:* Pain and stiffness of the foot and osteoarthritis are common. If the latter involves the calcaneocuboid joint only, a local fusion may be performed – otherwise a full triple fusion may be necessary. Rarely a medial plantar nerve palsy with intrinsic muscle wasting may be seen.

78. Isolated fractures of the navicular: (Do not mistake the common accessory centre of ossification for a fracture.) 1. The tuberosity may be fractured (Illus.) by avulsion of the tibialis posterior; this and other undisplaced fractures may be treated conservatively (e.g. by 6 weeks in plaster). 2. Body fractures may be accompanied by dorsal extrusion of a large fragment which should be accurately reduced and fixed surgically.

79. Tarsometatarsal dislocations (a): Injuries to the tarsometatarsal region are infrequent and the mechanism of injury is not always clear. Dislocation of one or more metatarsals may result from the following: (A) A fall on the plantar flexed foot or a blow to the forefoot as in road traffic accidents. (B) A blow on the heel when in the kneeling position, e.g. when a horse falls on top of a thrown rider. (C) Run-over kerb-side accidents.

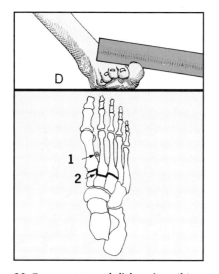

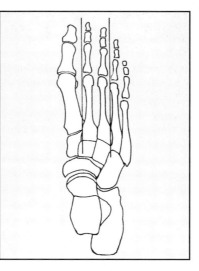

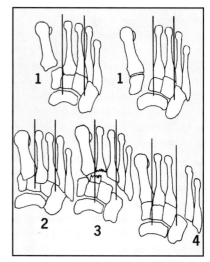

80. Tarsometatarsal dislocations (b): (D) Forced inversion, eversion or abduction of the forefoot as, for example, in a fall with the foot trapped. *Note:* (1) The dorsalis pedis/medial plantar anastomosis may be in jeopardy; (2) The metatarsal bases are keyed into the cuneiforms; the bony components are bound together by ligaments which, for mechanical reasons, are thick and strong on the plantar aspect; where there is much crushing of the soft tissues there is danger of compartment syndromes.

81. Classification: In the Myerson classification the foot is divided into three columns, one or more of which may be affected. The medial involves the joint between the 1st metatarsal and the medial cuneiform; the middle includes the joints between the 2nd and 3rd metatarsals and the intermediate and lateral cuneiforms; and the lateral involves the joints between the 4th and 5th metatarsals and the cuboid. The middle column is relatively fixed; there is slight mobility in the medial but most in the lateral.

82. Common patterns of injury: (1) 1st metatarsal or first ray (medial column). (2) Dorsal dislocation of all tarsometatarsal joints without fracture and with lateral drift (all three columns). (3) Dislocation of all tarsometatarsal joints with fracture of the base of the second metatarsal (three columns). (4) Dislocation and lateral drift of the lateral metatarsals (lateral column).

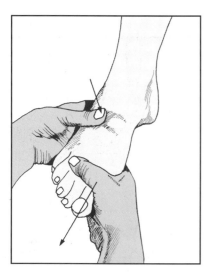

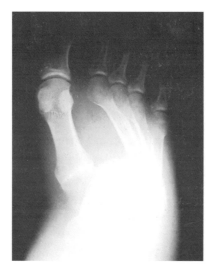

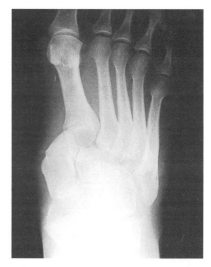

83. Treatment (a): Reduction should be attempted promptly (by applying traction in the line of the metatarsals and pressure over their bases) because of the risks of oedema and circulatory impairment. Even if several columns are involved but there is no fracture, the reduction may be stable. If so, use a padded cast for 8 weeks before weight bearing and mobilisation. There is however a tendency to late subluxation as the swelling subsides, and many prefer to internally fix most.

84. Treatment (b): *Unstable medial column injuries:* these may be stabilised by a K-wire with its end slipped beneath the skin to lessen the risks of infection. It is helpful to expose the affected joint through a short dorsal incision and carry out the reduction under vision. The entry point for the wire (medial cuneiform or navicular) is dependent on whether the dislocation is at the level of metatarsal/cuneiform joint or whether the whole of the first ray is involved.

85. Treatment (c): *Unstable middle column injuries:* These are often associated with a fracture through the base of the second metatarsal, and there may be lateral drift of all three columns (Illus.). The first aim of treatment should be to re-align the second metatarsal with the intermediate cuneiform. It is preferable if this can be achieved by manipulation, but if not it will be necessary to proceed to an open reduction.

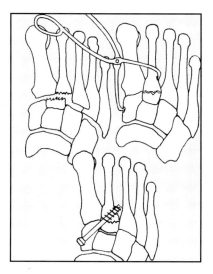

86. Treatment (c) cntd: To do so, use a longitudinal incision over the base of the second metatarsal, and apply a clamp between the second metatarsal and the medial cuneiform. If this fails, it is usually due to the presence of small bone fragments which may be picked out or pushed down into the sole. Once a reduction has been achieved it should be held with an obliquely placed cannulated screw (inserted percutaneously) and passed between the medial cuneiform and the second or third metatarsals.

87. Treatment (d): *Unstable lateral column injuries:* The affected metatarsals should be aligned with the cuboid and stabilised with K-wires.

Treatment (e): *Injuries associated with crushing of the cuboid:* Reduce the deformity with a distractor and make good the defect with a strut or cancellous bone graft. Occasionally a low profile plate may be required, or an external fixator, to maintain length.

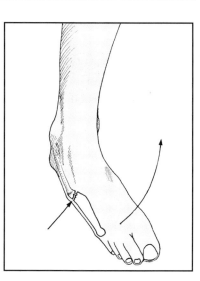

88. Fractures of the fifth metatarsal base: The commonest fracture of the lower limb is an avulsion fracture of the fifth metatarsal base: and it is often overlooked. It follows a sudden inversion strain (as, for example, from walking over uneven ground). In an effort to correct the progressive inversion of the foot, the peronei contract violently and the peroneus brevis avulses its bony attachment.

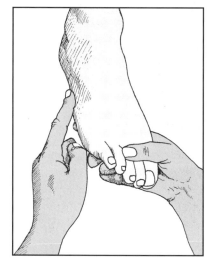

89. Diagnosis (a): Tenderness is marked and well localised over the fracture, so that diagnosis should be easy. As the fracture results from an inversion injury, the patient often complains of having sprained the ankle. If an adequate clinical examination is not carried out and radiographs taken of the ankle only, the *fracture line will not be visualised.* The diagnosis is confirmed by the correct radiographic projections.

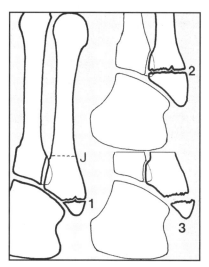

90. Diagnosis (b): Note in the radiographs that the fracture line runs at right angles to the axis of the metatarsal shaft. The fracture involves the joint (1) with the cuboid, if the fragment is small, and (2) that with the fourth metatarsal, if the fragment is large. In the former case (3) separation of the fragments may occur. (Note that the classical (unrelated) Jones fracture (J) is situated distal to the intermetatarsal joint.)

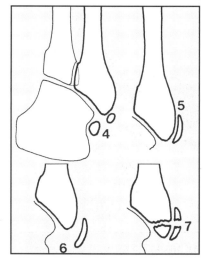

91. Diagnosis (c): Do not misinterpret the rounded shadows of accessory bones (e.g. the os peroneum in peroneus longus, the os vesalianum in peroneus brevis) (4). In children the epiphysis lying *parallel* to the shaft may also be wrongly taken for fracture (5). Nevertheless separation (6) or fracture of the epiphysis (7) may occur.

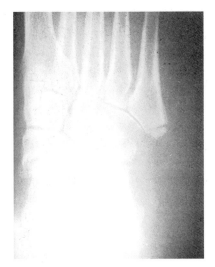

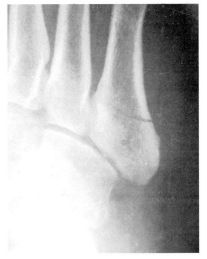

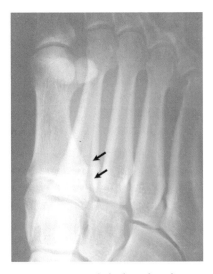

92. Treatment: Most fractures are undisplaced (Illus.) but even marked displacement does not merit reduction. If symptoms are slight, give a crepe or similar support for 2–3 weeks, and if marked a walking plaster for 5–7 weeks. Pain from the occasional non-union may be expected to resolve spontaneously, but Sudeck's atrophy is common and may require prolonged treatment.

93. Jones fracture: This fracture is not associated with inversion injuries, but tends to occur in athletes during training: it has some of the features of stress fractures. Non-union is common, and is most often associated with early weight bearing: because of this, treat with 7 weeks' fixation in a below-knee non-weight bearing cast. In the professional athlete, internal fixation with an intramedullary AO cancellous bone screw may be considered. Treat delayed or non-union with medullary curettage and bone grafting.

94. (a) Metatarsal shaft and neck fractures: These frequently result from crushing accidents, and any associated soft tissue injury will require careful surveillance (see Frame 104). Spiral fractures generally result from forced inversion or eversion of the forefoot. If the fracture is undisplaced (Illus.: 2nd metatarsal fracture) without soft tissue damage, treat symptomatically – a crepe bandage support, or a walking plaster if pain is severe.

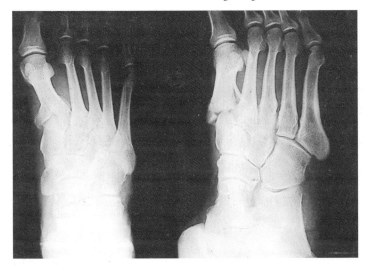

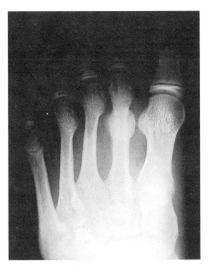

95. (b) First metatarsal: 1. AP and oblique projections illustrate a slightly displaced first metatarsal fracture. In this type of injury, damage to the peripheral circulation and post traumatic oedema may present problems. Admission for a short period of elevation and observation, with the limb supported in a well-padded split plaster is indicated. (Thereafter a below-knee walking plaster for 5–6 weeks.) 2. If there is marked displacement with off-ending, reduction should be carried out to avoid disturbance of the mechanics of the forefoot. Traction to the toe, with local pressure over the displaced metatarsal, may suffice, and stabilisation may be obtained with percutaneous K-wires transfixing the second and third metatarsals. Open reduction may be sometimes be necessary (aftercare as above). 3. Hairline fractures without soft tissue crushing may be treated without preliminary elevation, while, 4. Compound injuries will require the appropriate wound treatment.

96. (c) March fracture: Fatigue fractures, usually of the second metatarsal neck or shaft, are not often seen until callus formation has occurred; reassurance, with at most a light support for 2–3 weeks, is all that is indicated. If seen at an early stage, severe pain will occasionally merit treatment in a below-knee walking plaster until union has taken place.

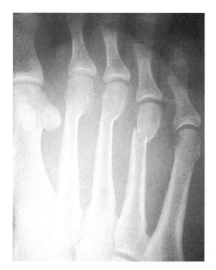

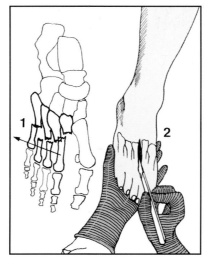

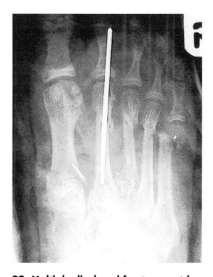

97. (d) Multiple undisplaced fractures:
The radiograph shows fractures of the necks of the 2nd, 3rd and 4th metatarsals (the clue to the second metatarsal fracture is the kinking of the cortical shadow). Multiple fractures of this type without much displacement may be treated conservatively by plaster support.

98. (e) Multiple displaced fractures:
Fractures of the four lesser metatarsals are frequently accompanied by lateral drift, an unstable situation (1). Open reduction and internal fixation are advisable; frequently reduction and stabilisation of the second metatarsal will suffice as the intermetatarsal alignment is preserved. An approach (2) between the second and third metatarsals gives access to both and avoids the arterial anastomosis.

99. Multiple displaced fractures cntd:
Stability may be preserved with an intramedullary wire and plaster fixation. *Displaced neck fractures* may be manipulated, but open reduction and K-wire fixation are often required. A second incision may be needed to gain access to the 4th and 5th metatarsals. Malunion may be treated by local trimming of any metatarsal head prominences in the sole.

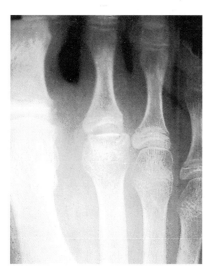

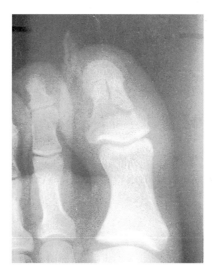

102. Treatment: 1. All wounds should be cleaned and the edges loosely approximated. 2. The nail should be retained unless virtually separated. Some advocate evacuation of any subungual haematoma. 3. Thereafter the fracture may be supported by:
    (a) Adhesive strapping to the adjacent toe;
    (b) A light dressing and the wearing of a stout shoe with, if necessary, a cut-out for the toe; or
    (c) A walking plaster with toe platform – all for 2–4 weeks.

Fractures of the terminal phalanges of the lesser toes may be treated in a similar manner.
    Fractures of the middle and proximal phalanges should be treated by strapping to the adjacent toe for 3–4 weeks; but if there is marked displacement with obvious deformity of the toes, they should first be reduced by traction.
    In the case of the great toe, a walking plaster with toe platform for 4 weeks may give greater relief of symptoms.
Note: In all cases the circulation must be carefully assessed and additional precautions taken where necessary (e.g. admission for elevation, etc.).

100. Freiberg's disease: Osteochondritis of a metatarsal head (usually the second) may cause confusion in diagnosis. Although this condition may result from local trauma, symptoms are usually of gradual onset. An osteochondritic segment may be present, or more commonly there is narrowing of the MP joint and widening and flattening of the head. Persistent symptoms may require excision of the metatarsal head.

101. Phalangeal fractures: Fractures of the terminal phalanx of the great toe are common in men and usually result from a heavy weight falling on the foot unprotected by industrial footwear. The fracture may involve the distal tuft only, but often runs into the IP joint. The fracture is often open.

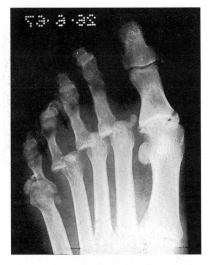

103. Toe dislocations: These should be reduced by traction. (Illus.: Dislocations of the four lateral MP joints, with fractures of all proximal phalanges except the third.) If there is instability K-wire fixation may be needed. Single dislocations may be reduced under local anaesthesia and supported by strapping to the adjacent toe; multiple dislocations will require general anaesthesia and a walking plaster with a toe platform for 4 weeks.

104. Crushing injuries of the foot without fracture: The foot is a resilient structure; it may be run over by a heavy vehicle or be severely crushed without sustaining any obvious fracture. If a history of this type of injury is obtained, admission is nevertheless advisable for:
(1) light pressure bandaging by crepe bandage over several layers of wool.
(2) elevation.
(3) observation of circulation and early detection of an impending compartment syndrome.

Sloughing of the skin over a heart-shaped area on the dorsum is not uncommon, but the area requiring desloughing and skin grafting will be minimised by prompt early care.

Degloving injuries of the foot: These are potentially serious, especially when sole skin is involved, and require prompt attention. Advice and possible treatment from an experienced plastic surgeon is highly desirable.

105. Compartment syndromes: These are most likely to develop after severe crushing injuries. Suspect if there is massive swelling of the foot and increased pain on passive dorsiflexion of the MP joints. Absence of the pulses is an unreliable sign. The diagnosis may be confirmed through pressure monitoring.

Decompression: There are 9 compartments in the foot, arranged in four groups. *Interosseous:* four groups of interossei lying between the metatarsal shafts. *Medial:* contains abductor hallucis and flexor hallucis brevis. *Central:* flexor digitorum brevis, quadratus plantae, adductor hallucis. *Lateral:* flexor digiti minimi, abductor digiti minimi.

Method: Two approaches are described. 1. Two longitudinal dorsal incisions are made slightly medial to the shafts of the 2nd and 4th metatarsals. The interossei are elevated from bone and blunt dissection carried into the sole to decompress the central and lateral groups of muscles. A separate medial incision may be needed to decompress the medial group. 2. Alternatively all compartments may be decompressed through a Henry medial longitudinal approach (with release of the so-called 'master knot').

SELF-TEST

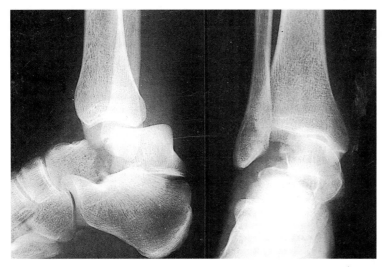

106. What is this injury? What complication is likely to develop?

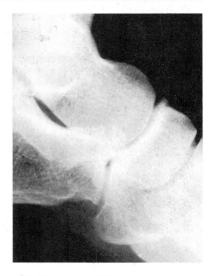

107. What abnormalities are shown on this radiograph?

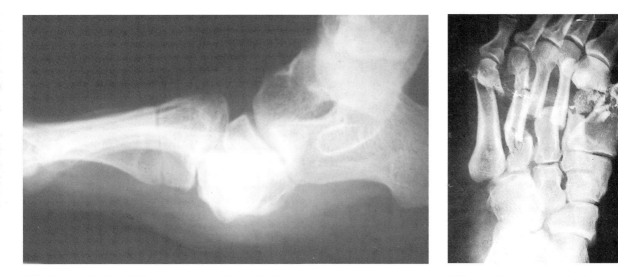

108. What is this injury? What treatment would be advised?

109. Describe this radiograph of a crushed foot. What would be the main principles of treatment?

ANSWERS TO SELF-TEST

106. Type 3 fracture of the neck of the talus. The incidence of avascular necrosis in this type of injury approximates to 85%.

107. There is an undisplaced fracture of the anterior process of the calcaneus as a result of recent trauma. In addition there is a small avulsion fracture of the dorsal aspect of the navicular, probably of long standing.

108. Tarsometatarsal dislocation: if a recent injury, open reduction would be advised; if an old injury, surgical wedge correction with a tarsometatarsal fusion might be indicated.

109. Comminuted fracture of the first metatarsal. Fractures of the shafts of the second and third metatarsals. Double fracture of the fourth metatarsal. Fracture of the neck of the fifth metatarsal. Lateral displacement. The injury is open (horizontal streaks of ingrained dirt can be seen). Treatment: if the foot is viable: 1. Debridement. 2. Reduction and K-wire fixation of the first and then the second metatarsals. 3. Plaster back shell or split padded plaster, elevation, observation, compartment pressure monitoring, infection prophylaxis (including antitetanus), etc.

CHAPTER

16
The fracture clinic

The organisation and running of fracture clinics varies from hospital to hospital. These differences are often dictated by the layout of the departments involved – records, appointments, secretarial, clinical, treatment, plaster, theatre and X-ray – and also by an established line of practice. A system which has worked for a number of years is difficult to change, as an apparently obvious improvement in one area may upset the smooth running of others – to the overall detriment; and change of any kind in an established system is unusual if it attracts universal acceptance. Those who work in fracture clinics have usually to do so within a framework imposed upon them, and it would be invidious to suggest a 'best way' of doing things. Nevertheless it might be helpful for the beginner who is confronted for the first time with a fracture clinic to offer a few guidelines on the handling of the actual consultation.

The newcomer to a fracture clinic is usually impressed by the number of cases dealt with in a short space of time. This speed often conceals the number of rather important decisions that are made about the patients' care. These decisions are, of course, determined by the basic principles of fracture treatment, but to ensure the smooth running of the clinic, the most professional and kindliest contact with the patient, and the avoidance of any error in management, the use of a simple system (at least at the beginning) may be of some help.

Assuming that the usual courtesies of greeting have been made, each consultation should start with asking the two questions – 'what?' and 'when?' – and end with asking 'when?' and 'what?'. In the middle, there are a number of things to go through which can be conveniently dealt with under three headings, each starting with the letter A – 'the three As'.

THE FRACTURE CONSULTATION

'WHAT?'

Every decision that is made, and everything that is done, is directly dependent on the diagnosis. *This must be clearly stated at the beginning of the notes on the first fracture clinic attendance*, where it will serve as a guide to everyone who sees the patient subsequently. It is a never-ending source of astonishment as to how difficult it may be to find this information, the time taken often varying directly in proportion to the size of the records. If there is a problem, a glance at the initial radiographs (they alone are helpful to label) may give the answer. Time spent establishing the diagnosis is essential. Recording it will prevent the effort having to be repeated at the patient's next attendance.

'WHEN?'

The point here is to establish the time that has passed since the patient's injury. While this can obviously be calculated on every occasion from the entries made on the day of injury and on the clinic visit, it is of greater practical value to give the elapsed time.

It is more professional to establish these primary facts before confronting the patient, rather than searching through the notes in their presence. When making the appropriate notes, where brevity should not compromise accuracy, the addition of a qualifier in the case of the diagnosis may be helpful, e.g.

Undisplaced L Colles 2/52 ago.

or

7/52: mid-shaft R femur, IM locked nailing.

On the solid basis of the knowledge of what you are dealing with, you can proceed to **Assessment, Action, and Advice**.

ASSESSMENT

1. The first step is to establish if the fracture to date has been treated *appropriately* and *adequately*, e.g. if a fracture has been manipulated, then it is necessary to consider whether this was the best method of treatment in the circumstances; the desirability of internal fixation or other methods of dealing with the condition should be reviewed. Then the check radiographs should be studied to assess the quality of the reduction, and an overall assessment made.

2. If a plaster cast has been applied, it should be seen to be appropriate to the injury. It should be checked for tightness, slackness or other inadequacy, and if it is only a backslab, a decision should be made as to whether it needs completion. The presence of swelling, the quality of the circulation, and any impairment of nerve supply in the limb should be noted.

3. If the fracture has been treated surgically, the need for inspection of the wound or removal of sutures should be assessed. If the fracture has been internally fixed, the quality of the fixation should be reviewed so that a decision may be made regarding the degree of mobilisation that may be permitted without the fracture coming adrift.

4. If some time has elapsed since the injury, an assessment should be made as to whether a greater degree of freedom may be permitted, e.g. whether a supporting sling may be discarded or whether a cast may be removed to allow joint mobilisation, or whether a walking heel may be applied to a leg plaster.

5. A decision when to remove all external splintage is not usually required until an appropriate length of time has elapsed since the injury, and in making the decision, radiographs may be required to check the state of union, and/or the cast may be removed so that a clinical assessment of the fracture may be made.

ACTION

Having assessed the fracture, the appropriate action should be taken. What should be done generally follows in a clear cut fashion from the assessment, e.g. if a plaster is too tight it should be split, or if there is complaint of local pressure the plaster should be windowed or trimmed.

The only difficulties that are likely to arise are those associated with the assessment of the treatment that has been carried out. This tends to present less of a problem as experience grows, although with the variety and vagaries of chance and changing opinion the need for the critical analysis of every case is one of the continuing delights of fracture clinics and one which prevents them ever becoming dull. *The point which is imperative to note is that if there is any doubt regarding the treatment or progress of a fracture, a more senior opinion should be sought without delay.*

Procrastination narrows the available treatment options, and will attract the criticism of why an earlier opinion was not sought. It is generally easy and a pleasure for a senior colleague to give timely advice on the treatment of a case, and gives him confidence in the reliability and common sense of his junior. Delay or failure in seeking advice may lead to an undesirable or even tragic outcome.

ADVICE

The patient should be given clear and appropriate advice. Some of the areas which might be considered include the following:

1. They should be told, or preferably shown, what exercises to do to encourage or preserve movements in the joints related to their fracture.
2. If they have been given an arm sling they should be advised when and if they may discard it, and how the limb may be exercised with and without it. If they have a leg in plaster they should be given clear advice on how much weight, if any, they should be allowed to transmit through the limb.
3. If appropriate, they should be given advice on their fitness to drive or return to work.
4. If they are being referred for physiotherapy they should be advised on what to do between visits to reinforce the treatment that they will receive.

It is important to explain to the patient, with repetition if necessary, the nature of their injury. It is equally important to keep them informed of their progress and to give, wherever possible, assurance regarding the position of a fracture, and what stage of healing it is at. They should be given some idea of when they can reasonably expect to reach the landmarks in their planned line of treatment, e.g. when they can hope to come out of a cast, when they might be able to weight bear, when they might be able to return to work.

If a complication arises, this should not be concealed. The proposed line of treatment should be clearly explained, and what result might be hoped for.

Frankness at all stages lessens the chances of misunderstanding, and may avert litigation which, in many cases, is embarked upon when a patient's anger at a less than perfect result is vented on an imagined lapse in management rather than the seriousness of an injury which has not been clearly explained.

'WHEN?'

The date and time of the next appointment is given, unless the patient is being discharged. In that event it is usually necessary to give a prognosis and advice regarding, for example, return to work or the procedure to follow should any complication arise. It may be necessary to give a recommendation about removal of an implant. It is usual to reinforce these points with the appropriate discharge letter to the patient's own doctor. Do not decide when to see a patient again by guesswork: instead, choose a date when you expect to have to make a further decision about the management of the case, e.g. whether a plaster will have to be changed or when union in a fracture might have to be assessed.

'WHAT?'

The purpose of the patient's next visit should be clearly stated so that the time and trouble that you have spent on assessing and treating the case can be pursued on the next attendance without any waste of precious time – of the patient or the clinic staff. For example, it may be helpful to indicate that on the next visit the patient should have their plaster removed, and an X-ray taken to assess union, as soon as they arrive at the clinic. Depending, of course, on how the clinic is organised this may save valuable time by avoiding the patient having to wait and be seen twice.

PATIENT'S NOTES

The smooth running of a clinic is dependent on the clinical notes, but these lose much of their value if they can only be read by the originator; and they become largely pointless if, as is not infrequent, even the writer has difficulty in interpreting them. If there is no facility for having *all* the notes typewritten, it is nevertheless strongly advised the notes should be typed on the first fracture clinic attendance *and* if there is any significant change in the line of treatment. Otherwise contractions in common usage, printed in upper case letters, may provide oases of understanding appreciated by every reader.

The following examples of two of the commonest conditions seen at fracture clinics are given to illustrate these points.

EXAMPLE 1 – A WRIST FRACTURE

A patient has had a Colles fracture which was only slightly displaced. The wrist was put in a plaster back shell without manipulation and the arm supported in a sling. Her plaster and the swelling and circulation were checked at a review clinic the following day. She is now attending her first fracture clinic 4 days later.

The post-fracture swelling has subsided and it would seem that the plaster backshell can be safely completed. Review of the initial radiographs indicate that the fracture was only slightly displaced, and the original decision not to manipulate the fracture seems quite correct. No radiographs have been taken to check the fracture, and while the chances of it having slipped are thought to be comparatively slight, it is desirable to have the position confirmed; for if the fracture has slipped and the position is not acceptable, it could be readily manipulated at this stage.

If check films are taken before the plaster is completed, there is the possibility that the position may alter during the course of that procedure. The action taken is therefore to complete the plaster and have check radiographs taken afterwards. These, in fact, show that the original position has been maintained, and it is thought that the risks of late slipping may now be judged to be slight.

The patient is assured that her fractured wrist is in good position, and that it is planned to see if it has joined in 5 weeks' time. She is warned that when she comes out of plaster her wrist will be rather stiff, but that it is anticipated that eventually she will regain a good range of movements and have little handicap. Her sling is removed, and she is advised (for what is hoped to be the second time) how she may exercise her shoulder and her fingers. She is asked to return in 2 weeks' time. The main purpose of that visit is to check her plaster.

Notes to cover this might be made along the following lines:

> **R Colles 4/7 ago. Circn OK, POP completed. Check X-ray satis.**
> **Discard sling. See 2/52 for POP check**.

When this next appointment is kept, no search has to be made (because of the content of the note above) for what is wrong or what would normally be expected at this visit. The plaster is checked and not found to be slack. It is decided on the basis of the original radiographs of this impacted fracture that if any slipping of the fracture has occurred this is likely to be minimal and not requiring correction; so there is no call for further radiographs. There has been some discomfort because of pressure in the region of the metacarpal of the little finger and the plaster is trimmed in this region. The fingers and shoulders are found to have a full range of movements, and the patient is encouraged to continue with the exercises she has been shown. She is told that her plaster will be removed on her next visit to see whether her fracture has joined; she is warned that if it transpires that union is not sufficiently far advanced she may have to go back into plaster for perhaps a further 2 weeks, although this is not particularly likely.

The note might read:

2/52+. POP trimmed. See 3/52, POP off on arrival.

On removal of her plaster 3 weeks later, no tenderness is found at the fracture site, and her fracture involving cancellous bone can be safely judged to have united. (Check radiographs are superfluous, and would not be indicated unless any complication were suspected.) There is no swelling, and the use of a Tubigrip or crepe bandage support is not considered necessary. She is advised to continue with her finger exercises, and shown what to do to mobilise her wrist. Her good progress is re-affirmed, and she is advised to return for review in 2 weeks' time when a decision will be made as to whether she needs to have any physiotherapy.

Note:

5/52+. POP off. No tenderness. Mobilise. See 2/52? physio.

Her next visit is her last as she had no complaints of pain, and has regained an excellent if not complete range of movements. She is told that as she has recovered such a good range of movements at this early stage physiotherapy is not necessary. She is advised that it is expected that she will regain almost full movements in the wrist, and that she will recover excellent if not quite complete strength, perhaps over the course of the next year. Should she develop any problems with pain, swelling or tingling sensations in the thumb or fingers (anticipating Sudeck's atrophy or carpal tunnel syndrome – now rather unlikely) she should make a review appointment. She should be told how this can be done.

A discharge letter would normally be written to her own doctor incorporating the diagnosis, her present state, and expected progress. The clinical note may be simply 'See discharge letter' or along the following lines:

7/52+. Lacks 20° dorsiflexion and 15° supination.
Full finger movements, good grip. Discharge.

EXAMPLE 2 – AN ANKLE FRACTURE

A 25-year-old man has sustained an undisplaced fracture of the lateral malleolus and this has been treated by the application of a below-knee non-weight bearing plaster cast. The notes record that, at the time of his initial attendance on the day of the injury 4 days ago, he had tenderness over both malleoli. The injury has been judged as being potentially unstable, and the decision to treat it conservatively by use of a cast would appear to be correct. A check radiograph taken after application of the plaster shows the fracture in anatomical position, and there is no talar shift.

The notes record that he was seen the day following the injury and the circulation was thought to be satisfactory. On his present attendance the toes are noted to be a little swollen, and he is complaining of pain in the little toe which is concealed by the cast which extends over it. This area must be inspected, and the excess plaster is trimmed back exposing the toe. Although the toe is red, it is judged that the relief of local pressure will allow a rapid return to normal. The degree of swelling of the toes suggests that it might be unwise to permit weight bearing at this stage.

The patient is told that, although his fracture is in excellent position, as is commonly the case he has too much swelling to allow him to take weight as yet through his plaster. He is advised to continue using his crutches, and to elevate the limb whenever possible. He is encouraged to exercise the toes.

His job is found to be that of a representative, and involves a mixture of driving, walking and sitting. He is advised that he will have to remain in a plaster cast for 6–8 weeks, and that while in his plaster he should not attempt to drive. Considering the nature of his job which cannot be adjusted to suit his circumstances, he must expect to be absent for at least 2 months. His actual time off will depend on his progress after coming out of plaster, but there is a good chance of his being able to get back to his particular job within 3 months of the injury.

His notes might read:

4/7 since R # lat. mall. POP trimmed. See 2/52? heel.

At his second fracture clinic appointment the toe swelling has subsided. The plaster is checked for slackness, and considered to be still offering adequate support. It is noted that the sole of the plaster is a little soft as a result of some weight having been put on it. The upper end of the cast at the back is a little high and is restricting knee flexion. The sole is reinforced, the calf of the plaster trimmed, and a walking heel or boot applied.

The patient is told that he may now start taking full weight through the limb; but that to begin with he should use his crutches until he has gained confidence, when he may or may not feel the need to use a single walking stick. He is asked to return in 4 weeks when it will be decided whether he can come out of plaster, or whether a short further period of plaster fixation will be needed. He is also advised to return in the interim if he has any problem with his plaster.

The note may read:

2/52. Sole reinforced. Heel. See 4/52 POP off and X-ray ankle on arrival.

On his third attendance the limb is inspected out of plaster. There is no swelling, and no tenderness in the region of the fracture. A check radiograph (which some would regard as being optional) shows some early callus formation in the region of the fracture whose position has been maintained. Movements of the ankle are restricted to 5° dorsiflexion and 10° plantar flexion.

Union of the fracture is assessed as being sufficient for the patient to remain out of plaster. It is anticipated that as he mobilises the ankle there will be some swelling, and he is given a Tubigrip or crepe bandage support. It is thought that he will rapidly regain most of his ankle and foot movements, and that although the need for physiotherapy will have to be kept in mind, this will probably not be required. He is shown how to exercise the foot and ankle on his own.

The patient is told that his fracture is progressing very well, but that he is likely to develop some rather persistent swelling of his ankle. The support he has been given to counteract this should be removed when in bed at night. He is advised to return in 2 weeks' time when he will be assessed regarding the need for further treatment or when he can return to work.

The note may read:

6/52. POP off. # uniting. Tubigrip. See 2/52? physio. ?discharge.

On his fourth visit a trace of swelling is noted, but he has recovered all but the last 5° of plantar flexion in the ankle, and foot movements are full. He has no complaint of pain and says he is anxious to return to work which he now thinks he will be able to manage. He wonders when he might return to playing golf and squash.

As he has no pain in the ankle and has recovered a good range of movements, no physiotherapy is necessary and it should be safe for him to drive and try going back to work. He is advised to continue wearing his support until any tendency to swelling has disappeared.

The presence of some swelling suggests that it would be wise not to overdo his weight bearing activities. A reasonable approach might be to recommend that after a further 2 weeks he might try a half round of golf, and be guided by any subsequent discomfort and swelling. As far as squash is concerned, where stress on the ankles is particularly high, it would be advisable to defer this until a full 3 months from the time of the original injury, and until all swelling of the ankle has subsided.

He should be told that at this stage, in view of his progress and the anticipation of a full recovery, there is no immediate need for him to reattend. Should however he become unhappy about his progress then he should make a review appointment. It should be mentioned that his doctor will be written to with a summary of the history, present findings and recommendations.

The final note then need only be: '**See discharge letter**'. The discharge letter itself need not be long, but should cover the main points in the history, the diagnosis, the treatment, and the prognosis. Such a letter might read:

> *Mr ——— attended the Casualty Department on ———*
> *with an undisplaced fracture of the right lateral*
> *malleolus sustained in a fall down some steps. It was*
> *treated by 6 weeks' fixation in POP and it has united in*
> *good position. He has regained a good range of*
> *movements in the ankle, but he has still a little swelling.*
> *He can now return to work, but should avoid contact*
> *sports for a further month at least. He has been*
> *discharged today, but I have advised him to return*
> *should he have any problem.*

Enjoy your clinics!

Index